W9-CMV-235

Source Book in

Bioethics

Source Book in Bioethics

EDITED BY

Albert R. Jonsen
Robert M. Veatch
LeRoy Walters

GEORGETOWN UNIVERSITY PRESS / WASHINGTON, D.C.

Georgetown University Press, Washington, D.C.

Printed in the United States of America

10 9 8 7 6 5 4 3 2 1 1998

THIS VOLUME IS PRINTED ON ACID-FREE OFFSET BOOK PAPER

Library of Congress Cataloging-in-Publication Data

Source book in bioethics : a documentary history / edited by Albert R.
Jonsen, Robert M. Veatch, LeRoy Walters.
p. cm.
Includes bibliographical references and index.
1. Medical ethics—History—Sources. I. Jonsen, Albert R.
II. Veatch, Robert M. III. Walters, LeRoy. IV. Title: Sourcebook
in bioethics.
R724,S599 1998
174'.2'09—DC21 97-41521
ISBN 0-87840-683-2 (cloth : alk. paper)

CONTENTS

PREFACE

The editors of this book have worked in the field of bioethics since its beginnings in the late 1960s. During the past thirty years, we have seen many public policy documents and legal decisions become landmarks in the development of the field. Contemporary students hear of these documents but often cannot find them to read and study. This Source Book will put at least some of them into their hands.

Albert Jonsen thanks his research assistant, Ms. Kelly Edwards, for her help. Robert Veatch thanks Kier Olsen and William Stempsey, S.J., for research assistance. LeRoy Walters thanks Karen Peterson-Iyer of Yale Graduate School for her research assistance.

The editors have divided their responsibilities as follows: Albert Jonsen edited Part I; Robert Veatch edited Parts II and V; and LeRoy Walters edited Parts III and IV.

INTRODUCTION

Albert R. Jonsen

BIOETHICS came into being in the early 1970s. As defined by the Encyclopedia of Bioethics (1995), bioethics is the "systematic study of the moral dimensions—including moral vision, decisions, conduct, and policies—of the life sciences and health care, employing a variety of ethical methodologies in an interdisciplinary setting."[1]

Today bioethics is a field of academic study. It has a discernible set of topics, a body of concepts, and a variety of analytic methods. A large body of literature is devoted to these topics, concepts, and methods.[2] Bioethics is taught in colleges and health professional schools and has its own professors, curricula, journals, conferences, and committees. Over a dozen institutions of higher learning offer degrees in bioethics, including the doctorate. Many questions that once aroused vigorous debate have been resolved, and policies and procedures are in place in health care institutions to assure that these broadly accepted resolutions are respected. Thus, the ethics of research with human subjects and many aspects of the use of life-sustaining treatments, once so controversial, now enjoy areas of broad consensus. At the same time, aspects of those issues remain problematic, such as research on the human embryo and assisted suicide. New issues continually arise. The advances in molecular biology have opened possibilities in genetic diagnosis and treatment that are ethically perplexing. Reproductive sciences make possible forms of human generation that challenge settled moral views. The curriculum of bioethics has a core of defined issues and an expanding margin of questions and quandaries.

During the past several decades, government bodies, such as the Department of Health and Human Services and special Commissions and Committees, have produced documents of great importance in bioethics. Courts have rendered decisions and legislatures passed laws that touch on bioethical issues. These reports, laws, and judicial decisions have often been pivotal in defining the issues and in establishing ways of managing them in American society. These documents sometimes reflect the thinking of scholars in bioethics and sometimes influence that thinking. They contain some of the fundamental concepts of the field, in association with significant events that have stimulated its formation. It would, for example, be unthinkable for a bioethics course in college or medical school not to refer to *Deciding to Forego Life Sustaining Treatment* from the President's Commission for the Study of Ethical Problems in Medicine and Biomedical and Behavioral Research, or the Supreme Court's decision on the legality of abortion (*Roe v. Wade*), or the *Policies and Regulations for the Protection of Research Subjects* from the Department of Health and Human Services.

Many of these important documents are difficult to find. Some, issuing from transitory governmental bodies, are out of print. Others exist in the arcane corners of law libraries and state archives. A few, produced outside the United States, have no natural home in this country. We believe that students of bioethics should have easier access to the classic sources of their field of study. Not content with a summary paragraph about Karen Ann Quinlan or about the Baby Doe Regulations, they should be able to study the language and logic of those documents. We are fortunate that many of these classic documents are in the public domain. They were issued by public bodies, such as commissions, legislatures, and courts, were the products of many minds, and had a wide public audience. Thus, we can present these documents as the history of bioethics and as part of its public heritage.

Although bioethics covers many fields, it has concentrated on several: experimentation with human subjects, care of the terminally ill, reproduction, and genetics. We have limited our selection of sources to these four fields, with a few important exceptions that are collected in Part 5: The Changing Health Care Scene. Since many of the documents are quite long, it was regrettably necessary to abbreviate them. In doing so, we have tried to preserve what we believe to be the essential arguments. We have added one or two secondary references to guide students to other literature or explain the background of the documents more fully. It is our hope that as the field of bioethics expands, its origins will not be forgotten or reduced to footnotes.

NOTES

1. Warren T. Reich, editor. *Encyclopedia of Bioethics*, 4 vols. (New York: Simon Schuster Macmillan, 1995), 1:xxi.
2. LeRoy Walters and Joy Kahn Tamar, editors. *Bibliography of Bioethics*. (Washington, D.C.: National Reference Center for Bioethics Literature, Kennedy Institute of Ethics, 1975, updated yearly).

Part I

THE ETHICS OF RESEARCH WITH HUMAN SUBJECTS

THE ETHICS OF RESEARCH WITH HUMAN SUBJECTS: A SHORT HISTORY

Albert R. Jonsen

ON JULY 19, 1947, the International Military Tribunal, sitting in Nuremberg, Germany, delivered its verdict in the case of *United States v. Karl Brandt et al.* This verdict convicted sixteen German physicians of crimes against humanity and sentenced seven of them to death. The crimes against humanity were acts of medical experimentation performed on prisoners in Nazi concentration camps. The verdict contained a ten-point code stating, "certain basic principles that must be observed in order to satisfy moral, ethical and legal concepts."[1] These ten points have become known as the Nuremberg Code.[2]

Two American physicians, Leo Alexander and Andrew Ivy, medical expert witnesses for the prosecution, are said to have devised the draft language for this famous document. In so doing, they drew on concepts that had been evolving within the world of medicine for at least 100 years. Although Drs. Ivy and Alexander invoked the Hippocratic Oath during their testimony—"I will follow that method of practice which, according to my ability and judgment, I consider for the benefit of my patients, and abstain from whatever is harmful and mischievous"—Hippocrates does not address the ethics of medical experimentation directly. From Hippocrates' time to the nineteenth century, experimentation was not clearly distinguished from practice. It was commonly understood that any medical intervention by drugs or surgery was "an experiment," in the sense that its outcome was uncertain. While there were bold experimenters, such as Paracelsus (1493–1541), who boldly, some would say rashly, ventured into the therapeutic unknown, nothing comparable to modern research existed before the nineteenth century.

In the first half of the nineteenth century, medicine began to reap the fruits of the previous century's scientific advances in chemistry and physics. The cellular basis of physiology and pathology, the germ theory of disease, the "numerical" (i.e., statistical) method of analyzing clinical experience, the invention of diagnostic instruments, such as the stethoscope and the thermometer, the initiation of clinical teaching, all led to the age of "experimental medicine." In 1865, the great French physiologist, Claude Bernard, published his groundbreaking work, *Introduction to the Study of Experimental Medicine.* This book argued that medicine must be placed on a solid scientific basis that has been established by experimentation, that is, on carefully designed and rigorously logical observations of the physiological conditions of health and disease.

Bernard proposed methods and rules of reasoning to reach this goal, which he illustrated with his own research. Thus, in considering whether one has a right "to perform experiments and vivisections on man," he writes:

> It is our duty and right to perform an experiment on man whenever it can save his life, cure him or gain him some personal benefit. The principle of medical and surgical morality, therefore, consists in never performing on man an experiment which might be harmful to him to any extent, even though the result might be highly advantageous to science, that is, to the health of others.[3]

Bernard makes no mention, however, of gaining the consent of experimental subjects and even commends an experiment in which a physician "had a condemned woman without her knowledge swallow the larvae of intestinal worms . . . to see whether the worms developed in the intestines after her death." He believed that this action involved "no suffering or harm [and] . . . Christian morals forbid only one thing, doing ill to one's neighbor."[3]

Despite Bernard's noble creed, experimental enthusiasm increased during the nineteenth century and with it our stock of horrendous stories of abuse, usually of hospitalized patients.[4] Among these tales was one about Sanarelli, the Italian bacteriologist who, searching for the causative agent of yellow fever, injected his candidate bacillus into five subjects without their knowledge and consent. The injections produced "typical yellow fever . . fever, congestions, hemorrhages, vomiting, steatosis of the liver, cephalalgia, rachialgia, nephritis, anuria, uremia, icterus, delirium, collapse." The patients recovered, reported Sanarelli, but the experiment provided "striking evidence in favor of the specific nature of the bacillus icteroides."[5] This experiment was widely criticized by other researchers. One scientist called it "ridiculous." The leading medical scholar of the day, William Osler, went further, exclaiming, "To deliberately inject a poison of a known degree of virulency into a human being, unless you obtain that man's sanction, is not ridiculous, it is criminal."[6]

Osler supplied a succinct statement about the ethics of human experimentation in testimony before a Royal Commission on Vivisection in 1908. In 1900, Major Walter Reed of the U.S. Army had supervised an experiment refuting Sanarelli's claim about the cause of yellow fever. He asked twenty-two volunteers to risk contracting yellow fever, half by exposure to supposedly infected materials and half by exposure to mosquitoes that had fed on the blood of yellow fever patients. Dr. Reed drew up a document detailing the risks, including death, and the benefit of potential immunity. It attested that the volunteer, "being in the enjoyment and exercise of his own free will, consents to submit himself to experiments for the purpose of determining the methods of transmission of yellow fever." At the conclusion of the experiment, $100 ($200, if they had became sick) would be given to all surviving subjects, or to their designates in case of death.

The Royal Commission questioned Dr. Osler about the Reed experiments, which had been famously successful.

COMMISSIONER: I understand that in the case of yellow fever the recent experiments have been on man.

OSLER: Yes, definitely with the specific consent of these individuals who went into this camp voluntarily. . . .

COMMISSIONER: We were told by a witness yesterday that, in his opinion, to experiment upon man with possible ill result was immoral. Would that be your view?

OSLER: It is always immoral, without a definite, specific statement from the individual himself, with a full knowledge of the circumstances. Under these circumstances, any man, I think, is at liberty to submit himself to experiments.

COMMISSIONER: Given voluntary consent, you think that entirely changes the question of morality or otherwise?

OSLER: Entirely.[7]

Thus, by the turn of this century, the leaders of medical science had acknowledged certain clear principles of the ethics of human experimentation: the integrity of the investigator, the consent of the subject, and a worthy scientific purpose. Ironically, these principles were stated for the first time in a government regulation by the Prussian Ministry of Health in 1900. That order forbade all nontherapeutic experimentation unless "the person concerned has . . . declared unequivocally that he consents to the intervention . . . on the basis of a proper explanation of the adverse consequences that may result from the intervention."[8] In 1931, the German government issued even stronger "Regulations on New Therapy and Experimentation." This document's fourteen points, "enumerate clear directives concerning the general, technical, and ethical standards of medicine, informed consent, documented justification of any deviation from protocol, a risk-benefit analysis, justification for the study of especially vulnerable populations, such as children, and the necessity to maintain written records. In many ways, these guidelines are more extensive than either the subsequent Nuremberg Code or the later Declaration of Helsinki."[9]

Ten years later, German physicians engaged in the most blatantly unethical experimentation. The Second World War not only produced the most horrendous examples of research malpractice; it also produced the first international ethical code and an intensification of scientific research. "The transforming event in the conduct of human experimentation," writes historian David Rothman, "was World War II." In 1941, President Roosevelt established the Committee on Medical Research to coordinate investigations in universities, hospitals, research institutes, and industrial firms dealing with military medicine. A tremendous volume of research was sponsored and supervised by this Committee. Much of its research, especially that concerning infectious diseases, was done in prisons, mental hospitals, and military camps, often with disregard for the rights and welfare of the subjects. Rothman suggests that for both researchers and the public, America was at that time a nation at war and "a sense of urgency pervaded the laboratories . . . [where] the rules of the battlefield seemed to apply. . . . Researchers were no more obliged to obtain the permission of their subjects than the Selective Service was to obtain the permission of civilians to become soldiers." Only in some instances, where there was risk of public outrage, did the Committee on Medical Research impose the safeguard of consent.[10]

The scientific sponsorship begun by the medical research committee had begun passed to the National Institutes of Health (NIH). After the war, interest in scientific research, having proven its public value, grew apace, and Congress bestowed federal support and largess on the NIH. Its intramural research expanded, and its grant program began to fund not only laboratory scientists but also clinical researchers in every medical school throughout the nation. University hospitals became major research centers, making thousands of patients available as subjects for physicians' scientific investigations. But while significant money flowed out of NIH into the nation's hospitals and laboratories, insufficient attention to the rights and welfare of human research subjects accompanied the dollars.

Articles about the Nuremberg trials appeared in major medical journals, including an editorial in the *Journal of the American Medical Association* (*JAMA*) that condemned the Nazi research and laid down three conditions for ethical research: the consent of the subject, the prerequisite of animal experiments, and proper medical supervision. These conditions were adopted by the American Medical Association's House of Delegates on December 28, 1947.[11] Simultaneously, many conferences were held, and many articles published on the problem of experimentation with human subjects.[12] A 1963 anthology, *Clinical Investigation in Medicine: Legal, Ethical and Moral Aspects*, collected 73 articles written in the previous decade and presented a bibliography of 500 others—and all had been published in significant English-language professional journals.[13] It can hardly be said that the problem of research with human subjects was ignored, or that the general outlines for ethical research were unknown.

Many individual researchers were aware of the problem. The common opinion, however, was that the research subject was best protected by the integrity of the researcher, who would assess whether an intervention might be, on balance, more harmful than helpful; and, if so, would refrain from doing it. The most vivid description of research activities in that era was a sociological study by Renée Fox. *Experiment Perilous* depicted researchers' concerns about the essential questions, particularly the uncertainty of the risks of research to their volunteers.[14] At the same time, however, the Atomic Energy Commission sponsored a number of radiation research projects that, forty years later, were strongly criticized.[15] In general, despite widespread recognition of the problem in postwar literature, many researchers apparently had little interest in the ethics of research, which they seemed to regard as an obstacle to social progress and personal success.

In 1953, the Clinical Center of the National Institutes of Health opened and, in addition to its research subject-patients, welcomed "normal volunteers." These persons, often coming from the traditional "peace" churches and colleges, offered themselves as healthy controls in drug studies. Investigators realized that these normal volunteers, not being patients, fell outside the fiduciary responsibilities that link physicians and their patients and therefore deserve special protection from risks and full information about those risks. However, the investigators failed to realize that even their research patients, insofar as they were subjects of investigations whose purpose was to generate new knowledge, also had a different relationship with the investigator physician than they would have had with a treating doctor. Dr. Otto Guttentag, speaking at a 1951 Symposium at the University of California, made the point clearly:

> . . . the relationship between the experimenter and the experimented on, entered upon not to help but to confirm or disprove some . . . biological generalization, is impersonal and objective. The original, basic patient-physician relationship implies the concept of solidarity, of life's finiteness. . . . Experimentation as just described is foreign to it.[16]

This conflict only gradually became clear at NIH over the next decade. Slowly, the leadership realized that attention must be paid to the rights and welfare of experimental subjects and that the good will of the investigator is not enough. An NIH-sponsored survey of its grantee institutions in 1962 showed that only nine of fifty-two departments of medicine had any policy regarding the rights of subjects; sixteen stated that they used written consent forms; and thirty-four departments did not bother to answer the survey questionnaire.[17] In 1964, Director James Shannon asked an internal NIH committee to review the issues involved in human experimentation. This committee came to a remarkable conclusion. Referring to a 1963 incident at the Jewish Chronic Disease Hospital in Brooklyn, the committee wrote that ". . . it clearly brought to the fore the basic issue that in the setting in which the patient is involved in an experimental effort, the judgment of the investigator is not sufficient as a basis for reaching a conclusion concerning the ethical and moral set of questions in that relationship."[18] In the Brooklyn case referred to here, two physician-researchers had obtained permission from the hospital to study the effects of injecting cancer cells under the skin of elderly, debilitated patients, who were not informed of the nature of the experiment. When the story became public, both physicians were professionally disciplined. The study had been funded by the National Institutes of Health.[19]

What makes the committee's conclusion so remarkable is the admission that the conscience of the investigator is an inadequate judge of the ethics of an experiment, an axiom on which research ethics had been firmly based for a century.[20] The Helsinki Declaration, adopted by the World Medical Association in 1964, had espoused the principles of voluntary consent and risk-benefit evaluation, but placed the responsibility for securing them on the investigator alone (although the revised Helsinki Declaration [1975] adds the requirement of "a specially appointed independent committee for consideration, comment and guidance").[21] Within a year of receiving the committee's report, Director Shannon concluded that the judgment of the investigator must be subject to prior peer review to ensure an independent determination of risks and benefits and the voluntary informed consent of the subject (such a committee had existed in the NIH Clinical Center since its beginning). In 1966, NIH issued an internal Policy and Procedure Order and extended it to affiliated research institutions several months later. This policy required the establishment of independent review bodies. Thus, the Institutional Review Board (IRB), as an official instrument of public policy, was born.

By coincidence, Henry Beecher's controversial article, "Ethics and Clinical Research," was published the same year, 1966, in the *New England Journal of Medicine*. The author, a distinguished professor of anesthesiology at Harvard Medical School, and the journal, the most prestigious medical publication in the nation, thus combined to cast a clear and disconcerting light on the practice of granting investigators almost unlimited discretion. Beecher presented twenty-two examples of unethical experimentation drawn from published articles by leading research scientists. He showed that they exposed patients to excessive risks, ignored the need for consent, used poor, mentally incapacitated persons, and withheld therapies of known efficacy. As valuable as this expose was, Beecher failed to transcend the conventional research ethic, namely, "the more reliable safeguard [is] provided by the presence of an intelligent, informed, conscientious, compassionate, responsible investigator."[22]

During these same decades, the quantitative increase in medical research was matched by significant qualitative improvement in research methods. The methods of controlled clinical trials and their statistical analysis, introduced only in the 1940s, were gradually becoming familiar to researchers and soon became standard practice. These methods, using techniques such as random selection of subjects between treatments or between experimental treatment and no treatment, and the "blinding" of researcher and subject to the nature of the intervention, raised significant ethical problems. The dilemmas posed by the new methods were clearly stated by the British statistician Sir Bradford Hill in 1951 and again in 1963.[23] Medical research was no longer doing something new merely to observe the results; it was the incorporation of doctor and patient in a carefully designed program to produce valid knowledge by methods that per se put subjects at risk.

The initiation of the Institutional Review Board was the beginning of the end of naive reliance on investigator integrity. Even those who recognized the importance of the investigator's integrity began to realize the intrinsic conflict of interest and different roles required of the physician as caregiver and the physician as researcher. The principle was dead, but the attitude survived. In 1968, at a congressional hearing sponsored by Senator Walter Mondale, leading medical researchers expressed their dismay that public or governmental oversight was deemed expedient. One witness stated that medical innovators "would be manacled by well-intentioned but meddlesome intruders. . . . I would urge you with all the strength I can muster, to leave this subject to conscionable people in the profession who are struggling valiantly to advance medicine."[24] Seven years later, at a conference sponsored by the National Academy of Science entitled *Experiments and Research with Humans: Values in Conflict*, the same sentiment was almost unanimous. One distinguished researcher after another asserted that ". . . human experimentation committees and all the rest, I think are fine . . . but there is no one who can relieve the investigator from assuming that responsibility and making the decision to put another person at risk." Others spoke even more strongly: "Nothing could be more unethical than critical judgment in this field made by persons who have not studied the biology of the field or the patient."[25] When one of the most perceptive and scholarly critics of the current research ethic, Dr. Jay Katz, suggested that "sorting out this value conflict cannot be left to the individual conscience of investigators," he was rebuffed by a noted scientist: "While Dr.Katz was talking, I was looking around the audience to see how many of my colleagues whom I know to be engaged . . . in human medical research had horns sticking out of their forehead."[26]

Change in the climate of research ethics was accelerated in 1972 when newspapers reported that from 1932 onward some 400 black men living in rural Macon County, Georgia, had been excluded from treatment for syphilis in order for the Public Health Service to study the untreated course of the disease.[27] In the volatile atmosphere of the civil rights movement, this revelation of the official exploitation of an already disadvantaged group could not be ignored. The Final Report of the Tuskegee Syphilis Study Ad Hoc Advisory Panel, issued in 1973, recommended establishment of a National Human Investigation Board, with authority to regulate all federally supported research with human subjects.[28]

This Board did not come into being. However, in the following year, Congress passed the National Research Act (Public Law 93-348, July 12, 1974), providing funding for the National Institutes of Health and establishing the National Commission for the Protection of Human Subjects of Biomedical and Behavioral Research. Congress charged the Commission with two tasks: to recommend to the Department of Health, Education and Welfare, regulations to protect the rights and welfare of human subjects of research, especially those with certain disabilities; and to develop principles to govern the ethical conduct of research. The twelve commissioners not only studied and debated these issues; they also invited a broad spectrum of scientists and scholars, particularly from philosophy and religion, to enlighten them. These scholars were themselves novices, but they quickly produced thoughtful reflections. Although several important conferences had explored the issues,[29] now a steady stream of insight and analysis from persons other than physician-researchers began to add to the social understanding of research and its moral dimensions. The Commission's work and resulting regulations significantly changed the climate of research in the United States.[30]

The climate before and after the Commission can be roughly described. In the decades before the Commission, from 1950 to 1970, clinical research activities greatly expanded the number of researchers and subjects, the sophistication of scientific methods, and financial resources. Many investigators seem to have been aware of certain special ethical duties, particularly the duties to avoid undue harm and to obtain consent, but the specifics of such duties were vague, and investigators alone determined their scope. A sense of social urgency, a remnant of wartime research, persisted; and a sense of social progress, fired by scientific enthusiasm, inspired researchers. As a result, it was easy to tip the balance between risks and benefits toward the benefit side and to define benefit, not in terms of the patient's needs, but in terms of the social goods that accrue from better medicine. It was also easy to see certain classes and groups as apt research subjects because they were less likely to reap any future benefits from treatment: the incurably ill, the severely retarded, and those who, like the incarcerated, had abused their social privileges.

After the Commission, the moral structure of research was much more clearly defined. Research was distinguished from therapy, and the essential features of the consent relationship were spelled out in detail. The easy assumptions about social progress as a rationale to override human rights was thoroughly demolished (a famous essay by philosopher Hans Jonas contributed mightily to its fall).[31] Sensitivity about exploiting the disadvantaged to benefit the advantaged was greatly heightened. Above all, research became a public enterprise. The review of research protocols by IRBs brought many outsiders to share in the ethical scrutiny of research proposals. Researchers began designing their protocols with greater attention to the rights and welfare of subjects precisely because they knew their projects would be reviewed. A new social institution, the review process with clearly articulated principles and procedures, was created. Over the last two decades, this institution has brought hundreds of scientists and citizens into the world of research ethics.

The resulting system, despite its faults and problems, has effected a major change in the climate of research. Ideas that had been abroad among scientists for a century were transformed in a decade from notions to practices, from ideals to established institutions, from occasional reference to habitual attention. Vague concepts have become specific practices. The culture of research after the 1970s is one in which researchers not only know about ethical constraints but have become accustomed to designing their research with those constraints in mind. They know that others, many as knowledgeable as themselves about scientific investigation, will review their efforts. Biomedical research has become a public enterprise.

NOTES

1. *Trials of War Criminals before the Nuremberg Military Tribunals under Control Council Law No. 10.* 2 vols. (Washington D.C.: Government Printing Office, 1950), pp. 181–182.
2. Michael A. Grodin. "Historical Origins of the Nuremberg Code," in George J. Annas and Michael A. Grodin, editors, *The Nazi Doctors and the Nuremberg Code* (New York: Oxford University Press, 1992).
3. Claude Bernard, *Introduction to Experimental Medicine* (New York: Dover, 1957), pp. 101–102.
4. Jay Katz, *Experimentation with Human Beings* (New York: Russell Sage, 1972), pp. 284–292; Susan Lederer, *Subjected to Science: Human Experimentation in America before the Second World War* (Baltimore: Johns Hopkins Press, 1995).
5. Sanarelli, "Etiologia e pathgenesi della febbra gialla." Quoted in W. Bean, "Walter Reed and the Ordeal of Human Experiments." *Bulletin of the History of Medicine* 51 (1977): 75–92, pp. 81–82. Originally reported in *Annales d'Igiene Sperimentale* n.s. 7 (1897): 345.
6. George Sternberg, "The bacillus icteroides (Sanarelli) and bacillus X (Sternberg)." *Transactions of the Association of American Physicians* 13 (1898): 71. Also quoted in W. Bean, "Walter Reed and the Ordeal," p. 83.
7. Harvey Cushing. *The Life of Sir William Osler* (Oxford: Clarendon Press, 1925), 2:109.
8. "Instructions to the Directors of Clinics, Out-Patient Clinics and Other Medical Facilities." *Centralblatt der gesamten Unterrichtsverwaltung in Preussen* (Prussian Ministry of Health, 1901), pp. 188–9; in Annas and Grodin, *The Nazi Doctors*, p. 127.
9. Michael Grodin, "Historical Origins," in *The Nazi Doctors*, pp. 131–132.
10. David Rothman, *Strangers at the Bedside* (New York: Basic Books, 1991), pp. 48–49.
11. "German Experiments at Auschwitz Camp," *Journal of the American Medical Association* 130 (1946): 892–893; Andrew C. Ivy, "History and Ethics of the Use of Human Subjects in Medical Experiments." *Science* 108 (1948): 1–5; W. L. Sperry, *New England Journal of Medicine* 239 (1946) 985; W.B. Bean, "Testament of Duty: Some Strictures on Moral Responsibility in Clinical Research." *Journal of Laboratory and Clinical Medicine* 39 (1952) 3; Otto E. Guttentag, *Annals of Internal Medicine* 31 (1949): 484; L. Alexander, "Medical Science and Dictatorship." *New England Journal of Medicine* 24 (1949): 39–47.
12. Otto E. Guttentag, "The Problem of Experimentation on Human Beings," *Science* 117 (1953): 205–214.
13. I. Ladimer, and R. W. Newman, *Clinical Investigation in Medicine: Legal, Ethical and Moral Aspects* (Boston: Boston University Law and Medicine Institute), 1963.
14. Renée Fox, *Experiment Perilous: Physicians and Patients Facing the Unknown* (Philadelphia: University of Pennsylvania Press, 1959).
15. Ruth Faden, editor. *The Human Radiation Experiments* (New York: Oxford, 1996).
16. Otto E. Guttentag, "The Physician's Point of View," *Science* 117 (1953): 205–214, at 209.

17. I. Ladimer, *Clinical Investigation in Medicine.*
18. R. B. Livingston, "Progress Report on Survey of Moral and Ethical Aspects of Clinical Investigation: Memorandum to Director, NIH," November 4, 1964. Quoted in Mark S. Frankel, "The Development of Policy Guidelines Governing Human Experimentation in the United States: A Case Study of Public Policy Making for Science and Technology," *Ethics in Science and Medicine* 2 (1975): 43–59, at 50.
19. Jay Katz, *Experimentation with Human Beings*, pp. 10–65.
20. M. B. Shimkin, "The researchers point of view." *Science* 117 (1953): 205–07, at 206.
21. World Medical Association, Declaration of Helsinki 1, June 1964; Declaration of Helsinki 2, October 1975. Reprinted in G. Annas and M. Grodin, *The Nazi Doctors*, pp. 331–342.
22. Henry Beecher, "Ethics and Clinical Research." *New England Journal of Medicine* 274 (1966): 1354–1360. Cf. David Rothman, *Strangers at the Bedside*, chap. 4.
23. A. B. Hill, "The Clinical Trial." *British Medical Bulletin* 7 (1951): 278–82; "Medical Ethics and Controlled Trials." *British Medical Journal* 1 (1963): 1043–49.
24. U.S. Senate. Committee on Government Operations, Hearing on the National Commission on Health Science and Society, 90th Congress, 2d session, 1968, p. 98; David Rothman, *Strangers at the Bedside*, p. 173.
25. W. McDermott, "The Risks of Research," in National Academy of Science, *Experiments and Research with Humans: Values in Conflict* (Washington D.C.: National Academy Press, 1975.), p. 42; and F. D. Moore, "A Cultural and Historical View," Ibid., p. 30.
26. Ibid., Jay Katz, p. 155; Sabin, p. 164. Cf. Jay Katz, "Ethics and Clinical Research Revisited," *Hastings Center Report* 23(5) (1993): 31–39.
27. J. Heller, "U.S. Testers Let Many Die of Syphilis." *Washington Post*, July 26, 1972, pp. A1 and A6.
28. James Jones, *Bad Blood* (New York: Free Press, 1981).
29. I. Ladimer and R. W. Newman, *Clinical Investigation in Medicine*; Paul Freund, editor, *Experimentation with Human Subjects* (New York: Braziller, 1969). Also published as *Daedalus* 98 (1969).
30. R. J. Levine, *Ethics and Regulation of Clinical Research*, 2d ed. (New Haven: Yale University Press, 1988).
31. Hans Jonas, "Philosophical Reflections on Experimenting with Human Subjects," in Paul Freund, editor, *Experimentation with Human Subjects.*

Editor's Suggestions for Further Reading

Frankel, Mark S. "The Development of Policy Guidelines Governing Human Experimentation in the United States: A Case Study of Public Policy-Making For Science and Technology." *Ethics in Science and Medicine* 2 (1975); 43–59.

Jonsen, Albert R. *The Birth of Bioethics. The Origin and Evolution of Bioethics in the United States: 1947–1987.* New York: Oxford University Press, 1998. Chapter 5.

Rothman, David J. *Strangers at the Bedside: A History of How Law and Bioethics Transformed Medical Decision Making.* New York: Basic Books, 1991. Chapters 3–5.

THE NUREMBERG CODE

INTRODUCTION. *In 1945, the Allied nations (United States, French Republic, United Kingdom, and Union of Soviet Socialist Republics) established an International Military Tribunal for the prosecution of German citizens accused of war crimes and crimes against humanity. At the end of the following year, an eight-month trial of twenty-three Nazi officials, twenty of them medical doctors, began. These defendants were accused of crimes against humanity by conducting criminal scientific and medical experiments on concentration camp prisoners. The "Doctors Trial" concluded on August 20, 1947, with a verdict of guilty imposed on sixteen defendants, of whom seven were sentenced to death. The final judgment concludes with a statement of ten points enumerating the principles for ethical research with human subjects. These ten points, subsequently known as the Nuremberg Code, have become part of International Law and serve as the basis for many formulations of the ethics of research with human subjects.*

THE PROOF AS TO WAR CRIMES AND CRIMES AGAINST HUMANITY

Judged by any standard of proof the record clearly shows the commission of war crimes and crimes against humanity substantially as alleged in counts two and three of the indictment.

Beginning with the outbreak of World War II, criminal medical experiments on non-German nationals, both prisoners of war and civilians, including Jews and "asocial" persons, were carried out on a large scale in Germany and the occupied countries. These experiments were not the isolated and casual acts of individual doctors and scientists working solely on their own responsibility, but were the product of coordinated policy-making and planning at high governmental, military, and Nazi Party levels, conducted as an integral part of the total war effort. They were ordered, sanctioned, permitted, or approved by persons in positions of authority who under all principles of law were under the duty to know about things and to take steps to terminate or prevent them.

Reprinted from *Trials of War Criminals before the Nuremberg Military Tribunals under Control Council Law No. 10: Nuremberg, October 1946–1949*, 2 vols. (Washington, D.C.: U.S. Government Printing Office, 1949), pp. 181–182. For additional information, see George J. Annas and Michael A. Grodin, editors, *The Nazi Doctors and the Nuremberg Code: Human Rights in Human Experimentation* (New York: Oxford University Press, 1992).

PERMISSIBLE MEDICAL EXPERIMENTS

The great weight of evidence before us is to the effect that certain types of medical experiments on human beings, when kept within reasonable well-defined bounds, conform to the ethics of the medical profession generally. The protagonists of the practice of human experimentation justify their views on the basis that such experiments yield results for the good of society that are unprocurable by other methods or means of study. All agree, however, that certain basic principles must be observed in order to satisfy moral, ethical and legal concepts:

1. The voluntary consent of the human subject is absolutely essential.

   This means that the person involved should have legal capacity to give consent; should be so situated as to be able to exercise free power of choice, without the intervention of any element of force, fraud, deceit, duress, overreaching, or other ulterior form of constraint or coercion; and should have sufficient knowledge and comprehension of the elements of the subject matter involved as to enable him to make an understanding and enlightened decision. This latter element requires that before the acceptance of an affirmative decision by the experimental subject there should be made known to him the nature, duration, and purpose of the experiment; the method and means by which it is to be conducted; all inconveniences and hazards reasonably to be expected; and the effects upon his health or person which may possibly come from his participation in the experiment.

The duty and responsibility for ascertaining the quality of the consent rests upon each individual who initiates, directs or engages in the experiment. It is a personal duty and responsibility which may not be delegated to another with impunity.

2. The experiment should be such as to yield fruitful results for the good of society, unprocurable by other methods or means of study, and not random and unnecessary in nature.
3. The experiment should be so designed and based on the results of animal experimentation and a knowledge of the natural history of the disease or other problem under study that the anticipated results will justify the performance of the experiment.
4. The experiment should be so conducted as to avoid all unnecessary physical and mental suffering and injury.
5. No experiment should be conducted where there is an *a priori* reason to believe that death or disabling injury will occur; except, perhaps, in those experiments where the experimental physicians also serve as subjects.
6. The degree of risk to be taken should never exceed that determined by the humanitarian importance of the problem to be solved by the experiment.
7. Proper preparations should be made and adequate facilities provided to protect the experimental subject against even remote possibilities of injury, disability, or death.
8. The experiment should be conducted only by scientifically qualified persons. The highest degree of skill and care should be required through all stages of the experiment of those who conduct or engage in the experiment.
9. During the course of the experiment the human subject should be at liberty to bring the experiment to an end if he has reached the physical or mental state where continuation of the experiment seems to him to be impossible.
10. During the course of the experiment the scientist in charge must be prepared to terminate the experiment at any stage, if he has probable cause to believe, in the exercise of the good faith, superior skill and careful judgment required of him that a continuation of the experiment is likely to result in injury, disability, or death to the experimental subject.

DECLARATION OF HELSINKI: RECOMMENDATIONS GUIDING MEDICAL DOCTORS IN BIOMEDICAL RESEARCH INVOLVING HUMAN SUBJECTS

Introduction. *The World Medical Association, founded in 1946, approved a statement of* Principles for Those in Research and Experimentation *at its eighth general assembly, in Rome, Italy, in 1954. In June 1964, the 18th World Medical Assembly meeting in Helsinki, Finland, adopted an expanded version of this statement, which became widely known as the* Helsinki Declaration. *It, too, was amended: at Tokyo in 1975, Venice in 1983 and Hong Kong in 1989. Alterations made after 1975 (Tokyo's "Declaration II") have been minor.*

It is the mission of the medical doctor to safeguard the health of the people. His or her knowledge and conscience are dedicated to the fulfillment of this mission.

The Declaration of Geneva of the World Medical Association binds the doctor with the words, "The health of my patient will be my first consideration," and the International Code of Medical Ethics declares that, "Any act or advice which could weaken physical or mental resistance of a human being may be used only in his interest."

The purpose of biomedical research involving human subjects must be to improve diagnostic, therapeutic and prophylactic procedures and the understanding of the aetiology and pathogenesis of disease.

In current medical practice most diagnostic, therapeutic or prophylactic procedures involve hazards. This applies *a fortiori* to biomedical research.

Medical progress is based on research which ultimately must rest in part on experimentation involving human subjects.

In the field of biomedical research a fundamental distinction must be recognized between medical research in which the aim is essentially diagnostic or therapeutic for a patient, and medical research, the essential object of which is purely scientific and without direct diagnostic or therapeutic value to the person subjected to the research.

Special caution must be exercised in the conduct of research which may affect the environment, and the welfare of animals used for research must be respected.

Because it is essential that the results of laboratory experiments be applied to human beings to further scientific knowledge and to help suffering humanity, the World Medical Association has prepared the following recommendations as a guide to every doctor in biomedical research involving human subjects. They should be kept under review in the future. It must be stressed that the standards as drafted are only a guide to physicians all over the world. Doctors are not relieved from criminal, civil and ethical responsibilities under the laws of their own countries.

I. BASIC PRINCIPLES

1. Biomedical research involving human subjects must conform to generally accepted scientific principles and should be based on adequately performed laboratory and animal experimentation and on a thorough knowledge of the scientific literature.
2. The design and performance of each experimental procedure involving human subjects should be clearly for-

World Medical Association, Recommendations Guiding Medical Doctors in Biomedical Research Involving Human Subjects (Helsinki: 18th World Medical Assembly, 1964; revised Tokyo: 29th World Medical Assembly, 1975).

mulated in an experimental protocol which should be transmitted to a specially appointed independent committee for consideration, comment and guidance.

3. Biomedical research involving human subjects should be conducted only by scientifically qualified persons and under the supervision of a clinically competent medical person. The responsibility for the human subject must always rest with a medically qualified person and never rest on the subject of the research, even though the subject has given his or her consent.
4. Biomedical research involving human subjects cannot legitimately be carried out unless the importance of the objectives is in proportion to the inherent risk to the subject.
5. Every biomedical research project involving human subjects should be preceded by careful assessment of predictable risks in comparison with foreseeable benefits to the subject or to others. Concern for the interests of the subject must always prevail over the interest of science and society.
6. The right of the research subject to safeguard his or her integrity must always be respected. Every precaution should be taken to respect the privacy of the subject and to minimize the impact of the study on the subject's physical and mental integrity and on the personality of the subject.
7. Doctors should abstain from engaging in research projects involving human subjects unless they are satisfied that the hazards involved are believed to be predictable. Doctors should cease any investigation if the hazards are found to outweigh the potential benefits.
8. In publication of the results of his or her research, the doctor is obliged to preserve the accuracy of the results. Reports of experimentation not in accordance with the principles laid down in this Declaration should not be accepted for publication.
9. In any research on human beings, each potential subject must be adequately informed of the aims, methods, anticipated benefits and potential hazards of the study and the discomfort it may entail. He or she should be informed that he or she is at liberty to abstain from participation in the study and that he or she is free to withdraw his or her consent to participation at any time. The doctor should then obtain the subject's freely given informed consent, preferably in writing.
10. When obtaining informed consent for the research project the doctor should be particularly cautious if the subject is in a dependent relationship to him or her or may consent under duress. In that case the informed consent should be obtained by a doctor who is not engaged in the investigation and who is completely independent of this official relationship.
11. In case of legal incompetence, informed consent should be obtained from the legal guardian in accordance with national legislation. Where physical or mental incapacity makes it impossible to obtain informed consent, or when the subject is a minor, permission from the responsible relative replaces that of the subject in accordance with national legislation.
12. The research protocol should always contain a statement of the ethical considerations involved and should indicate that the principles enunciated in the present Declaration are complied with.

II. MEDICAL RESEARCH COMBINED WITH PROFESSIONAL CARE (Clinical Research)

1. In the treatment of the sick person, the doctor must be free to use a new diagnostic and therapeutic measure, if in his or her judgment it offers hope of saving life, reestablishing health or alleviating suffering.
2. The potential benefits, hazards and discomforts of a new method should be weighed against the advantages of the best current diagnostic and therapeutic methods.
3. In any medical study, every patient—including those of a control group, if any—should be assured of the best proven diagnostic and therapeutic method.
4. The refusal of the patient to participate in a study must never interfere with the doctor-patient relationship.
5. If the doctor considers it essential not to obtain informed consent, the specific reasons for this proposal should be stated in the experimental protocol for transmission to the independent committee (I, 2).
6. The doctor can combine medical research with professional care, the objective being the acquisition of new medical knowledge, only to the extent that medical research is justified by its potential diagnostic or therapeutic value for the patient.

III. NON-THERAPEUTIC BIOMEDICAL RESEARCH INVOLVING HUMAN SUBJECTS (Non-clinical Biomedical Research)

1. In the purely scientific application of medical research carried out on a human being, it is the duty of the doctor to remain the protector of the life and health of that person on whom biomedical research is being carried out.

2. The subjects should be volunteers - either healthy persons or patients for whom the experimental design is not related to the patient's illness.
3. The investigator or the investigating team should discontinue the research if in his/her or their judgment it may, if continued, be harmful to the individual.
4. In research on man, the interest of science and society should never take precedence over considerations related to the well-being of the subject.

ON THE PROTECTION OF HUMAN SUBJECTS: U.S. DEPARTMENT OF HEALTH, EDUCATION AND WELFARE'S INSTITUTIONAL GUIDE

INTRODUCTION. *In 1971, the Department of Health, Education and Welfare (DHEW), now known as the Department of Health and Human Services (HHS), issued institutional guidance designed to safeguard the rights and welfare of human subjects of federally funded medical research. This document expanded and formalized guidelines that the National Institutes of Health had published in 1966 and revised in 1969. The policies in the DHEW document were also reviewed, and a revised version was published in the Code of Federal Regulations (45 CFR 46) in May 1974. These regulations, the 1974 version of the Guide, were likewise reviewed and revised—this time on the basis of recommendations from the National Commission for the Protection of Human Subjects of Biomedical and Behavioral Research (1974–1978)—and officially promulgated in 1981. The DHEW guidance document remains the bedrock of federal regulations governing the protection of human subjects in research.*

Policy

Safeguarding the rights and welfare of human subjects involved in activities supported by grants or contracts from the Department of Health, Education, and Welfare is the responsibility of the institution which receives or is accountable to the DHEW for the funds awarded for the support of the activity. In order to provide for the adequate discharge of this institutional responsibility, it is the policy of the Department that no grant or contract for an activity involving human subjects shall be made unless the application for such support has been reviewed and approved by an appropriate institutional committee.

This review shall determine that the rights and welfare of the subjects involved are adequately protected, that the risks to an individual are outweighed by the potential benefits to him or by the importance of the knowledge to be gained, and that informed consent is to be obtained by methods that are adequate and appropriate.

In addition the committee must establish a basis for continuing review of the activity in keeping with these determinations.

The institution must submit to the DHEW, for its review, approval, and official acceptance, an assurance of its compliance with this policy. The institution must also provide with each proposal involving human subjects a certification that it has been or will be reviewed in accordance with the institution's assurance.

No grant or contract involving human subjects at risk will be made to an individual unless he is affiliated with or sponsored by an institution which can and does assume responsibility for the protection of the subjects involved.

Since the welfare of subjects is a matter of concern to the Department of Health, Education, and Welfare as well as to the institution, no grant or contract involving human subjects shall be made unless the proposal for such support has been reviewed and approved by an appropriate professional committee within the responsible component of the Department. As a result of this review, the committee may recommend to the operating agency, and the operating agency may require, the imposition of specific grant or contract terms providing for the protection of human subjects, including requirements for informed consent.

Reprinted from *The Institutional Guide to DHEW Policy on Protection of Human Subjects.* DHEW Publication No. NIH 72-102, December 1, 1971 (Washington, D.C.: U.S. Government Printing Office, 1971), pp. 2–11.

Applicability

A. General This policy applies to all grants and contracts which support activities in which subjects may be at risk.

B. Subject This term describes any individual who may be at risk as a consequence of participation as a subject in research, development, demonstration, or other activities supported by DHEW funds.

This may include patients; outpatients; donors of organs, tissues, and services; informants; and normal volunteers, including students who are placed at risk during training in medical, psychological, sociological, educational, and other types of activities supported by DHEW.

Of particular concern are those subjects in groups with limited civil freedom. These include prisoners, residents or clients of institutions for the mentally ill and mentally retarded, and persons subject to military discipline.

The unborn and the dead should be considered subjects to the extent that they have rights which can be exercised by their next of kin or legally authorized representatives.

C. At Risk An individual is considered to be "at risk" if he may be exposed to the possibility of harm—physical, psychological, sociological, or other—as a consequence of any activity which goes beyond the application of those established and accepted methods necessary to meet his needs. The determination of when an individual is at risk is a matter of the application of common sense and sound professional judgment to the circumstances of the activity in question. Responsibility for this determination resides at all levels of institutional and departmental review. Definitive determination will be made by the operating agency.

D. Types of Risks and Applicability of the Policy

1. Certain risks are inherent in life itself, at the time and in the places where life runs its course. This policy is not concerned with the ordinary risks of public or private living, or those risks associated with admission to a school or hospital. It is not concerned with the risks inherent in professional practice as long as these do not exceed the bounds of established and accepted procedures, including innovative practices applied in the interest of the individual patient, student or client.

Risk and the applicability of this policy are most obvious in medical and behavioral science research projects involving procedures that may induce a potentially harmful altered physical state or condition. Surgical and biopsy procedures; the removal of organs or tissues for study, reference, transplantation, or banking; the administration of drugs or radiation; the use of indwelling catheters or electrodes; the requirement of strenuous physical exertion; subjection to deceit, public embarrassment, and humiliation are all examples of procedures which require thorough scrutiny by both the Department of Health, Education, and Welfare and institutional committees. In general those projects which involve risk of physical or psychological injury require prior written consent.

2. There is a wide range of medical, social, and behavioral projects and activities in which no immediate physical risk to the subject is involved; e.g., those utilizing personality inventories, interviews, questionnaires, or the use of observation, photographs, taped records, or stored data. However, some of these procedures may involve varying degrees of discomfort, harassment, invasion of privacy, or may constitute a threat to the subject's dignity through the imposition of demeaning or dehumanizing conditions.

3. There are also medical and biomedical projects concerned solely with organs, tissues, body fluids, and other materials obtained in the course of the routine performance of medical services such as diagnosis, treatment and care, or at autopsy. The use of these materials obviously involves no element of physical risk to the subject. However, their use for many research, training, and service purposes may present psychological, sociological, or legal risks to the subject or his authorized representatives. In these instances, application of the policy requires review to determine that the circumstances under which the materials were procured were appropriate and that adequate and appropriate consent was, or can be, obtained for the use of these materials for project purposes.

4. Similarly, some studies depend upon stored data or information which was often obtained for quite different purposes. Here, the reviews should also determine whether the use of these materials is within the scope of the original consent, or whether consent can be obtained.

E. Established and Accepted Methods Some methods become established through rigorous standardization procedures prescribed, as in the case of drugs or biologicals, by law or, as in the case of many educational tests, through the aegis of professional societies or nonprofit agencies. Acceptance is a matter of professional response, and determination as to when a method passes from the experimental stage and becomes "established and accepted" is a matter of judgment.

In determining what constitutes an established and accepted method, consideration should be given to both national and local standards of practice. A management procedure may become temporarily established in the routine of a local institution but still fail to win acceptance at the national level. A psychological inventory may be accepted nationally, but still contain questions which are disturbing or offensive to a local population. Surgical procedures which are established and accepted in one part of the country may be considered experimental in another, not due to inherent deficiencies, but because of the lack of proper facilities and trained personnel. Diagnostic procedures which are routine in the United States may pose serious hazards to an undernourished, heavily infected, overseas population.

If doubt exists as to whether the procedures to be employed are established and accepted, the activity should be subject to review and approval by the institutional committee.

F. Necessity to Meet Needs Even if considered established and accepted, the method may place the subject at risk if it is being employed for purposes other than to meet the needs of the subject. Determination by an attending professional that a particular treatment, test, regimen, or curriculum is appropriate for a particular subject to meet his needs limits the attendant risks to those inherent in the delivery of services, or in training.

On the other hand, arbitrary, random, or other assignment of subjects to differing treatment or study groups in the interests of a DHEW supported activity, rather than in the strict interests of the subject, introduces the possibility of exposing him to additional risk. Even comparisons of two or more established and accepted methods may potentially involve exposure of at least some of the subjects to additional risks. Any alteration of the choice, scope, or timing of an otherwise established and accepted method, primarily in the interests of a DHEW activity, also raises the issue of additional risk.

If doubt exists as to whether the procedures are intended solely to meet the needs of the subject, the activity should be subject to review and approval by the institutional committee.

Institutional Review

A. Initial Review of Projects 1. Review must be carried out by an appropriate institutional committee. The committee may be an existing one, such as a board of trustees, medical staff committee, utilization committee, or research committee, or it may be specially constituted for the purpose of this review. Institutions may utilize subcommittees to represent major administrative or subordinate components in those instances where establishment of a single committee is impracticable or inadvisable. The institution may utilize staff, consultants, or both.

The committee must be composed of sufficient members with varying backgrounds to assure complete and adequate review of projects and activities commonly conducted by the institution. The committee's membership, maturity, experience, and expertise should be such as to justify respect for its advice and counsel. No member of an institutional committee shall be involved in either the initial or continuing review of an activity in which he has a professional responsibility, except to provide information requested by the committee. In addition to possessing the professional competence to review specific activities, the committee should be able to determine acceptability of the proposal in terms of institutional commitments and regulations, applicable law, standards of professional conduct and practice, and community attitudes [note to 21 CFR 130 omitted]. The committee may therefore need to include persons whose primary concerns lie in these areas rather than in the conduct of research, development, and service programs of the types supported by the DHEW.

If an institution is so small that it cannot appoint a suitable committee from its own staff, it should appoint members from outside the institution.

Committee members shall be identified by name, occupation or position, and by other pertinent indications of experience and competence in areas pertinent to the areas of review such as earned degrees, board certifications, licensures, memberships, etc.

Temporary replacement of a committee member by an alternate of comparable experience and competence is permitted in the event a member is momentarily unable to fulfill committee responsibility. The DHEW should be notified of any permanent replacement or additions.

2. The institution should adopt a statement of principles that will assist it in the discharge of its responsibilities for protecting the rights and welfare of subjects. This may be an appropriate existing code or declaration or one formulated by the institution itself [note omitted]. It is to be understood that no such principles supersede DHEW policy or applicable law.

3. Review begins with the identification of those projects or activities which involve subjects who may be at risk. In institutions with large grant and contract programs, administrative staff may be delegated the responsibility of separating those projects which do not involve human subjects in any degree; i.e., animal and nonhuman materials studies. However, determinations as to whether any project or activity involves human subjects at risk is a professional responsibility to be discharged through review by the committee, or by subcommittees.

If review determines that the procedures to be applied are to be limited to those considered by the committee to be established, accepted, and necessary to the needs of the subject, review need go no further; and the application should be certified as approved by the committee. Such projects involve human subjects, but these subjects are not considered to be at risk.

If review determines that the procedures to be applied will place the subject at risk, review should be expanded to include the issues of the protection of the subject's rights and welfare, of the relative weight of risks and benefits, and of the provision of adequate and appropriate consent procedures.

Where required by workload considerations or by geographic separation of operating units, subcommittees or mail review may be utilized to provide preliminary review of applications.

Final review of projects involving subjects at risk should be carried out by a quorum of the committee. . . . Such review should determine, through review of reports by subcommittees, or through its own examination of applications or of protocols, or through interviews with those individuals who will have professional responsibility for the proposal project or activity, or through other acceptable procedures that the requirements of the institutional assurance and of DHEW policy have been met, specifically that:

a. The rights and welfare of the subjects are adequately protected.

Institutional committees should carefully examine applications, protocols, or descriptions of work to arrive at an independent determination of possible risks. The committee must be alert to the possibility that investigators, program directors, or contractors may, quite unintentionally, introduce unnecessary or unacceptable hazards, or fail to provide adequate safeguards. This possibility is particularly true if the project crosses disciplinary lines, involves new and untried procedures, or involves established and accepted procedures which are new to the personnel applying them. Committees must also assure themselves that proper precautions will be taken to deal with emergencies that may develop even in the course of seemingly routine activities.

When appropriate, provision should be made for safeguarding information that could be traced to, or identified with, subjects. The committee may require the project or activity director to take steps to insure the confidentiality and security of data, particularly if it may not always remain under his direct control.

Safeguards include, initially, the careful design of questionnaires, inventories, interview schedules, and other data gathering instruments and procedures to limit the personal information to be acquired to that absolutely essential to the project or activity. Additional safeguards include the encoding or enciphering of names, addresses, serial numbers, and of data transferred to tapes, discs, and printouts. Secure, locked spaces and cabinets may be necessary for handling and storing documents and files. Codes and ciphers should always be kept in secure places, distinctly separate from encoded and enciphered data. The shipment, delivery, and transfer of all data, printouts, and files between offices and institutions may require careful controls. Computer to computer transmission of data may be restricted or forbidden.

Provision should also be made for the destruction of all edited, obsolete or depleted data on punched cards, tapes, discs, and other records. The committee may also determine a future date for destruction of all stored primary data pertaining to a project or activity.

Particularly relevant to the decision of the committees are those rights of the subject that are defined by law. The committee should familiarize itself through consultation with legal counsel with these statutes and common law precedents which may bear on its decisions. The provisions of this policy may not be construed in any manner or sense that would abrogate, supersede, or moderate more restrictive applicable law or precedential legal decisions.

Laws may define what constitutes consent and who may give consent, prescribe or proscribe the performance of certain medical and surgical procedures, protect confidential communications, define negligence, define invasion of privacy, require disclosure of records pursuant to legal process, and limit charitable and governmental immunity.

b. The risks to an individual are outweighed by the potential benefits to him or by the importance of the knowledge to be gained.

The committee should carefully weigh the known or foreseeable risks to be encountered by subjects, the probable benefits that may accrue to them, and the probable benefits to humanity that may result from the subject's participation in the project or activity. If it seems probable that participation will confer substantial benefits on the subjects, the committee may be justified in permitting them to accept commensurate or lesser risks. If the potential benefits are insubstantial, or are outweighed by risks, the committee may be justified in permitting the subjects to accept these risks in the interests of humanity. The committee should consider the possibility that subjects, or those authorized to represent subjects, may be motivated to accept risks for unsuitable or inadequate reasons. In such instances the consent procedures adopted should incorporate adequate safeguards.

Compensation to volunteers should never be such as to constitute an undue inducement.

No subject can be expected to understand the issues of risks and benefits as fully as the committee. Its agreement that consent can reasonably be sought for subject participation in a project or activity is of paramount practical importance.

> The informed consent of the subject, while often a legal necessity is a goal toward which we must strive, but hardly ever achieve except in the simplest cases.
>
> Henry K. Beecher, M.D.

c. The informed consent of subjects will be obtained by methods that are adequate and appropriate [note to 21 CFR 130 omitted].

Informed consent is the agreement obtained from a subject, or from his authorized representative, to the subject's participation in an activity.

The basic elements of informed consent are:

1. A fair explanation of the procedures to be followed, including an identification of those which are experimental;
2. A description of the attendant discomforts and risks;
3. A description of the benefits to be expected;
4. A disclosure of appropriate alternative procedures that would be advantageous for the subject;

5. An offer to answer any inquiries concerning the procedures;
6. An instruction that the subject is free to withdraw his consent and to discontinue participation in the project or activity at any time.

In addition, the agreement, written or oral, entered into by the subject, should include no exculpatory language through which the subject is made to waive, or to appear to waive, any of his legal rights, or to release the institution or its agents from liability for negligence (the use of exculpatory clauses is contrary to public policy [*Tunkl v. Regents of University of California*]).

Informed consent must be documented. . . .

Consent should be obtained, whenever practicable, from the subjects themselves. When the subject group will include individuals who are not legally or physically capable of giving informed consent, because of age, mental incapacity, or inability to communicate, the review committee should consider the validity of consent by next of kin, legal guardians, or by other qualified third parties representative of the subjects' interests. In such instances, careful consideration should be given by the committee not only to whether these third parties can be presumed to have the necessary depth of interest and concern with the subjects' rights and welfare, but also to whether these third parties will be legally authorized to expose the subjects to the risks involved.

The review committee will determine if the consent required, whether to be secured before the fact, in writing or orally, or after the fact following debriefing, or whether implicit in voluntary participation in an adequately advertised activity, is appropriate in the light of the risks to the subject, and the circumstances of the project.

The review committee will also determine if the information to be given to the subject, or to qualified third parties, in writing or orally, is a fair explanation of the project or activity, of its possible benefits, and of its attendant hazards.

Where an activity involves therapy, diagnosis, or management, and a professional/patient relationship exists, it is necessary "to recognize that each patient's mental and emotional condition is important . . . and that in discussing the element of risk, a certain amount of discretion must be employed consistent with full disclosure of fact necessary to any informed consent" (*Salgo v. Leland Stanford Jr. University Board of Trustees* [154C.A.2nd 560; 317 P. 2d 1701]).

Where an activity does not involve therapy, diagnosis, or management, and a professional/subject rather than a professional/patient relationship exists, "the subject is entitled to a full and frank disclosure of all the facts, probabilities, and opinions which a reasonable man might be expected to consider before giving his consent" (*Halushka v. University of Saskatchewan* [1965] 53 D.L.R. [2d]).

When debriefing procedures are considered as a necessary part of the plan, the committee should ascertain that these will be complete and prompt.

B. Continuing Review This is an essential part of the review process. While procedures for continuing review of ongoing projects and activities should be based in principle on the initial review criteria, they should also be adapted to the size and administrative structure of the institution. Institutions which are small and compact and in which the committee members are in day-to-day contact with professional staff may be able to function effectively with some informality. Institutions which have placed responsibility for review in boards of trustees, utilization committees, and similar groups that meet on frequent schedules may find it possible to have projects reviewed during these meetings.

In larger institutions with more complex administrative structures and specially appointed committees, these committees may adopt a variety of continuing review mechanisms. They may involve systematic review of projects at fixed intervals, or at intervals set by the committee commensurate with the project's risk. Thus, a project involving an untried procedure may initially require reconsideration as each subject completes his involvement. A highly routine project may need no more than annual review. Routine diagnostic service procedures, such as biopsy and autopsy, which contribute to research and demonstration activities generally require no more than annual review. Spot checks may be used to supplement scheduled reviews.

Actual review may involve interviews with the responsible staff, or review of written reports and supporting documents and forms. In any event, such review must be completed at least annually to permit certifications of review on noncompeting continuation applications.

C. Communication of the Committee's Action, Advice, and Counsel If the committee's overall recommendation is favorable, it may simultaneously prescribe restrictions or conditions under which the activity may be conducted, define substantial changes in the research plans which should be brought to its attention, and determine the nature and frequency of interim review procedures to insure continued acceptable conduct of the research.

Favorable recommendations by an institutional committee are, of course, always subject to further appropriate review and rejection by institution officials.

Unfavorable recommendations, restrictions, or conditions cannot be removed except by the committee or by the action of another appropriate review group described in the assurance filed with the Department of Health, Education, and Welfare.

Staff with supervisory responsibility for investigators and program directors whose projects or activities have been disapproved or restricted, and institutional administrative and financial officers should be informed of the committee's recommendations. Responsible professional staff should be informed of the reasons for any adverse actions taken by the institutional committee.

The committee should be prepared at all times to provide advice and counsel to staff developing new projects or activities or contemplating revision of ongoing projects or disapproved proposals.

D. Maintenance of an Active and Effective Committee Institutions should establish policy determining overall committee composition, including provisions for rotation of memberships and appointment of chairmen. Channels of responsibility should be established for implementation of committee recommendations as they may affect the actions of responsible professional staff, grants and contracts officers, business officers, and other responsible staff. Provisions should be made for remedial action in the event of disregard of committee recommendations. . . .

THE BELMONT REPORT: ETHICAL PRINCIPLES AND GUIDELINES FOR THE PROTECTION OF HUMAN SUBJECTS OF RESEARCH

INTRODUCTION. *In 1974, the U.S. Congress passed Public Law 93-348, establishing the National Commission for the Protection of Human Subjects of Biomedical and Behavioral Research. This body, made up of twelve citizens drawn from science, law, ethics, and the lay public, was required to make recommendations to the Secretary of Health, Education and Welfare for protecting the rights and welfare of human subjects of research. Sections of the Commission's report involving research on the human fetus, children, prisoners, and on the functions of Institutional Review Boards (IRBs) were published separately and are included in this book. The Commission was also asked to distinguish between medical research and practice and to develop the basic ethical principles that should govern research with human subjects. The Belmont Report, issued on April 18, 1979, fulfilled the latter mandate. It has since become a document of considerable importance, not only in research ethics, but in bioethics generally.*

SCIENTIFIC RESEARCH has produced substantial social benefits. It has also posed some troubling ethical questions. Public attention was drawn to these questions by reported abuses of human subjects in biomedical experiments, especially during the Second World War. During the the Nuremberg War Crime Trials, the Nuremberg code was drafted as a set of standards for judging physicians and scientists who had conducted biomedical experiments on concentration camp prisoners. This code became the prototype of many later codes[1] intended to assure that research involving human subjects would be carried out in an ethical manner.

The codes consist of rules, some general, others specific, that guide the investigators or the reviewers of research in their work. Such rules often are inadequate to cover complex situations; at times they come into conflict, and they are frequently difficult to interpret or apply. Broader ethical principles will provide a basis on which specific rules may be formulated, criticized and interpreted.

Three principles, or general prescriptive judgments, that are relevant to research involving human subjects are identified in this statement. Other principles may also be relevant. These three are comprehensive, however, and are stated at a level of generalization that should assist scientists, subjects, reviewers and interested citizens to understand the ethical issues inherent in research involving human subjects. These principles cannot always be applied so as to resolve beyond dispute particular ethical problems. The objective is to provide an analytical framework that will guide the resolution of ethical problems arising from research involving human subjects.

This statement consists of a distinction between research and practice, a discussion of the three basic ethical principles, and remarks about the application of these principles.

A. Boundaries Between Practice and Research

It is important to distinguish between biomedical and behavioral research, on the one hand, and the practice of

National Commission for the Protection of Human Subjects of Biomedical and Behavioral Research, *The Belmont Report: Ethical Principles and Guidelines for the Protection of Human Subjects of Research* (Washington, D.C.: U.S. Government Printing Office, 1979). For additional information, see Robert J. Levine, *Ethics and Regulation of Clinical Research* (New Haven: Yale University Press, 1988), Chapter 1.

accepted therapy on the other, in order to know what activities ought to undergo review for the protection of human subjects of research. The distinction between research and practice is blurred partly because both often occur together (as in research designed to evaluate a therapy) and partly because notable departures from standard practice are often called "experimental" when the terms "experimental" and "research" are not carefully defined.

For the most part, the term "practice" refers to interventions that are designed solely to enhance the well-being of an individual patient or client and that have a reasonable expectation of success. The purpose of medical or behavioral practice is to provide diagnosis, preventive treatment or therapy to particular individuals.[2] By contrast, the term "research" designates an activity designed to test an hypothesis, permit conclusions to be drawn, and thereby to develop or contribute to generalizable knowledge (expressed, for example, in theories, principles, and statements of relationships). Research is usually described in a formal protocol that sets forth an objective and a set of procedures designed to reach that objective.

When a clinician departs in a significant way from standard or accepted practice, the innovation does not, in and of itself, constitute research. The fact that a procedure is "experimental," in the sense of new, untested or different, does not automatically place it in the category of research. Radically new procedures of this description should, however, be made the object of formal research at an early stage in order to determine whether they are safe and effective. Thus, it is the responsibility of medical practice committees, for example, to insist that a major innovation be incorporated into a formal research project.[3]

Research and practice may be carried on together when research is designed to evaluate the safety and efficacy of a therapy. This need not cause any confusion regarding whether or not the activity requires review; the general rule is that if there is any element of research in an activity, that activity should undergo review for the protection of human subjects.

B. Basic Ethical Principles

The expression "basic ethical principles" refers to those general judgments that serve as a basic justification for the many particular ethical prescriptions and evaluations of human actions. Three basic principles, among those generally accepted in our cultural tradition, are particularly relevant to the ethics of research involving human subjects: the principles of respect for persons, beneficence and justice.

1. Respect for Persons Respect for persons incorporates at least two ethical convictions: first, that individuals should be treated as autonomous agents, and second, that persons with diminished autonomy are entitled to protection. The principle of respect for persons thus divides into two separate moral requirements: the requirement to acknowledge autonomy and the requirement to protect those with diminished autonomy.

An autonomous person is an individual capable of deliberation about personal goals and of acting under the direction of such deliberation. To respect autonomy is to give weight to autonomous persons' considered opinions and choices while refraining from obstructing their actions unless they are clearly detrimental to others. To show lack of respect for an autonomous agent is to repudiate that person's considered judgments, to deny an individual the freedom to act on those considered judgments, or to withhold information necessary to make a considered judgment, when there are no compelling reasons to do so.

However, not every human being is capable of self-determination. The capacity for self-determination matures during an individual's life, and some individuals lose this capacity wholly or in part because of illness, mental disability, or circumstances that severely restrict liberty. Respect for the immature and the incapacitated may require protecting them as they mature or while they are incapacitated.

Some persons are in need of extensive protection, even to the point of excluding them from activities which may harm them; other persons require little protection beyond making sure they undertake activities freely and with awareness of possible adverse consequences. The extent of protection afforded should depend upon the risk of harm and the likelihood of benefit. The judgment that any individual lacks autonomy should be periodically reevaluated and will vary in different situations.

In most cases of research involving human subjects, respect for persons demands that subjects enter into the research voluntarily and with adequate information. In some situations, however, application of the principle is not obvious. The involvement of prisoners as subjects of research provides an instructive example. On the one hand, it would seem that the principle of respect for persons requires that prisoners not be deprived of the opportunity to volunteer for research. On the other hand, under prison conditions they may be subtly coerced or unduly influenced to engage in research activities for which they would not otherwise volunteer. Respect for persons would then dictate that prisoners be protected. Whether to allow prisoners to "volunteer" or to "protect" them presents a dilemma. Respecting persons, in most hard cases, is often a matter of balancing competing claims urged by the principle of respect itself.

2. Beneficence Persons are treated in an ethical manner not only by respecting their decisions and protecting them from harm, but also by making efforts to secure their well-being. Such treatment falls under the principle of beneficence. The term "beneficence" is often understood to cover acts of kindness or charity that go beyond strict obligation. In this document, beneficence is understood in a stronger sense, as an obligation. Two general rules have been formulated as complementary expressions of beneficent actions in this sense: (1) do not harm and (2) maximize possible benefits and minimize possible harms.

The Hippocratic maxim "do no harm" has long been a fundamental principle of medical ethics. Claude Bernard extended it to the realm of research, saying that one should not injure one person regardless of the benefits that might come to others. However, even avoiding harm requires learning what is harmful; and, in the process of obtaining this information, persons may be exposed to risk of harm. Further, the Hippocratic Oath requires physicians to benefit their patients "according to their best judgment." Learning what will in fact benefit may require exposing persons to risk. The problem posed by these imperatives is to decide when it is justifiable to seek certain benefits despite the risks involved, and when the benefits should be foregone because of the risks.

The obligations of beneficence affect both individual investigators and society at large, because they extend both to particular research projects and to the entire enterprise of research. In the case of particular projects, investigators and members of their institutions are obliged to give forethought to the maximization of benefits and the reduction of risk that might occur from the research investigation. In the case of scientific research in general, members of the larger society are obliged to recognize the longer term benefits and risks that may result from the improvement of knowledge and from the development of novel medical, psychotherapeutic, and social procedures.

The principle of beneficence often occupies a well-defined justifying role in many areas of research involving human subjects. An example is found in research involving children. Effective ways of treating childhood diseases and fostering healthy development are benefits that serve to justify research involving children—even when individual research subjects are not direct beneficiaries. Research also makes is possible to avoid the harm that may result from the application of previously accepted routine practices that on closer investigation turn out to be dangerous. But the role of the principle of beneficence is not always so unambiguous. A difficult ethical problem remains, for example, about research that presents more than minimal risk without immediate prospect of direct benefit to the children involved. Some have argued that such research is inadmissible, while others have pointed out that this limit would rule out much research promising great benefit to children in the future. Here again, as with all hard cases, the different claims covered by the principle of beneficence may come into conflict and force difficult choices.

3. Justice Who ought to receive the benefits of research and bear its burdens? This is a question of justice, in the sense of "fairness in distribution" or "what is deserved." An injustice occurs when some benefit to which a person is entitled is denied without good reason or when some burden is imposed unduly. Another way of conceiving the principle of justice is that equals ought to be treated equally. However, this statement requires explication. Who is equal and who is unequal? What considerations justify departure from equal distribution? Almost all commentators allow that distinctions based on experience, age, deprivation, competence, merit and position do sometimes constitute criteria justifying differential treatment for certain purposes. It is necessary, then, to explain in what respects people should be treated equally. There are several widely accepted formulations of just ways to distribute burdens and benefits. Each formulation mentions some relevant property on the basis of which burdens and benefits should be distributed. These formulations are (1) to each person an equal share, (2) to each person according to individual need, (3) to each person according to individual effort, (4) to each person according to societal contribution, and (5) to each person according to merit.

Questions of justice have long been associated with social practices such as punishment, taxation and political representation. Until recently these questions have not generally been associated with scientific research. However, they are foreshadowed even in the earliest reflections on the ethics of research involving human subjects. For example, during the 19th and early 20th centuries the burdens of serving as research subjects fell largely upon poor ward patients, while the benefits of improved medical care flowed primarily to private patients. Subsequently, the exploitation of unwilling prisoners as research subjects in Nazi concentration camps was condemned as a particularly flagrant injustice. In this country, in the 1940s, the Tuskegee syphilis study used disadvantaged, rural black men to study the untreated course of a disease that is by no means confined to that population. These subjects were deprived of demonstrably effective treatment in order not to interrupt the project, long after such treatment became generally available.

Against this historical background, it can be seen how conceptions of justice are relevant to research involving human subjects. For example, the selection of research subjects needs to be scrutinized in order to determine whether some classes (e.g., welfare patients, particular racial and ethnic minorities, or persons confined to institutions) are being systematically selected simply because of their easy availability, their compromised position, or their manipulability, rather than for reasons directly related to the problem being studied. Finally, whenever research supported by public funds leads to the development of therapeutic devices and procedures, justice demands both that these not provide advantages only to those who can afford them and that such research should not unduly involve persons from groups unlikely to be among the beneficiaries of subsequent applications of the research.

C. Applications

Applications of the general principles to the conduct of research leads to consideration of the following requirements: informed consent, risk/benefit assessment, and the selection of subjects of research.

1. Informed Consent Respect for persons requires that subjects, to the degree that they are capable, be given the opportunity to choose what shall or shall not happen to them. This opportunity is provided when adequate standards for informed consent are satisfied.

While the importance of informed consent is unquestioned, controversy prevails over the nature and possibility of an informed consent. Nonetheless, there is widespread agreement that the consent process can be analyzed as containing three elements: information, comprehension and voluntariness.

Information. Most codes of research establish specific items for disclosure intended to assure that subjects are given sufficient information. These items generally include: the research procedure, their purposes, risks and anticipated benefits, alternative procedures (where therapy is involved), and a statement offering the subject the opportunity to ask questions and to withdraw at any time from the research. Additional items have been proposed, including how subjects are selected, the person responsible for the research, etc.

However, a simple listing of items does not answer the question of what the standard should be for judging how much and what sort of information should be provided. One standard frequently invoked in medical practice, namely the information commonly provided by practitioners in the field or in the locale, is inadequate since research takes place precisely when a common understanding does not exist. Another standard, currently popular in malpractice law, requires the practitioner to reveal the information that reasonable persons would wish to know in order to make a decision regarding their care. This, too, seems insufficient since the research subject, being in essence a volunteer, may wish to know considerably more about risks gratuitously undertaken than do patients who deliver themselves into the hand of a clinician for needed care. It may be that a standard of "the reasonable volunteer" should be proposed: the extent and nature of information should be such that persons, knowing that the procedure is neither necessary for their care nor perhaps fully understood, can decide whether they wish to participate in the furthering of knowledge. Even when some direct benefit to them is anticipated, the subjects should understand clearly the range of risk and the voluntary nature of participation.

A special problem of consent arises where informing subjects of some pertinent aspect of the research is likely to impair the validity of the research. In many cases, it is sufficient to indicate to subjects that they are being invited to participate in research of which some features will not be revealed until the research is concluded. In all cases of research involving incomplete disclosure, such research is justified only if it is clear that (1) incomplete disclosure is truly necessary to accomplish the goals of the research, (2) there are no undisclosed risks to subjects that are more than minimal, and (3) there is an adequate plan for debriefing subjects, when appropriate, and for dissemination of research results to them. Information about risks should never be withheld for the purpose of eliciting the cooperation of subjects, and truthful answers should always be given to direct questions about the research. Care should be taken to distinguish cases in which disclosure would destroy or invalidate the research from cases in which disclosure would simply inconvenience the investigator.

Comprehension. The manner and context in which information is conveyed is as important as the information itself. For example, presenting information in a disorganized and rapid fashion, allowing too little time for consideration or curtailing opportunities for questioning, all may adversely affect a subject's ability to make an informed choice.

Because the subject's ability to understand is a function of intelligence, rationality, maturity and language, it is necessary to adapt the presentation of the information to the subject's capacities. Investigators are responsible for ascertaining that the subject has comprehended the information. While there is always an obligation to ascertain that the information about risk to subjects is complete and adequately comprehended, when the risks are more serious, that obligation increases. On occasion, it may be suitable to give some oral or written tests of comprehension.

Special provision may need to be made when comprehension is severely limited—for example, by conditions of immaturity or mental disability. Each class of subjects that one might consider as incompetent (e.g., infants and young children, mentally disabled patients, the terminally ill and the comatose) should be considered on its own terms. Even for these persons, however, respect requires giving them the opportunity to choose to the extent they are able, whether or not to participate in research. The objections of these subjects to involvement should be honored, unless the research entails providing them a therapy unavailable elsewhere. Respect for persons also requires seeking the permission of other parties in order to protect the subjects from harm. Such persons are thus respected both by acknowledging their own wishes and by the use of third parties to protect them from harm.

The third parties chosen should be those who are most likely to understand the incompetent subject's situation and to act in that person's best interest. The person authorized to act on behalf of the subject should be given an opportunity to observe the research as it proceeds in order to be able to withdraw the subject from the research, if such action appears in the subject's best interest.

Voluntariness. An agreement to participate in research constitutes a valid consent only if voluntarily given. This element of informed consent requires conditions free of coercion and undue influence. Coercion occurs when an overt threat of harm is intentionally presented by one person to another in order to obtain compliance. Undue influence, by contrast, occurs through an offer of an excessive, unwarranted, inappropriate or improper reward or other overture in order to obtain compliance. Also, inducements that would ordinarily be acceptable may become undue influences if the subject is especially vulnerable.

Unjustifiable pressures usually occur when persons in positions of authority or commanding influence—especially where possible sanctions are involved—urge a course of action for a subject. A continuum of such influencing factors exists, however, and it is impossible to state precisely where justifiable persuasion ends and undue influence begins. But undue influence would include actions such as manipulating a person's choice through the controlling influence of a close relative and threatening to withdraw health services to which an individual would otherwise be entitled.

2. Assessment of Risks and Benefits The assessment of risks and benefits requires a careful arrayal of relevant data, including, in some cases, alternative ways of obtaining the benefits sought in the research. Thus, the assessment presents both an opportunity and a responsibility to gather systematic and comprehensive information about proposed research. For the investigator, it is a means to examine whether the proposed research is properly designed. For a review committee, it is a method for determining whether the risks that will be presented to subjects are justified. For prospective subjects, the assessment will assist the determination whether or not to participate.

The nature and scope of risks and benefits. The requirement that research be justified on the basis of a favorable risk/benefit assessment bears a close relation to the principle of beneficence, just as the moral requirement that informed consent be obtained is derived primarily from the principle of respect for persons. The term "risk" refers to a possibility that harm may occur. However, when expressions such as "small risk" or "high risk" are used, they usually refer (often ambiguously) both to the chance (probability) of experiencing a harm and the severity (magnitude) of the envisioned harm.

The term "benefit" is used in the research context to refer to something of positive value related to health or welfare. Unlike "risk," "benefit" is not a term that expresses probabilities. Risk is properly contrasted to probability of benefits, and benefits are properly contrasted with harms rather than risks of harm. Accordingly, so-called risk/benefit assessments are concerned with the probabilities and magnitudes of possible harms and anticipated benefits. Many kinds of possible harms and benefits need to be taken into account. There are, for example, risks of psychological harm, physical harm, legal harm, social harm and economic harm and the corresponding benefits. While the most likely types of harms to research subjects are those of psychological or physical pain or injury, other possible kinds should not be overlooked.

Risks and benefits of research may affect the individual subjects, the families of the individual subjects, and society at large (or special groups of subjects in society). Previous codes and Federal regulations have required that risks to subjects be outweighed by the sum of both the anticipated benefit to the subject, if any, and the anticipated benefit to society in the form of knowledge to be gained from the research. In balancing these different elements, the risks and benefits affecting the immediate research subject will normally carry special weight. On the other hand, interests other than those of the subject may on some occasions be sufficient by themselves to justify the risks involved in the research, so long as the subjects' rights have been protected. Beneficence thus requires that we protect against risk of harm to subjects and also that we be concerned about the loss of the substantial benefits that might be gained from research.

The systematic assessment of risks and benefits. It is commonly said that benefits and risks must be "balanced" and shown to be "in a favorable ratio." The metaphorical character of these terms draws attention to the difficulty of making precise judgments. Only on rare occasions will quantitative techniques be available for the scrutiny of research protocols. However, the idea of systematic, nonarbitrary analysis of risks and benefits should be emulated insofar as possible. This ideal requires those making decisions about the justifiability of research to be thorough in the accumulation and assessment of information about all aspects of the research, and to consider alternatives systematically. This procedure renders the assessment of research more rigorous and precise, while making communication between review board members and investigators less subject to misinterpretation, misinformation and conflicting judgments. Thus, there should first be a determination of the validity of the presuppositions of the research; then the nature, probability and magnitude of risk should be distinguished with as much clarity as possible. The method of ascertaining risks should be explicit, especially where there is no alternative to the use of such vague categories as small or slight risk. It should also be determined whether an investigator's estimates of the probability of harm or benefits are reasonable, as judged by known facts or other available studies.

Finally, assessment of the justifiability of research should reflect at least the following considerations: (i) Brutal or inhumane treatment of human subjects is never morally justified. (ii) Risks should be reduced to those necessary to achieve the research objective. It should be determined whether it is in fact necessary to use human subjects at all. Risk can perhaps never be entirely eliminated, but it can often be reduced by careful attention to alternative procedures. (iii) When research involves significant risk of serious impairment, review committees should be extraordinarily insistent on the justification of the risk (looking usually to the likelihood of benefit to the subject—or, in some rare cases, to the manifest voluntariness of the participation). (iv) When vulnerable populations are involved in research, the appropriateness of involving them should itself be demonstrated. A number of variables go into such judgments, including the nature and degree of risk, the condition of the particular population involved, and the nature and level of the anticipated benefits. (v) Relevant risks and benefits must be thoroughly arrayed in documents and procedures used in the informed consent process.

3. Selection of Subjects Just as the principle of respect for persons finds expression in the requirements for consent, and the principle of beneficence in risk/benefit assessment, the principle of justice gives rise to moral requirements that there be fair procedures and outcomes in the selection of research subjects.

Justice is relevant to the selection of subjects of research at two levels: the social and the individual. Individual justice in the selection of subjects would require that researchers exhibit fairness: thus, they should not offer potentially beneficial research only to some patients who are in their favor or select only "undesirable" persons for risky research. Social justice requires that distinction be drawn between classes of subjects that ought, and ought not, to participate in any particular kind of research, based on the ability of members of that class to bear burdens and on the appropriateness of placing further burdens on already burdened persons. Thus, it can be considered a matter of social justice that there is an order of preference in the selection of classes of subjects (e.g., adults before children) and that some classes of potential subjects (e.g., the institutionalized mentally infirm or prisoners) may be involved as research subjects, if at all, only on certain conditions.

Injustice may appear in the selection of subjects, even if individual subjects are selected fairly by investigators and treated fairly in the course of research. Thus injustice arises from social, racial, sexual and cultural biases institutionalized in society. Thus, even if individual researchers are treating their research subjects fairly, and even if IRBs are taking care to assure that subjects are selected fairly within a particular institution, unjust social patterns may nevertheless appear in the overall distribution of the burdens and benefits of research. Although individual institutions or investigators may not be able to resolve a problem that is pervasive in their social setting, they can consider distributive justice in selecting research subjects.

Some populations, especially institutionalized ones, are already burdened in many ways by their infirmities and environments. When research is proposed that involves risks and does not include a therapeutic component, other less burdened classes of persons should be called upon first to accept these risks of research, except where the research is directly related to the specific conditions of the class involved. Also, even though public funds for research may often flow in the same directions as public funds for health care, it seems unfair that populations dependent on public health care constitute a pool of preferred research subjects if more advantaged populations are likely to be the recipients of the benefits.

One special instance of injustice results from the involvement of vulnerable subjects. Certain groups, such as racial minorities, the economically disadvantaged, the very sick, and the institutionalized may continually be sought as research subjects, owing to their ready availability in settings where research is conducted. Given their dependent status and their frequently compromised capacity for free consent, they should be protected against the danger of being involved in research solely for administrative convenience, or because they are easy to manipulate as a result of their illness or socioeconomic condition.

NOTES

1. Since 1945, various codes for the proper and responsible conduct of human experimentation in medical research have been adopted by different organizations. The best known of these codes are the Nuremberg Code of 1947, the Helsinki Declaration of 1964 (revised in 1975), and the 1971 Guidelines (codified into Federal Regulations in 1974) issued by the U.S. Department of Health, Education, and Welfare. Codes for the conduct of social and behavioral research have also been adopted, the best known being that of the American Psychological Association, published in 1973.
2. Although practice usually involves interventions designed solely to enhance the well-being of a particular individual, interventions are sometimes applied to one individual for the enhancement of the well-being of another (e.g., blood donation, skin grafts, organ transplants) or an intervention may have the dual purpose of enhancing the well-being of a particular individual, and, at the same time, providing some benefit to others (e.g., vaccination, which protects both the person who is vaccinated and society generally). The fact that some forms of practice have elements other than immediate benefit to the individual receiving an intervention, however, should not confuse the general distinction between research and practice. Even when a procedure applied in practice may benefit some other per-

son, it remains an intervention designed to enhance the well-being of a particular individual or groups of individuals; thus, it is practice and need not be reviewed as research.

3. Because the problems related to social experimentation may differ substantially from those of biomedical and behavioral research, the Commission specifically declines to make any policy determination regarding such research at this time. Rather, the Commission believes that the problem ought to be addressed by one of its successor bodies.

RESEARCH ON THE FETUS

INTRODUCTION. *The National Commission for Protection of Human Subjects of Biomedical and Behavioral Research was charged by Congress with several specific tasks in addition to its general charge to develop fundamental ethical principles of research. Among these, the first was to recommend to the Secretary of Health, Education and Welfare, "policies defining the circumstances (if any), under which research regarding the living fetus could be conducted and supported." It completed that report within four months, notwithstanding that it had to conduct extensive studies on the nature of fetal research and the ethical and legal considerations it raised. Materials related to its investigation were published in an appendix following the report.*

SECTION 8: DELIBERATIONS AND CONCLUSIONS

The charge to the Commission is to investigate and study research involving the living fetus and to make recommendations to the Secretary, DHEW, on "policies defining the circumstances (if any) under which such research may be conducted or supported." The Commission has attempted to fulfill that duty by conducting investigations into research on the fetus and by providing a public forum for the presentation and analysis of views on this subject. It must be recognized that the Commission was placed under severe limitations of time by its congressional mandate. As a result, these considerations on research involving fetuses have necessarily been developed prior to the Commission's larger task of studying the nature of research, the basic ethical principles which should guide it, the problem of informed consent and the review process.

After the Commission identified the information that was required for adequate consideration of the charge, a compendium of pertinent scientific literature and medical experience was prepared by consultants and contractors. In addition, a broad range of views was presented in letters, reports and testimony by theologians, philosophers, physicians, scientists, lawyers, public officials and private citizens. The Commission then undertook critical analysis of the studies and presentations, and conducted public deliberations on the issues involved. Finally, the Commission formulated its Recommendations.

This section of the Commission's report summarizes the reasoning and conclusions that emerged during the deliberations. Section nine of the report sets forth the Commission's Recommendations to the Secretary, DHEW. These Recommendations arise from and are consistent with the Deliberations and Conclusions of the Commission. The Recommendations should be considered only within the context of the Deliberations that precede them.

Preface to Deliberations and Conclusions

Throughout the deliberations of the Commission, the belief has been affirmed that the fetus as a human subject is deserving of care and respect. Although the Commission has not addressed directly the issues of the personhood and the civil status of the fetus, the members of the Commission are convinced that moral concern should extend to all who share human genetic heritage, and that the fetus, regardless of life prospects, should be treated respectfully and with dignity.

The members of the Commission are also convinced that medical research has resulted in significant improvements in the care of the unborn threatened by death or disease, and they recognize that further progress is anticipated. Within the broad category of medical research, however, public concern has been expressed with regard to the nature and necessity of research on the human fetus. The evidence pre-

Excerpts from the National Commission for Protection of Human Subjects of Biomedical and Behavioral Research, *Report and Recommendations: Research on the Fetus*, DHEW (OS) 76-127 (Washington, D.C.: U.S. Government Printing Office, 1975). For additional information, see also the Appendix to Research on the Fetus, DHEW (OS) 76-128; "Excerpts from the philosophical and theological essays in the Appendix to Research on the Fetus," *Hastings Center Report* (June 1975); and Robert J. Levine, *Ethics and Regulation of Clinical Research* (New Haven: Yale University Press, 1988), Chapter 13.

sented to the Commission was based upon a comprehensive search of the world's literature and a review of more than 3000 communications in scientific periodicals. The preponderance of all research involved experimental procedures designed to benefit directly a fetus threatened by premature delivery, disease or death, or to elucidate normal processes or development. Some research constituted an element in the health care of pregnant women. Other research involved only observation or the use of noninvasive procedures bearing little or no risk. A final class of investigation (falling outside the present mandate of the Commission) has made use of tissues of the dead fetus, in accordance with accepted standards for treatment of the human cadaver. The Commission finds that, to the best of its knowledge, these types of research have not contravened accepted ethical standards.

Nonetheless, the Commission notes that there have been instances of abuse in the area of fetal research. Moreover, differences of opinion exist as to whether desired results could have been attained without the use of the human fetus in nontherapeutic research.

Concern has also been expressed that the poor and minority groups may bear an inequitable burden as research subjects. The Commission believes that those groups which are most vulnerable to inequitable treatment should receive special protection.

The Commission concludes that some information which is in the public interest and which provides significant advances in health care can be attained only through the use of the human fetus as a research subject. The Recommendations which follow express the Commission's belief that, while the exigencies of research and the moral imperatives of fair and respectful treatment may appear to be mutually limiting, they are not incompatible.

Ethical Principles and Requirements Governing Research on Human Subjects with Special Reference to the Fetus and the Pregnant Woman

The Commission has a mandate to develop the ethical principles underlying the conduct of all research involving human subjects. Until it can adequately fulfill this charge, its statement of principles is necessarily limited. In the interim, it proposes the following as basic ethical principles for use of human subjects in general, and research involving the fetus and the pregnant woman in particular.

Scientific inquiry is a distinctly human endeavor. So, too, is the protection of individual integrity. Freedom of inquiry and the social benefits derived therefrom, as well as protection of the individual are valued highly and are to be encouraged. For the most part, they are compatible pursuits. When occasionally they appear to be in conflict, efforts must be made through public deliberation to effect a resolution.

In effecting this resolution, the integrity of the individual is preeminent. It is therefore the duty of the Commission to specify the boundaries that respect for the fetus must impose upon freedom of scientific inquiry. The Commission has considered the principles proposed by ethicists in relation to the exigencies of scientific inquiry, the requirements and present limitations of medical practice, and legal commentary. Among the general principles for research on human subjects judged to be valid and binding are: (1) to avoid harm whenever possible, or at least to minimize harm; (2) to provide for fair treatment by avoiding discrimination between classes or among members of the same class; and (3) to respect the integrity of human subjects by requiring informed consent. An additional principle pertinent to the issue at hand is to respect the human character of the fetus.

To this end, the Commission concludes that in order to be considered ethically acceptable, research involving the fetus should be determined by adequate review to meet certain general requirements:

(1) Appropriate prior investigations using animal models and nonpregnant humans must have been completed.
(2) The knowledge to be gained must be important and obtainable by no reasonable alternative means.
(3) Risks and benefits to both the mother and the fetus must have been fully evaluated and described.
(4) Informed consent must be sought and granted under proper conditions.
(5) Subjects must be selected so that risks and benefits will not fall inequitably among economic, racial, ethnic and social classes.

These requirements apply to all research on the human fetus. In the application of these principles, however, the Commission found it helpful to consider the following distinctions: (1) therapeutic and nontherapeutic research; (2) research directed toward the pregnant woman and that directed toward the fetus; (3) research involving the fetus-going-to-term and the fetus-to-be-aborted; (4) research occurring before, during or after an abortion procedure; and (5) research which involves the nonviable fetus ex utero and that which involves the possibly viable infant. The first two distinctions encompass the entire period of the pregnancy through delivery; the latter three refer to different portions of the developmental continuum.

The Commission observes that the fetus is sometimes an unintended subject of research when a woman participating in an investigation is incorrectly presumed not to be pregnant. Care should be taken to minimize this possibility.

Application to Research Involving the Fetus

The application of the general principles enumerated above to the use of the human fetus as a research subject presents problems because the fetus cannot be a willing participant in experimentation. As with children, the comatose and other subjects unable to consent, difficult questions arise regarding the balance of risk and benefit and the validity of proxy consent.

In particular, some would question whether subjects unable to consent should ever be subjected to risk in scientific research. However, there is general agreement that where the benefits as well as the risks of research accrue to the subject, proxy consent may be presumed adequate to protect the subject's interests. The more difficult case is that where the subject must bear risks without direct benefit.

The Commission has not yet studied the issues surrounding informed consent and the validity of proxy consent for nontherapeutic research (including the difficult issue of consent by a pregnant minor). These problems will be explored under the broader mandate of the Commission. In the interim, the Commission has taken various perspectives into consideration in its deliberations about the use of the fetus as a subject in different research settings. The Deliberations and Conclusions of the Commission regarding the application of general principles to the use of the fetus as a human subject in scientific research are as follows:

1. In therapeutic research directed toward the fetus, the fetal subject is selected on the basis of its health condition, benefits and risks accrue to that fetus, and proxy consent is directed toward that subject's own welfare. Hence, with adequate review to assess scientific merit, prior research, the balance of risks and benefits, and the sufficiency of the consent process, such research conforms with all relevant principles and is both ethically acceptable and laudable. In view of the necessary involvement of the woman in such research, her consent is considered mandatory; in view of the father's possible ongoing responsibility, his objection is considered sufficient to veto.

2. Therapeutic research directed toward the pregnant woman may expose the fetus to risk for the benefit of another subject and thus is at first glance more problematic. Recognizing the woman's priority regarding her own health care, however, the Commission concludes that such research is ethically acceptable provided that the woman has been fully informed of the possible impact on the fetus and that other general requirements have been met. Protection for the fetus is further provided by requiring that research put the fetus at minimum risk consistent with the provision of health care for the woman. Moreover, therapeutic research directed toward the pregnant woman frequently benefits the fetus, though it need not necessarily do so. In view of the woman's right to privacy regarding her own health care, the Commission concludes that the informed consent of the woman is both necessary and sufficient.

In general, the Commission concludes that therapeutic research directed toward the health condition of either the fetus or the pregnant woman is, in principle, ethical. Such research benefits not only the individual woman or fetus but also women and fetuses as a class, and should therefore be encouraged actively.

The Commission, in making recommendations on therapeutic and nontherapeutic research directed toward the pregnant woman, (Recommendations 2 and 3), in no way intends to preclude research on improving abortion techniques otherwise permitted by law and government regulation.

3. Nontherapeutic research directed toward the fetus *in utero* or toward the pregnant woman poses difficult problems because the fetus may be exposed to risk for the benefit of others.

Here, the Commission concludes that where no additional risks are imposed on the fetus (e.g., where fluid withdrawn during the course of treatment is used additionally for nontherapeutic research), or where risks are so minimal as to be negligible, proxy consent by the parent(s) is sufficient to provide protection. (Hence, the consent of the woman is sufficient provided the father does not object.) The Commission recognizes that the term "minimal" involves a value judgment and acknowledges that medical opinion will differ regarding what constitutes "minimal risk." Determination of acceptable minimal risk is a function of the review process.

When the risks cannot be fully assessed, or are more than minimal, the situation is more problematic. The Commission affirms as a general principle that manifest risks imposed upon nonconsenting subjects cannot be tolerated. Therefore, the Commission concludes that only minimal risk can be accepted as permissible for nonconsenting subjects in nontherapeutic research.

The Commission affirms that the woman's decision for abortion does not, in itself, change the status of the fetus for purposes of protection. Thus, the same principles apply whether or not abortion is contemplated; in both cases, only minimal risk is acceptable.

Differences of opinion have arisen in the Commission, however, regarding the interpretation of risk to the fetus-to-be-aborted and thus whether some experiments that would not be permissible on a fetus-going-to-term might be permissible on a fetus-to-be-aborted. Some members hold that no procedures should be applied to a fetus-to-be-aborted that would not be applied to a fetus-going-to-term. Indeed, it was also suggested that any research involving fetuses-to-be-aborted must also involve fetuses-going-to-term. Others argue that, while a woman's decision for abortion does not change the status of the fetus per se, it does make a significant difference in one respect—namely, in the risk of harm to the fetus. For example, the injection of a drug which crosses the placenta may not injure the fetus which is aborted within two weeks of injection, where it might injure the fetus two months after injection. There is always, of course, the possibility that a woman might change her mind about the abortion. Even taking this into account, however, some members argue that risks to the fetus-to-be-aborted may be considered "minimal" in research which would entail more than minimal risk for a fetus-going-to-term.

There is basic agreement among Commission members as to the validity of the equality principle. There is disagreement as to its application to individual fetuses and classes of fetuses. Anticipating that differences of interpretation will arise over the application of the basic principles of equality and the determination of "minimal risk," the Commission recommends review at the national level. The Commission believes that such review would provide the appropriate forum for determination of the scientific and public merit of such research. In addition, such review would facilitate public discussion of the sensitive issues surrounding the use of vulnerable nonconsenting subjects in research.

The question of consent is a complicated one in this area of research. The Commission holds that procedures that are part of the research design should be fully disclosed and clearly distinguished from those which are dictated by the health care needs of the pregnant woman or her fetus. Questions have been raised regarding the validity of parental proxy consent where the parent(s) have made a decision for abortion. The Commission recognizes that unresolved problems both of law and of fact surround this question. It is the considered opinion, however, that women who have decided to abort should not be presumed to abandon thereby all interest in and concern for the fetus. In view of the close relationship between the woman and the fetus, therefore, and the necessary involvement of the woman in the research process, the woman's consent is considered necessary. The Commission is divided on the question of whether her consent alone is sufficient. Assignment of an advocate for the fetus was proposed as an additional safeguard; this issue will be thoroughly explored in connection with the Commission's review of the consent process. Most of the Commissioners agree that in view of the father's possible responsibility for the child, should it be brought to term, the objection of the father should be sufficient to veto. Several Commissioners, however, hold that for nontherapeutic research directed toward the pregnant woman, the woman's consent alone should be sufficient and the father should have no veto.

4. Research on the fetus during the abortion procedure or on the nonviable fetus *ex utero* raises sensitive problems because such a fetus must be considered a dying subject. By definition, therefore, the research is nontherapeutic in that the benefits will not accrue to the subject. Moreover, the question of consent is complicated because of the special vulnerability of the dying subject.

The Commission considers that the status of the fetus as dying alters the situation in two ways. First, the question of risk becomes less relevant, since the dying fetus cannot be "harmed" in the sense of "injured for life." Once the abortion procedure has begun, or after it is completed, there is no chance of a change of mind on the woman's part which will result in a living, injured subject. Second, however, while questions of risk become less relevant, considerations of respect for the dignity of the fetus continue to be of paramount importance, and require that the fetus be treated with the respect due to dying subjects. While dying subjects may not be "harmed" in the sense of "injured for life," issues of violation of integrity are nonetheless central. The Commission concludes, therefore, that out of respect for the dying subjects, no nontherapeutic interventions are permissible which would alter the duration of life of the nonviable fetus *ex utero*.

Additional protection is provided by requiring that no significant changes are made in the abortion procedure strictly for purposes of research. The Commission was divided on the question of whether a woman has a right to accept modifications in the timing or method of the abortion procedure in the interest of research, and whether the investigator could ethically request her to do so. Some Commission members desired that neither the research nor the investigator in any way influence the abortion procedure; others felt that modifications in timing or method of abortion were acceptable provided no new elements of risk were introduced. Still others held that even if modifications increased the risk, they would be acceptable provided the woman had been fully informed of all risks, and provided such modifications did not postpone the abortion beyond the twentieth week of gestational age (five lunar months, four and one-half calendar months). Despite this division of opinion, the Recommendation of the Commission on this matter is that the design and conduct of a nontherapeutic research protocol should not determine the recommendations by a physician regarding the advisability, timing or method of abortion. No members of the Commission desired less stringent measures.

Furthermore, it is possible that, due to mistaken estimation of gestational age, an abortion may issue in a possibly viable infant. If there is any danger that this might happen, research which would entail more than minimal risk would be absolutely prohibited. In order to avoid that possibility the Commission recommends that, should research during abortion be approved by national review, it be always on condition that estimated gestational age be below 20 weeks. There is, of course, a moral and legal obligation to attempt to save the life of a possibly viable infant.

Finally, the Commission has been made aware that certain research, particularly that involving the living nonviable fetus, has disturbed the moral sensitivity of many persons. While it believes that its Recommendations would preclude objectionable research by adherence to strict review processes, problems of interpretation or application of the Commission's Recommendations may still arise. In that event, the Commission proposes ethical review at a national level in which informed public disclosure and assessment of the problems, the type of proposed research and the scientific and public importance of the expected results can take place.

Review Procedures

The Commission will conduct comprehensive studies of existing review mechanisms in connection with its broad mandate to develop guidelines and make recommendations concerning ethical issues involved in research on human subjects. Until the Commission has completed these studies, it can offer only tentative conclusions and recommendations regarding review mechanisms.

In the interim, the Commission finds that existing review procedures required by statute (P.L. 93-348) and DHEW regulations (45 CFR 46) suffice for all therapeutic research involving the pregnant woman and the fetus, and for all nontherapeutic research which imposes minimal or no risk and which would be acceptable for conduct on a fetus *in utero* to be carried to term or on an infant. Guidelines to be employed under the existing review procedures include: (1) importance of the knowledge to be gained; (2) completion of appropriate studies on animal models and nonpregnant humans and existence of no reasonable alternative; (3) full evaluation and disclosure of the risks and benefits that are involved; and (4) supervision of the conditions under which consent is sought and granted, and of the information that is disclosed during that process.

The case is different, however, for nontherapeutic research directed toward a pregnant woman or a fetus if it involves more than minimal risk or would not be acceptable for application to an infant. Questions may arise concerning the definition of risk or the assessment of scientific and public importance of the research. In such cases, the Commission considers current review procedures insufficient. It recommends these categories be reviewed by a national review body to determine whether the proposed research could be conducted within the spirit of the Commission's recommendations. It would interpret these recommendations and apply them to the proposed research, and in addition, assess the scientific and public value of the anticipated results of the investigation.

The national review panel should be composed of individuals having diverse backgrounds, experience and interests, and be so constituted as to be able to deal with the legal, ethical, and medical issues involved in research on the human fetus. In addition to the professions of law, medicine, and the research sciences, there should be adequate representation of women, members of minority groups, and individuals conversant with the various ethical persuasions of the general community.

Inasmuch as even such a panel cannot always judge public attitudes, panel meetings should be open to the public, and, in addition, public participation through written and oral submissions should be sought.

Compensation

The Commission expressed a strong conviction that considerable attention be given to the issue of provision of compensation to those who may be injured as a consequence of their participation as research subjects.

Concerns regarding the use of inducements for participation in research are only partially met by the Commission's Recommendation (14) on the prohibition of the procurement of an abortion for research purposes. Compensation not only for injury from research but for participation in research as a normal volunteer or in a therapeutic situation will be part of later Commission deliberations.

Research Conducted Outside the United States

The Commission has considered the advisability of modifying its standards for research which is supported by the Secretary, DHEW, and is conducted outside the United States. It has concluded that its recommendations should apply as a single minimal standard, but that research should also comply with any more stringent limitations imposed by statutes or standards of the country in which the research will be conducted.

The Moratorium on Fetal Research

The Commission notes that the restrictions on fetal research (imposed by Section 213 of P.L. 93-348) have been construed broadly throughout the research community, with the result that ethically acceptable research, which might yield important biomedical information, has been halted. For this reason, it is considered in the public interest that the moratorium be lifted immediately, that the Secretary take special care thereafter that the Commission's concerns for the protection of the fetus as a research subject are met, and appropriate regulations based upon the Commission's recommendations be implemented within a year from the date of submission of this report to the Secretary, DHEW. Until final regulations are published, the existing review panels at the agency and institutional levels should utilize the Deliberations and Recommendations of the Commission in evaluating the acceptability of all grant and contract proposals submitted for funding.

Synthesis

The Commission concludes that certain prior conditions apply broadly to all research involving the fetus, if ethical considerations are to be met. These requirements include evidence of pertinent investigations in animal models and nonpregnant humans, lack of alternative means to obtain the information, careful assessment of the risks and benefits of the research, and procedures to ensure that informed consent has been sought and granted under proper conditions. Determinations as to whether these essential requirements have been met may be made under existing review procedures, pending study by the Commission of the entire review process.

In the judgment of the Commission, therapeutic research directed toward the health care of the pregnant woman or the fetus raises little concern, provided it meets the essential requirements for research involving the fetus, and is conducted under appropriate medical and legal safeguards.

For the most part, nontherapeutic research involving the fetus to be carried to term or the fetus before, during or after abortion is acceptable so long as it imposes minimal or no risk to the fetus and, when abortion is involved, imposes no change in the timing or procedure for terminating pregnancy which would add any significant risk. When a research protocol or procedure presents special problems of interpretation or application of these guidelines, it should be subject to national ethical review; and it should be approved only if the knowledge to be gained is of medical importance, can be obtained in no other way, and the research proposal does not offend community sensibilities.

SECTION 9: RECOMMENDATIONS

1. Therapeutic research directed toward the fetus may be conducted or supported, and should be encouraged, by the Secretary, DHEW, provided such research (a) conforms to appropriate medical standards, (b) has received the informed consent of the mother, the father not dissenting, and (c) has been approved by existing review procedures with adequate provision for the monitoring of the consent process. (Adopted unanimously.)

2. Therapeutic research directed toward the pregnant woman may be conducted or supported, and should be encouraged, by the Secretary, DHEW, provided such research (a) has been evaluated for possible impact on the fetus, (b) will place the fetus at risk to the minimum extent consistent with meeting the health needs of the pregnant woman, (c) has been approved by existing review procedures with adequate provision for the monitoring of the consent process, and (d) the pregnant woman has given her informed consent. (Adopted unanimously.)

3. Nontherapeutic research directed toward the pregnant woman may be conducted or supported by the Secretary, DHEW, provided such research (a) has been evaluated for possible impact on the fetus, (b) will impose minimal or no risk to the well-being of the fetus, (c) has been approved by existing review procedures with adequate provision for the monitoring of the consent process, (d) special care has been taken to assure that the woman has been fully informed regarding possible impact on the fetus, and (e) the woman has given informed consent. (Adopted unanimously.)

It is further provided that nontherapeutic research directed at the pregnant woman may be conducted or supported (f) only if the father has not objected, both where abortion is not at issue (adopted by a vote of 8 to 1) and where an abortion is anticipated (adopted by a vote of 5 to 4).

4. Nontherapeutic research directed toward the fetus *in utero* (other than research in anticipation of, or during, abortion) may be conducted or supported by the Secretary, DHEW, provided (a) the purpose of such research is the development of important biomedical knowledge that cannot be obtained by alternative means, (b) investigation on pertinent animal models and nonpregnant humans has preceded such research, (c) minimal or no risk to the well-being of the fetus will be imposed by the research, (d) the research has been approved by existing review procedures with adequate provision for the monitoring of the consent process, (e) the informed consent of the mother has been obtained, and (f) the father has not objected to the research. (Adopted unanimously.)

5. Nontherapeutic research directed toward the fetus in anticipation of abortion may be conducted or supported by the Secretary, DHEW, provided such research is carried out within the guidelines for all other nontherapeutic research directed toward the fetus *in utero*. Such research presenting special problems related to the interpretation or application of these guidelines may be conducted or supported by the Secretary, DHEW, provided such research has been approved by a national ethical review body. (Adopted by a vote of 8 to 1.)

6. Nontherapeutic research directed toward the fetus during the abortion procedure and nontherapeutic research directed toward the nonviable fetus *ex utero* may be conducted or supported by the Secretary, DHEW, provided (a) the purpose of such research is the development of important biomedical knowledge that cannot be obtained by alternative means, (b) investigation on pertinent animal models and nonpregnant humans (when appropriate) has preceded such research, (c) the research has been approved by existing review procedures with adequate provision for the monitoring of the consent process, (d) the informed consent of the mother has been obtained, and (e) the father has not objected to the research; and provided further that (f) the fetus is less than 20 weeks gestational age, (g) no significant procedural changes are introduced into the abortion procedure in the interest of research alone, and (h) no intrusion into the fetus is made which alters the duration of life. Such research presenting special problems related to the interpretation or application of these guidelines may be conducted or supported by the Secretary, DHEW, provided such research has been approved by a national ethical review body. (Adopted by a vote of 8 to 1.)

7. Nontherapeutic research directed toward the possibly viable infant may be conducted or supported by the Secre-

tary, DHEW, provided (a) the purpose of such research is the development of important biomedical knowledge that cannot be obtained by alternative means, (b) investigation on pertinent animal models and nonpregnant humans (when appropriate) has preceded such research, (c) no additional risk to the well-being of the infant will be imposed by the research, (d) the research has been approved by existing review procedures with adequate provision for the monitoring of the consent process, and (e) informed consent of either parent has been given and neither parent has objected. (Adopted unanimously.)

8. Review Procedures. Until the Commission makes its recommendations regarding review and consent procedures, the review procedures mentioned above are to be those presently required by the Department of Health, Education, and Welfare. In addition, provision for monitoring the consent process shall be required in order to ensure adequacy of the consent process and to prevent unfair discrimination in the selection of research subjects, for all categories of research mentioned above. A national ethical review, as required in Recommendations (5) and (6), shall be carried out by an appropriate body designated by the Secretary, DHEW, until the establishment of the National Advisory Council for the Protection of Subjects of Biomedical and Behavioral Research. In order to facilitate public understanding and the presentation of public attitudes toward special problems reviewed by the national review body, appropriate provision should be made for public attendance and public participation in the national review process. (Adopted unanimously, one abstention.)

9. Research on the Dead Fetus and Fetal Tissue. The Commission recommends that use of the dead fetus, fetal tissue and fetal material for research purposes be permitted, consistent with local law, the Uniform Anatomical Gift Act and commonly held convictions about respect for the dead. (Adopted unanimously, one abstention.)

10. The design and conduct of a nontherapeutic research protocol should not determine recommendations by a physician regarding the advisability, timing or method of abortion. (Adopted by a vote of 6 to 2.)

11. Decisions made by a personal physician concerning the health care of a pregnant woman or fetus should not be compromised for research purposes, and when a physician of record is involved in a prospective research protocol, independent medical judgment on these issues is required. In such cases, review panels should assure that procedures for such independent medical judgment are adequate, and all conflict of interest or appearance thereof between appropriate health care and research objectives should be avoided. (Adopted unanimously.)

12. The Commission recommends that research on abortion techniques continue as permitted by law and government regulation. (Adopted by a vote of 6 to 2.)

13. The Commission recommends that attention be drawn to Section 214(d) of the National Research Act (P.L. 93-348) which provides that

> No individual shall be required to perform or assist in the performance of any part of a health service program or research activity funded in whole or in part by the Secretary of Health, Education, and Welfare if his performance or assistance in the performance of such part of such program or activity would be contrary to his religious beliefs or moral convictions.
> (Adopted unanimously.)

14. No inducements, monetary or otherwise, should be offered to procure an abortion for research purposes. (Adopted unanimously.)

15. Research which is supported by the Secretary, DHEW, to be conducted outside the United States should at the minimum comply in full with the standards and procedures recommended herein. (Adopted unanimously.)

16. The moratorium which is currently in effect should be lifted immediately, allowing research to proceed under current regulations but with the application of the Commission's Recommendations to the review process. All the foregoing Recommendations of the Commission should be implemented as soon as the Secretary, DHEW, is able to promulgate regulations based upon these Recommendations and the public response to them. (Adopted by a vote of 9 to 1.)

DISSENTING STATEMENT OF COMMISSIONER DAVID W. LOUISELL

I am compelled to disagree with the Commission's Recommendations (and the reasoning and definitions on which they are based) insofar as they succumb to the error of sacrificing the interests of innocent human life to a postulated social need. I fear this is the inevitable result of Recommendations 5 and 6. These would permit nontherapeutic research on the fetus in anticipation of abortion and during the abortion procedure, and on a living infant after abortion when the infant is considered nonviable, even though such research is precluded by recognized norms governing human research in general. Although the Commission uses adroit language to minimize the appearance of violating standard norms, no facile verbal formula can avoid the reality that under these Recommendations the fetus and nonviable infant will be subjected to nontherapeutic research from which other humans are protected.

I disagree with regret, not only because of the Commission's zealous efforts but also because there is significant good in its Report, especially its showing that much of the research in this area is therapeutic for the individuals involved, both born and unborn, and hence of unquestioned morality when based on prudent medical judgment. The Report also makes clear that some research, even though nontherapeutic, is merely observational or otherwise without significant risk to the subject, and therefore is within standard human research norms and as unexceptional morally as it is useful scientifically.

But the good in much of the Report cannot blind me to its departure from our society's most basic moral commitment: the essential equality of all human beings. For me the lessons of history are too poignant, and those of this century too fresh, to ignore another violation of human integrity and autonomy by subjecting unconsenting human beings, whether or not viable, to harmful research even for laudable scientific purposes.

Admittedly, the Supreme Court's rationale in its abortion decisions of 1973—*Roe v. Wade* and *Doe v. Bolton*, 310 U.S. 113, 179—has given this Commission an all but impossible task. For many see in that rationale a total negation of fetal rights, absolutely so for the first two trimesters and substantially so for the third. The confusion is understandable, rooted as it is in the Court's invocation of the specially constructed legal fiction of "potential" human life, its acceptance of the notion that human life must be "meaningful" in order to be deserving of legal protection, and its resuscitation of the concept of partial human personhood, which had been thought dead in American society since the demise of the *Dredd Scott* decision. Little wonder that intelligent people are asking: how can one who has no right to life itself have the lesser right of precluding experimentation on his or her person?

It seems to me that there are at least two compelling answers to the notion that *Roe* and *Doe* have placed fetal experimentation, and experimentation on nonviable infants, altogether outside the established protections for human experimentation. First, while we must abide the Court's mandate in a particular case on the issues actually decided even though the decision is wrong and in fact only an exercise of "raw judicial power" (White, J., dissenting in *Roe* and *Doe*), this does not mean we should extend an erroneous rationale to other situations. To the contrary, while seeking to have the wrong corrected by the Court itself, or by the public, the citizen should resist its extension to other contexts. As Abraham Lincoln, discussing the *Dredd Scott* decision, put it:

> (T)he candid citizen must confess that if the policy of the government upon vital questions affecting the whole people, is to be irrevocably fixed by decisions of the Supreme Court, the instant that they are made, in ordinary litigation between parties in personal actions, the people will have ceased to be their own rulers, having, to that extent, practically resigned their government, into the hands of that eminent tribunal (4 Basler, *The Collected Works of Abraham Lincoln* 262, 268 [1963]).

Thus even if the Court had intended by its *Roe* and *Doe* rationale to exclude the unborn, and newly born nonviable infants, from all legal protection including that against harmful experimentation, I can see no legal principle which would justify, let alone require, passive submission to such a breach of our moral tradition and commitment.

Secondly, the Court in *Roe* and *Doe* did not have before it, and presumably did not intend to pass upon and did not in fact pass upon, the question of experimentation on the fetus or born infant. Certainly that question was not directly involved in those cases. Granting the fullest intendment to those decisions possibly arguable, it seems to me that the woman's new-found constitutional right of privacy is fulfilled upon having the fetus aborted. If an infant survives the abortion, there is hardly an additional right of privacy to then have him or her killed or harmed in any way, including harm by experimentation impermissible under standard norms. At least *Roe* and *Doe* should not be assumed to recognize such a right. And while the Court's unfortunate language respecting "potential" and "meaningful" life is thought by some to imply a total abandonment of *in utero* life for all legal purposes, at least for the first two trimesters, such a conclusion would so starkly confront our social, legal, and moral traditions that I think we should not assume it. To the contrary we should assume that the language was limited by the abortion context in which used and was not intended to effect a departure from the limits on human experimentation universally recognized at least in principle.

A shorthand way, developed during the Commission's deliberations, of stating the principle that would adhere to recognized human experimentation norms and that should be recommended in place of Recommendation (5) is: No research should be permitted on a fetus-to-be-aborted that would not be permitted on one to go to term. This principle is essential if all of the unborn are to have the protection of recognized limits on human experimentation. Any lesser protection violates the autonomy and integrity of the fetus, and even a decision to have an abortion cannot justify ignoring this fact. There is not only the practical problem of a possible change of mind by the pregnant woman. For me, the chief vice of Recommendation 5 is that it permits an escape hatch from human experimentation principles merely by decision of a national ethical review body. No principled basis for an exception has been, nor in my judgment can be, formulated. The argument that the fetus-to-be-aborted "will die anyway" proves too much. All of us "will die anyway." A woman's decision to have an abortion, however protected by *Roe* and *Doe* in the interests of her privacy or freedom of her own body, does not change the nature or quality of fetal life.

Recommendation 6 concerns what is now called the "nonviable fetus *ex utero*" but which up to now has been known by the law, and I think by society generally, as an infant, however premature. This Recommendation is unacceptable to me because, on approval of a national review body, it makes certain infants up to five months gestational age potential research material, provided the mother who has of course consented to the abortion, also consents to the experimentation and the father has not objected. In my judgment all infants, however premature or inevitable their death, are within the norms governing human experimentation generally. We do not subject the aged dying to unconsented experimentation, nor should we the youthful dying.

Both Recommendations 5 and 6 have the additional vice of giving the researcher a vested interest in the actual effectuation of a particular abortion, and society a vested interest in permissive abortion in general.

I would, therefore, turn aside any approval, even in science's name, that would by euphemism or other verbal device, subject any unconsenting human being, born or unborn, to harmful research, even that intended to be good for society. Scientific purposes might be served by nontherapeutic research on retarded children, or brain dissection of the old who have ceased to lead "meaningful" lives, but such research is not proposed—at least not yet. As George Bernard Shaw put it in *The Doctor's Dilemma*: "No man is allowed to put his mother in the stove because he desires to know how long an adult woman will survive the temperature of 500 degrees Fahrenheit, no matter how important or interesting that particular addition to the store of human knowledge may be." Is it the mere youth of the fetus that is thought to foreclose the full protection of established human experimentation norms? Such reasoning would imply that a child is less deserving of protection than an adult. But reason, our tradition, and the U.N. Declaration of Human Rights all speak to the contrary, emphasizing the need of special protection for the young.

Even if I were to approach my task as a Commissioner from a utilitarian viewpoint only, I would have to say that on the record here I am not convinced that an adequate showing has been made of the necessity for nontherapeutic fetal experimentation in the scientific or social interest. The Commission's reliance is on the Battelle Report and its reliance is misplaced. The relevant Congressional mandate was to conduct an investigation and study of the alternative means for achieving the purposes of fetal research (P.L. 93-348, July 12, 1974, Sec. 202(b); National Research Act).

As Commissioner Robert E. Cooke, M.D., who is sophisticated in research procedures, pointed out in his Critique of the Battelle Report: "The only true objective approach beyond question, since scientists make [the analysis of the necessity for nontherapeutic fetal research], is to collect information and analyze past research accomplishments with the intention of *disproving, not proving* the hypothesis that research utilizing the living human fetus nonbeneficially is necessary." The Battelle Report seems to me not in accord with the Congressional intention in that it proceeds from a viewpoint opposite to that quoted, and is really an effort to prove the indispensability of nontherapeutic research. In any event, if that is its purpose, it fails to achieve it, for most of what it claims to have been necessary could be justified as therapeutic research or at least as noninvasive of the fetus (e.g., probably amniocentesis). In view of the haste with which this statement must be prepared if it is to accompany the Commission's report, rather than enlarge upon these views now I refer both to the Cooke Critique and the Battelle Report itself, both of which I am informed will be a part of or appended to the Commission's Report.

An emotional plea was made at the Commission's hearings not to acknowledge limitations on experimentation that would inhibit the court-granted permissive abortion. However, until its last meeting, I think the Commission for the most part admirably resisted the temptation to distort its purpose by pro-abortion advocacy. But at the last meeting, without prior preparation or discussion, it adopted Recommendation 12 promotive of research on abortion techniques. This I feel is not germane to our task, is imprudent and certainly was not adequately considered.

Finally, I do not think that the Commission should urge lifting the moratorium on fetal research as stated in Recommendation 16. To the extent that duration of the moratorium is controlled by Section 213 of the National Research Act, the subject is beyond our control and we ought not assume authority that is not ours. This is matter not for us and not, ultimately, for any administrative official, but for Congress. If the American people as a democratic society really intend to withdraw from the fetus and nonviable infant the protection of the established principles governing human experimentation, that action I feel should come from the Congress of the United States, in the absence of a practical way to have a national vote. Assuming that any representative voice is adequate to bespeak so basic and drastic a change in the public philosophy of the United States, it could only be the voice of Congress. Of course there is no reason why the Secretary of DHEW cannot immediately make clear that no researcher need stand in fear of therapeutic research.

As noted at the outset, the Commission's work has achieved some good results in reducing the possibilities of manifest abuses and thereby according a measure of protection to humans at risk by reason of research. That it has not been more successful is in my judgment not due so much to the Commission's failings as to the harsh and pervasive reality that American society is itself at risk—the risk of losing its dedication "to the proposition that all men are created equal." We may have to learn once again that when the bell tolls for the lost rights of any human being, even the politically weakest, it tolls for all.

STATEMENT OF COMMISSIONER KAREN LEBACQZ WITH COMMISSIONER ALBERT R. JONSEN'S CONCURRENCE ON THE FIRST ITEM

The following comments include some points of dissent from the Recommendations of the Commission. For the most part, however, these comments are intended as elaborations on the Report rather than dissent from it.

1. At several points, the Commission established as a criterion for permissible research an acceptable level of risk—e.g., "no risk" or "minimal risk." I support the Com-

mission's Recommendations regarding such criteria, but I wish to make several interpretative comments.

First, I think it should be stressed that in the first trials on human subjects or on a new class of human subjects, the risks are almost always unknown. The Commission heard compelling evidence that differences in physiology and pharmacology between human and other mammalian fetuses are such that even with substantial trials in animal models it is often not possible to assess the risks for the first trials with human fetuses. For example, evidence from animal trials in the testing of thalidomide provided grounds for an estimation of low risk to human subjects; the initial trials in the human fetus resulted in massive teratogenic effects.

I would therefore urge review boards to exercise caution in the interpretation of "risk" and to avoid the temptation to consider the risks "minimal" when in fact they cannot be fully assessed.

Second, I think it important to emphasize the evaluative nature of judgments of risk. The term "risk" means *chance of harm*. Interpretation of risk involves both an assessment of statistical *chance* of injury and an assessment of the *nature* of the injury. Value judgments about what constitutes a "harm" and what percentage chance of harm is acceptable are both involved in the determination of acceptable risk. A small chance of great harm may be considered unacceptable where a greater chance of a smaller harm would be acceptable. For example, it is commonly accepted that a 1–2 percent chance of having a child with Down's syndrome is a "high" risk, where the same chance of minor infection from amniocentesis would be considered a "low" risk. Opinions will differ both about what constitutes "harm" or injury and also about what chance of a particular harm is acceptable.

For all these reasons, the interpretation of risk and the designation of acceptable "minimal risk" merit considerable attention by the scientific community and the lay public. The provision of national review in problematic instances should engender serious deliberation on these critical issues.

Third, the establishment of criteria for "no risk" or "minimal risk" is obviously related to the interpretation of "harm." In general, the Commission has discussed "harm" in terms of two indices: (1) injury or diminished faculty, and (2) pain. A third commonly accepted definition of "harm" is "offense against right or morality"; this meaning of harm has been subsumed under the rubric of violation of dignity or integrity of the fetus, and thus is separated out of the Commission's deliberations on acceptable levels of risk. In establishing acceptable levels of risk, therefore, the Commission has been concerned with injury and pain to the fetus.

Several ethicists argued cogently before the Commission that the ability to experience pain is morally relevant to decisions regarding research. Indeed, the argument was advanced that the ability to experience pain is a more appropriate consideration than is viability for purposes of establishing the limits of intervention into fetal life.

However, scientific opinion is divided on the question of whether the fetus can experience pain—and on the appropriate indices on which to measure the experience of pain. Several experts argue that the fetus does not feel pain.

I believe that the Commission has implicitly accepted this view in making Recommendation (6) regarding research on the fetus during the abortion procedure and on the nonviable fetus *ex utero*. Should this view not be correct, and should the fetus indeed be able to experience pain before the twentieth week of gestation, I would modify Recommendation (6) in two ways:

First, the Recommendation as it now stands does not specify an acceptable level of risk. The reason for this omission is essentially as follows: in a dying subject prior to viability, "diminution of faculties" does not appear to be a meaningful index of harm since this index refers largely to future life expectations. Therefore, the critical meaning of "harm" for such a subject lies in the possibility of experiencing pain. If the fetus does not feel pain it cannot be "harmed" in this sense, and thus there is no risk of harm for such a fetus. It is for this reason that the Commission has not specified an acceptable level of "risk" for fetuses in this category, although it has been careful to protect the dignity of the fetus.

Clearly, however, if the fetus does indeed feel pain, then it can be "harmed" by the above definition of harm. If so, then I would argue that an acceptable level of risk should be established at the same level as that considered acceptable for fetuses *in utero*—namely, "no risk" or "minimal risk."

Second, the Commission has concluded that out of respect for the dying subject, no interventions are permissible which would alter the duration of life of the subject—i.e., by shortening or lengthening the dying process (item 6). I find the prohibition against shortening the life of the dying fetus to be acceptable provided the fetus does not feel pain. If the fetus does feel pain, however, then its dying may be painful and respect for the dying subject may require that its pain be minimized even if its life-span is shortened in so doing.

2. The Commission has stated that its provisions regarding therapeutic and nontherapeutic research directed toward the pregnant woman are not intended to limit research on improving abortion techniques. I support this stand and wish to clarify the reasons for my support.

In supporting this statement, I neither condone nor encourage widespread abortion. However, I do believe that some abortions are both legally and morally justifiable. It is therefore consonant with the principle of minimizing harm to develop techniques of abortion that are least harmful. Indeed, under the present climate of legal freedom to abort and widespread practice of abortion, adherence to the principle of not-harming may impose an obligation on us to research abortion technology in order to minimize harm. This obligation arises not only out of consideration of the health and well-being of the woman but also from a concern for possible pain or discomfort of the fetus during the abortion procedure.

3. Evidence presented to the Commission indicates that there is a strong emphasis in the law on avoiding possible injury to a child to be born. This evidence, coupled with the uncertainty of risks in a new class of human subjects, suggests that considerable importance ought to be attached to the question of compensation for injury incurred during research.

The Commission will study this question in depth at a later time, and therefore has not made any recommendations on compensation at this time. As a matter of personal opinion, I would like to note that I am reluctant to allow any research on the living human fetus unless provision has been made for adequate compensation of subjects injured during research.

4. The Commission's Recommendation on research during the abortion procedure and on the nonviable fetus *ex utero* prevents prolongation of the dying process for purposes of research. This prohibition may appear to have the effect of preventing research on the development of an artificial placenta.

It is my understanding that such an effect does not necessarily follow. Steps toward the development of an artificial placenta are prohibited only through *nontherapeutic* research; innovative therapy or therapeutic research on the possibly viable infant is not only condoned but encouraged. Thus, the development of an artificial placenta may proceed, but under more restricted circumstances in which it is limited to therapeutic research or to nontherapeutic research which does not alter the duration of life. I do not believe that it was the intention of the Commission to curtail all research toward the development of an artificial placenta, nor do I believe that such will be the effect of the Commission's Recommendations.

Were the Recommendations to have such an effect, however, I would dissent. Indeed, I would argue that a prematurely delivered fetus that is unable to survive, given the support of available medical technology, would have an interest in the development of an artificial placenta that would allow others like it to survive. Thus, it would not be contrary to the interests of that fetus for it to be subjected to nontherapeutic research in the development of an artificial placenta.

In making such an argument, I invoke a principle that I call the "principle of proximity": namely, that research is ethically more acceptable the more closely it approximates what the considered interests of the subject would reasonably be. For example, Hans Jonas has argued that dying subjects should not be used in nontherapeutic research, even when they have consented, unless the research deals directly with the cause from which they are dying; that is, it is presumed that a dying subject has an interest in his/her own disease which legitimates research on that disease where research in general would not be legitimate.

Such a principle is, of course, open to wide interpretation. But I think it not unreasonable to suggest that the dying fetus would have an interest in the cause of its dying or in the development of technology which would allow others like it to survive. On such a principle, one might argue that it is more ethically acceptable to use dying fetuses with Tay-Sachs disease as subjects in nontherapeutic research on Tay-Sachs disease than in nontherapeutic research on general fetal pharmacology. Similarly, one might argue that it is ethically acceptable to use nonviable fetuses *ex utero* as subjects in nontherapeutic research on the development of an artificial placenta. The development of a full rationale for such a position would require an analysis along the lines suggested by McCormick and Toulmin, and I cannot attempt that here. At this point I simply wish to suggest that I believe it is possible to argue for both therapeutic and nontherapeutic research directed toward the development of an artificial placenta.

5. Finally, members of the Commission disagreed about changes in the timing or method of abortion in relation to research. Recommendation (10) states clearly that the recommendations of a physician regarding timing and method of abortion should not be determined by the design or conduct of nontherapeutic research. I am in full agreement with this Recommendation.

The provision in Recommendation 6, item g, however, is more ambiguous. I would argue that changes in timing or method of abortion are ethically acceptable provided that they are freely chosen by the woman and that she has been fully informed of all possible risks from such changes. I base this argument on the right of any patient to be informed about alternative courses of treatment and to choose between them. It seems to me that the pregnant woman, as a patient, may choose the timing and method of abortion, provided that she has been fully informed of the following: 1) the relation of alternative methods of abortion to possible research on the fetus; 2) risks to herself and to possible future children of alternative possible methods of abortion; and 3) procedures which would be introduced into the abortion as part of the research design which would not be medically indicated.

Some members of the Commission have argued that a woman might choose such changes provided that they entail no additional risk. While I appreciate the concern to protect the woman's health and well-being, such a restriction seems to me a violation of her right to freedom of choice as a patient. Thus, I would allow a woman to choose to delay her abortion until the second trimester for purposes of research, *provided that* she has been fully informed of all risks in so doing. One restriction seems imperative to me, however: in no case, should she be allowed to delay the abortion beyond the twentieth week of gestation *for research purposes*. This position is reflected in the Deliberations and Conclusions of the Commission's Report.

RESEARCH INVOLVING CHILDREN

INTRODUCTION. *In 1977, Congress charged the National Commission for Protection of Human Subjects of Biomedical and Behavioral Research to report on the ethical issues involved in using children as research subjects. Several reports about the use of retarded children in medical research had raised concerns about this issue with added urgency. The Commission's report, issued in September 1977, contained eight recommendations and a review of the major ethical considerations that had led to them. Several commissioners preferred an alternative version of this chapter, that is, of part 8; and their concerns were likewise included in the report (see part 9). The excerpt that follows includes all of the Commission's recommendations and most of the theoretical discussions that accompanied them. The essays referred to in the latter were printed as an appendix to the report. They are listed at the end of this excerpt as resources for further reading.*

Recommendations

The National Commission for the Protection of Human Subjects of Biomedical and Behavioral Research makes the following recommendations for research involving children to the Secretary of Health, Education, and Welfare, with respect to research that is subject to his regulation, i.e., research conducted or supported under programs administered by him and research reported to him in fulfillment of regulatory requirements; and the Congress, with respect to research that is not subject to regulation by the Secretary of Health, Education, and Welfare.

Recommendation 1 Since the Commission finds that research involving children is important for the health and well-being of all children and can be conducted in an ethical manner, the Commission recommends that such research be conducted and supported, subject to the conditions set forth in the following recommendations.

Comment: The Commission recognizes the importance of safeguarding and improving the health and well-being of children, because they deserve the best care that society can reasonably provide. It is necessary to learn more about normal development as well as disease states in order to develop methods of diagnosis, treatment and prevention of conditions that jeopardize the health of children, interfere with optimal development, or adversely affect well-being in later years. Accepted practices must be studied as well, for although infants cannot survive without continual support, the effects of many routine practices are unknown and some have been shown to be harmful.

Much research on childhood disorders or conditions necessarily involves children as subjects. The benefits of this research may accrue to the subjects directly or to children as a class. The Commission considers, therefore, that the participation of children in research related to their conditions should receive the encouragement and support of the federal government.

The Commission recognizes, however, that the vulnerability of children, which arises out of their dependence and immaturity, raises questions about the ethical acceptability of involving them in research. Such ethical problems can be offset, the Commission believes, by establishing conditions that research must satisfy to be appropriate for the involvement of children. Such conditions are set forth in the following recommendations.

Recommendation 2 Research involving children may be conducted or supported provided an institutional review board has determined that (a) the research is scientifically sound and significant; (b) where appropriate, studies have been conducted first on animals and adult humans, then on older children, prior to involving infants;

Excerpts from the National Commission for the Protection of Human Subjects of Biomedical and Behavioral Research, *Research Involving Children.* DHEW (OS)77-0004 (Washington, D.C.: U.S. Government Printing Office, 1977). The format varies somewhat from the original; the notes have been edited for clarity and recast as endnotes (appearing at the end of this document).

(c) risks are minimized by using the safest procedures consistent with sound research design and by using procedures performed for diagnostic or treatment purposes whenever feasible; (d) adequate provisions are made to protect the privacy of children and their parents, and to maintain confidentiality of data; (e) subjects will be selected in an equitable manner; and (f) the conditions of all applicable subsequent recommendations are met.

Comment: This recommendation sets forth general conditions that should apply to all research involving children. Such research must also satisfy the conditions of one or more of recommendations 3 through 6, as applicable; recommendation 7; recommendation 8, if permission of parents or guardians is not a reasonable requirement; recommendation 9, if the subjects are wards of the state; and recommendation 10, if the subjects are institutionalized.

Respect for human subjects requires the use of sound methodology appropriate to the discipline. The time and inconvenience requested of subjects should be justified by the soundness of the research and its design, even if no more than minimal risk is involved. In addition, research involving children should satisfy a standard of scientific significance, since these subjects are less capable than adults of determining for themselves whether to participate. If necessary, the IRB should obtain the advice of consultants to assist in determining scientific soundness and significance. (The Commission will consider problems related to the determination of scientific soundness and significance in a future report on the performance of IRBs.)

Whenever possible, research involving risk should be conducted first on animals and adult humans in order to ascertain the degree of risk and the likelihood of generating useful knowledge. Sometimes this is not relevant or possible, as when the research is designed to study disorders or functions that have no parallel in animals or adults. In such cases, studies involving risk should be initiated on older children to the extent feasible prior to including infants, because older children are less vulnerable and they are better able to understand and to assent to participation. In addition, they are more able to communicate about any physical or psychological effects of such participation.

In order to minimize risk, investigators should use the safest procedures consistent with good research design and should make use of information or materials obtained for diagnostic or treatment purposes whenever feasible. For example, if a blood sample is needed, it should be obtained from samples drawn for diagnostic purposes whenever it is consistent with research requirements to do so.

Adequate measures should be taken to protect the privacy of children and their families, and to maintain the confidentiality of data. The adequacy of procedures for protecting confidentiality should be considered in light of the sensitivity of the data to be collected (i.e., the extent to which disclosure could reasonably be expected to be harmful or embarrassing).

Subjects should be selected in an equitable manner, avoiding overutilization of any one group of children based solely upon administrative convenience or availability of a population living in conditions of social or economic deprivation. The burdens of participation in research should be equitably distributed among the segments of our society, no matter how large or small those burdens may be.

In addition to the foregoing requirements, research must satisfy the conditions of the following recommendations, as applicable.

Recommendation 3 Research that does not involve greater than minimal risk to children may be conducted or supported provided an institutional review board has determined that (a) the conditions of recommendation 2 are met; and (b) adequate provisions are made for assent of the children and permission of their parents or guardians, as set forth in recommendations 7 and 8.

Comment: If the IRB determines that proposed research will present no more than minimal risk to children, the research may be conducted or supported provided the conditions of recommendation 2 are met and appropriate provisions are made for parental permission and the children's assent, as described in recommendations 7 and 8 below. If the IRB is unable to determine that the proposed research will present no more than minimal risk to children, the research should be reviewed under recommendations 4, 5, and 6, as applicable.

Recommendation 4 Research in which more than minimal risk to children is presented by an intervention that holds out the prospect of direct benefit for the individual subjects, or by a monitoring procedure required for the well-being of the subjects, may be conducted or supported provided an institutional review board has determined that (a) such risk is justified by the anticipated benefit to the subjects; (b) the relation of anticipated benefit to such risk is at least as favorable to the subjects as that presented by available alternative approaches; (c) the conditions of recommendation 2 are met; and (d) adequate provisions are made for assent of the children and permission of their parents or guardians, as set forth in recommendations 7 and 8.

Comment: The Commission emphasizes that the purely investigative procedures in research encompassed by recommendation 4 should entail no more than minimal risk to children. Greater risk is permissible under this recommendation only if it is presented by an intervention that holds out the prospect of direct benefit to the individual subjects or by a procedure necessary to monitor the effects of such intervention in order to maintain the well-being of these subjects (e.g., obtaining samples of blood or spinal fluid in order to determine drug levels that are safe and effective for the subjects). Such risk is acceptable, for example, when all available treatments for a serious illness or disability have been tried without success, and the remaining option is a new intervention under investigation. The expectation of success should be scientifically sound to justify undertaking whatever risk is involved. It is also appropriate to involve children in research when accepted therapeutic, diagnostic or preventive methods involve risk or are not entirely successful, and new biomedical or behavioral procedures under investigation present at least an equally favorable risk-benefit ratio. The IRB should evaluate research protocols of this sort in the same way that comparable decisions are made in clinical practice. It should compare the risk and anticipated benefit of the intervention under investigation (including the monitoring procedures necessary for care of the child) with those of available alternative methods for achieving the same goal, and should also consider the risk and possible benefit of attempting no intervention whatsoever.

To determine the overall acceptability of the research, the risk and anticipated benefit of activities described in a protocol must be evaluated individually as well as collectively, as is done in clinical practice. Research protocols meeting the criteria regarding risk and benefit may be conducted or supported provided the conditions of recommendation 2 are fulfilled and the requirements for assent of the children and for permission and participation of their parents or guardians, as set forth in recommendations 7 and 8 will be met. If the research also includes a purely investigative procedure presenting more than minimal risk, the research should be reviewed under recommendation 5 with respect to such procedure.

Recommendation 5 Research in which more than minimal risk to children is presented by an intervention that does not hold out the prospect of direct benefit for the individual subjects, or by a monitoring procedure not required for the well-being of the subjects, may be conducted or supported provided an institutional review board has determined that (a) such risk represents a minor increase over minimal risk; (b) such intervention or procedure presents experiences to subjects that are reasonably commensurate with those inherent in their actual or expected medical, psychological or social situations, and is likely to yield generalizable knowledge about the subjects' disorder or condition; (c) the anticipated knowledge is of vital importance for understanding or amelioration of the subjects' disorder or condition; (d) the conditions of recommendation 2 are met; and (e) adequate provisions are made for assent of the children and permission of their parents or guardians, as set forth in recommendations 7 and 8.

Comment: An IRB must determine that three special criteria are met in order to approve research presenting more than minimal risk but no direct benefit to the individual subjects. First, the increment in risk must be no more than a minor increase over minimal risk. The IRB should consider the degree of risk presented by the research from at least the following four perspectives: a common-sense estimation of the risk; an estimation based upon investigators' experience with similar interventions or procedures; any statistical information that is available regarding such interventions or procedures; and the situation of the proposed subjects. Second, the research activity must be commensurate with (i.e., reasonably similar to) procedures that the prospective subjects and others with the specific disorder or condition ordinarily experience (by virtue of having or being treated for that disorder or condition). Finally, the research must hold out the promise of significant benefit in the future to children suffering from or at risk for the disorder or condition (including, possibly, the subjects themselves). If necessary, the advice of scientific consultants should be obtained to assist in determining whether the research is likely to provide knowledge of vital importance to understanding the etiology or pathogenesis, or developing methods for the prevention, diagnosis or treatment, of the disorder or condition affecting the subjects.

The requirement of commensurability of experience should assist children who can assent to make a knowledgeable decision about their participation in research, based on some familiarity with the intervention or procedure and its effects. More generally, commensurability is intended to assure that participation in research will be closer to the ordinary experience of the subjects. The use of procedures that are familiar or similar to those used in treatment of the subjects should not, however, be used as a major justification for their participation in research, but rather as one of several criteria regarding the acceptability of such participation.

In addition to these special criteria, the IRB should assure that the conditions of recommendation 2 are fulfilled and the requirements for assent of the children and permission and participation of their parents or guardians, as set forth in recommendations 7 and 8 will be met. If the proposed research includes an intervention or procedure from which the subjects may derive direct benefit, it should also be reviewed under recommendation 4 with respect to that intervention or procedure.

Recommendation 6 Research that cannot be approved by an institutional review board under recommendations 3, 4, and 5, as applicable, may be conducted or supported provided an institutional review board has determined that the research presents an opportunity to understand, prevent or alleviate a serious problem affecting the health or welfare of children and, in addition, a national ethical advisory board and, following opportunity for public review and comment, the Secretary of the responsible federal department (or highest official of the responsible federal agency) have determined either (a) that the research satisfies the conditions of recommendations 3, 4, and 5, as applicable, or (b) [that it satisfies] the following: (i) the research presents an opportunity to understand, prevent or alleviate a serious problem affecting the health or welfare of children; (ii) the conduct of the research would not violate the principles of respect for persons, beneficence and justice; (iii) the conditions of recommendation 2 are met; and (iv) adequate provisions are made for assent of the children and permission of their parents or guardians, as set forth in recommendations 7 and 8.

Comment: If an IRB is unable for any reason to determine that proposed research satisfies the conditions of recommendations 3, 4, and 5, as applicable, the IRB may nevertheless certify the research for review and possible approval by a national ethical advisory board and the Secretary of the responsible department. Such review is contingent upon an IRB's determination that the research presents an opportunity to understand, prevent or alleviate a serious problem affecting the health or welfare of children. Thereafter, the research should be reviewed by the national board and Secretary, with opportunity for public comment, to determine whether the conditions of recommendations 3, 4, and 5, as applicable, are satisfied, or, alternatively, the research is justified by the importance of the knowledge sought and would not contravene principles of respect for persons, beneficence and justice that underlie these recommendations. In the latter instance, commencement of the research should be delayed pending congressional notification and a reasonable opportunity for Congress to take action regarding the proposed research.

The provision for national review and approval under recommendations 3, 4, and 5 is intended to fit the situation where an IRB has difficulty in applying those recommendations but considers the research of sufficient importance to warrant national review. Such difficulty may be resolved by a determination on the national level pursuant to recommendation 6a: that the research does satisfy the conditions of the applicable earlier recommendations. Alternatively, the national review may determine either that the research satisfies the conditions of recommendation 6b or that it should not be conducted.

The Commission believes that only research of major significance, in the presence of a serious health problem, would justify the approval of research under recommendation 6b. The problem addressed must be a grave one, the expected benefit should be significant, the hypothesis regarding the expected benefit must be scientifically sound, and an equitable method should be used for selecting subjects who will be invited to participate. Finally, appropriate provisions should be made for assent of the subjects and permission and participation of parents or guardians.

Recommendation 7 In addition to the determinations required under the foregoing recommendations, as applicable, the institutional review board should determine that adequate provisions are made for (a) soliciting the assent of the children (when capable) and the permission of their parents or guardians; and, when appropriate, (b) monitoring the solicitation of assent and permission, and involving at least one parent or guardian in the conduct of the research. A child's objection to participation in research should be binding unless the intervention holds out a prospect of direct benefit that is important to the health or well-being of the child and is available only in the context of the research.

Comment: The Commission uses the term parental or guardian "permission," rather than "consent," in order to distinguish what a person may do autonomously (consent) from what one may do on behalf of another (grant permission). Parental permission normally will be required for the participation of children in research. In addition, assent of the children should be required when they are seven years of age or older. The Commission uses the term "assent" rather than "consent" in this context, to distinguish a child's agreement from a legally valid consent.

Parental or guardian permission, as used in this recommendation, refers to the permission of parents, legally appointed guardians, and others who care for a child in a reasonably normal family setting. The last category might include, for example, stepparents or relatives such as aunts, uncles or grandparents who have established a continuing, close relationship with the child. Recommendation 8 describes circumstances in which the IRB may determine that the permission of parents or guardians is not appropriate because of the nature of the subject under investigation (e.g., contraception, drug abuse) or because of a failure in the relationship with the child (e.g., child abuse, neglect).

Parental or guardian permission should reflect the collective judgment of the family that an infant or child may participate in research. There are some research projects for which documented permission of one parent or guardian should be sufficient, such as research involving no more than minimal risk (as described in recommendation 3), or research in which risks or discomforts are related to a therapeutic, diagnostic or preventive intervention (as described in recommendation 4). In such cases, it may be assumed that the person giving formal permission is reflecting a family consensus. For research that is described in recommendations 5 and 6, the permission of both parents should be documented unless one parent is deceased, unknown, incompetent or not reasonably available, or the child has a guardian or belongs to a single-parent family (i.e., when only one person has legal responsibility for the care, custody and financial support of the child). The IRB should determine for each project whether permission of one or both parents should be required, a substitute mechanism may be used, or the provision may be waived. In making such determination, the IRB should consider the nature of the activities described in the research protocol and the age, status and condition of the subjects.

The IRB should assure that children who will be asked to participate in research described in recommendation 5 are those with good relationships with their parents or guardians and their physician, and who are receiving care in supportive surroundings. Projects approved under recommendations 4 and 6 may also require scrutiny of this sort. The IRB may wish to appoint someone to assist in the selection of subjects and to review the quality of interaction between parents or guardian and child. A member of the board or a consultant such as the child's pediatrician, a psychologist, a social worker, a pediatric nurse, or other experienced and perceptive person would be appropriate. The IRB should be particularly sensitive to the difficulties surrounding permission when the investigator is the treating physician to whom the parents or guardian may feel an obligation.

Because of the dependence of infants, the traditional role of parents as protectors, and the general authority of parents to determine the care and upbringing of their children, the IRB may determine that small children should participate in certain research only if the parents or guardians participate themselves by being present during some or all of the conduct of the research. This role will vary according to the nature of the research, the risk involved, the extent to which the research entails possibly disturbing deviations from normal routine, and the age and condition of the children. As a general rule, when infants participate in research that may cause physical discomfort or emotional stress and involves a significant departure from normal routine, a parent or guardian should be present. However, if discomfort arises only as a result of therapeutic interventions that must continue over a considerable period of time, the continual presence of parents need not be required. Parental presence during the conduct of much behavioral research may not be feasible or warranted, especially with older children. Generally, parents or guardians should be sufficiently involved in the research to understand its effects on their children and be able to intervene, if necessary.

The Commission believes that children who are seven years of age or older are generally capable of understanding the procedures and general purpose of research and of indicating their wishes regarding participation. Their assent should be required in addition to parental permission. However, if any child over six years of age is incapacitated so that he or she cannot reasonably be consulted, then parental permission should be sufficient, as it is for infants. The objection of a child of any age to participation in research should be binding except as noted below.

If the research protocol includes an intervention from which the subjects might derive significant benefit to their health or welfare, and that intervention is available only in a research context, the objection of a small child may be overridden. Such would be the case, for example, with a new drug that is not approved by the Food and Drug Administration for general distribution until safety and efficacy have been demonstrated in controlled clinical trials. Access to a drug under investigation generally requires participation in the research. Similar restrictions may be placed on other innovative therapies as a precaution. As children mature, their ability to perceive and act in their own best interest increases; thus, their wishes with respect to such research should carry increasingly more weight. When school-age children disagree with their parents regarding participation in such research, the IRB may wish to have a third party discuss the matter with all concerned and be present during the consent process. Although parents may legally override the objections of school-age children in such cases, the burden of that decision becomes heavier in relation to the maturity of the particular child.

Disclosure requirements for assent and permission are the same as those for informed consent. Similarly, children and parents or guardians should be free from duress. In order to assure understanding and freedom of choice, the IRB may determine that there is a need for an advocate to be present during the decision-making process. The need for third-party involvement in this process will vary according to the risk presented by the research and the autonomy of the subjects. The advocate should be an individual who has the experience and perceptiveness to fulfill such a role and who is not related in any way (except in the role as advocate or member of the IRB) to the research or the investigators.

Finally, the IRB should pay particular attention to the explanation and consent form, if any, to assure that appropriate language is used.

Recommendation 8 If the institutional review board determines that a research protocol is designed for conditions or a subject population for which parental or guardian permission is not a reasonable requirement to protect the subjects, it may waive such requirement provided an appropriate mechanism for protecting the children who will participate as subjects in the research is substituted. The choice of an appropriate mechanism should depend upon the nature and purpose of the activities described in the protocol, the risk and anticipated benefit to the research subjects, and their age, status and condition.

Comment: Circumstances that would justify modification or waiver of the requirement for parental or guardian permission includes: (1) research designed to identify factors related to the incidence or treatment of certain conditions in adolescents for which, in certain jurisdictions, they legally may receive treatment without parental consent; (2) research in which the subjects are "mature minors" and the procedures involved entail essentially no more than minimal risk that such individuals might reasonably assume on their own; (3) research designed to understand and meet the needs of neglected or abused children, or children designated by their parents as "in need of supervision"; and (4) research involving children whose parents are legally or functionally incompetent.

There is no single mechanism that can be substituted for parental permission in every instance. In some cases the consent of mature minors should be sufficient. In other cases court approval may be required. The mechanism invoked will vary with the research and the age, status and condition of the prospective subjects.

A number of states have specific legislation permitting minors to consent to treatment for certain conditions (e.g., pregnancy, drug addiction, venereal diseases) without the permission (or knowledge) of their parents. If parental permission were required for research about such conditions, it would be difficult to develop improved methods of prevention and therapy that meet the special needs of adolescents. Therefore, assent of such mature minors should be considered sufficient with respect to research about conditions for which they have legal authority to consent on their own to treatment. An appropriate mechanism for protecting such subjects might be to require that a clinic nurse or physician, unrelated to the research, explain the nature and the purpose of the research to prospective subjects, emphasizing that participation is unrelated to provision of care.

Another alternative might be to appoint a social worker, pediatric nurse, or physician to act as surrogate parent when the research is designed, for example, to study neglected or battered children. Such surrogate parents would be expected to participate not only in the process of soliciting the children's cooperation but also in the conduct of the research, in order to provide reassurance for the subjects and to intervene or support their desires to withdraw if participation becomes too stressful.

Recommendation 9 Children who are wards of the state should not be included in research approved under recommendations 5 or 6 unless such research is (a) related to their status as orphans, abandoned children, and the like; or (b) conducted in a school or similar group setting in which the majority of children involved as subjects are not wards of the state. If such research is approved, the institutional review board should require that an advocate for each child be appointed, with an opportunity to intercede that would normally be provided by parents.

Comment: It is important to learn more about the effects of various settings in which children who are wards of the state may be placed, as well as about the circumstances surrounding child abuse and neglect, in order to improve the care that is provided for such children by the community. Also, it is important to avoid embarrassment or psychological harm that might result from excluding wards of the state from research projects in which their peers in a school, camp or other group setting will be participating. Provision must be made to permit the conduct of such studies in ways that will protect the children involved, even though no parents or guardians are available to act in their behalf.

To this end, the IRB reviewing such research should evaluate the reasons for including wards of the state as research subjects and assure that such children are not the sole participants in a research project unless the research is related to their status as orphans, abandoned children, and the like. The IRB should require, as a minimum, that an advocate for each child be appointed to intercede, when appropriate, on the child's behalf. The IRB may also require additional protections, such as prior court approval.

Recommendation 10 Children who reside in institutions for the mentally infirm or who are confined in correctional facilities should participate in research only if the conditions regarding research on the institutionalized mentally infirm or on prisoners (as applicable) are fulfilled in addition to the conditions set forth herein.

Note: The foregoing recommendations were adopted unanimously with the exception of recommendation 5, from which Commissioners Cooke and Turtle dissented.

CHAPTER 8—ETHICAL ISSUES

The general purpose of research involving children is to obtain scientific information about them. Often the research provides some direct benefit to the subjects involved in the research. However, some research may produce benefits only for other children, and frequently it is quite uncertain whether the subjects themselves will ultimately benefit from the research. In some cases benefits are long-range or unpredictable, and the major objective is to develop a body of knowledge. Ethical issues about the involvement of children arise because of competing answers to the following question: Under what conditions (if any) are these various types of research justified? When the objective of procedures is that of directly benefiting the subjects, the research is generally agreed to be justifiable, under certain limiting conditions, if there is a reasonable prospect that the subjects will benefit. However, research in which procedures present no prospect of direct benefit to the subjects raises a variety of ethical problems about the protection and the rights of children and about the authority of parents. Although only alluded to in classical ethical codes and regulations, these problems have received extensive attention in recent ethical literature.

Codes and Regulations

The Nuremberg Code (1949) has seemed to some to preclude the participation of children in research. The first principle of that code states explicitly:

> The voluntary consent of the human subject is absolutely essential. This means that the person involved should have the legal capacity to give consent.[1]

The apparent clarity of this statement, however, is clouded by the written statements of two individuals who participated in the drafting of the Code. Leo Alexander, whose first draft of principles formed the basis of the Code, has written that the original draft contained provisions for consent by next of kin on behalf of incompetent patients, but that the judges omitted those provisions in the final version "probably because they did not apply in the specific cases under trial."[2] Similarly, Andrew Ivy, chief medical consultant to the War Crimes Trials, wrote (in the same year the Code was published) that

> The ethical principles involved in the use of the mentally incompetent are the same as for mentally competent persons. The only difference involves the matter of consent. Since mental cases are likened to children in an ethical and legal sense, the consent of the guardian is required.[3]

The record does not show whether the judges at Nuremberg disagreed with their medical consultants on this matter or whether, as Alexander suggests, they simply followed judicial custom by limiting their opinion to the facts of the case at bar.

The Medical Research Council of Great Britain took the position in 1963 that young children should not be subjects of "nontherapeutic" research if that research "may carry some risk of harm."[4] Their general rule is that if a child is under 12 years of age: "information requiring the performance of any procedure involving his body would need to be obtained incidentally to and without altering the nature of a procedure intended for his individual benefit."[5] If the child is over age 12, his or her consent should be obtained, and its validity would depend upon a showing that the child understood the implications of the procedures involved.

The Declaration of Helsinki,[6] published by the World Medical Association in 1964, provides, with respect to "nontherapeutic" research, that "if [the subject] is legally incompetent the consent of the legal guardian should be secured." [The 1975 revision states, as a basic ethical principle, that "when the subject is a minor, permission from the responsible relative replaces that of the subject in accordance with national legislation" (unnumbered footnote in original)]. The acceptance of this code by the American Society for Clinical Investigation, the American College of Physicians, the American College of Surgeons, and particularly the American Medical Association[7] resulted in the general acceptance throughout this country of third-party permission for research employing interventions that are not for an incompetent subject's direct benefit.

The 1971 Institutional Guide to DHEW Policy for the Protection of Human Subjects required the consent of a subject "or his authorized representative." It did not define "authorized representative," but cautioned that

> The review committee should consider the validity of consent by next of kin, legal guardians, or by other qualified third parties representative of the subjects' interests. In such instances, careful consideration should be given by the committee not only to whether these third parties can be presumed to have the necessary depth of interest and concern with the subjects' rights and welfare, but also to whether these third parties will be legally authorized to expose the subjects to the risks involved.[8]

DHEW invited comments in 1973 on the proposal that parental or guardian consent be supplemented both by the judgment of a consent committee and by requirements for the assent of the child or incompetent.[9] The following approach was taken regarding the refusal and consent of children:

> Although children might not have the capacity to consent on their own to participate in research activities, they must be given the opportunity (so far as they are able) to refuse to participate. The traditional requirement of parental consent for medical procedures is intended to be protective rather than coercive. Thus, while it was held to be unlawful to proceed merely with the consent of the child, but without consent of the parent or legal guardian, the reverse should also hold.[10]

This proposal to require assent of the child was adopted for intramural research by the NIH Clinical Center on July 14, 1975.[11]

Current DHEW regulations provide that consent may be obtained from an individual's "legally authorized representative," which is defined as "an individual or judicial or other body authorized under applicable law to consent on behalf of a prospective subject to such subject's participation in the particular activity or procedure."[12] Strictly construed, this provision would permit third-party permission only in those jurisdictions which specifically authorize a third party to consent for another's participation in research. While parental authority to consent for medical care is clear, there is no statute or judicial decision granting such authority for nonbeneficial procedures.

Ethical Positions in Recent Literature

At least five different positions on the involvement of children in research can be found in recent literature.

(1) The most restrictive position is found in the writings of Paul Ramsey. He argues that research which does not directly benefit individual children is always ethically impermissible. His argument rests on the general viewpoint that "nontherapeutic" research should never be performed

without the informed consent of the subject. Since young children are not capable of giving informed consent, it is a short step to the conclusion that no research ought to be performed on them unless the research holds out the possibility of direct benefit. In his book, *The Patient as Person*, Ramsey argues as follows:

> A parent's decisive concern is for the care and protection of the child, to whom he owes the highest fiduciary loyalty, even when he also appreciates the benefits to come to others from the investigation and might submit his own person to experiment in order to obtain them.
>
> This is simply the minimum claim of childhood upon the adult community, whose members may make themselves joint adventurers or partners in the enterprise of medical advancement at cost to themselves if they will.[13]

Ramsey distinguishes "beneficial research," for which parental consent is a proper fulfillment of the fiduciary duty, from "nonbeneficial research," for which he considers third-party permission a breach of the fiduciary duty. It is not merely the exposure to possible risk that he finds unacceptable. Rather, it is the abrogation of "the right of each of us to determine for ourselves, not alone the extent to which we will share ourselves with others, but the timing and the nature of any such sharing."[14] It is thus a claimed violation of respect for persons (by treating others as a means to one's own end) which is morally unacceptable to Ramsey: "where there is no possible relation to the child's recovery, a child is not to be made a mere object in medical experimentation."[15] Still, Ramsey is concerned with the risk of harm as well as with the violation of autonomy. He argues that the imperative to avoid evil has a moral primacy in biomedical research over the imperative to do good, and he takes this priority as one more support for his general position.[16] Nonetheless, it is the alleged use of human beings merely as means to others' ends that most deeply informs Ramsey's polemic against "nontherapeutic" research.

Ramsey proposes to give ethical primacy to the protection of nonconsenting subjects against wrongful treatment. While this general position must be commended, Ramsey's views are subject to a number of objections. First, it is important to distinguish those who refuse to consent to participation in research from those who are not fully qualified to consent to participation. It would be generally conceded that children who refuse to agree to participate in "nonbeneficial" research should not be involved. But it appears to be increasingly the case that most children are willingly involved in research and give their assent (when capable). Second, Ramsey neglects discussion of the low level of risk involved in most research involving children. His conclusions (though not his actual arguments) would be more supportable if there were a widespread risk of serious harm. In fact, however, much biomedical and behavioral research involves no more risk to children than those risks encountered in their daily lives. Ramsey's proposals for curbing research in general, if acted upon, would render impermissible research that is only observational, or merely uses questions, or involves only paper and pencil tests or procedures of a routine medical examination. While everyone would agree that the line specifying permissible risk must be drawn somewhere, Ramsey's absolute prohibition seems too restrictive. Ramsey's argument is internally consistent on these matters, in that he would prohibit all research without regard to risk or to the assent of children. It is his treatment of these relevant factors (risk and assent) as irrelevant which is unacceptable.[17]

Third, Ramsey's position rests on a false dichotomy between research intended to benefit subjects directly—which he concedes is permissible—and research intended to develop more knowledge. Much research does not fit neatly into either category, since the outcome is uncertain and the research may or may not benefit the subjects involved. Research on chronic diseases, for example, may or may not directly benefit those involved in the research, contingent upon the results of the research. Indeed, the possibility of (even remote) future benefits for the subjects can seldom be ruled out from the beginning.[18]

This problem introduces a further problem about the meaning and scope of the term "research," as Ramsey employs it. Research, by definition, is intended to develop general knowledge. Therapy, by definition, is for the benefit of an individual and therefore does not inherently involve any generalizable component. The term "therapeutic research" thus mixes together two quite different ingredients, and it remains unclear what "therapeutic research" could mean. There are dangers in this unclarity. On the one hand, there is the danger that simply because a benefit (therapy) is included in a "therapeutic" research protocol, all sorts of additional interventions not germane to the therapeutic intervention but useful for general knowledge can be regarded as justified (under Ramsey's scheme). On the other hand, if a quite narrow but nonetheless reasonable interpretation of "research" is accepted, then one literally could never do any "research" at all, because the research itself (e.g., data analysis) is not therapeutic. Ramsey can perhaps introduce further distinctions to handle some of these problems—for example by arguing that "therapeutic research" is a certain kind of mixture of controlled studies of alternative therapies, when all treatments are thought to be equally efficacious. But as his work now stands there remain conceptual unclarities which introduce needless confusion.

Ramsey at one point acknowledges that even if there were powerful moral reasons for doing "nontherapeutic research with uncomprehending subjects" such as children, "it is better to leave [this] research imperative in incorrigible conflict with the principle that protects the individual human person from being used for research purposes without either his expressed or correctly construed consent."[19] Ramsey argues that it would be "immoral" either to do or not to do the research, but he maintains that one should "sin bravely" in the face of this dilemma by sinning on the side of avoiding harm rather than attempting to promote welfare. But why must a calculation of benefits and harms always fall on the side of preventing research? In those cases where potentially great therapeutic benefits may well result from research and only minimal risk is involved, it may be reasonably argued that the calculus of morally right actions has shifted.

Ramsey attempts to support his view by appeal to the Kantian maxim that persons ought to be treated as ends only, and never merely as means. But what is it, in the context of research, to be treated merely as a means? When a soldier is conscripted, he is treated as a means (even against his will, in some cases). But he is not treated merely as a means, for none in the military hierarchy is free to do anything with a soldier he wishes. Similarly, a child involved in research may be used as a means, but not merely as a means; for no investigator is free to use a child in any way he wishes. The question remains whether the child is being used in such a way that the treatment qualifies as immoral treatment. And if the child is exposed only to minimal risk (with judicious parental permission and the child's agreement), while substantial benefit may accrue to others, it is far from obvious that any immoral treatment is present. If there were some reason for supposing that children would regard themselves as being violated or as being used as mere means, Ramsey's argument would be strengthened; but in a world where many adults feel themselves morally obliged to help those in need, there is no reason to attribute an unduly selfish attitude to children, as Ramsey's argument often seems to presuppose. Moreover, as Benjamin Freedman has argued, even if children occupy a dependent, morally different status from that of adults—as Ramsey contends—it does not follow that parents are derelict in their duty in consenting for children to participate in research. Even though children have some claims upon us for protection, participation in research does not seem to violate their rights unless such participation constitutes a harmful invasion.[20]

(2) The fact that some research on children involves minimal risk and holds out the prospect of benefit for the class of children (but presumably not direct benefit to the research subjects themselves) has been the decisive factor in motivating some writers to accept less stringent criteria than Ramsey's. One example is Richard McCormick, who has written in opposition to Ramsey from the perspective that children have obligations to participate in research. McCormick employs a natural law foundation for his arguments. He maintains that a child ought to do something if that action is expressive of basic values of human nature or purposes of human life. In the case of therapy, for example, it is a reasonable presumption that the child would consent because (in light of the normative ideal of health) the child ought to promote his own health. Similarly in the "nontherapeutic" case, according to McCormick, it is a reasonable presumption that the child would consent because (in light of the normative ideal of contributing to the health of others) the child ought to choose to participate in research. There is a general moral obligation to help others when there is little cost to oneself. Because children (like all individuals in society) ought to benefit others by their actions and would so act if they had a proper moral perspective, it is legitimate to involve them in research (provided it is of no more than minimal risk). McCormick's presumption is not that someone would actually act in a certain way but only that another may validly presume consent because the act is right. Parental consent is said to be morally valid for both "therapeutic" and "nontherapeutic" contexts, because it is based on a reasonable presumption of the child's obligations:

> . . . there are things we ought to do for others simply because we are members of the human community. . . . If it can be argued that it is good for all of us to share in these experiments, and hence that we ought to do so (social justice), then a presumption of consent where children are involved is reasonable and proxy consent becomes legitimate.[21]

In sum: the parent is the vehicle for choosing what the child should rightly choose if he were so situated that he knew what he ought to do.

McCormick's position is subject to a variety of objections. There are at least two possible problems with his claim that we can presume consent because a child ought to consent. First, natural law arguments have been subjected to sharp criticism in ethical theory. In particular, one common objection to natural law theory is that it does not follow from the wide or even universal sharing by human beings of certain values or purposes (e.g., health, happiness, etc.) that human beings ought to promote those values or purposes. For example, from the value human beings place on propagation of the species it does not follow that all persons ought to propagate at will or even that they should propagate at all. It does not follow even if such a value is basic to human nature. This apparent deficiency in McCormick's position is important, since if his natural law foundation is insupportable, the entire position on children is groundless.

A second possible problem with McCormick's position resides in the claim that consent may validly be presumed where there is an underlying obligation. There are probably numerous activities in which adults ought to participate, but to which many would not consent. The whole point of obtaining a person's consent is to protect his autonomy. What one person will consent to may vary significantly from what another will consent to because of basic differences of value. To respect persons is to respect their right to their own evaluative choices, including their right not to perform certain actions which other persons believe, with some justification, that they ought to perform. While we have a moral right to demand that individuals fulfill their obligations, some obligations are created only by an individual's own commitments, and we often have no right to demand the commitment itself. Consent is such a commitment, and absent the commitment, no valid consent can be presumed (this much is true in Ramsey's position).

Accordingly, it seems certain that we could never validly presume consent on the part of a competent adult subject merely because the person ought to consent. How, then, can consent of the child be validly presumed? As Ramsey has argued, McCormick's position "amounts to the destruction of the protections consent-language was designed to afford."[22] Consent can rarely be presumed, and there seems no way it can be presumed on the part of a child. In short, perhaps the gravest deficiency in McCormick's position is its very core: the notion that the child's consent can be validly presumed.

Ramsey has generalized this conclusion in the following way: if McCormick's standard is used

> . . . then anyone—and not only children—may legitimately be entered into human experimentation *without* his will or unwillingly. . . . If a child may be treated as an adult who would will what he should, then any other nonvolunteer may be treated simply as a child who . . . *would* will what he *should*. Any nonvolunteer may be treated as a child who does not will as he ought.[23]

Ramsey's point is that if consent can validly be presumed because of what persons ought to do, then (1) it is hard to find a principled basis for the claim that there is any morally relevant difference between adults and children, and (2) it would follow that the general conscription of adults is permissible. Ramsey's argument does not constitute an objection to McCormick, from one perspective, since McCormick actually favors the conscription of adults. The pertinent point, however, is about consent, not about conscription. The form of McCormick's argument is if one ought to do it, then consent may be validly assumed. But consent is precisely what may not be assumed even if one ought to do it. One reason why the requirement of informed consent has become so important in recent years is that the consent of some subjects was never solicited, because a prior judgment had been made that they ought to participate.

Moreover, it is not even clear, based on McCormick's arguments, that consent should be a relevant consideration. If a child ought to do something and the obligation justifies the child's doing that thing, then the consent of his parents could neither validate nor invalidate his participation. Parental consent is simply irrelevant to the justification for involving the child in research. To put this point another way, McCormick operates with two levels for the justification of involving children: natural law and consent by third parties. If the natural law justification is correct, it actually undermines the consent model by rendering it gratuitous.

A possible response by McCormick to some of these arguments is considered at the end of the next section (3). But it is worth mentioning at this point that an alternative interpretation of McCormick's arguments to the one presented above might be offered. In his later writings McCormick's major conclusions appear anchored in the argument that all members of society, including children, have minimal obligations to benefit other members of society. These obligations are created by social circumstances (rather than by some general property of human nature). Among these obligations is that of participating in minimal risk biomedical or behavioral research. Because of these social obligations the child should be willing to participate in research; and parents may be empowered to consent for the child's participation whenever the child *should* be willing to be involved in the research if the child *could* comprehend and consent. On this alternative interpretation, "proxy consent" is merely a device to protect the child, and plays no more substantive role in the argument. That is, the obligations children have justify using them, and consent is merely a protective device that plays no role in the justification. McCormick's position is thus turned into a "presumed duty" rather than a "presumed consent" position. If this alternative reading of McCormick is preferable, then his position is perhaps closer to the one that is presented in section 5, below.

(3) A variant of McCormick's stance might be developed along lines proposed by Stephen Toulmin[24] in the course of considering the justification of fetal research. He suggests that instead of beginning with what children ought to do, we might ask whether it may be presumed that they could not reasonably object if they were capable of understanding what is at stake and of making a decision in their own right. This strategy is thought by Toulmin to free the theory of the objection of imputing obligations to children and to reconcile McCormick's approach with common public policy judgments about the validity of involving children in research. Toulmin's proposal is distinguishable from the two positions previously outlined by its philosophical basis. Rather than using a theory of informed consent or natural law, Toulmin makes an appeal to what the reasonable person would agree to choose—or, as he states it negatively—what the child could not reasonably object to. . . .

(4) Some writers have attempted to mediate between Ramsey's entire exclusion of the class of children and McCormick's (and others') apparent entire inclusion of the class. These writers have suggested that children old enough to be educated can be aided in their education by participation in research, but not at earlier ages. The justification for participation, then, is moral development; and if there can be no moral development through participation, the justification is lost. Perhaps the first to suggest this approach was Henry Beecher. In *Research and the Individual* he suggested, without further elaboration, that

> Parents have the obligation to inculcate into their children attitudes of unselfish service. One could hope that this might be extended to include participation in research for the public welfare, when it is important and there is no discernible risk.[25]

This kind of position has been defended in a paper written for the Commission by William Bartholome.[26] He discusses the involvement of children from age five to seven through age 14 to 16 in research activities. He criticizes Ramsey's total exclusion of children from "nontherapeutic" research as harsh, and suggests that to focus exclusively on informed consent (as Ramsey does) as the moral basis for including subjects in research is to prejudge the answer to the question whether children may participate in "nontherapeutic" research. At the same time Bartholome agrees with Ramsey that interventions in the lives of children can be justified only if they are to benefit the child. These two authors largely differ over what shall count as a benefit. While Ramsey considers only therapy to be beneficial, Beecher and Bartholome consider improved moral character to be a benefit.

Bartholome criticizes McCormick for presuming that adults are able to know what a child should want and rejects McCormick's suggestion that there are certain things a child "ought to do." Children are not morally "transparent," he argues, and thus no adult can know what a particular child should choose. And since it cannot be asked what they would choose, only their *needs* should be considered in asking about their participation in research. Even if there are certain things that a child ought to want to do for others, Bartholome claims, no one has the right to determine how, when and in what manner such obligations should be fulfilled. Bartholome also disputes what he takes to be McCormick's argument that we owe to future generations the cure or prevention of certain diseases and that, in general, involvement in "nontherapeutic" research is obligatory for everyone. Bartholome prefers to see such rewards for future generations as "gifts" rather than as obligations required by justice or by social need.

To resolve the conflict between the two polar positions exemplified by the writings of Ramsey and McCormick, Bartholome suggests that children may be assisted in their moral education by participating in "nontherapeutic" research, once (at age five to seven) they are able to appreciate the importance of helping others. As part of their general obligation to enhance the moral development of such children, parents should encourage them to take advantage of opportunities for moral growth; and Bartholome contends that involvement in research is one of many activities which parents might select to this end. He distinguishes between the parental duty to encourage such behavior and McCormick's notion that parents have a right to force children to engage in charitable acts. Bartholome disagrees both with Ramsey's position that "children are not capable by nature or grace of charitable acts" and with McCormick's position that parents have a right to see that their children undertake such acts. Instead, Bartholome considers the parental obligation to be one of moral instruction, which may include encouragement but also requires that the child be a willing participant. Assent by the child should be mandatory, he maintains, and parents should be involved in the process both by deciding whether or not participation in research would be a beneficial learning experience for their child and by participating with their child as "joint-subjects" when the experimental design provides an opportunity for such collaboration.

In an accompanying paper on "The Infant as Person," Bartholome takes the position that infants (i.e., children below the age of understanding) have a right to be treated as persons but, because they have no awareness even of themselves, do not have a moral obligation to the human community. For this reason he would reject "nontherapeutic" research involving infants below the age of five, at least where research requires serious invasive procedures. . . .

(5) A position with a conclusion similar to the presumed consent and reasonable consent positions, but with a somewhat different theoretical foundation, is that some research on children is justified because of the beneficial consequences to the class of children in general. If this position were stated in extreme form, it would be the unqualified utilitarian position that such research ought to be done whenever it maximizes social welfare to do so (whether or not the subjects assent or dissent). While no writer seems to hold this unqualified position, two papers done for the Commission give weight to the consideration of benefit to others as the theoretical justification for research. The first paper was done by H. Tristram Engelhardt, Jr.,[27] and the second by Robert Veatch.[28] (Neither paper, however, deals solely or even primarily with research involving children.)

Engelhardt recognizes the absolutely fundamental character of both the principle of respect for individual human subjects and the principle of beneficence (which involves the concern to maximize benefits for society in general), though he considers the protection of autonomy and promotion of individual self-determination to be primary. Accordingly, he rejects the involvement of unwilling subjects in research, even if the results of the research would be of considerable utility.[29] With respect to children clearly too young to consent, he argues that "infants, though often willful, have no free will and are not the object of respect as adults are." Since infants are nonautonomous, there is no obligation to respect autonomy; there is only an obligation to protect them from harm. He further contends that the function of third-party consent in such contexts is not to respect the child as an autonomous moral agent but to safeguard the child's best interest by preserving his or her physiological and psychological integrity. But he regards the notion of third-party consent to be less appropriate than other substitute language might be, since the third-party feature contravenes the purpose of consent. The point of informed consent, he argues, is to respect the freedom of individuals by asking their permission before involving them in research, yet for many children such treatment is impossible and inappropriate.

Engelhardt advances two sorts of arguments bearing on the use of children in research. He first argues that research is nonallowable if it would leave a residual amount of damage to the child. This argument stakes out his restraining conditions on appeals to beneficial consequences. Although his argument justifies research by appeal to beneficial consequences, Engelhardt also advances one consequentialist argument which actually restricts research. He contends that investigators and parents should always act in the best interest of children in order to provide general support for social practices of attention and kindness to the defenseless and powerless (a larger class than the class of children). Nonetheless, Engelhardt concludes that experiments which may involve minor discomforts but which would not expose children to physical or psychological risks greater than "in the usual ambience," are justifiable "in terms of an appeal to the minimal duties that each of us owe(s) to society."[30] In this argument, his usually strong emphasis on individual self-determination does not apply, and his argument turns on the duties owed to society. These duties are grounded in beneficence rather than respect for persons.[31]

Veatch agrees that "for the most part, it is a mistake to speak of proxy consent for experiments in children";[32] however, parents may approve a child's participation in "therapeutic" research because, as guardians, they rightly serve to protect the best interests of the child, and as parents they are given limited authority to exercise their own self-determination about their offspring, to the extent that their determination does not substantially deviate from the social consensus.[33] He argues that parents may also encourage their children to make minor contributions to the general welfare or to the welfare of specific others. He further maintains that if "the individual is seen as a member of the social community, then certain obligations to the common welfare may be presupposed even in cases where consent is not obtained."[34] This formulation expresses the common thread of argument from beneficence running through the positions of McCormick, Engelhardt and Veatch. This condition would apply, he says, only in very special cases where there would be no risk or only minimal risk to the subject and when the information to be obtained would be of great social value and could be obtained in no other way. The subject's participation in such research is justified, he contends, because of the substantial contribution to the general welfare which may be made—a contribution which, even without consent, the "reasonable person would find required."[35] (Veatch, however, adds that proceeding without consent is valid only in the case of very young children where self-determination is impossible. And he is always careful to add that his position does not entail that social benefits can be used to justify a cancellation of individual rights.) Veatch also argues in favor of retaining age 18 as the age of consent for medical treatment, and favors adjudicating on a case-by-case basis when, in the case of "therapeutic" research, children and their parents disagree. Finally, he proposes that a national committee review all research protocols involving children, using the same review criteria applied by IRBs.[36]

The qualified beneficial consequences position taken by Veatch and Engelhardt would obviously be found deficient by Ramsey and Bartholome, for example, on grounds that it justifies too much. In particular they would argue that it fails to respect persons by subjecting them to risk without consent and without obvious beneficial consequences for the subjects. However, perhaps the largest potential deficit in the positions taken by Veatch and Engelhardt rests in the lack of specificity concerning the scope of research justified by their principles. For example, how much research (if any) which involves more than minimal risk is acceptable in "nontherapeutic" cases? It is hard to see how an answer could be derived from their theory. Without further argument minimal risk seems a purely arbitrary cut-off point when, in very special cases, substantial benefit for others is in prospect. Both Veatch and Engelhardt are appropriately engaged in the attempt to balance the obligation to protect individuals against the obligation to provide substantial social benefits. While this balancing must be done, it is doubtful that their theories satisfactorily show how and at what point the individual rights of children properly limit their social obligations. Relatedly, it is one thing to argue that some research on infants may be allowed, and another to develop the precise conditions under which it is justified. Neither Veatch nor Engelhardt delineates a rigorous set of such conditions.

Among the well-known dangers of social benefit approaches is that they may justify so much on grounds of the principle of beneficence that the principle of respect for persons fails to be applied.[37] That is, the obligation to benefit others (perhaps by developing therapies which avoid harm to them) might be employed in such a way that the obligation to protect subjects is not fulfilled. Both Veatch and Engelhardt attempt to guard against this possibility, because, as Veatch puts it, there are such "great dangers" in unqualified appeals to the benefit of others. Accordingly, what must be said to be lacking in the Veatch and Engelhardt papers is not that they make no appeal to the principle of respect for persons. What seems in need of development is an explanation of the proper balance to be struck between the competing obligations to respect persons and to benefit those in need of help.

CHAPTER 9—DELIBERATIONS AND CONCLUSIONS

. . . The most difficult ethical issues for the Commission arose with respect to research presenting more than minimal risk but no immediate prospect of direct benefit to the individual children involved. Some members of the Commission urged that the limit for such research remain at the level of minimal risk; others pointed out that such a limit might eliminate much research that has great scientific significance and the promise of substantial long-term benefit to children in general, while possibly avoiding only minor additional risk to the research subjects. Much of the Commission's later debate was focused on this class of research projects. The Commission was seeking to determine the circumstances (if any) under which such research might be ethically acceptable, and, if so, what review procedures would be appropriate to assure proper protection of the research subjects.

In their resolution of this question, the Commission relied largely upon two considerations. It noted, first, that the scope of parental authority routinely covers a child's participation in many activities in which risk is more than minimal, and yet benefit is questionable. (Involvement in skiing and contact sports are two examples among many.) The Commission was also impressed by reported examples of diagnostic, therapeutic and preventive measures that might well have been derived from research involving risk that, while minor, would be considered more than minimal.

Most of the Commissioners agreed that a minor increase in risk would be permissible in order to attain substantial future benefits to children other than the subject. "Minor increase" refers to a risk which, while it goes beyond the narrow boundaries of minimal risk determined by the Commission, poses no significant threat to the child's health or well-being. Moreover, the Commission requires that the research activities presenting such risks be similar to the experiences familiar to the children who would be the subjects of the research. Such activities, then, would be considered normal for these children. Given this conservative limit, the Commission concluded that promise of substantial benefit does justify research which goes beyond, but only slightly beyond, the minimal risk. The Commission considers that, as in the question of "no more than minimal risk," permission to allow such research lies within the scope of parental responsibility. In addition, children capable of more mature judgment may wish to volunteer for research of this sort.

Ultimately, the Commission decided (with two members dissenting) that if three conditions are satisfied, research in this most difficult class of cases could be justified (recommendation 5). First, the risk involved must be only a minor increment beyond minimal. In addition, the procedures to be used must be reasonably commensurate with (similar to) those with which prospective subjects have had experience. Finally, the research must be likely to yield knowledge important for the understanding or amelioration of the subject's specific disorder or condition from which the subject suffers, even though the subject may not actually benefit. Thus, foreseeable benefit to an identifiable class of children may justify a minor increment of risk to research subjects.

The Commission acknowledged that exceptional situations may arise in which considerable dangers to children or to the community at large might be avoided or prevented by exposing children to research attended by more than minimal risk. Some might offer the ethical argument that avoidance of great danger or disaster outweighs the injunction against exposing children to risk of more than minimal harm. For instance, they may say the threat of an epidemic that could be offset by developing a safe and effective vaccine might justify research involving risk greater than otherwise acceptable to establish safety, efficacy and dosage levels for children of different ages. The outright prohibition of such research on grounds of risk might have consequences which themselves appear unethical.

Faced with such a hypothetical situation, the Commission found itself confronted by a common dilemma: regardless of whatever course is chosen, some benefit may be foregone and some harm may be done. Rather than attempt to resolve the dilemma in the abstract, the Commission has chosen to recommend that the ethical argument should be made, not over a hypothetical case, but over an actual situation, in which the real issues and the likely costs of any solution can be more clearly discerned. The ethical principles at stake are the moral obligation to protect the community or to come to the aid of certain sufferers within it and the moral prohibition against using unconsenting persons, at considerable risk to their well-being, for the promotion of the common good. . . .

NOTES TO CHAPTER 8

1. *Trials of War Criminals Before the Nuremberg Military Tribunals, U.S. v. Karl Brandt*, vol. II, U.S. Government Printing Office, 1949, p. 181.
2. Leo Alexander, "Psychiatry: Methods and Processes for Investigation of Drugs," *Annals of the New York Academy of Science*, 169 (1970): 347.
3. Andrew Ivy, "The History of the Use of Human Subjects in Medical Experiments," 108 *Science* 1948, p. 1. For an extended discussion of this matter see Beecher, *Research and the Individual: Human Studies*, Little, Brown & Co., Boston, 1970, p. 277.
4. Medical Research Council, Great Britain, "Responsibility in Investigations on Human Subjects" (1963) in Beecher, op. cit., pp. 262, 265.
5. Ibid.
6. World Medical Association, "Declaration of Helsinki," 1964, in Beecher, op. cit., p. 277.
7. Ibid., p. 279.
8. DHEW, *The Institutional Guide to DHEW Policy on Protection of Human Subjects*, DHEW Publication No. (NIH) 72-102, December 1, 1971, p. 7.
9. DHEW, Protection of Human Subjects, Policies and Procedures, 39 *Federal Register* 31742, November 16, 1973.
10. Ibid.
11. *Policy and Communications Bulletin*, The Clinical Center, No. 75-5 (July 14, 1975).
12. 45 CFR 46.103 (1975).

13. Paul Ramsey, *The Patient as Person*, Yale University Press, New Haven, 1970, p. 25.
14. Ibid., p. 39 (quoting Oscar M. Ruebhausen, Experiments with Human Subjects, 23 *Records of N.Y. Bar Association*, Feb., 1968, p. 93).
15. Ibid., p. 12.
16. Ramsey, "Children as Research Subjects: A Reply," *Hastings Center Report*, April 1977, pp. 40f.
17. See Chapter 3 [of this report; not reprinted here].
18. Ramsey does say, however, that benefits are sometimes unclear and would make a difference in emergency situations. Cf. *The Patient as Person*, p. 15.
19. Ramsey, "The Enforcement of Morals: Nontherapeutic Research on Children," *Hastings Center Report*, August 1976, p. 21.
20. Benjamin Freedman, "A Moral Theory of Informed Consent," *Hastings Center Report* 5, August 1975, pp. 29–39. Cf. esp. p. 38.
21. Richard McCormick, "Experimentation on the Fetus: Policy Proposals," Report Submitted to the National Commission for the Protection of Human Subjects of Biomedical and Behavioral Research, 1975. In *Appendix: Research on the Fetus*, DHEW Publication No. (OS) 76-128, 1976, pp. 5-3 and 5-4.

    For a fuller discussion by the same author, see "Proxy Consent in the Experimentation Situation," 18 *Perspectives in Biology and Medicine*, Autumn, 1974, and "Experimentation in Children: Sharing in Sociality," *Hastings Center Report*, December 1976.
22. "Children as Research Subjects: A Reply," p. 40.
23. [Ramsey], The Enforcement of Morals: Nontherapeutic Research on Children, p. 24.
24. Stephen Toulmin, Fetal Experimentation: Moral Issues and Institutional Controls, Report to the National Commission for the Protection of Human Subjects of Biomedical and Behavioral Research, 1975. In *Appendix: Research on the Fetus*, DHEW Publication No. (OS) 76-128, 1976, pp. 10-7 and 10-8.
25. [Beecher, *Research and the Individual*] (Boston: Little, Brown & Co., 1970), p. 63. Cf. W. J. Curran and H. K. Beecher, "Experimentation with Children," *Journal of the American Medical Association* 10 (October 10, 1969): 77ff.
26. [William Bartholome] "The Ethics of Non-Therapeutic Clinical Research on Children."
27. [Paper by H. Tristram Engelhardt, Jr., done for the Commission], "Basic Ethical Principles in the Conduct of Biomedical and Behavioral Research Involving Human Subjects" (December 1975).
28. [Paper by Robert Veatch, done for the Commission], "Three Theories of Informed Consent: Philosophical Foundations and Policy Implications" (February 2, 1976).
29. Engelhardt ["Basic ethical Principles"], p. 7.
30. Ibid., pp. 36–37.
31. Ibid., pp. 35–37.
32. Veatch ["Three Theories"], p. 35.
33. Ibid., p. 36.
34. Ibid., p. 37.
35. Ibid., p. 38.
36. Ibid., p. 49.
37. This form of reply to the Veatch and Engelhardt type of approach is found in Hans Jonas's essay, "Philosophical Reflections on Experimenting with Human Subjects," in Paul A. Freund, ed., *Experimentation with Human Subjects* (New York: George Braziller, Inc., 1970). [Jonas] construes such research as a duty only in emergency situations.

INSTITUTIONAL REVIEW BOARDS

INTRODUCTION. *The National Commission for the Protection of Human Subjects of Biomedical and Behavioral Research was required by Congress to study the method for reviewing proposals to use human subjects in research. The review process had been established by NIH policies of 1966 and 1977. That method consisted of review by a committee or board of appropriate members established by each institution that received federal funds for the conduct of research. The Commission carefully reviewed and evaluated this system, later designated as the IRB or Institutional Review Board system, and endorsed it with many suggestions for modification. It has been the centerpiece of the ethics of human subject research in the United States since that time.*

RECOMMENDATIONS

The ethical conduct of research involving human subjects requires a balancing of society's interests in protecting the rights of the subjects and in developing knowledge that can benefit the subjects or society as a whole. The elements that must be considered in this balancing of interests are identified and analyzed in the Commission's separate report on the basic ethical principles that should underlie the conduct of research involving human subjects. In the recommendations that follow, the Commission expresses its judgment about the ways in which those elements ought to be brought to bear on research practices, so that a reasonable and ethical balance of society's interests may be attained.

The Commission's deliberations begin with the premise that investigators should not have sole responsibility for determining whether research involving human subjects fulfills ethical standards. Others, who are independent of the research, must share this responsibility, because investigators are always in positions of potential conflict by virtue of their concern with the pursuit of knowledge as well as the welfare of the human subjects of their research.

The Commission believes that the rights of subjects should be protected by local review committees operating pursuant to federal regulations and located in institutions where research involving human subjects is conducted. Compared to the possible alternatives of a regional or national review process, local committees have the advantage of greater familiarity with the actual conditions surrounding the conduct of research. Such committees can work closely with investigators to assure that the rights and welfare of human subjects are protected and, at the same time, that the application of policies is fair to the investigators. They can contribute to the education of the research community and the public regarding the ethical conduct of research. The committees can become resource centers for information concerning ethical standards and federal requirements and can communicate with federal officials and with other local committees about matters of common concern.

The Commission further believes that institutions receiving federal support for the conduct of research involving human subjects should be governed by uniform federal regulations applicable to the review of all such research, whether it is supported by one federal department or another, or is not federally supported. The regulations should also apply to research conducted intramurally by federal departments and to research conducted by private organizations that is otherwise subject to federal regulations (e.g., research conducted to meet the regulatory requirements of the Food and Drug Administration).

The Institutional Review Boards (IRBs) that have existed for some years at institutions that conduct research involving human subjects have been closely examined by the Commission. The Commission finds on the basis of its study that IRBs play an essential role in the protection of human subjects. However, the existing system may be improved. The following recommendations are made to

---

Excerpts from the National Commission for the Protection of Human Subjects of Biomedical and Behavioral Research, *Report and Recommendations on Institutional Review Boards.* DHEW Publication No. (OS) 78-0012 with two Appendices, 78-0013 and 78-0014. (Washington, D.C.: U.S. Government Printing Office, 1978). For additional information, see Robert J. Levine, *Ethics and Regulation of Clinical Research.* New Haven: Yale University Press, 1988, Chapter 14.

strengthen, simplify and broaden the coverage of this system.

Recommendation 1 (A) Federal law should be enacted or amended to authorize the Secretary of Health, Education, and Welfare to promulgate regulations governing ethical review of all research involving human subjects that is subject to federal regulation.

(B) Federal law should be enacted or amended to provide that each institution which sponsors or conducts research involving human subjects that is supported by any federal department or agency or otherwise subject to federal regulation, and each federal department or agency which itself conducts research involving human subjects, shall give assurances satisfactory to the Secretary of Health, Education, and Welfare that all research involving human subjects sponsored or conducted by such institution, or conducted by such department or agency, will be reviewed by and conducted in accordance with the determinations of a review board established and operated in accordance with the regulations promulgated by the Secretary under the authority recommended in paragraph A of this recommendation.

(C) Federal law should be enacted or amended to provide that all research involving human subjects sponsored or conducted by an institution that receives funds from any federal department or agency to provide health care or conduct health-related research shall be subject to federal regulation regarding the review and conduct of such research, as provided under paragraphs A and B of this recommendation.

(D) Federal law should be enacted or amended to authorize and appropriate funds to support the operation of institutional review boards by direct cost funding.

Comment: (A) Recommendation 1A would establish DHEW as the single cognizant agency for the promulgation of regulations relating to the protection of human research subjects. Such regulations, dealing with the composition, functions and procedures of IRBs, would apply to all entities that receive financial support from the federal government to conduct research involving human subjects. Entities conducting such research to fulfill federal regulatory requirements (e.g., of the Food and Drug Administration or the Environmental Protection Agency) would be covered by the same regulations. Thus, all entities under federal jurisdiction would be subject to a single set of regulations relating to review of research involving human subjects, without regard to the particular federal department(s) that support or regulate their research. An alternative to the enactment of federal law might be the issuance by the President of an executive order establishing DHEW as the single cognizant agency for the promulgation of regulations to protect human subjects.

Implementation of Recommendation 1A, by law or executive order, is necessary to assure government-wide uniformity in the review requirements that are imposed on entities subject to federal regulation. A survey by the Commission has shown that virtually all federal agencies with policies for the protection of human subjects currently adopt DHEW standards and procedures to a substantial degree. However, there are many variations arising out of differences in wording, imposition of additional requirements, introduction of minor changes, etc. Establishing DHEW as the sole authority for the issuance of regulations in this area would not substantially change current practice but would reduce the burden on IRBs to interpret and apply the regulations to which they are subject. Moreover, uniformity would assure a minimum level of protection to human subjects of research, no matter which federal agency is supporting the research or which entity is conducting it. . . .

(B) Recommendation 1B would establish DHEW as the single cognizant agency for the accreditation of all IRBs, including IRBs established by nonfederal entities and IRBs that are established within federal departments and agencies. DHEW would also carry out compliance and educational activities to assure that the quality of performance of all IRBs is high. Although some nonfederal entities may receive support for research involving human subjects from federal departments other than DHEW, the Commission recommends centralization of accreditation and compliance responsibility in DHEW as a means of promoting uniform treatment and administrative efficiency. Similarly, the Commission recommends that DHEW accredit and review the compliance of IRBs established by other federal entities, to assure uniform review, throughout government, of proposed research involving human subjects. As an alternative to enactment of law, Recommendation 1B might be accomplished by the issuance of an executive order.

Establishment of DHEW as the sole authority for accreditation and compliance activities would recognize that department's initiation of the requirements of IRBs and its extensive experience in supervising their operation. As with the promulgation of regulations (Recommendation 1A), centralizing authority to conduct these activities would also assist in standardizing the review of research with human subjects and reducing the burden on nonfederal IRBs that is imposed by federal enforcement activities. . . .

Recommendation 2 (A) Federal law should be enacted or amended to authorize the Secretary of Health, Education, and Welfare to establish a single office to carry out the following duties: (i) accreditation of institutional review boards based upon the submission of assurances containing descriptions of their membership, authority, staff, meeting facilities, review and monitoring procedures and provisions for record-keeping; (ii) compliance activities, including site visits and audits of institutional review board records, to examine the performance of the boards and their fulfillment of institutional assurances and regulatory requirements; and (iii) educational activities to assist members of institutional review boards in recognizing and considering the ethical issues that are presented by research involving human subjects.

(B) Federal law should be enacted or amended to authorize and appropriate funds to support the duties described in paragraph A of this recommendation.

Comment: Recommendation 2 requires that DHEW consolidate and expand its accreditation and compliance activities to provide within the federal government a single supervising authority for all IRBs that are required under recommendation 1 to review research involving human subjects. In addition, this DHEW office should conduct educational activities to assist IRB members in discharging their review responsibilities. The Commission suggests that the office be established outside of any subdivision of DHEW and that funds be appropriated to support its operation.

Institutions should be required to submit information such as the following to enable accreditation determinations to be made:

- The names and qualifications of members of the IRB and the process by which members are selected;
- The resources (e.g., meeting room, staff, office facilities, release of IRB members from other responsibilities) that will be devoted to the review function;
- The general operating procedures of the IRB, and the number and types of proposals that are expected to be reviewed by it;
- Expedited review procedures, if any, and the categories of research for which such procedures will be used; and
- Procedures to assure that all research involving human subjects conducted by or at the institution will be reviewed by an IRB and, if approved, will be conducted in accordance with any restrictions or conditions imposed by the IRB.

Site visits, audits of IRB records, and other compliance activities should be conducted routinely to assure continuing quality control of the performance of IRBs. The compliance effort should be aimed at educating, improving performance of IRBs, and providing needed advice. Where necessary, however, failure by investigators, institutions or IRBs to meet their responsibilities should be subject to sanctions ranging from warnings to loss of IRB accreditation and consequent ineligibility to receive federal funds for research involving human subjects or refusal by a regulatory agency to accept data.

DHEW should develop materials to assist in the orientation of new members of IRBs and mechanisms for dissemination of information about ethical issues and key IRB decisions to promote uniform treatment of similar protocols. Caution should be exercised, however, to avoid usurping the IRBs' decision-making authority. The accreditation and compliance, as well as the educational functions, of DHEW should be aimed at assuring and promoting the effective operation of IRBs, but not as a forum or mechanism for questioning the substantive decisions of IRBs. DHEW should assure that IRBs have appropriate authorities, membership, and rules and standards of operation, and that useful materials are provided for the information of IRB members; these functions should not include any activities intended directly to influence or alter IRB decisions.

The generation of information about the various topics in its mandate has been essential to the operation of the Commission. Similarly, a program of research in the ethical issues that arise in research involving human subjects would greatly assist the compliance and educational activities of DHEW in this area.

Recommendation 3 The Secretary of Health, Education, and Welfare should require by regulation that an institutional review board (A) consist of at least five men and women of diverse backgrounds and sufficient maturity, experience and competence to assure that the board will be able to discharge its responsibilities and that its determinations will be accorded respect by investigators and the community served by the institution or in which it is located; (B) include at least one member who is not otherwise affiliated with the institution; (C) have the authority to review and approve, require modifications in, or disapprove all research involving human subjects conducted at the institution; (D) have the authority to conduct continuing review of research involving human subjects and to suspend approval of research that is not being conducted in accordance with the determinations of the board or in which there is unexpected serious harm to subjects; (E) maintain appropriate records, including copies of proposals reviewed, approved consent forms, minutes of board meetings, progress reports submitted by investigators, reports of injuries to subjects, and records of continuing review activities; (F) be provided with meeting space and sufficient staff to support its review and recordkeeping duties; (G) be authorized and directed to report to institutional authorities and the Secretary any serious or continuing noncompliance by investigators with the requirements and determinations of the board; (H) be provided with protection for members in connection with any liability arising out of their performance of duties on the board.

Comment: (A) IRB members should be appointed by a governing body or chief executive officer of the institution, who should consult widely to find persons who will serve on the IRB with distinction and commitment. The IRB should include persons who are familiar with the ethical issues in research involving human subjects. The IRB should also include persons with the scientific competence necessary to analyze accurately and thoroughly the risks and benefits of the types of proposals generally reviewed by the IRB, since this analysis is essential to the review process. To assure the IRB's access to such expertise, yet guard against self-interest influencing or appearing to influence IRB determinations, at least one-third but no more than two-thirds of the IRB members should be scientists, including members of the disciplines in which research is customarily reviewed by the IRB. The expertise of IRB members should be supplemented, when necessary, by the use of consultants.

In its deliberations, it is desirable that the IRB show awareness and appreciation of the various qualities, values and needs of the diverse elements of the community served by the institution or in which it is located. A diverse membership will enhance the IRB's credibility as well as the likelihood that its determinations will be sensitive to the concerns of those who conduct or participate in the research and other interested parties.

If an IRB regularly reviews research that has an impact on a broad category of vulnerable subjects (e.g., residents of an institution for the retarded), the IRB should include persons who are primarily concerned with the welfare of those subjects (e.g., parents of retarded children). The IRB should establish formal or informal consultation with community and other bodies that have interests in areas affected by or involved in the conduct of proposed research.

The institution should provide suitable orientation to new IRB members, in order to familiarize them with the purpose and authority of the IRB, the standards it applies, the ethical and legal principles that apply to research involving human subjects, and the main ethical dilemmas that arise in research. IRB members should be appointed for a fixed term of at least a year and should not be removed during this term except for good cause. An IRB's membership should be relatively stable from year to year in order to enhance the experience of the IRB and to introduce stability into standards applied by the IRB. Some degree of turnover of members and chairmen is desirable, however, as a way both of exposing more members of the institution to the issues considered by the IRB and of introducing into the IRB a variety of viewpoints.

The institution should encourage service on the IRB and indicate the importance of such service by giving IRB members appropriate relief from other duties, by giving recognition for service on the IRB (e.g., in decisions regarding promotions) and by providing remuneration to nonemployees.

(B) A member of the immediate family of a person who is affiliated with the institution should not be appointed to serve as the unaffiliated member of an IRB.

(C) Institutional support is necessary for the successful operation of an IRB and can be expressed most directly in rules, procedures, etc., that are formally adopted by the institution to assure that the IRB is lawfully established and that all research involving human subjects will be reviewed and conducted in accordance with its determinations.

(D) The IRB should adopt procedures for the continuing review of approved research, such as examination of records, requiring reports from investigators, soliciting information from subjects, and observing the recruitment of subjects and conduct of the research. As a basic requirement, all investigators should be directed to report immediately to the IRB any substantial changes in the research activity, unanticipated problems, or adverse reactions by subjects. In research that presents more than minimal risk to subjects (i.e., more than the risk of harm or discomfort that is normally encountered in the daily lives, or in the routine medical or psychological examination, of normal persons) or involves vulnerable subjects (e.g., children, institutionalized or hospitalized persons), investigators should be required, in addition, to make periodic reports to the IRB on the progress of the research. The frequency of such periodic reports should depend upon the degree of risk presented to subjects, but at a minimum should be on an annual basis.

The justification for undertaking some studies rests, in part, on uncertainty about the relative safety and efficacy of alternative therapies. New knowledge, however, is continually being developed, and uncertainties that play a role in prompting a study may be reduced over time as new information is developed in the study or elsewhere. Subjects should not be excluded from known benefits simply because those benefits were unknown or uncertain at the time the research began. An important aspect of the continuing review of research, particularly in studies that involve the evaluation of a therapeutic procedure for a chronic condition, is to assure that subjects are not excluded from the benefits of newly developed knowledge by continuing in a protocol after the superiority of a particular therapy for their condition has been demonstrated.

At the discretion of the IRB, the consent process or the research itself may be observed on a sample or routine basis, subjects may be interviewed about their experience in research, and research records (including consent forms) may be reviewed. Also at the discretion of the IRB, investigators may be required to provide subjects with a form on which they can report to the IRB their experiences in research. The form could be given to subjects at the time consent is obtained and be completed by subjects who wish to do so during or after their participation.

Observation of the consent process or conduct of research is both a difficult and delicate task. The designation of staff or members of the IRB to observe research activities can impose a substantial strain on the limited resources of the IRB. Further, such observation may intrude on confidential relationships or the privacy of individual subjects. IRBs should take these factors into account when determining appropriate means for continuing review of a protocol, and alternatives such as investigator reporting requirements should be considered. However, certain research will warrant observation to assure the protection of subjects, and in such cases IRBs have an obligation to take suitable measures.

In cases in which the investigator is responsible for the care of the subjects, the IRB may require that a neutral person, not otherwise associated with the research or the investigator, be present when consent is sought, to explain the research to prospective subjects, or to observe the conduct of the research. The involvement of a physician or therapist as an investigator may have significant advantages for patients and make available to them new forms of therapy. However, research interests may compromise the therapist's sound judgments regarding therapeutic goals. The involvement of a neutral third party may reduce the possibility of such a conflict of interest occurring, particularly in research that presents more than minimal risk. Such a person may be designated to play a role in informing subjects of their rights and the details of protocols, assuring that there is continuing assent to participation, determining the advisability of continued participation, receiving complaints from subjects, and bringing grievances to the attention of the IRB as part of its continuing review of research.

(E) Records regarding research protocols reviewed by IRBs should be retained for five years after completion of the research. Minutes should be in sufficient detail to show the basis of actions taken by the IRB.

(F) An IRB should have an identifiable meeting space and designated staff to support its function. Although the staff may be part-time, their effort should be identified and placed on a continuing basis.

(G) Any knowledge of serious or continuing noncompliance by investigators with the requirements and determinations of the IRB should be transmitted by the IRB to institutional authorities and to the Secretary of Health, Education, and Welfare. Institutions should take such steps as are necessary and appropriate to assure compliance by all investigators with IRB requirements and determinations.

(H) Protection against liability arising out of their performance of duties on the IRB may be provided to members in any of several ways, including sovereign immunity, insurance, indemnification by the institution, or specific provisions of state law. The institution should assure that such protection is provided either by law or by means of institutional arrangements.

Recommendation 4 The Secretary of Health, Education, and Welfare should require by regulation that all research involving human subjects that is subject to federal regulation shall be reviewed by an institutional review board and that the approval of such research shall be based upon affirmative determinations by the board that

(A) the research methods are appropriate to the objectives of the research and the field of study;

(B) selection of subjects is equitable;

(C) risks to subjects are minimized by using the safest procedures consistent with sound research design and, whenever appropriate, by using procedures being performed for diagnostic or treatment purposes;

(D) risks to subjects are reasonable in relation to anticipated benefits to subjects and importance of the knowledge to be gained;

(E) informed consent will be sought under circumstances that provide sufficient opportunity for subjects to consider whether or not to participate and that minimize the possibility of coercion or undue influence;

(F) informed consent will be based upon communicating to subjects, in language they can understand, information that the subjects may reasonably be expected to desire in considering whether or not to participate, generally including:

(i) that an institutional review board has approved the solicitation of subjects to participate in the research, that such participation is voluntary, that refusal to participate will involve no penalties or loss of benefits to which subjects are otherwise entitled, that participation can be terminated at any time, and that the conditions of such termination are stated;

(ii) the aims and specific purposes of the research, whether it includes procedures designed to provide direct benefit to subjects, and available alternative ways to pursue any such benefit;

(iii) what will happen to subjects in the research, and what they will be expected to do;

(iv) any reasonably foreseeable risks to subjects, and whether treatment or compensation is available if harm occurs;

(v) who is conducting the study, who is funding it, and who should be contacted if harm occurs or there are complaints; and

(vi) any additional costs to subjects or third parties that may result from participation.

(G) informed consent will be appropriately documented, unless the board determines that written consent is not necessary or appropriate because (i) the existence of signed consent forms would place subjects at risk, or (ii) the research presents no more than minimal risk and involves no procedures for which written consent is normally required;

(H) notwithstanding the requirements of paragraphs E, F and G above, informed consent is unnecessary (i) where the subjects' interests are determined to be adequately protected in studies of documents, records or pathological specimens and the importance of the research justifies such invasion of the subjects' privacy, or (ii) in studies of public behavior where the research presents no more than minimal risk, is unlikely to cause embarrassment, and has scientific merit;

(I) there are adequate provisions to protect the privacy of subjects and to maintain the confidentiality of data; and

(J) applicable regulatory provisions for the protection of fetuses, pregnant women, prisoners, children and those institutionalized as mentally infirm will be fulfilled.

Comment: (A) Subjects should not be exposed to risk in research that is so inadequately designed that its stated purpose cannot be achieved. It must be recognized, however, that equally rigorous standards of scientific methodology are not suitable in all disciplines or necessarily appropriate for all research purposes. Not all research is intended to provide a definitive test of a hypothesis, and much research, such as research done by students, has modest aims. The Commission's statements in previous reports that all research should be scientifically sound should be interpreted as requiring that the proposed methods be suited to the discipline and the objectives of the research.

(B) The proposed involvement of hospitalized patients, other institutionalized persons, or disproportionate numbers of racial or ethnic minorities or persons of low socioeconomic status should be justified.

(C) Materials or information that are obtained for diagnostic or therapeutic purposes should be used whenever possible, provided such use will not unjustifiably increase the burdens of the ill. Where appropriate, screening should be employed to eliminate from participation in research persons who would be at particularly high risk. The number of subjects exposed to risk in research should be no larger than required by considerations of scientific soundness.

(D) The possible harms and benefits from proposed research involving human subjects may not be quantifiable but should be evaluated systematically to assure a reasonable relation between the harms that are risked and the benefits that may be anticipated for the subjects or the gains in knowledge that may result from the research. This evaluation should include an arrayal of alternatives to the procedures under review and the possible harms and benefits associated with each alternative.

The evaluation of possible harms in relation to expected benefits or gains in knowledge may provide sufficient grounds on which to disapprove proposed research, when this relation is found to be unreasonable. This would be the case, for example, where research includes an intervention that presents a high degree of risk to subjects and no great likelihood of producing direct benefit to them, or where an alternative to the intervention would present less risk but the same likelihood of benefit. Even when, as in most cases, the relation between possible harms and benefits or gains in knowledge is not found to be unreasonable, the evaluation will serve an important purpose of exposing fully the ethical and other issues that may be involved and thereby aiding in decision making by all parties concerned. The evaluation aids the IRB not only in judging whether it is reasonable to invite the participation of subjects in the research, but also in determining whether the information that will be given to subjects is sufficient for their own determination whether or not to participate.

In evaluating risks and benefits to subjects, an IRB should consider only those risks and benefits that may result from the conduct of the research. For example, the risks and benefits of therapies that subjects would receive even if not participating in the research should not be considered as risks and benefits of the research. (However, the risks and benefits of established therapies provide a point of comparison for the risks and benefits of new therapies that are the object of research.) The possible long-range effects of applying knowledge gained in the research (e.g., the possible effects of the research on public policy affecting a segment of the population) should not be considered as among those research risks falling within the purview of the IRB, although such consequences may be relevant to a policy decision by an institution as to the desirability of approving the research at that institution. The IRB may advise institutional authorities in such cases.

As risk increases and, similarly, as the vulnerability of patients increases (by virtue of illness, institutionalization, etc.), it becomes more important to evaluate risks of harm and possible benefits and to require a reasonable relation between them. In effect, the IRB should assume more of the burden of determining whether subjects ultimately should be allowed to participate. In research that does not present significant risk to subjects, however, an IRB should not prevent an investigator from inviting subjects to participate in research because of its judgment that the research appears to be of marginal scientific importance or does not include an intervention that may benefit the subjects. Also, if the prospective subjects are normal adults, the primary responsibility of the IRB should be to assure that sufficient information will be disclosed in the informed consent process, provided the research does not present an extreme case of unreasonable risk.

(E) Circumstances in which prospective subjects might be coerced or unduly influenced should be avoided in the consent process. The need for concern about coercion or undue influence will depend upon the nature of the particular studies and the amount of risk they present. Protective steps may include the following:

- Providing subjects with an interval of time (consistent with the nature of the protocol) in which to weigh risks and benefits, consider alternatives, and ask questions or consult with others;
- Avoiding, whenever possible, seeking consent in physical settings in which subjects may feel coerced or unduly influenced to participate;
- Avoiding, whenever possible, seeking consent when subjects are in a vulnerable emotional state;
- Limiting remuneration to payment for the time and inconvenience of participation and compensation for any injury resulting from participation; and
- If students in a course will be requested to participate in research, assuring that this is understood at the outset and that reasonable alternatives are offered.

(F) Informed consent requires that all information relevant to a decision regarding participation be properly communicated to subjects. The information must be presented in a manner likely to result in its being understood. Thus, for example, medical or technical terms should be explained in lay language when they must be used. Written statements should be straightforward and easily readable. The specific information to be communicated should include those items that it is reasonable to expect that the subjects would want to know in making a decision regarding participation in the research. While recommendation 4F contains a list of topics about which it can generally be presumed that subjects would want to be informed, it should be recognized that no such list is wholly adequate for this purpose. Thus, there may be research in which it is not reasonable to expect that subjects would want to be informed of some item on the list (e.g., who is funding the research). More frequently, it can be expected that research will involve an element that is not on the list but about which it can be expected that subjects would want to be informed. Such information should, of course, be communicated to subjects. In addition, the investigator should indicate to subjects that questions are appropriate and be prepared to answer such questions. The investigator should also indicate whether the results of the research will be made available to subjects.

In some research there is concern that disclosure to subjects or providing an accurate description of certain information, such as the purpose of the research or the procedures to be used, would affect the data and the validity of the research. The IRB can approve withholding or altering such information provided it determines that the incomplete disclosure or deception is not likely to be harmful in and of itself and that sufficient information will be disclosed to give subjects a fair opportunity to decide whether they want to participate in the research. The IRB should also consider whether the research could be done without incomplete disclosure or deception. If the procedures involved in the study present risk of harm or discomfort, this must always be disclosed to subjects. In seeking consent, information should not be withheld for the purpose of eliciting the cooperation of subjects, and investigators should always give truthful answers to questions, even if this means that a prospective subject thereby becomes unsuitable for participation. In general, where participants have been deceived in the course of research, it is desirable that they be debriefed after their participation.

(G) As a rule it is desirable that there be documentation of consent to provide the investigator with evidence thereof and the subjects with a readily available source of information about the research. However, consent forms should not be considered the only method by which information about the research is communicated to subjects. Usually an oral presentation will be an effective method of communicating with subjects. The documentation of consent (i.e., the consent form) should never be confused with the substance of informed consent.

Because a consent form documents an agreement between two parties, both the subject and the investigator should retain a copy. The form should contain the address and phone number of the investigator and indicate how to contact the IRB.

In some studies of illegal or stigmatizing characteristics or behavior, subjects would be placed at risk by the creation of documents linking them with the research. The most secure method of protecting confidentiality of subjects in such studies is to create no written record of their identity, since such records may be vulnerable to subpoena. Confidentiality assurances are available from the Department of Justice and the Department of Health, Education, and Welfare that may effectively protect such documents from subpoena in certain studies of illegal behavior or drug abuse. When such protection is not available in studies in which a breach of confidentiality may be harmful to subjects, and subjects might prefer that there be no documentation linking them with the research, the IRB may waive the requirement for documentation of consent in the interest of protecting the subjects.

In other studies, the requirement for documentation may place an undue burden on the research while adding little protection to the subjects. Such burdens might include a negative impact on the validity of a survey sample or introduction of an element that is incongruent with the social relationships involved in the research (e.g., in anthropological research). For research that would be burdened by a requirement of written documentation of consent, such documentation may be waived, provided that the research presents no more than minimal risk of harm to subjects and involves no procedures for which written consent is normally required outside of the research context. (For example, a physical intrusion into the body may generally require written consent, whether or not the intrusion is performed for purposes of research.) In many cases (e.g., a survey using mailed questionnaires) it would be appropriate for the investigator to provide subjects with a written statement regarding the research, but not to request their signature. In other cases (e.g., a telephone survey) an oral explanation might be sufficient because subjects can readily terminate their involvement in the research.

In all research, but particularly when a short form or no written consent will be used, it is important for the IRB to review the investigator's plans regarding information that is to be provided orally.

(H) In studies of documents, records or pathological specimens, where the subjects are identified, informed consent may be deemed unnecessary but the IRB must assure that subjects' interests are protected. (If the subjects are not identified or identifiable, the research need not be considered to involve human subjects.) The Privacy Protection Study Commission concluded that medical records can legitimately be used for biomedical or epidemiological research, without the individual's explicit authorization:

"provided that the medical-care provider maintaining the medical record:

(i) determines that such use or disclosure does not violate any limitations under which the record or information was collected;

(ii) ascertains that use of disclosure in individually identifiable form is necessary to accomplish the research or statistical purpose for which use of disclosure is to be made;

(iii) determines that the importance of the research or statistical purpose for which any use of disclosure is to be made is such as to warrant the risk to the individual from additional exposure of the record or information contained therein;

(iv) requires that adequate safeguards to protect the record or information from unauthorized disclosure be established and maintained by the user or recipient, including a program for removal or destruction of identifiers; and

(v) consents in writing before any further use or redisclosure of the record or information in individually identifiable form is permitted."

The IRB should assure that such conditions exist before approving proposed research in which documents, records or pathology specimens are used for research purposes without explicit consent, and that the importance of the research justifies such use.

When the conduct of research using documents, records or pathology specimens without explicit consent is anticipated, incoming patients or other potential subjects should be informed of the potential use of such materials upon admission into the institution or program in which the materials will be developed, and given an opportunity to provide a general consent or to object to such research. The IRB should scrutinize with care any proposal to isolate and use materials about persons with particular problems or conditions, to assure compliance with the foregoing provisions regarding the use of private information.

Other situations in which informed consent might not be necessary arise in field research in the social sciences. Sometimes in such research, purely observational methods are supplemented by interaction with the persons being studied and therefore come within the Commission's definition of research involving human subjects. An IRB may waive the informed consent requirement in such research when it finds a number of factors to be present. The behavior to be studied must in some sense be public, e.g., responses of businesses or institutions to members of the public, or social behavior in public places. Nondisclosure must be essential to the methodological soundness of the research, and must be justified by the importance or scientific merit of the research. Further, the research must present no more than minimal risk and be unlikely to cause embarrassment to the subjects.

(I) When proposed research involves the collection of data that might be harmful to subjects if disclosed to third parties in an individually identifiable form, the IRB should be particularly attentive to the adequacy of provisions to protect the confidentiality of the data. Depending upon the degree of sensitivity of the data, appropriate methods for protecting the confidentiality of the data may include the coding or removal of identifiers as soon as possible, limitation of access to the data, or the use of locked file cabinets. IRBs should be aware of the general vulnerability of research data to subpoena, particularly in studies that collect data that would put subjects in legal jeopardy if disclosed. When the identity of subjects who may have committed crimes or abused drugs is to be recorded in a research investigation, the IRB should see that the study, if it is eligible, is conducted under the appropriate assurances of confidentiality available from the Department of Health, Education, and Welfare and the Department of Justice.

(J) The Commission has transmitted recommendations for regulatory guidelines governing the conduct of research involving various subject populations with reduced capacity to give informed consent. IRBs should assure that research involving these populations complies with the guidelines that are adopted by DHEW.

FEDERAL REGULATIONS REGARDING THE PROTECTION OF HUMAN SUBJECTS OF RESEARCH

INTRODUCTION. *When the National Commission for Protection of Human Subjects of Biomedical and Behavioral Research completed its work in 1978, its recommendations were published in the* Federal Register *for public commentary and deliberation by the Secretary of Health, Education and Welfare. The recommendations were then recast as Title 45 of the Code of Federal Regulations, Part 46 (45 CFR 46). The "proposed regulations" were announced in the* Federal Register, *January 16, 1981, and a period of public commentary commenced. After several revisions, and after all federal agencies that sponsor human research agreed, a uniform policy was adopted and published in the June 18, 1991 edition of the* Federal Register. *These regulations are now the official policy governing research with human subjects in the United States. The regulations have four subparts: a basic policy; additional protections for fetuses, pregnant women, and in vitro fertilization; additional protections for prisoners; and additional protections for children. Title 45, part 46 begins with a detailed table of contents; that section has been omitted here.*

SUBPART A—BASIC HHS POLICY FOR PROTECTION OF HUMAN RESEARCH SUBJECTS

§ 46.101—To what do these regulations apply?

(a) Except as provided in paragraph (b) of this section, this subpart applies to all research involving human subjects conducted by the Department of Health and Human Services or funded in whole or in part by a Department grant, contract, cooperative agreement or fellowship.

(1) This includes research conducted by Department employees, except each Principal Operating Component head may adopt such nonsubstantive, procedural modifications as may be appropriate from an administrative standpoint.

(2) It also includes research conducted or funded by the Department of Health and Human Services outside the United States, but in appropriate circumstances, the Secretary may, under paragraph (e) of this section waive the applicability of some or all of the requirements of these regulations for research of this type.

(b) Research activities in which the only involvement of human subjects will be in one or more of the following categories are exempt from these regulations unless the research is covered by other subparts of this part:

(1) Research conducted in established or commonly accepted educational settings, involving normal educational practices, such as (i) research on regular and special education instructional strategies, or (ii) research on the effectiveness of or the comparison among instructional techniques, curricula, or classroom management methods.

(2) Research involving the use of educational tests (cognitive, diagnostic, aptitude, achievement), if information taken from these sources is recorded in such a manner that subjects cannot be identified, directly or through identifiers linked to the subjects.

45 CRF 46. Source for Subpart A, 46 *Federal Register* 8386, January 26, 1981, revised 48 *Federal Register* 9269, March 4, 1983; other subparts are also documented as they appear in the text.

(3) Research involving survey or interview procedures, except where all of the following conditions exist: (i) responses are recorded in such a manner that the human subjects can be identified, directly or through identifiers linked to the subjects, (ii) the subject's responses, if they became known outside the research, could reasonably place the subject at risk of criminal or civil liability or be damaging to the subject's financial standing or employability, and (iii) the research deals with sensitive aspects of the subject's own behavior, such as illegal conduct, drug use, sexual behavior, or use of alcohol. All research involving survey or interview procedures is exempt, without exception, when the respondents are elected or appointed public officials or candidates for public office.

(4) Research involving the observation (including observation by participants) of public behavior, except where all of the following conditions exist: (i) observations are recorded in such a manner that the human subjects can be identified, directly or through identifiers linked to the subjects, (ii) the observations recorded about the individual, if they became known outside the research, could reasonably place the subject at risk of criminal or civil liability or be damaging to the subject's financial standing or employability, and (iii) the research deals with sensitive aspects of the subject's own behavior such as illegal conduct, drug use, sexual behavior, or use of alcohol.

(5) Research involving the collection or study of existing data, documents, records, pathological specimens, or diagnostic specimens, if these sources are publicly available or if the information is recorded by the investigator in such a manner that subjects cannot be identified, directly or through identifiers linked to the subjects.

(6) Unless specifically required by statute (and except to the extent specified in paragraph [i]), research and demonstration projects which are conducted by or subject to the approval of the Department of Health and Human Services, and which are designed to study, evaluate, or otherwise examine: (i) programs under the Social Security Act, or other public benefit or service programs; (ii) procedures for obtaining benefits or services under those programs; (iii) possible changes in or alternatives to those programs or procedures; or (iv) possible changes in methods or levels of payment for benefits or services under those programs.

(c) The Secretary has final authority to determine whether a particular activity is covered by these regulations.

(d) The Secretary may require that specific research activities or classes of research activities conducted or funded by the Department, but not otherwise covered by these regulations, comply with some or all of these regulations.

(e) The Secretary may also waive applicability of these regulations to specific research activities or classes of research activities, otherwise covered by these regulations. Notices of these actions will be published in the *Federal Register* as they occur.

(f) No individual may receive Department funding for research covered by these regulations unless the individual is affiliated with or sponsored by an institution which assumes responsibility for the research under an assurance satisfying the requirements of this part, or the individual makes other arrangements with the Department.

(g) Compliance with these regulations will in no way render inapplicable pertinent federal, state, or local laws or regulations.

(h) Each subpart of these regulations contains a separate section describing to what the subpart applies. Research which is covered by more than one subpart shall comply with all applicable subparts.

(i) If, following review of proposed research activities that are exempt from these regulations under paragraph (b)(6), the Secretary determines that a research or demonstration project presents a danger to the physical, mental, or emotional well-being of a participant or subject of the research or demonstration project, then federal funds may not be expended for such a project without the written, informed consent of each participant or subject.

§ 46.102—Definitions

(a) "Secretary" means the Secretary of Health and Human Services and any other officer or employee of the Department of Health and Human Services to whom authority has been delegated.

(b) "Department" or "HHS" means the Department of Health and Human Services.

(c) "Institution" means any public or private entity or agency (including federal, state, and other agencies).

(d) "Legally authorized representative" means an individual or judicial or other body authorized under applicable law to consent on behalf of a prospective subject to the subject's participation in the procedure(s) involved in the research.

(e) "Research" means a systematic investigation designed to develop or contribute to generalizable knowledge. Activities which meet this definition constitute "research" for purposes of these regulations, whether or not they are supported or funded under a program which is considered research for other purposes. For example, some "demonstration" and "service" programs may include research activities.

(f) "Human subject" means a living individual about whom an investigator (whether professional or student) conducting research obtains (1) data through intervention or interaction with the individual, or (2) identifiable private information. "Intervention" includes both physical procedures by which data are gathered (for example, venipuncture) and manipulations of the subject or the subject's environment that are performed for research purposes. "Interaction" includes communication or interpersonal contact between investigator and subject. "Private information" includes information about behavior that occurs in a context in which an individual can reasonably expect that no observation or recording is taking place, and information which has been provided for specific purposes by an individual and which the individual can reasonably expect will not be made public (for example, a medical record). Private information must be individually identifiable (i.e., the identity of the subject is or may readily be ascertained by the investigator or associated with the information) in order for obtaining the information to constitute research involving human subjects.

(g) "Minimal risk" means that the risks of harm anticipated in the proposed research are not greater, considering probability and magnitude, than those ordinarily encountered in daily life or during the performance of routine physical or psychological examinations or tests.

(h) "Certification" means the official notification by the institution to the Department in accordance with the requirements of this part that a research project or activity involving human subjects has been reviewed and approved by the Institutional Review Board (IRB) in accordance with the approved assurance on file at HHS. (Certification is required when the research is funded by the Department and not otherwise exempt in accordance with § 46.101(b)).

§ 46.103—Assurances

(a) Each institution engaged in research covered by these regulations shall provide written assurance satisfactory to the Secretary that it will comply with the requirements set forth in these regulations.

(b) The Department will conduct or fund research covered by these regulations only if the institution has an assurance approved as provided in this section, and only if the institution has certified to the Secretary that the research has been reviewed and approved by an IRB provided for in the assurance, and will be subject to continuing review by the IRB. This assurance shall at a minimum include:

(1) A statement of principles governing the institution in the discharge of its responsibilities for protecting the rights and welfare of human subjects of research conducted at or sponsored by the institution, regardless of source of funding. This may include an appropriate existing code, declaration, or statement of ethical principles, or a statement formulated by the institution itself. This requirement does not preempt provisions of these regulations applicable to Department funded research and is not applicable to any research in an exempt category listed in § 46.101.

(2) Designation of one or more IRBs established in accordance with the requirements of this subpart, and for which provisions are made for meeting space and sufficient staff to support the IRB's review and recordkeeping duties.

(3) A list of the IRB members identified by name; earned degrees; representative capacity; indications of experience such as board certifications, licenses, etc., sufficient to describe each member's chief anticipated contributions to IRB deliberations; and any employment or other relationship between each member and the institution; for example: full-time employee, part-time employee, member of governing panel or board, stockholder, paid or unpaid consultant. Changes in IRB membership shall be reported to the Secretary. (Footnote deleted.)

(4) Written procedures which the IRB will follow (i) for conducting its initial and continuing review of research and for reporting its findings and actions to the investigator and the institution; (ii) for determining which projects require review more often than annually and which projects need verification from sources other than the investigators that no material changes have occurred since previous IRB review; (iii) for insuring prompt reporting to the IRB of proposed changes in a research activity, and for insuring that changes in approved research, during the period for which IRB approval has already been given, may not be initiated without IRB review and approval except where necessary to eliminate apparent immediate hazards to the subject; and (iv) for insuring prompt reporting to the IRB and to the Secretary [footnote deleted] of unanticipated problems involving risks to subjects or others.

(c) The assurance shall be executed by an individual authorized to act for the institution and to assume on behalf of the institution the obligations imposed by these regulations, and shall be filed in such form and manner as the Secretary may prescribe.

(d) The Secretary will evaluate all assurances submitted in accordance with these regulations through such officers and employees of the Department and such experts or consultants engaged for this purpose as the Secretary determines to be appropriate. The Secretary's evaluation will take into consideration the adequacy of the proposed IRB in light of the anticipated scope of the institution's research activities and the types of subject populations likely to be involved, the appropriateness of the proposed initial and continuing review procedures in light of the probable risks, and the size and complexity of the institution.

(e) On the basis of this evaluation, the Secretary may approve or disapprove the assurance, or enter into negotiations to develop an approvable one. The Secretary may limit the period during which any particular approved assurance or class of approved assurances shall remain effective or otherwise condition or restrict approval.

(f) Within 60 days after the date of submission to HHS of an application or proposal, an institution with an approved assurance covering the proposed research shall certify that the application or proposal has been reviewed and approved by the IRB. Other institutions shall certify that the application or proposal has been approved by the IRB within 30 days after receipt of a request for such a certification from the Department. If the certification is not submitted within these time limits, the application or proposal may be returned to the institution.

§§ 46.104 - 46.106 [reserved]

§ 46.107—IRB Membership

(a) Each IRB shall have at least five members, with varying backgrounds to promote complete and adequate review of research activities commonly conducted by the institution. The IRB shall be sufficiently qualified through the experience and expertise of its members, and the diversity of the members' backgrounds including consideration of the racial and cultural backgrounds of members and sensitivity to such issues as community attitudes, to promote respect for its advice and counsel in safeguarding the rights and welfare of human subjects. In addition to possessing the professional competence necessary to review specific research activities, the IRB shall be able to ascertain the acceptability of proposed research in terms of institutional commitments and regulations, applicable law, and standards of professional conduct and practice. The IRB shall therefore include persons knowledgeable in these areas. If an IRB regularly reviews research that involves a vulnerable category of subjects, including but not limited to subjects covered by other subparts of this part, the IRB shall include one or more individuals who are primarily concerned with the welfare of these subjects.

(b) No IRB may consist entirely of men or entirely of women, or entirely of members of one profession.

(c) Each IRB shall include at least one member whose primary concerns are in nonscientific areas; for example, lawyers, ethicists, members of the clergy.

(d) Each IRB shall include at least one member who is not otherwise affiliated with the institution and who is not part of the immediate family of a person who is affiliated with the institution.

(e) No IRB may have a member participating in the IRB's initial or continuing review of any project in which the member has a conflicting interest, except to provide information requested by the IRB.

(f) An IRB may, in its discretion, invite individuals with competence in special areas to assist in the review of complex issues which require expertise beyond or in addition to that available on the IRB. These individuals may not vote with the IRB.

§ 46.108—IRB Functions and Operations

In order to fulfill the requirements of these regulations each IRB shall:

(a) Follow written procedures as provided in § 46.103(b)(4).

(b) Except when an expedited review procedure is used (see § 46.110), review proposed research at convened meetings at which a majority of the members of the IRB are present, including at least one member whose primary concerns are in nonscientific areas. In order for the research to be approved, it shall receive the approval of a majority of those members present at the meeting.

(c) Be responsible for reporting to the appropriate institutional officials and the Secretary [footnote deleted] any serious or continuing noncompliance by investigators with the requirements and determinations of the IRB.

§ 46.109—IRB Review of Research

(a) An IRB shall review and have authority to approve, require modifications in (to secure approval), or disapprove all research activities covered by these regulations.

(b) An IRB shall require that information given to subjects as part of informed consent is in accordance with § 46.116. The IRB may require that information, in addition to that specifically mentioned in § 46.116, be given to the subjects when in the IRB's judgment the information would meaningfully add to the protection of the rights and welfare of subjects.

(c) An IRB shall require documentation of informed consent or may waive documentation in accordance with § 46.117.

(d) An IRB shall notify investigators and the institution in writing of its decision to approve or disapprove the proposed research activity, or of modifications required to secure IRB approval of the research activity. If the IRB decides to disapprove a research activity, it shall include in its written notification a statement of the reasons for its decision and give the investigator an opportunity to respond in person or in writing.

(e) An IRB shall conduct continuing review of research covered by these regulations at intervals appropriate to the degree of risk, but not less than once per year, and shall have authority to observe or have a third party observe the consent process and the research.

§ 46.110—Expedited review procedures for certain kinds of research involving no more than minimal risk, and for minor changes in approved research

(a) The Secretary has established, and published in the *Federal Register*, a list of categories of research that may be reviewed by the IRB through an expedited review procedure. The list will be amended, as appropriate, through periodic republication in the *Federal Register*.

(b) An IRB may review some or all of the research appearing on the list through an expedited review procedure, if the research involves no more than minimal risk. The IRB may also use the expedited review procedure to review minor changes in previously approved research during the period for which approval is authorized. Under an expedited review procedure, the review may be carried out by the IRB chairperson or by one or more experienced reviewers designated by the chairperson from among members of the IRB. In reviewing the research, the reviewers may exercise all of the authorities of the IRB except that the reviewers may not disapprove the research. A research activity may be disapproved only after review in accordance with the nonexpedited procedure set forth in § 46.108(b).

(c) Each IRB which uses an expedited review procedure shall adopt a method for keeping all members advised of research proposals which have been approved under the procedure.

(d) The Secretary may restrict, suspend, or terminate an institution's or IRB's use of the expedited review procedure when necessary to protect the rights or welfare of subjects.

§ 46.111—Criteria for IRB approval of research

(a) In order to approve research covered by these regulations the IRB shall determine that all of the following requirements are satisfied:

(1) Risks to subjects are minimized: (i) By using procedures which are consistent with sound research design and which do not unnecessarily expose subjects to risk, and (ii) whenever appropriate, by using procedures already being performed on the subjects for diagnostic or treatment purposes.

(2) Risks to subjects are reasonable in relation to anticipated benefits, if any, to subjects, and the importance of the knowledge that may reasonably be expected to result. In evaluating risks and benefits, the IRB should consider only those risks and benefits that may result from the research (as distinguished from risks and benefits of therapies subjects would receive even if not participating in the research). The IRB should not consider possible long-range effects of applying knowledge gained in the research (for example, the possible effects of the research on public policy) as among those research risks that fall within the purview of its responsibility.

(3) Selection of subjects is equitable. In making this assessment the IRB should take into account the purposes of the research and the setting in which the research will be conducted.

(4) Informed consent will be sought from each prospective subject or the subject's legally authorized representative, in accordance with, and to the extent required by § 46.116.

(5) Informed consent will be appropriately documented, in accordance with, and to the extent required by § 46.117.

(6) Where appropriate, the research plan makes adequate provision for monitoring the data collected to insure the safety of subjects.

(7) Where appropriate, there are adequate provisions to protect the privacy of subjects and to maintain the confidentiality of data.

(b) Where some or all of the subjects are likely to be vulnerable to coercion or undue influence, such as persons with acute or severe physical or mental illness, or persons who are economically or educationally disadvantaged, appropriate additional safeguards have been included in the study to protect the rights and welfare of these subjects.

§ 46.112—Review by institution

Research covered by these regulations that has been approved by an IRB may be subject to further appropriate review and approval or disapproval by officials of the institution. However, those officials may not approve the research if it has not been approved by an IRB.

§ 46.113—Suspension or termination of IRB approval of research

An IRB shall have authority to suspend or terminate approval of research that is not being conducted in accordance with the IRB's requirements or that has been associated with unexpected serious harm to subjects. Any suspension or termination of approval shall include a statement of the reasons for the IRB's action and shall be reported promptly to the investigator, appropriate institutional officials, and the Secretary. (Footnote deleted.)

§ 46.114—Cooperative research

Cooperative research projects are those projects, normally supported through grants, contracts, or similar arrangements, which involve institutions in addition to the grantee or prime contractor (such as a contractor with the grantee, or a subcontractor with the prime contractor). In such instances, the grantee or prime contractor remains responsible to the Department for safeguarding the rights and welfare of human subjects. Also, when cooperating institutions conduct some or all of the research involving some or all of these subjects, each cooperating institution shall comply with these regulations as though it received funds for its participation in the project directly from the

Department, except that in complying with these regulations institutions may use joint review, reliance upon the review of another qualified IRB, or similar arrangements aimed at avoidance of duplication of effort.

§ 46.115—IRB Records

(a) An institution, or where appropriate an IRB, shall prepare and maintain adequate documentation of IRB activities, including the following:

(1) Copies of all research proposals reviewed, scientific evaluations, if any, that accompany the proposals, approved sample consent documents, progress reports submitted by investigators, and reports of injuries to subjects.
(2) Minutes of IRB meetings which shall be in sufficient detail to show attendance at the meetings; actions taken by the IRB; the vote on these actions including the number of members voting for, against, and abstaining; the basis for requiring changes in or disapproving research; and a written summary of the discussion of controverted issues and their resolution.
(3) Records of continuing review activities.
(4) Copies of all correspondence between the IRB and the investigators.
(5) A list of IRB members as required by § 46.103(b)(3).
(6) Written procedures for the IRB as required by § 46.103(b)(4).
(7) Statements of significant new findings provided to subjects, as required by § 46.116(b)(5).

(b) The records required by this regulation shall be retained for at least 3 years after completion of the research, and the records shall be accessible for inspection and copying by authorized representatives of the Department at reasonable times and in a reasonable manner.

§ 46.116—General requirements for informed consent

Except as provided elsewhere in this or other subparts, no investigator may involve a human being as a subject in research covered by these regulations unless the investigator has obtained the legally effective informed consent of the subject or the subject's legally authorized representative. An investigator shall seek such consent only under circumstances that provide the prospective subject or the representative sufficient opportunity to consider whether or not to participate and that minimize the possibility of coercion or undue influence. The information that is given to the subject or the representative shall be in language understandable to the subject or the representative. No informed consent, whether oral or written, may include any exculpatory language through which the subject or the representative is made to waive or appear to waive any of the subject's legal rights, or releases or appears to release the investigator, the sponsor, the institution or its agents from liability for negligence.

(a) Basic elements of informed consent. Except as provided in paragraph (c) or (d) of this section, in seeking informed consent the following information shall be provided to each subject:

(1) A statement that the study involves research, an explanation of the purposes of the research and the expected duration of the subject's participation, a description of the procedures to be followed, and identification of any procedures which are experimental;
(2) A description of any reasonably foreseeable risks or discomforts to the subject;
(3) A description of any benefits to the subject or to others which may reasonably be expected from the research;
(4) A disclosure of appropriate alternative procedures or courses of treatment, if any, that might be advantageous to the subject;
(5) A statement describing the extent, if any, to which confidentiality of records identifying the subject will be maintained;
(6) For research involving more than minimal risk, an explanation as to whether any compensation and an explanation as to whether any medical treatments are available if injury occurs and, if so, what they consist of, or where further information may be obtained;
(7) An explanation of whom to contact for answers to pertinent questions about the research and research subjects' rights, and whom to contact in the event of a research-related injury to the subject; and
(8) A statement that participation is voluntary, refusal to participate will involve no penalty or loss of benefits to which the subject is otherwise entitled, and the subject may discontinue participation at any time without penalty or loss of benefits to which the subject is otherwise entitled.

(b) Additional elements of informed consent. When appropriate, one or more of the following elements of information shall also be provided to each subject:

(1) A statement that the particular treatment or procedure may involve risks to the subject (or to the embryo or fetus, if the subject is or may become pregnant) which are currently unforeseeable;
(2) Anticipated circumstances under which the subject's participation may be terminated by the investigator without regard to the subject's consent;
(3) Any additional costs to the subject that may result from participation in the research;
(4) The consequences of a subject's decision to withdraw from the research and procedures for orderly termination of participation by the subject;

(5) A statement that significant new findings developed during the course of the research which may relate to the subject's willingness to continue participation will be provided to the subject; and
(6) The approximate number of subjects involved in the study.

(c) An IRB may approve a consent procedure which does not include, or which alters, some or all of the elements of informed consent set forth above, or waive the requirement to obtain informed consent provided the IRB finds and documents that:

(1) The research or demonstration project is to be conducted by or subject to the approval of state or local government officials and is designed to study, evaluate, or otherwise examine: (i) programs under the Social Security Act, or other public benefit or service programs; (ii) procedures for obtaining benefits or services under those programs; (iii) possible changes in or alternatives to those programs or procedures; or (iv) possible changes in methods or levels of payment for benefits or services under those programs; and
(2) The research could not practicably be carried out without the waiver or alteration.

(d) An IRB may approve a consent procedure which does not include, or which alters, some or all of the elements of informed consent set forth above, or waive the requirements to obtain informed consent provided the IRB finds and documents that:

(1) The research involves no more than minimal risk to the subjects;
(2) The waiver or alteration will not adversely affect the rights and welfare of the subjects;
(3) The research could not practicably be carried out without the waiver or alteration; and
(4) whenever appropriate, the subjects will be provided with additional pertinent information after participation.

(e) The informed consent requirements in these regulations are not intended to preempt any applicable federal, state, or local laws which require additional information to be disclosed in order for informed consent to be legally effective.

(f) Nothing in these regulations is intended to limit the authority of a physician to provide emergency medical care, to the extent the physician is permitted to do so under applicable federal, state, or local law.

§ 46.117—Documentation of informed consent

(a) Except as provided in paragraph (c) of this section, informed consent shall be documented by the use of a written consent form approved by the IRB and signed by the subject or the subject's legally authorized representative. A copy shall be given to the person signing the form.

(b) Except as provided in paragraph (c) of this section, the consent form may be either of the following:

(1) A written consent document that embodies the elements of informed consent required by § 46.116. This form may be read to the subject or the subject's legally authorized representative, but in any event, the investigator shall give either the subject or the representative adequate opportunity to read it before it is signed; or
(2) A "short form" written consent document stating that the elements of informed consent required by § 46.116 have been presented orally to the subject or the subject's legally authorized representative. When this method is used, there shall be a witness to the oral presentation. Also, the IRB shall approve a written summary of what is to be said to the subject or the representative. Only the short form itself is to be signed by the subject or the representative. However, the witness shall sign both the short form and a copy of the summary, and the person actually obtaining consent shall sign a copy of the summary. A copy of the summary shall be given to the subject or the representative, in addition to a copy of the "short form."

(c) An IRB may waive the requirement for the investigator to obtain a signed consent form for some or all subjects if it finds either:

(1) That the only record linking the subject and the research would be the consent document and the principal risk would be potential harm resulting from a breach of confidentiality. Each subject will be asked whether the subject wants documentation linking the subject with the research, and the subject's wishes will govern; or
(2) That the research presents no more than minimal risk of harm to subjects and involves no procedures for which written consent is normally required outside of the research context.

In cases where the documentation requirement is waived, the IRB may require the investigator to provide subjects with a written statement regarding the research.

* * *

§ 46.123—Early termination of research funding; evaluation of subsequent applications and proposals

(a) The Secretary may require that Department funding for any project be terminated or suspended in the manner prescribed in applicable program requirements, when the

Secretary finds an institution has materially failed to comply with the terms of these regulations. . . .

SUBPART B—ADDITIONAL PROTECTIONS PERTAINING TO RESEARCH DEVELOPMENT AND RELATED ACTIVITIES INVOLVING FETUSES, PREGNANT WOMEN, AND HUMAN IN VITRO FERTILIZATION

Source: 40 FR 33528, Aug. 8, 1975, 43 FR 1758, January 11, 1978, 43 FR 51559, November 3, 1978

§ 46.201—Applicability

(a) The regulations in this subpart are applicable to all Department of Health, Education, and Welfare grants and contract supporting research, development, and related activities involving: (1) The fetus, (2) pregnant women, and (3) human *in vitro* fertilization.

(b) Nothing in this subpart shall be construed as indicating that compliance with the procedures set forth herein will in any way render inapplicable pertinent State or local laws bearing upon activities covered by this subpart.

(c) The requirements of this subpart are in addition to those imposed under the other subparts of this part.

§ 46.202—Purpose

It is the purpose of this subpart to provide additional safeguards in reviewing activities to which this subpart is applicable to assure that they conform to appropriate ethical standards and relate to important societal needs.

§ 46.203—Definitions

As used in this subpart:

(a) "Secretary" means the Secretary of Health, Education, and Welfare and any other officer or employee of the Department of Health, Education, and Welfare to whom authority has been delegated.

(b) "Pregnancy" encompasses the period of time from confirmation of implantation (through any of the presumptive signs of pregnancy, such as missed menses, or by a medically acceptable pregnancy test), until expulsion or extraction of the fetus.

(c) "Fetus" means the product of conception from the time of implantation (as evidenced by any of the presumptive signs of pregnancy, such as missed menses, or a medically acceptable pregnancy test), until a determination is made, following expulsion or extraction of the fetus, that it is viable.

(d) "Viable" as it pertains to the fetus means being able, after either spontaneous or induced delivery, to survive (given the benefit of available medical therapy) to the point of independently maintaining heart beat and respiration. The Secretary may from time to time, taking into account medical advances, publish in the *Federal Register* guidelines to assist in determining whether a fetus is viable for purposes of this subpart. If a fetus is viable after delivery, it is a premature infant.

(e) "Nonviable fetus" means a fetus *ex utero* which, although living, is not viable.

(f) "Dead fetus" means a fetus *ex utero* which exhibits neither heartbeat, spontaneous respiratory activity, spontaneous movement of voluntary muscles, nor pulsation of the umbilical cord (if still attached).

(g) "*In vitro* fertilization" means any fertilization of human ova which occurs outside the body of a female, either through admixture of donor human sperm and ova or by any other means.

§ 46.204—Ethical Advisory Boards

(a) One or more Ethical Advisory Boards shall be established by the Secretary. Members of these board(s) shall be so selected that the board(s) will be competent to deal with medical, legal, social, ethical, and related issues and may include, for example, research scientists, physicians, psychologists, sociologists, educators, lawyers, and ethicists, as well as representatives of the general public. No board member may be a regular, full-time employee of the Department of Health, Education, and Welfare.

(b) At the request of the Secretary, the Ethical Advisory Board shall render advice consistent with the policies and requirements of this Part as to ethical issues, involving activities covered by this subpart, raised by individual applications or proposals. In addition, upon request by the Secretary, the Board shall render advice as to classes of applications or proposals and general policies, guidelines, and procedures.

(c) A Board may establish, with the approval of the Secretary, classes of applications or proposals which: (1) must be submitted to the Board, or (2) need not be submitted to the Board. Where the Board so establishes a class of applications or proposals which must be submitted, no application or proposal within the class may be funded by the Department or any component thereof until the application or proposal has been reviewed by the Board and the Board has rendered advice as to its acceptability from an ethical standpoint.

(d) No application or proposal involving human *in vitro* fertilization may be funded by the Department or any component thereof until the application or proposal has been reviewed by the Ethical Advisory Board and the Board has rendered advice as to its acceptability from an ethical standpoint.

§ 46.205—Additional duties of the Institutional Review Boards in connection with activities involving fetuses, pregnant women, or human in vitro fertilization

(a) In addition to the responsibilities prescribed for Institutional Review Boards under Subpart A or this part, the applicant's or offeror's Board shall, with respect to activities covered by this subpart, carry out the following additional duties:

(1) Determine that all aspects of the activity meet the requirements of this subpart;
(2) Determine that adequate consideration has been given to the manner in which potential subjects will be selected, and adequate provision has been made by the applicant or offeror for monitoring the actual informed consent process (e.g., through such mechanisms, when appropriate, as participation by the Institutional Review Board or subject advocates in: (i) Overseeing the actual process by which individual consents required by this subpart are secured either by approving induction of each individual into the activity or verifying, perhaps through sampling, that approved procedures for induction of individuals into the activity are being followed, and (ii) monitoring the progress of the activity and intervening as necessary through such steps as visits to the activity site and continuing evaluation to determine if any unanticipated risks have arisen);
(3) Carry out such other responsibilities as may be assigned by the Secretary.

(b) No award may be issued until the applicant or offeror has certified to the Secretary that the Institutional Review Board has made the determinations required under paragraph (a) of this section and the Secretary has approved these determinations, as provided in § 46.120 of Subpart A of this part.

(c) Applicants or offerors seeking support for activities covered by this subpart must provide for the designation of an Institutional Review Board, subject to approval by the Secretary, where no such Board has been established under Subpart A of this part.

§ 46.206—General limitations

(a) No activity to which this subpart is applicable may be undertaken unless:

(1) Appropriate studies on animals and nonpregnant individuals have been completed;
(2) Except where the purpose of the activity is to meet the health needs of the mother or the particular fetus, the risk to the fetus is minimal and, in all cases, is the least possible risk for achieving the objectives of the activity.
(3) Individuals engaged in the activity will have no part in: (i) Any decisions as to the timing, method, and procedures used to terminate the pregnancy, and (ii) determining the viability of the fetus at the termination of the pregnancy; and
(4) No procedural changes which may cause greater than minimal risk to the fetus or the pregnant woman will be introduced in the procedure for terminating the pregnancy solely in the interest of the activity.

(b) No inducements, monetary or otherwise, may be offered to terminate pregnancy for purposes of the activity.

[40 FR 33528, Aug. 8, 1975, as amended at 40 FR 51638, Nov. 6, 1975]

§ 46.207—Activities directed toward pregnant women as subjects

(a) No pregnant woman may be involved as a subject in an activity covered by this subpart unless: (1) The purpose of the activity is to meet the health needs of the mother and the fetus will be placed at risk only to the minimum extent necessary to meet such needs, or (2) the risk to the fetus is minimal.

(b) An activity permitted under paragraph (a) of this section may be conducted only if the mother and father are legally competent and have given their informed consent after having been fully informed regarding possible impact on the fetus, except that the father's informed consent need not be secured if: (1) The purpose of the activity is to meet the health needs of the mother; (2) his identity or whereabouts cannot reasonably be ascertained; (3) he is not reasonably available; or (4) the pregnancy resulted from rape.

§ 46.208—Activities directed toward fetuses in utero as subjects

(a) No fetus *in utero* may be involved as a subject in any activity covered by this subpart unless: (1) the purpose of the activity is to meet the health needs of the particular fetus and the fetus will be placed at risk only to the minimum extent necessary to meet such needs, or (2) the risk to the fetus imposed by the research is minimal and the purpose of the activity is the development of important biomedical knowledge which cannot be obtained by other means.

(b) An activity permitted under paragraph (a) of this section may be conducted only if the mother and father are legally competent and have given their informed consent, except that the father's consent need not be secured if: (1) His identity or whereabouts cannot reasonably be ascertained, (2) he is not reasonably available, or (3) the pregnancy resulted from rape.

§ 46.209—Activities directed toward fetuses *ex utero*, including nonviable fetuses, as subjects

(a) Until it has been ascertained whether or not a fetus ex utero is viable, a fetus ex utero may not be involved as a subject in an activity covered by this subpart unless:

(1) There will be no added risk to the fetus resulting from the activity, and the purpose of the activity is the development of important biomedical knowledge which cannot be obtained by other means, or
(2) The purpose of the activity is to enhance the possibility of survival of the particular fetus to the point of viability.

(b) No nonviable fetus may be involved as a subject in an activity covered by this subpart unless:

(1) Vital functions of the fetus will not be artificially maintained,
(2) Experimental activities which of themselves would terminate the heartbeat or respiration of the fetus will not be employed, and
(3) The purpose of the activity is the development of important biomedical knowledge which cannot be obtained by other means.

(c) In the event the fetus *ex utero* is found to be viable, it may be included as a subject in the activity only to the extent permitted by and in accordance with the requirements of other subparts of this part.

(d) An activity permitted under paragraph (a) or (b) of this section may be conducted only if the mother and father are legally competent and have given their informed consent, except that the father's informed consent need not be secured if: (1) his identity or whereabouts cannot reasonably be ascertained, (2) he is not reasonably available, or (3) the pregnancy resulted from rape.

§ 46.210—Activities involving the dead fetus, fetal material, or the placenta

Activities involving the dead fetus, macerated fetal material, or cells, tissue, or organs excised from a dead fetus shall be conducted only in accordance with any applicable State or local laws regarding such activities.

§ 46.211—Modification or waiver of specific requirements

Upon the request of an applicant or offeror (with the approval of its Institutional Review Board), the Secretary may modify or waive specific requirements of this subpart, with the approval of the Ethical Advisory Board after such opportunity for public comment as the Ethical Advisory Board considers appropriate in the particular instance. In making such decisions, the Secretary will consider whether the risks to the subject are so outweighed by the sum of the benefit to the subject and the importance of the knowledge to be gained as to warrant such modification or waiver and that such benefits cannot be gained except through a modification or waiver. Any such modifications or waivers will be published as notices in the *Federal Register*.

SUBPART C—ADDITIONAL PROTECTIONS PERTAINING TO BIOMEDICAL AND BEHAVIORAL RESEARCH INVOLVING PRISONERS AS SUBJECTS

Source: 43 FR 53655, Nov. 16, 1978

§ 46.301—Applicability

(a) The regulations in this subpart are applicable to all biomedical and behavioral research conducted or supported by the Department of Health, Education, and Welfare involving prisoners as subjects.

(b) Nothing in this subpart shall be construed as indicating that compliance with the procedures set forth herein will authorize research involving prisoners as subjects, to the extent such research is limited or barred by applicable State or local law.

(c) The requirements of this subpart are in addition to those imposed under the other subparts of this part.

§ 46.302—Purpose

Inasmuch as prisoners may be under constraints because of their incarceration which could affect their ability to make a truly voluntary and uncoerced decision whether or not to participate as subjects in research, it is the purpose of this subpart to provide additional safeguards for the protection of prisoners involved in activities to which this subpart is applicable.

§ 46.303—Definitions

As used in this subpart:

(a) "Secretary" means the Secretary of Health, Education, and Welfare and any other officer or employee of the Department of Health, Education, and Welfare to whom authority has been delegated.

(b) "DHEW" means the Department of Health, Education, and Welfare.

(c) "Prisoner" means any individual involuntarily confined or detained in a penal institution. The term is intended to encompass individuals sentenced to such an institution under a criminal or civil statute, individuals detained in other facilities by virtue of statutes or commitment procedures which provide alternatives to criminal prosecution or incarceration in a penal institution, and individuals detained pending arraignment, trial or sentencing.

(d) "Minimal risk" is the probability and magnitude of physical or psychological harm that is normally encountered in the daily lives, or in the routine medical, dental, or psychological examination of healthy persons.

§ 46.304—Composition Of Institutional Review Boards where prisoners are involved

In addition to satisfying the requirements in § 46.107 of this part, an Institutional Review Board, carrying out responsibilities under this part with respect to research covered by this subpart, shall also meet the following specific requirements:

(a) A majority of the Board (exclusive of prisoner members) shall have no association with the prison(s) involved, apart from their membership on the Board.

(b) At least one member of the Board shall be a prisoner, or a prisoner representative with appropriate background and experience to serve in that capacity, except that where a particular research project is reviewed by more than one Board only one Board need satisfy this requirement.

§ 46.305—Additional duties of the Institutional Review Boards where prisoners are involved

(a) In addition to all other responsibilities prescribed for Institutional Review Boards under this part, the Board shall review research covered by this subpart and approve such research only if it finds that:

(1) The research under review represents one of the categories of research permissible under § 46.306(a)(2);

(2) Any possible advantages accruing to the prisoner through his or her participation in the research, when compared to the general living conditions, medical care, quality of food, amenities and opportunity for earnings in the prison, are not of such a magnitude that his or her ability to weigh the risks of the research against the value of such advantages in the limited choice environment of the prison is impaired;

(3) The risks involved in the research are commensurate with risks that would be accepted by nonprisoner volunteers;

(4) Procedures for the selection of subjects within the prison are fair to all prisoners and immune from arbitrary intervention by prison authorities or prisoners. Unless the principal investigator provides to the Board justification in writing for following some other procedures, control subjects must be selected randomly from the group of available prisoners who meet the characteristics needed for that particular research project;

(5) The information is presented in language which is understandable to the subject population;

(6) Adequate assurance exists that parole boards will not take into account a prisoner's participation in the research in making decisions regarding parole, and each prisoner is clearly informed in advance that participation in the research will have no effect on his or her parole; and

(7) Where the Board finds there may be a need for follow-up examination or care of participants after the end of their participation, adequate provision has been made for such examination or care, taking into account the varying lengths of individual prisoners' sentences, and for informing participants of this fact.

(b) The Board shall carry out such other duties as may be assigned by the Secretary.

(c) The institution shall certify to the Secretary, in such form and manner as the Secretary may require, that the duties of the Board under this section have been fulfilled.

§ 46.306—Permitted research involving prisoners

(a) Biomedical or behavioral research conducted or supported by DHEW may involve prisoners as subjects only if:

(1) The institution responsible for the conduct of the research has certified to the Secretary that the Institutional Review Board has approved the research under § 46.305 of this subpart; and

(2) In the judgment of the Secretary the proposed research involves solely the following:

(A) Study of the possible causes, effects, and processes of incarceration, and of criminal behavior, provided that the study presents no more than minimal risk and no more than inconvenience to the subject:

(B) Study of prisons as institutional structures or of prisoners as incarcerated persons, provided that the study presents no more than minimal risk and no more than inconvenience to the subjects;

(C) Research on conditions particularly affecting prisoners as a class (for example, vaccine trials and other research on hepatitis which is much more prevalent in prisons than elsewhere; and research on social and psychological problems such as alcoholism, drug addiction and sexual assaults) provided that the study may proceed only after the Secretary has consulted with appropriate experts including experts in penology, medicine and ethics, and published notice, in the *Federal Register*, of his intent to approve such research; or

(D) Research on practices, both innovative and accepted, which have the intent and reasonable probability of improving the health or well-being of the subject. In cases in which those studies require the assignment of prisoners in a manner consistent with protocols approved by the IRB to control groups which may not benefit from the research, the study may proceed only after the Secretary has consulted with appropriate experts, including experts in penology, medicine and ethics, and published notice, in the *Federal Register*, of his intent to approve such research.

(b) Except as provided in paragraph (a) of this section, biomedical or behavioral research conducted or supported by DHEW shall not involve prisoners as subjects.

SUBPART D—ADDITIONAL PROTECTIONS FOR CHILDREN INVOLVED AS SUBJECTS IN RESEARCH

Source: 48 FR 9818, March 8, 1983

§ 46.401—To what do these regulations apply?

(a) This subpart applies to all research involving children as subjects, conducted or supported by the Department of Health and Human Services.

(1) This includes research conducted by Department employees, except that each head of an Operating Division of the Department may adopt such nonsubstantive, procedural modifications as may be appropriate from an administrative standpoint.

(2) It also includes research conducted or supported by the Department of Health and Human Services outside the United States, but in appropriate circumstances, the Secretary may, under paragraph (3) of § 46.101 of Subpart A, waive the applicability of some or all of the requirements of these regulations for research of this type. . . .

§ 46.402—Definitions

The definitions in § 46.102 of Subpart A shall be applicable to this subpart as well. In addition, as used in this subpart:

(a) "Children" are persons who have not attained the legal age for consent to treatments or procedures involved in the research, under the applicable law of the jurisdiction in which the research will be conducted.

(b) "Assent" means a child's affirmative agreement to participate in research. Mere failure to object should not, absent affirmative agreement, be construed as assent.

(c) "Permission" means the agreement of parent(s) or guardian to the participation of their child or ward in research.

(d) "Parent" means a child's biological or adoptive parent.

(e) "Guardian" means an individual who is authorized under applicable state or local law to consent on behalf of a child to general medical care.

§ 46.403—IRB duties

In addition to other responsibilities assigned to IRBs under this part, each IRB shall review research covered by this subpart and approve only research which satisfies the conditions of all applicable sections of this subpart.

§ 46.404—Research not involving greater than minimal risk

HHS will conduct or fund research in which the IRB finds that no greater than minimal risk to children is presented, only if the IRB finds that adequate provisions are made for soliciting the assent of the children and the permission of their parents or guardians, as set forth in § 46.606.

§ 46.405—Research involving greater than minimal risk but presenting the prospect of direct benefit to the individual subjects

HHS will conduct or fund research in which the IRB finds that more than minimal risk to children is presented by an intervention or procedure that holds out the prospect of direct benefit for the individual subject, or by a monitoring procedure that is likely to contribute to the subject's well-being only if the IRB finds that:

(a) The risk is justified by the anticipated benefit to the subjects;

(b) The relation of the anticipated benefit to the risk is at least as favorable to the subjects as that presented by available alternative approaches; and

(c) Adequate provisions are made for soliciting the assent of the children and permission of their parents or guardians, as set forth in § 46.408.

§ 46.406—Research involving greater than minimal risk and no prospect of direct benefit to individual subjects, but likely to yield generalizable knowledge about the subject's disorder or condition

HHS will conduct or fund research in which the IRB finds that more than minimal risk to children is presented by an intervention or procedure that does not hold out the prospect of direct benefit for the individual subject, or by a monitoring procedure which is not likely to contribute to the well-being of the subject, only if the IRB finds that:

(a) The risk represents a minor increase over minimal risk;

(b) The intervention or procedure presents experiences to subjects that are reasonably commensurate with those inherent in their actual or expected medical, dental, psychological, social or educational situations;

(c) The intervention or procedure is likely to yield generalizable knowledge about the subjects' disorder or condition which is of vital importance for the understanding or amelioration of the subjects' disorder or condition; and

(d) Adequate provisions are made for soliciting assent of the children and permission of their parents or guardians, as set forth in § 46.408.

§ 46.407—Research not otherwise approvable which presents an opportunity to understand, prevent, or alleviate a serious problem affecting the health or welfare of children

HHS will conduct or fund research that the IRB does not believe meets the requirements of §§ 46.404, 46.405, or 46.406 only if:

(a) The IRB finds that the research presents a reasonable opportunity to further understanding, prevention, or alleviation of a serious problem affecting the health or welfare of children; and

(b) The Secretary, after consultation with a panel of experts in pertinent disciplines (for example: science, medicine, education, ethics, law) and following opportunity for public review and comment, has determined either: (1) That the research in fact satisfies the conditions of §§ 46.404, 46.405, or 46.406, as applicable, or (2) the following:

(i) The research presents a reasonable opportunity to further the understanding, prevention, or alleviation of a serious problem affecting the health or welfare of children;

(ii) The research will be conducted in accordance with sound ethical principles;

(iii) Adequate provisions are made for soliciting the assent of children and the permission of their parents or guardians, as set forth in § 46.408.

§ 46.408—Requirements for permission by parents or guardians and for assent by children

(a) In addition to the determinations required under other applicable sections of this subpart, the IRB shall determine that adequate provisions are made for soliciting the assent of the children, when in the judgment of the IRB the children are capable of providing assent. In determining whether children are capable of assenting, the IRB shall take into account the ages, maturity, and psychological state of the children involved. This judgment may be made for all children to be involved in research under a particular protocol, or for each child, as the IRB deems appropriate. If the IRB determines that the capability of some or all of the children is so limited that they cannot reasonably be consulted or that the intervention or procedure involved in the research holds out a prospect of direct benefit that is important to the health or well-being of the children and is available only in the context of the research, the assent of the children is not a necessary condition for proceeding with the research. Even where the IRB determines that the subjects are capable of assenting, the IRB may still waive the assent requirement under circumstances in which consent may be waived in accord with § 46.116 of Subpart A.

(b) In addition to the determinations required under other applicable sections of this subpart, the IRB shall determine, in accordance with and to the extent that consent is required by § 46.116 of Subpart A, that adequate provisions are made for soliciting the permission of each child's parents or guardian. Where parental permission is to be obtained, the IRB may find that the permission of one parent is sufficient for research to be conducted under §§ 46.404 or 46.405. Where research is covered by §§ 46.406 and 46.407 and permission is to be obtained from parents, both parents must give their permission unless one parent is deceased, unknown, incompetent, or not reasonably available, or when only one parent has legal responsibility for the care and custody of the child.

(c) In addition to the provisions for waiver contained in § 46.116 of Subpart A, if the IRB determines that a research protocol is designed for conditions or for a subject population for which parental or guardian permission is not a reasonable requirement to protect the subjects (for example, neglected or abused children), it may waive the consent requirements in Subpart A of this part and paragraph (b) of this section, provided an appropriate mechanism for protecting the children who will participate as subjects in the research is substituted, and provided further that the waiver is not inconsistent with federal state or local law. The choice of an appropriate mechanism would depend upon the nature and purpose of the activities described in the protocol, the risk and anticipated benefit to the research subjects, and their age, maturity, status, and condition.

(d) Permission by parents or guardians shall be documented in accordance with and to the extent required by § 46.117 of Subpart A.

(e) When the IRB determines that assent is required, it shall also determine whether and how assent must be documented.

§ 46.409—Wards

(a) Children who are wards of the state or any other agency, institution, or entity can be included in research approved under §§ 46.406 or 46.407 only if such research is:

(1) Related to their status as wards; or
(2) Conducted in schools, camps, hospitals, institutions, or similar settings in which the majority of children involved as subjects are not wards.

(b) If the research is approved under paragraph (a) of this section, the IRB shall require appointment of an advocate for each child who is a ward, in addition to any other individual acting on behalf of the child as guardian or in loco parentis. One individual may serve as advocate for more than one child. The advocate shall be an individual who has the background and experience to act in, and agrees to act in, the best interests of the child for the duration of the child's participation in the research and who is not associated in any way (except in the role as advocate or member of the IRB) with the research, the investigator(s), or the guardian organization.

RESEARCH ACTIVITIES WHICH MAY BE REVIEWED THROUGH EXPEDITED REVIEW PROCEDURES

Source: 46 Federal Register 8392 January 26,1981

Research activities involving no more than minimal risk *and* in which the only involvement of human subjects will be in one or more of the following categories (carried out through standard methods) may be reviewed by the Institutional Review Board through the expedited review procedure authorized in 46.110 of 45 CFR Part 46.

(1) Collection of: hair and nail clippings, in a nondisfiguring manner; deciduous teeth; and permanent teeth if patient care indicates a need for extraction.
(2) Collection of excreta and external secretions including sweat, uncannulated saliva, placenta removed at delivery, and amniotic fluid at the time of rupture of the membrane prior to or during labor.
(3) Recording of data from subjects 18 years of age or older using noninvasive procedures routinely employed in clinical practice. This includes the use of physical sensors that are applied either to the surface of the body or at a distance and do not involve input of matter or significant amounts of energy into the subject or an invasion of the subject's privacy. It also includes such procedures as weighing, testing sensory acuity, electrocardiography, electroencephalography, thermography, detection of naturally occurring radioactivity, diagnostic echography, and electroretinography. It does not include exposure to electromagnetic radiation outside the visible range (for example, x-rays, microwaves).
(4) Collection of blood samples by venipuncture, in amounts not exceeding 450 milliliters in an eight-week period and no more often than two times per week, from subjects 18 years of age or older and who are in good health and not pregnant.
(5) Collection of both supra and subgingival dental plaque and calculus, provided the procedure is not more invasive than routine prophylactic scaling of the teeth and the process is accomplished in accordance with accepted prophylactic techniques.
(6) Voice recordings made for research purposes such as investigations of speech defects.
(7) Moderate exercise by healthy volunteers.
(8) The study of existing data, documents, records, pathological specimens, or diagnostic specimens.
(9) Research on individual or group behavior or characteristics of individuals, such as studies of perception, cognition, game theory, or test development, where the investigator does not manipulate subjects' behavior and the research will not involve stress to subjects.
(10) Research on drugs or devices for which an investigational new drug exemption or an investigational device exemption is not required.

FINAL REPORT OF THE TUSKEGEE SYPHILIS STUDY AD HOC ADVISORY PANEL

INTRODUCTION. *From the early 1930s to the 1970s, the U.S. Public Health Service conducted research to determine the ways in which syphilis affects the human body. The study involved some 400 rural, black males living in Macon County, Georgia (of which Tuskegee is the county seat). They were not told of their disease or about the research, and were left untreated until their death. The public revelation of this long episode, in July 1972, prompted public outrage. A month later, the Secretary of Health, Education and Welfare appointed a panel of distinguished persons to investigate the episode and make recommendations preventing future similar events. The Final Report of the Tuskegee Syphilis Study Ad Hoc Advisory Panel appeared in 1973, its format reflecting the panel's charge to respond to specific questions set by the Secretary. The Report also includes two letters from Dr. Jay Katz, one of the panel members.*

REPORT ON CHARGE I-A

Statement of Charge I-A: Determine whether the study was justified in 1932

BACKGROUND DATA

The Tuskegee Study was one of several investigations that were taking place in the 1930's with the ultimate objective of venereal disease control in the United States. Beginning in 1926, the United States Public Health Service, with the cooperation of other organizations, actively engaged in venereal disease control work.[1] In 1929, the United States Public Health Service entered into a cooperative demonstration study with the Julius Rosenwald Fund and state and local departments of health in the control of venereal disease in six southern states[2]: Mississippi (Bolivar County); Tennessee (Tipton County); Georgia (Glynn County); Alabama (Macon County); North Carolina (Pitt County); Virginia (Albermarle County). These syphilis control demonstrations took place from 1930–1932 and disclosed a high prevalence of syphilis (35%) in the Macon County survey. Macon County was 82.4% Negro. The cultural status of this Negro population was low and the illiteracy rate was high.

During the years 1928–1942 the Cooperative Clinical Studies in the Treatment of Syphilis[3] were taking place in the syphilis clinics of Western Reserve University, Johns Hopkins University, Mayo Clinic, University of Pennsylvania, and the University of Michigan. The Division of Venereal Disease, [of the United States Public Health Service; hereafter] USPHS provided statistical support, and financial support was provided by the USPHS and a grant from the Milbank Memorial Fund. These studies included a focus on effects of treatment in latent syphilis which had not been clinically documented before 1932. A report issued in 1932 indicated a satisfactory clinical outcome in 35% of untreated latent syphilitics.

The findings of Bruusgaard of Oslo on the results of untreated syphilis became available in 1929.[4] The Oslo study was a classic retrospective study involving the analysis of 473 patients at three to forty years after infection. For the first time, as a result of the Oslo study, clinical data were available to suggest the probability of spontaneous cure, continued latency, or serious or fatal outcome. Of the 473 patients included in the Oslo study, 309 were living and examined and 164 were deceased. Among the 473 patients, 27.7 percent were clinically free from symptoms

Excerpts from the *Final Report of the Tuskegee Syphilis Study Ad Hoc Advisory Panel*. (Washington, D.C.: U.S. Government Printing Office, 1973). The superscripts in the Report on Charges I-A and I-B refer to a numbered list of references, and particular references are cited more than once. Superscripts in the report on Charge III are simple footnotes (reprinted here as endnotes and renumbered to include a first unnumbered note). All references and notes have been printed following the final excerpt. For additional information on the Tuskegee episode, see James Jones, *Bad Blood. The Tuskegee Syphilis Experiment* (New York: The Free Press, 1981).

and Wassermann negative; 14.8 percent had no clinical symptoms with Wassermann positive; 14.1 percent had heart and vessel disease; 2.76 percent had general paresis and 1.27 percent had tabes dorsalis. Thus in 1932, as the Public Health Service put forth a major effort toward control and treatment, much was still unknown regarding the latent stages of the disease especially pertaining to its natural course and the epidemiology of late and latent syphilis.

Facts and Documentation Pertaining to Charge I-A

1. There is no protocol which documents the original intent of the study. None of the literature searches or interviews with participants in the study gave any evidence that a written protocol ever existed for this study. The theories postulated from time to time include the following purposes either by direct statement or implication:[5–7]

a. Study of the natural history of the disease.
b. Study of the course of treated and untreated syphilis (Annual Report of the Surgeon General of the Public Health Service of the United States 1935–36).
c. Study of the differences in histological and clinical course of the disease in black versus white subjects.
d. Study with an "acceptance" of the postulate that there was a benign course of the disease in later stages vis-a-vis the dangers of available therapy.
e. Short term study (6 months or longer) of the incidence and clinical course of late latent syphilis in the Negro male (From letter of correspondence from T. Clark, Assistant Surgeon General, to M.M. Davis of the Rosenwald Fund, October 29, 1932)—Original plan of procedure is stated herein.
f. A study which would provide valuable data for a syphilis control program for a rural impoverished community.

In the absence of an original protocol, it can only be assumed that between 1932 and 1936 (when the first report[5] of the study was made) the decision was made to continue the study as a long-term study. The Annual Report of the Surgeon General for 1935–36 included the statement: "Plans for the continuation of this study are underway. During the last 12 months, success has been obtained in gaining permission for the performance of autopsies on 11 of 15 individuals who died."

2. There is no evidence that informed consent was gained from the human participants in this study. Such consent would and should have included knowledge of the risk of human life for the involved parties and information re possible infections of innocent, nonparticipating parties such as friends and relatives. Reports such as "Only individuals giving a history of infection who submitted voluntarily to examination were included in the 399 cases" are the only ones that are documentable.[5] Submitting voluntarily is not informed consent.

3. In 1932, there was a known risk to human life and transmission of the disease in latent and late syphilis was believed to be possible [see memorandum of Vonderlehr to T. Clark, June 10, 1932]. Moore[3] [in] 1932 reported satisfactory clinical outcome in 85% of patients with latent syphilis that were treated in contrast to 35% if no treatment is given.

4. The study as announced and continually described as involving "untreated" male Negro subjects was not a study of "untreated" subjects. Caldwell[8] in 1971 reported that: All but one of the originally untreated syphilitics seen in 1968–1970 have received therapy, although heavy metals and/or antibiotics were given for a variety of reasons by many non-study physicians and not necessarily in doses considered curative for syphilis. Heller[6] in 1946 reported "about one-fourth of the syphilitic individuals received treatment for their infection. Most of these, however, received no more than 1 or 2 arsenical injections; only 12 received as many as 10." The "untreated" group in this study is therefore a group of treated *and* untreated male subjects.

5. There is evidence that control subjects who became syphilitic were transferred to the "untreated" group. This data is present in the patient files at the Center for Disease Control in Atlanta. Caldwell[8] reports 12 original controls either acquired syphilis or were found to have reactive treponemal tests (unavailable prior to 1953). Heller[6] also reported that "It is known that some of the control group have acquired syphilis although the exact number cannot be accurately determined at present." Since this transfer of patients from the control group to the syphilitic group did occur, the study is not one of late latent syphilis. Also, it is not certain that this group of patients did in fact receive adequate therapy.

6. In the absence of a definitive protocol, there is no evidence or assurance that standardization of evaluative procedures, which are essential to the validity and reliability of a scientific study, existed at any time. This fact leaves open to question the true scientific merits of a longitudinal study of this nature. Standardization of evaluative procedures and clinical judgment of the investigators are considered essential to the valid interpretation of clinical data.[9] It should be noted that, in 1932, orderly and well planned research related to latent syphilis was justifiable since

a. Morbidity and mortality had not been documented for this population and the significance of the survey procedure had just been reported in findings of the prevalence studies for 6 southern counties;[1]
b. Epidemiologic knowledge of syphilis at the time had not produced facts so that it could be scientifically documented "just how and at what stage the disease is

spread" [see the letter from L. Usilton, VD Program 1930–32 and memorandum from Vonderlehr to T. Clark (Assistant Surgeon General) June 10, 1932].

c. There was a paucity of knowledge re clinical aspects and spontaneous cure in latent syphilis[3] and the Oslo study[4] had just reported spontaneous remission of the disease in 27.7% of the patients studied. If perhaps a higher "cure" rate could have been documented for the latent syphilitics, then the treatment priorities and recommendations may have been altered for this community where funds and medical services were already inadequate.

The retrospective summary of the "Scientific Contributions of the Tuskegee Study" from the Chief, Venereal Disease Branch, USPHS (dated November 21, 1972) includes the following merits of the study:

> Knowledge already gained or potentially able to be gained from this study may be categorized as contributing to improvements in the following areas:
>
> 1. Care of the surviving participants,
> 2. Care of all persons with latent syphilis,
> 3. The operation of a national syphilis control program,
> 4. Understanding of the disease of syphilis,
> 5. Understanding of basic disease producing mechanisms.

Panel Judgments on Charge 1-A

1. In retrospect, the Public Health Service Study of Untreated Syphilis in the Male Negro in Macon County, Alabama, was ethically unjustified in 1932. This judgment made in 1973 about the conduct of the study in 1932 is made with the advantage of hindsight acutely sharpened over some forty years, concerning an activity in a different age with different social standards. Nevertheless one fundamental ethical rule is that a person should not be subjected to avoidable risk of death or physical harm unless he freely and intelligently consents. There is no evidence that such consent was obtained from the participants in this study.

2. Because of the paucity of information available today on the manner in which the study was conceived, designed and sustained, a scientific justification for a short term demonstration study cannot be ruled out. However, the conduct of the longitudinal study as initially reported in 1936 and through the years is judged to be scientifically unsound and its results are disproportionately meager compared with known risks to human subjects involved. Outstanding weaknesses of this study, supported by the lack of written protocol, include lack of validity and reliability assurances; lack of calibration of investigator responses; uncertain quality of clinical judgments between various investigators; questionable data base validity and questionable value of the experimental design for a long term study of this nature.

The position of the Panel must not be construed to be a general repudiation of scientific research with human subjects. It is possible that a scientific study in 1932 of untreated syphilis, properly conceived with a clear protocol and conducted with suitable subjects who fully understood the implications of their involvement, might have been justified in the pre-penicillin era. This is especially true when one considers the uncertain nature of the results of treatment of late latent syphilis and the highly toxic nature of therapeutic agents then available.

REPORT ON CHARGE I-B

Statement of Charge I-B: Determine whether the study should have been continued when penicillin became generally available

BACKGROUND DATA

In 1932, treatment of syphilis in all stages was being provided through the use of a variety of chemotherapeutic agents including mercury, bismuth, arsphenamine, neoarsphenamine, iodides and various combinations thereof. Treatment procedures being used in the early 1930's extended over long periods of time (up to two years) and were not without hazard to the patient.[10] As of 1932, also, treatment was widely recommended and treatment schedules specifically for late latent syphilis were published and in use.[3–10] The rationale for treatment at that time was based on the clinical judgment "that the latent syphilitic patient must be regarded as a potential carrier of the disease and should be treated for the sake of the Community's health."[3] The aims of treatment in the treatment of latent syphilis were stated to be: (1) to increase the probability of "cure" or arrest, (2) to decrease the probability of progression or relapse over the probable result if no treatment were given and (3) the control of potential infectiousness from contact of the patient with adults of either sex, or in the case of women with latent syphilis, for unborn children.

According to Pfeiffer (1935)[11] treatment of late syphilis is quite individualistic and requires the physician's best judgment based upon sound fundamental knowledge of internal medicine and experience, and should not be undertaken as a routine procedure. Thus, treatment was being recommended in the United States for all stages of syphilis as of 1932 despite the "spontaneous" cure concept that was being justified by interpretations of the Oslo study, the potential hazards of treatment due to drug toxicity and to possible Jarisch-Herxheimer reactions in acute late syphilis.[12]

Documented reports of the effects of penicillin in the 1940's and early 1950's vary from outright support and endorsement of the use of penicillin in late and latent syphilis,[13–15] to statements of possible little or no value,[16–17] to expressions of doubts and uncertainty[18–19] related to its value, the potency of penicillin, absence of control of the rate of absorption, and potential hazard related to severe Herxheimer effects.

Although the mechanism of action of penicillin is not clear from available scientific reports of late latent syphilis, the therapeutic benefits were clinically documented by the early 1950's and have been widely reported from the mid 1950's to the present. In fact, the Center for Disease Control of the USPHS has reported treatment of syphilitic mothers in all stages of infection with penicillin as of 1953[20] and has demonstrated that penicillin is the most effective treatment yet known for neurosyphilis (1960).[21]

Facts and Documentation re Charge I-B

1. Treatment schedules recommending the use of arsenicals and bismuth in the treatment of late latent syphilis were available in 1932.[3] Penicillin therapy was recommended for treatment of late latent syphilis in the late 1940's[14–15] which was *before* it became readily available for public use (estimated to have been 1952–53).

2. It was "known as early as 1932 that 85% of patients treated in late latent syphilis would enjoy prolonged maintenance of good health and freedom from disease as opposed to 35 percent if left untreated."[3] Scientists in this study,[5] reported in 1936, that morbidity in male Negroes with untreated syphilis far exceeds that in a comparable nonsyphilitic group and that cardiovascular and central nervous system involvements were two to three times as common. Moreover, Wenger,[22] in 1950, reported: "We know now, where we could only surmise before, that we have contributed to their ailments and shortened their lives. I think the least we can say is that we have a high moral obligation to those that have died to make this the best study possible." The effect of syphilis in shortening life was published from observations made by Usilton et al. in 1937.[23] The study by Rosahn[24] at Yale in 1947 reported strong clinical evidence that syphilis ran a more fatal course in Negroes than in Caucasians.

3. Reports regarding the withholding of treatment from patients in this study are varied and are still subject to controversy. Statements received from personal interviews conducted by Panel members with participants in this study cannot be considered as conclusive since there are varied opinions concerning what actually happened. In written letters and in open interviews, the panel received reports that treatment was deliberately withheld on the one hand and on the other, we were told that individuals seeking treatment were not denied treatment (in transcript and correspondence documents).

What is clearly documentable (in a series of letters between Vonderlehr and Health officials in Tuskegee taking place between February 1941 and August 1942) is that known seropositive, untreated males under 45 years of age from the Tuskegee Study had been called for army duty and rejected on account of a positive blood. The local board was furnished with a list of 256 names of men under 45 years of age and asked that these men be excluded from the list of draftees needing treatment! According to the letters, the board agreed with this arrangement in order to make it possible to continue this study on an effective basis. It should be noted that some of these patients had already received notices from the Local Selective Service Board "to begin their antisyphilitic treatment immediately."

According to Wenger,[22] the patients in the study "received no treatment on our recommendation." At the present time, we know that most of the participants in this study received some form of treatment with heavy metals and/or antibiotics.[8] Although the adequacy of treatment received is not known, it is clear that the treatment received was provided by physicians who were not a part of the study and who were individually sought by the individual patients related to their own medical symptoms and pursuit of treatment.

4. The five survey periods in this study occurred in 1932, 1938–39, 1948, 1952–53 and 1968–70.[8–25] This study lacks continuity except through the public health nurse and at these isolated survey periods. In 1969 an Ad Hoc Committee reviewed the Tuskegee Study with the purpose: to examine data from the Tuskegee Study and offer advice on continuance of this study. . . .

Panel Judgments on Charge I-B

The ethical, legal and scientific implications which are evoked from the facts presented in the previous section led the Panel to the following judgment:

> That penicillin therapy should have been made available to the participants in this study especially as of 1953 when penicillin became generally available.

Withholding of penicillin, after it became generally available, amplified the injustice to which this group of human beings had already been subjected. The scientific merits of the Tuskegee Study are vastly overshadowed by the violation of basic ethical principles pertaining to human dignity and human life imposed on the experimental subjects. . . .

REPORT ON CHARGE I

SUMMARY

This section of the Advisory Panel's report deals specifically with Charge Codes I-A and I-B.

STATEMENT OF CHARGE CODES

Charge I-A. Determine whether the study was justified in 1932, and

Charge I-B. Determine whether it should have been continued when penicillin became generally available.

INTRODUCTION

The Background Paper on the Tuskegee Study, prepared by the Venereal Disease Branch of the Center for Disease Control, July 27, 1972, included the following statements:

> Because of the lack of knowledge of the pathogenesis of syphilis, a long-term study of untreated syphilis was considered desirable in establishing a more knowledgeable syphilis control program.

A prospective study was begun late in 1932 in Macon County, Alabama, a rural area with a static population and a high rate of untreated syphilis. An untreated population such as this offered an unusual opportunity to follow and study the disease over a long period of time. In 1932, a total of 26 percent of the male population tested, who were 25 years of age or older, were serologically reactive for syphilis by at least two tests, usually on two occasions. The original study group was composed of 399 of these men who had received no therapy and who gave historical and laboratory evidence of syphilis which had progressed beyond the infectious stages. A total of 201 men comparable in age and environment and judged by serology, history, and physical examination to be free of syphilis were selected to be the control group.

Panel Conclusions re Charge I-A and I-B of the Tuskegee Study

After extensive review of the available documents, interviews with associated parties and pursuit of various other avenues of documentation, the Panel concludes that:

1. In retrospect, the Public Health Service Study of Untreated Syphilis in the Male Negro in Macon County, Alabama, was ethically unjustified in 1932.
2. Because of the paucity of information available today on the manner in which the study was conceived, designed and sustained, scientific justification for a short-term demonstration study in 1932 cannot be ruled out. However, the conduct of the longitudinal study as initially reported in 1936 and through the years is judged to be scientifically unsound and its results are disproportionately meager compared with known risks to the human subjects involved.
3. Penicillin therapy should have been made available to the participants in this study not later than 1953.

The Panel qualifies its conclusions with several position statements summarized as follows:

a. The judgments in 1973 about the conduct of the Tuskegee Study in 1932 are made with the advantage of hindsight, acutely sharpened over some forty years concerning an activity in a different age with different social standards. Nevertheless one fundamental ethical rule is that a person should not be subjected to avoidable risk of death or physical harm unless he freely and intelligently consents. There was no evidence that such consent was obtained from the participants in this study.
b. History has shown that certain people under psychological, social or economic duress are particularly acquiescent. These are the young, the mentally impaired, the institutionalized, the poor and persons of racial minority and other disadvantaged groups. These are the people who may be selected for human experimentation and who, because of their station in life, may not have an equal chance to withhold consent.
c. The Tuskegee Syphilis Study, placed in the perspective of its early years, is not an isolated event in terms of the generally accepted conditions and practices that prevailed in the 1930's.
d. The position of the Panel must not be construed to be a general repudiation of scientific research with human subjects. It is possible that a scientific study in 1932 of untreated syphilis, properly conceived with a clear protocol and conducted with suitable subjects who fully understood the implications of their involvement, might have been justified in the prepenicillin era because of the uncertain nature of results of treatment of late latent syphilis with the highly toxic therapeutic agents then available.

LETTER FROM JAY KATZ, M.D.

To the Assistant Secretary for Health and Scientific Affairs Concerning Reservations about the Panel Report on Charge I

I should like to add the following findings and observations to the majority opinion:

(1) There is ample evidence in the records available to us that the consent to participation was not obtained from the Tuskegee Syphilis Study subjects, but that instead they were exploited, manipulated, and deceived. They were treated not as human subjects but as objects of research. The most fundamental reason for condemning the Tuskegee Study at its inception and throughout its continuation is not that all the subjects should have been treated, for some might not have wished to be treated, but rather that they were never fairly consulted about the research project, its consequences for them, and the alternatives available to them. Those who for reasons of intellectual incapacity could not have been so consulted should not have been invited to participate in the study in the first place.

(2) It was already known before the Tuskegee Syphilis Study was begun, and reconfirmed by the study itself, that persons with

untreated syphilis have a higher death rate than those who have been treated. The life expectancy of at least forty subjects in the study was markedly decreased for lack of treatment.

(3) In addition, the untreated and the "inadvertently" (using the word frequently employed by the investigators) but inadequately treated subjects suffered many complications which could have been ameliorated with treatment. This fact was noted on occasion in the published reports of the Tuskegee Syphilis Study and as late as 1971. However the subjects were not apprised of this possibility.

(4) One of the senior investigators wrote in 1936 that since "a considerable portion of the infected Negro population remained untreated during the entire course of syphilis . . . an unusual opportunity (arose) to study the untreated syphilitic patient from the beginning of the disease to the death of the infected person." Throughout, the investigators seem to have confused the study with an "experiment in nature." But syphilis was not a condition for which no beneficial treatment was available, calling for experimentation to learn more about the condition in the hope of finding a remedy. The persistence of the syphilitic disease from which the victims of the Tuskegee Study suffered resulted from the unwillingness or incapacity of society to mobilize the necessary resources for treatment. The investigators, the USPHS, and the private foundations who gave support to this study should not have exploited this situation in the fashion they did. Unless they could have guaranteed knowledgeable participation by the subjects, they all should have disappeared from the research scene or else utilized their limited research resources for therapeutic ends. Instead, the investigators believed that the persons involved in the Tuskegee Study would *never* seek out treatment; a completely unwarranted assumption which ultimately led the investigators deliberately to obstruct the opportunity for treatment of a number of the participants.

(5) In theory if not in practice, it has long been "a principle of medical and surgical morality (never to perform) on man an experiment which might be harmful to him to any extent, even though the result might be highly advantageous to science" (Claude Bernard 1865), at least without the knowledgeable consent of the subject. This was one basis on which the German physicians who had conducted medical experiments in concentration camps were tried by the Nuremberg Military Tribunal for crimes against humanity. Testimony at their trial by official representatives of the American Medical Association clearly suggested that research like the Tuskegee Syphilis Study would have been intolerable in this country or anywhere in the civilized world. Yet the Tuskegee study was continued after the Nuremberg findings and the Nuremberg Code had been widely disseminated to the medical community. Moreover, the study was not reviewed in 1966 after the Surgeon General of the USPHS promulgated his guidelines for the ethical conduct of research, even though this study was carried on within the purview of his department.

(6) The Tuskegee Syphilis Study finally was reviewed in 1969. A lengthier transcript of the proceedings, not quoted by the majority, reveals that one of the five members of the reviewing committee repeatedly emphasized that a moral obligation existed to provide treatment for the "patients." His plea remained unheeded. Instead the Committee, which was in part concerned with the possibility of adverse criticism, seemed to be reassured by the observation that "if we established good liaison with the local medical society, there would be no need to answer criticism."

(7) The controversy over the effectiveness and the dangers of arsenic and heavy metal treatment in 1932 and of penicillin treatment when it was introduced as a method of therapy is beside the point. For the real issue is that the participants in this study were never informed of the availability of treatment because the investigators were never in favor of such treatment. Throughout the study the responsibility rested heavily on the shoulders of the investigators to make every effort to apprise the subjects of what could be done for them if they so wished. In 1937 the then Surgeon General of the USPHS wrote: "(f) or late syphilis no blanket prescription can be written. Each patient is a law unto himself. For every syphilis patient, late and early, a careful physical examination is necessary before starting treatment and should be repeated frequently during its course." Even prior to that, in 1932, ranking USPHS physicians stated in a series of articles that adequate treatment "will afford a practical, if not complete guaranty of freedom from the development of any late lesions. . . ."

In conclusion, I note sadly that the medical profession, through its national association, its many individual societies, and its journals, has on the whole not reacted to this study except by ignoring it. One lengthy editorial appeared in the October 1972 issue of the Southern Medical Journal which exonerated the study and chastised the "irresponsible press" for bringing it to public attention. When will we take seriously our responsibilities, particularly to the disadvantaged in our midst who so consistently throughout history have been the first to be selected for human research? . . . (sgd.) Jay Katz, M.D.

October 25, 1972

Initial Recommendation of the Tuskegee Syphilis Study Ad Hoc Advisory Panel

The Charter of the Tuskegee Syphilis Study Ad Hoc Advisory Panel, issued on August 28, 1972, mandates advice on three specific aspects of the study of untreated syphilis initiated by the Public Health Service in 1932. Item two of the three charges requires the Panel to:

> Recommend whether the study should be continued at this point in time, and if not, how it should be terminated in a way consistent with the rights and health needs of its remaining participants.

Initially, the Panel has limited its deliberations and recommendations exclusively to this charge, and the recommendations contained in this report are intended to respond solely to this specific issue.

In determining our initial recommendations, the Panel has made inquiries which have led us to accept certain evidence outlined here. Though our research on the background and conduct of the Tuskegee Syphilis Study has not been completed, the Panel is satisfied that in the light of its preliminary findings, which will be fully documented at a later date, the recommendations set forth below are fully justified.

BACKGROUND

Since 1932, under the leadership, direction and guidance of the United States Public Health Service, there has been a continuing study, centered in Macon County, Alabama, of the effect of untreated syphilitic infection in approximately 400 Black male human beings previously infected with syphilis as subjects. In the pursuit of this study approximately 200 Black male human beings without syphilis were followed as controls. No convincing evidence has been presented to this Panel that participants in this study were adequately informed about the nature of the experiment, either at its inception or subsequently.

The United States Public Health Service from the onset of the study has maintained a continuous policy of withholding treatment for syphilis from the infected subjects. There was common medical knowledge, before this study, that untreated syphilitic infection produces disability and premature mortality. To date, including its earliest reports, this study has confirmed that untreated syphilitic infection produces disability and premature mortality. Since the late 1940's numerous medical authorities have recommended treatment for syphilis with penicillin in all stages of the disease, including late latent syphilis and tertiary syphilis.

A technical and medical advisory panel convened in 1969 by the United States Public Health Service is reported to have recommended with some ambiguity, that the participants surviving at that time should not be treated. It is estimated that approximately 125 of the participants, including 50 of the controls, are still alive; and the current health status of the participants in the Tuskegee Study is not known.

RECOMMENDATIONS

I. Termination The study of *untreated* syphilis in Black males in Macon County, Alabama, now known as the "Tuskegee Syphilis Study," should be terminated immediately. With this most basic recommendation, the participants involved in this study are to be given the care now required to treat any disabilities resulting from their participation. In furtherance of this goal we recommend:

A. That a Select Specialists Group, composed of competent doctors and other appropriate persons, with experience in the problems arising from this study, be appointed by the Assistant Secretary for Health and Scientific Affairs, DHEW, no later than fifteen days after the adoption of these recommendations.
B. That the members of the Select Specialists Group have had no prior involvement in the Tuskegee Syphilis Study.
C. That the Select Specialists Group be composed of, but not necessarily be limited to, a dermatologist with experience in syphilology who will serve as Chairman, two internists (at least one of whom shall be a cardiologist), a radiologist, a neurologist, an ophthalmologist, a psychiatrist, a doctor of dental surgery, and a social worker.
D. That the Select Specialists Group be solely charged to apply its expert diagnostic and therapeutic skills in order to safeguard the best interests of the participants and of others who may have been infected as a result of the withholding of treatment from the participants.
E. That the Select Specialists Group be vested with the full legally permissible medical authority, medical supervision and medical judgment with regard to the treatment or referral of all of the surviving participants and others within and outside Macon County who may be identified, in cooperation with the appropriate medical societies and Health Departments.
F. That the Public Health Service immediately inform all surviving participants of the nature of their participation in the study, and the desire of the Public Health Service to assess their current health status.
G. That the members of the "Subcommittee on Medical Care" of the Tuskegee Syphilis Study Ad Hoc Advisory Panel be ex-officio members of the Select Specialists Group to function primarily as liaison between the Select Specialists Group and the entire Panel.
H. That on completion of its charge, the Select Specialists Group submit a detailed report about its activities to the Tuskegee Syphilis Study Ad Hoc Advisory Panel through its Chairman. This report shall include, but by no means be limited to, the reasons for administering or withholding penicillin and other drug treatment for syphilis from untreated participants who are infected with syphilis.
I. That the highest priorities be given to this mission so that the charge to the Select Specialists Group shall be completed at the earliest possible date consistent with the best interests of the participants and the ethical responsibilities of the Department of Health, Education, and Welfare.

II. Assessment, Treatment and Care

A. That arrangements be made with *all speed* for the immediate health assessment, treatment and care of all persons included in the study in a suitably adequate facility easily accessible to the surviving participants. That whenever a participant expresses the wish to be cared for or treated by physicians of his own choice, such choices be respected and given all necessary support.
B. That every effort be made to preserve confidentiality with respect to the identification of any participant.
C. That the United States Public Health Service's epidemiologists be mobilized, on a highest priority basis, to assist in locating all surviving participants as well as

others who may have been infected as a result of the withholding of treatment from the participants.

III. Encouragement of Participation

A. That adequate arrangements be provided for maintaining present standards of living during the evaluation and treatment periods in order to minimize any economic barriers to the cooperation of the participants.

B. That at a minimum, any benefits which have been promised to the participants in the past continue to remain in effect.

LETTER FROM JAY KATZ, M.D.

To the Assistant Secretary for Health and Scientific Affairs Concerning Addendum to the Panel Report on Charge II

I entirely concur in the Panel's recommendations and in the reasons given therefor. However, one additional piece of evidence lends even greater conviction, if any is still needed, to the decision to terminate the Tuskegee Syphilis Study. We have been informed that no scientific knowledge of any consequence would be derived from its continuation. The Panel felt that recording this fact might create the impression that it was *the* major reason for terminating the study. I believe that its inclusion should not, and would not, be so construed.

There are cogent reasons for not dismissing the issue of scientific merit. As long as society continues to favor the pursuit of medical knowledge for the possible benefit of the patients participating in research or for the benefit of future patients, a balancing of risks and benefits is inevitable. We must acknowledge this reality in order to confront such questions as: Do we wish to preserve this balancing process and, if we do, how might we learn to minimize inevitable harm to subjects and science? We urgently need to establish an orderly process which will permit the assessment of the conflicting claims inherent in decisions to initiate, continue or terminate research projects. Such an assessment might proceed in four steps: (1) a relentless inquiry into the harmful consequences to the participants; (2) an appraisal of the benefits which may accrue to science as well as to society; (3) a balancing of the risks to the participants against the benefits to them and/or science; and (4) an anticipatory rebuttal to the charge that either the interests of the participants or of science have not been sufficiently considered. In the light of the finding that no interests of science are surrendered by terminating the Tuskegee Syphilis Study, there is nothing to balance and nothing to rebut, and continuance of the study would for this reason alone be inadmissible.

I appreciate that had the conclusion been otherwise, the study would in all probability still have to be terminated because of the other findings set forth in the Panel's report, findings which will be further explored in our deliberations with respect to Charge One ("whether the study was justified"). Moreover, I should note that the four factors, listed above, do not directly address themselves to such other important considerations as: who should be selected for research, what disclosures must be made to participants in research, etc. This will surely be considered in our response to Charge Three ("whether existing [research] policies are adequate and effective"). Finally, I also leave unconsidered for now another question which emerges from the finding of "no scientific merit": why was the study not terminated at a time prior to the appointment of this Panel? One of the benefits of including a finding of scientific merit in every assessment is that many more projects might be terminated sooner, because the reviewer would be hard pressed to make an affirmative finding on this issue. . . (sgd.) Jay Katz, M.D.

REPORT ON CHARGE III

To the Assistant Secretary for Health
From the Tuskegee Syphilis Study Ad Hoc Advisory Panel

I. INTRODUCTION

In his third charge to the Tuskegee Syphilis Study Ad Hoc Advisory Panel, Dr. Merlin K. DuVal, the HEW Assistant Secretary for Health and Scientific Affairs, has asked us to determine

> whether existing policies to protect the rights of patients participating in health research conducted or supported by the Department of Health, Education, and Welfare are adequate and effective and to recommend improvements in these policies, if needed.

Our response to this charge, embodied in this report,[1] should not be viewed simply as a reaction to a single ethically objectionable research project. For the Tuskegee Syphilis Study, despite its widespread publicity was not an isolated phenomenon. We believe that the revelations from Macon County merely brought to the surface once again the unresolved problems which have long plagued medical research activities. Indeed, we hasten to add that although we refer in this report almost exclusively to physicians and to biomedical investigations, the issues we explore also arise in the context of non-medical investigations with human beings, conducted by psychologists, sociologists, educators, lawyers and others. The scope of the DHEW Policy on Protection of Human Subjects, broadened in 1971 to encompass such research, attests to the increasing significance of non-medical investigations with human beings.

Our initial determination that the protection of human research subjects is a current and widespread problem should not be surprising, especially in light of the recent Congressional hearings and bills focusing on the regulation of experimentation. In the past decade the press has publicized and debated a number of experiments which raised ethical questions: for example, the injection of cancer cells into aged patients at the Jewish Chronic Disease Hospital in Brooklyn, the deliberate infection of mentally retarded children with hepatitis at Willowbrook, the development of heart transplantation techniques, the enormous amount of drug research conducted in American prisons, the whole-body irradiation treatment of cancer patients at the University of Cincinnati, the advent and spread of "psychosurgery," and the Tuskegee Syphilis Study itself.

With so many dramatic projects coming to the attention of the general public, more must lie beneath the surface. Evidence for this too has been forthcoming. In 1966, Dr. Henry K. Beecher, the eminent Dorr Professor of Research in Anesthesia at the Harvard Medical School, charged in the prestigious New England Journal of Medicine that "many of the patients (used in experiments which Dr. Beecher investigated and reported) never had the risk satisfactorily explained to them, and . . . further hundreds have not known that they were the subjects of an experiment although grave consequences have been suffered as the direct result. . . ."[2] Dr. Beecher concluded that "unethical or questionably ethical procedures are not uncommon."[3] Quite recently this charge has been corroborated by the sociologist Bernard Barber and his associates, who interviewed biomedical researchers about their own research practices.[4] Despite the expected tendency of researchers to minimize ethical problems in their own work, Barber *et al.* were able to conclude that "while the large majority of our samples of biomedical researchers seems to hold and live up to high ethical standards, a significant minority may not."[5]

The problem of ethical experimentation is the product of the unresolved conflict between two strongly held values: the dignity and integrity of the individual, and the freedom of scientific inquiry. Professionals of many disciplines, and researchers especially, exercise unexamined discretion to intervene in the lives of their subjects for the sake of scientific progress. Although exposure to needless harm and neglect of the duty to obtain the subject's consent have generally been frowned upon in theory, the infliction of unnecessary harm and infringements on informed consent are frequently accepted, in practice, as the price to be paid for the advancement of knowledge. How have investigators come to claim this sweeping prerogative? If the answer to this question is that "society" has authorized professionals to choose between scientific progress and individual human dignity and welfare, should not "society" retain some control over the research enterprise? We agree with philosopher Hans Jonas that

> a slower progress in the conquest of disease would not threaten society, grievous as it is to those who have to deplore that their particular disease be not yet conquered, but that society would indeed be threatened by the erosion of those moral values whose loss, possibly caused by too ruthless a pursuit of scientific progress, would make its most dazzling triumphs not worth having.[6]

We have, as will be seen, made far-reaching recommendations for change. We do not propose these changes lightly. But throughout, in accordance with our mandate, our concern has not been just to define the ethical issues, but also to examine the structures and policies thus far devised to deal with those issues. In urging greater societal involvement in the research enterprise, we believe that the goal of scientific progress can be harmonized with the need to assure the protection of human subjects.

II. SUMMARY OF CONCLUSIONS AND RECOMMENDATIONS

A. Evaluation of Current DHEW Policies for the Protection of Human Research Subjects

1. No uniform Departmental policy for the protection of research subjects exists. Instead one policy governs "extramural" research—research supported by DHEW grants or contracts to institutions outside the Federal Government and conducted by private researchers—and another policy governs "intramural" research—research conducted by personnel of the Public Health Service. Furthermore, Food and Drug Administration (FDA) regulations promulgated to protect subjects in drug research, whether or not supported by DHEW or conducted by the PHS, incorporate variations of their own. The lack of uniformity in DHEW policies creates confusion, and denies some subjects the protection they deserve.

Moving to the next higher level, no uniform Federal policies exist for the protection of subjects in Government-sponsored research. Other agencies wholly separate from DHEW most notably the Department of Defense support or conduct human research. DHEW policies do not govern such research. Here too, the Federal Government's failure to develop a uniform policy has been detrimental to the welfare of research subjects.

2. Under current DHEW policies for the protection of research subjects, regulation of research practices is largely left to the biomedical professions. Since the conduct of human experimentation raises important issues of social policy, greater participation in decision-making by representatives of other professions and of the general public is required.

3. The present reliance by DHEW on the institutional review committee as the primary mechanism for the protection of research subjects was an important advance in the continuing effort to guarantee ethical experimentation. Prior peer review of research protocols is a requirement which should be retained.

4. The existing review committee system suffers from basic defects which seriously undermine the accomplishment of the task assigned to the committees:

a. The governing standards promulgated by DHEW which are intended to guide review committee decisions in specific cases are vague and overly general.
b. No provisions are made for the dissemination or publication of review committee decisions. Their low level of visibility hampers efforts to evaluate and learn from

committee attempts to resolve the complex problems of human research.

c. Although the informed consent of the research subject is one of the most important requirements of research ethics, DHEW policies for obtaining consent are poorly drafted and contain critical loopholes. As a result, one crucial task of institutional review committees—the implementation of the informed consent requirement—is commonly performed inadequately. In particular, consent is far too often obtained in form alone and not in substance.
d. DHEW policies do not give sufficient attention to the protection of such special research subjects as children, prisoners and the mentally incompetent. The use of these subjects in human experimentation presents grave dangers of abuse.
e. The obligation of institutional review committees to conduct continuing review of research projects after their initial approval is undefined and as a consequence often neglected.
f. Inefficient utilization of institutional review committees contributes to their ineffectiveness. Committees are overburdened with a variety of separate functions, and could operate best if their tasks were narrowly defined to encompass mainly the implementation of research policies adequately formulated by others.
g. Effective procedures for enforcing DHEW policies, when those policies are disregarded, have not been devised.

5. No policy for the compensation of research subjects harmed as a consequence of their participation in research has been formulated, despite the fact that no matter how careful investigators may be, unavoidable injury to a few is the price society must pay for the privilege of engaging in research which ultimately benefits the many. Remitting injured subjects to the uncertainties of the law court is not a solution.

B. Policy Recommendations

1. Congress should establish a permanent body with the authority to regulate *at least* all Federally supported research involving human subjects, whether it is conducted in intramural or extramural settings, or sponsored by DHEW or other government agencies, such as the Department of Defense. Ideally, the authority of this body should extend to all research activities, even those not Federally supported. But such a proposal may raise major jurisdictional problems. This body could be called the National Human Investigation Board. The Board should be independent of DHEW, for we do not believe that the agency which both conducts a great deal of research itself and supports much of the research that is carried on elsewhere is in a position to carry out dispassionately the functions we have in mind. The members of the Board should be appointed from diverse professional and scientific disciplines, and should include representatives from the public at large.

2. The primary responsibility of the National Human Investigation Board should be to formulate research policies, in much greater detail and with much more clarity than is presently the case. The Board must promulgate detailed procedures to govern the implementation of its policies by institutional review committees. It must also promulgate procedures for the review of research decisions and their consequences. In particular, this Board should establish procedures for the publication of important institutional committee and Board decisions. Publication of such decisions would permit their intensive study both inside and outside the medical profession and would be a first step toward the case-by-case development of policies governing human experimentation. We regard such a development, analogous to the experience of the common law, as the best hope for ultimately providing workable standards for the regulation of the human experimentation process.

3. The National Human Investigation Board should develop appeals procedures for the adjudication of disagreements between investigators and the institutional review committees.

4. The National Human Investigation Board should also develop a "no fault" clinical research insurance plan to assure compensation for subjects harmed as a result of their participation in research. Institutions which sponsor Federally supported research activities should be required to participate in such a plan.

5. With the establishment of adequate policy formulation and review mechanisms, the structure and functions of the institutional review committees should be altered to enhance the effectiveness of prior review. In place of the amorphous institutional review committee as it now exists, we propose the creation of an Institutional Human Investigation Committee (IHIC) with two distinct subcommittees. The IHIC should be the direct link between the institution and the National Human Investigation Board, and should establish local regulations consistent with national policies. The IHIC should also assume an educational role in its institutions, informing participants in the research enterprise of their rights and obligations. The implementation of research policies should be left to the two subcommittees of the IHIC:

a. A Protocol Review Group (PRG) should be responsible for the prior review of research protocols. The PRG should be composed mainly of competent biomedical professionals.
b. A Subject Advisory Group (SAG) should be responsible for aiding subjects in their decision-making whenever they request its services. Subject must be made aware of the existence of the SAG. The primary concern of the SAG should be with procedures for obtaining con-

sent, and with the quality of consents obtained. The SAG should be composed of both professionals and laymen.

* * *

VI. CONCLUSION

Human experimentation reflects the recurrent societal dilemma of reconciling respect for human rights and individual dignity with the felt needs of society to overrule individual autonomy for the common good. Throughout this report we have expressed our concern for the lack of attention which has been given to the protection of the rights and welfare of human subjects in research. Society can no longer afford to leave the balancing of individual rights against scientific progress to the scientific community alone. The revelations of the Tuskegee Syphilis Study once again dramatically confirmed this conclusion.

We offer our far-reaching proposals in the hope that the decision-making process for human research will become more open and more effectively regulated. We have amply documented the need for implementing this most basic recommendation. Precise rules and efficient procedures, however, are not by themselves proof against a repetition of Tuskegee. For, however well designed the system of regulation, the danger of token adherence to ethical standards and evasion in the guise of flexibility will persist. Ultimately, the spirit in which an aware society undertakes to use human beings for research ends will determine the protection which those human beings will receive. Therefore, we have urged throughout a greater participation by society in the decisions which affect so many human lives.

REFERENCES TO THE FINAL REPORT ON CHARGES 1-A AND 1-B

1. Clark, T. *The Control of Syphilis in Southern Rural Areas.* Julius Rosenwald Fund, Chicago, 1932, p. 27.
2. Ibid., pp. 6–36.
3. Moore, Joseph Earle. "Latent Syphilis Cooperative Clinical Studies in the Treatment of Syphilis." Reprint No. 45 from *Venereal Disease Information*, vols. 13(8–12) 1932 and 14(1), 1933, pp. 1–56.
4. Bruusgaard, E. "The Fate of Syphilitics Who Are not Given Specific Treatment." *Archiv fur Dermatologie und Syphilis* 1929, 157, p. 309.
5. Vonderlehr, R.A. et al. "Untreated Syphilis in the Male Negro." *Venereal Disease Information* 17:260–265, 1936.
6. Heller, J.R. and Bruyere, P.T.: "Untreated Syphilis in the Male Negro: II. Mortality During 12 Years of Observation." *Venereal Disease Information* 27: 34–38, 1946.
7. Shafer, J.K., Usilton, L.J., and Gleason, G.A. "Untreated Syphilis in the Male Negro: Prospective Study of Effect on Life Expectancy." *Public Health Reports* 69:684–690, 1954; *Milbank Memorial Fund Quarterly.* 32:262–274, July 1954.
8. Caldwell, J.G., Price, E.V., Shroeter, A.L., and Fletcher, G.F. "Aortic Regurgitation in a Study of Aged Males with Previous Syphilis." Presented in part at American Venereal Disease Association Annual Meeting, 22 June 1971.
9. Feinstein, A.R. *Clinical Judgment.* Baltimore, Williams and Wilkins Co., 1967, pp. 45–48.
10. Gaupin, C. E. "The Treatment of Latent Syphilis." *Kentucky Medical Journal* 30:74–77, February 1932.
11. Pfeiffer, A. "Medical Aspects in the Prevention and Management of Late and Latent Syphilis." *Psychiatric Quarterly* 9: 185–193, April 1935.
12. Greenbaum, S.C. "The 'Bismuth Approach' in the Treatment of Acute (Late) Syphilis." *Journal of Chemotherapy* 13: 5–8, April 1936.
13. Stokes, J.H., et al. "The Action of Penicillin in Late Syphilis." *J.A.M.A.* 126: 73–79, September 1944.
14. Dexter, D.C. and Tucker, H.A. "Penicillin Treatment of Benign Late Gummatous Syphilis, Report of Twenty-one Cases." *American Journal of Syphilis, Gonorrhea, and Venereal Disease* 30:211–226, May 1946.
15. Committee on Medical Research: "The Changing Character of Commercial Penicillin with Suggestions as to the Use of Penicillin in Syphilis." U.S. Health Service and Food and Drug Administration. *J.A.M.A.* 131: 271–275, May 1946.
16. Barnett, C.W. "The Public Health Aspects of Late Latent Syphilis." *Stanford Medical Bulletin* 10: 152–156, August 1952.
17. Reynolds, F.W. "Treatment Failures Following the Use of Penicillin in Late Syphilis." *American Journal of Syphilis, Gonorrhea, and Venereal Disease* 32:233–242, May 1948.
18. McElligott, G.L.M. "The Management of Late and Latent Syphilis." *British Medical Journal* 1:829–830, April 1953.
19. Barnett, C.W., Epstein, N.J., Brewer, A.F. et al. "Effect of Treatment in Late Latent Syphilis." *Arch Dermat Syph* 69:91–99, January 1954.
20. *VD Fact Sheet.* No. 10. U.S. Public Health Service Publication, December 1953, p. 20.
21. *VD Fact Sheet.* No. 17. U.S. Public Health Service Publication, December 1960, p. 19.
22. Wenger, O.C. "Untreated Syphilis in the Negro Male." Hot Springs Seminar, 9-18-50 (from CDC Files).
23. Usilton, L. et al. "A Tentative Death Curve for Acquired Syphilis in White and Colored Males in the United States." *Venereal Disease Information* 18:231–234, 1937.
24. Rosahn, P.D. "Autopsy Studies in Syphilis." *Journal of Venereal Disease Information* 28(Supplement No. 21): 32–39, 1949.
25. Rivers, E., Schuman, S., Simpson, L., and Olansky, S. "Twenty Years of Follow-up Experience in a Long-Range Medical Study." *Public Health Reports* 68(4): 391–395, April 1953.

NOTES TO THE FINAL REPORT ON CHARGE III

1. This report was prepared by the Subcommittee on Charge III (Jay Katz, M.D., chairman, Ronald H. Brown, J.D.,

Seward Hiltner, Ph.D. and Fred Speaker, J.D.). The subcommittee chairman wishes to thank his research assistant Stephen H. Glickman, a third year law student at Yale University, for his valuable contributions to this report. Special thanks go also to Dr. Robert C. Backus, Mrs. Bernice M. Lee and Ms. Jackie Eagle who in many ways facilitated the work of the subcommittee.

2. Henry K. Beecher, "Ethics and Clinical Research," 274 *New Eng. J. Med.* 1354 (1966).
3. Ibid., p. 1355.
4. Barber, Lally, Makarushka, and Sullivan, *Research on Human Subjects: Problems of Social Control in Medical Experimentation* (Russell Sage Foundation 1973).
5. Barber et al. (see note 3), p. 52.
6. Jonas, "Philosophical Reflections on Experimenting with Human Subjects," *Daedalus* 98:219, 245 (1969).

RESEARCH ON *IN VITRO* FERTILIZATION

INTRODUCTION. *The National Commission for the Protection of Human Subjects of Biomedical and Behavioral Research recommended that an Ethics Advisory Board be established within the Department of Health, Education and Welfare to review special classes of research, for example, research that involves "more than minimal risk to children" and research involving the human fetus. The Secretary of the Department established this Board in 1977. Although the National Commission did not address the issue of research on reproductive technology, Federal Regulations require that research on in vitro fertilization be submitted to the Ethical Advisory Board (45 CFR 46, subpart B). In 1979, the Ethical Advisory Board was asked to review a proposal to do such research. Its report appeared in the* Federal Register *on June 18, 1979, but no action was ever taken on the recommendations and the Board itself was dissolved in 1980. Clinical applications of assisted reproduction, based on in vitro fertilization, have proceeded.*

PREFACE

Current regulations of the Department of Health, Education, and Welfare (HEW) prohibit the support of research involving the fertilization of a woman's egg (ovum) outside her body (*in vitro* fertilization) until the Ethics Advisory Board has advised the Secretary as to its ethical acceptability. In 1977, the Department received an application for support of such research and, after it had been approved from a scientific point of view, forwarded it to the Board. At its meeting in May 1978, the Board agreed to review the research proposal.

Over the summer, the announcement of the birth of a baby following *in vitro* fertilization in England aroused great public interest; it appears that a number of couples are ready and eager to avail themselves of such procedures in order to overcome infertility. Therefore, in September, Secretary Califano asked the Board to broaden its consideration of the pending application to include the scientific, ethical, legal and social issues surrounding human *in vitro* fertilization and embryo transfer in general.

This report is the result of over a half year of study during which the Board asked scholars and experts in the fields of reproductive science, ethics, theology, law, and the social sciences, to prepare reports and discuss the issues with Board members in public meetings. In addition, the Board held a series of eleven public hearings throughout the country in which private individuals, professional societies and public interest groups had an opportunity to present their views. The Board also received over 2,000 pieces of correspondence including letters, postcards and formal testimony, all of which were copied and distributed to each of the members.

Chapter 1 of the Report provides background information about the human reproductive process and research involving *in vitro* fertilization and embryo transfer. Chapter 2 explores the technical and ethical issues surrounding such research in humans and Chapter 3 addresses the technical and ethical issues surrounding the use of the procedures in clinical practice. Chapter 4 presents a review of the legal issues, and Chapter 5 summarizes public attitudes as presented to the board and as determined by recent public opinion polls. The Board's conclusions are set forth in Chapter 6.

The Board hopes that its deliberations and conclusions will be useful to the Secretary and staff of the Department in making decisions regarding the support and conduct of research involving human *in vitro* fertilization and embryo transfer. . . .

CHAPTER 1

* * *

D. The Evolution of HEW Involvement

HEW involvement in setting guidelines for research involving *in vitro* fertilization and/or embryo transfer has

44 *Federal Register* (118), 35033-35058, 1979. Footnotes have been renumbered and edited for clarity; where feasible, they have been supplied in brackets within the text.

resulted in the publication of three documents: a "draft working document of proposed policy" ([38 FR 31743] November 16, 1973); a set of proposed regulations ([39 FR 30650] August 23, 1974); and final regulations ([40 FR 33527] August 8, 1975). It is perhaps worthy of note that the questions of fetal research, research with pregnant women, and research involving children received substantially greater attention in the three HEW documents than did the issue of *in vitro* fertilization. This differential allocation of attention accurately reflected the public-policy setting of 1973, when fetal research, in particular, was a matter of significant public controversy. The relative deemphasis of *in vitro* fertilization in the HEW guidelines also reflected the view that successful embryo transfer in humans was not likely to be technically feasible in the near future.

The successive versions of HEW guidelines and rules published between 1973 and 1975 tended toward less detail in their stipulations and toward a greater emphasis on a review procedure for proposed research with human *in vitro* fertilization and/or embryo transfer. The 1973 draft policy stipulated that

1. Care must be taken not to bring human ova fertilized *in vitro* to viability. . . .
2. All proposals for research involving human *in vitro* fertilization must be reviewed by the Ethical Review Board.
3. No research involving the implantation of human ova fertilized in the laboratory into recipient women should be supported until the appropriate scientific review boards are satisfied that there has been sufficient work in animals (including subhuman primates) to demonstrate the safety of the technique. It is recommended that this determination of safety include studies of natural born offspring of the products of *in vitro* fertilization.
4. No implantation of human ova fertilized in the laboratory should be attempted until guidelines are developed governing the responsibilities of the donor and recipient "parents" and of research institutions and personnel [38 FR 31743 November 16, 1973].

In August 1974, subsequent to the passage of legislation establishing the National Commission for the Protection of Human Subjects but prior to the Commission's first meeting, HEW published proposed rule-making on research with several specific groups of human subjects. This document responded to comments on the November 16, 1973 preliminary draft regarding *in vitro* fertilization research, clarified the definition of a fetus, and suggested issues to be considered by the Ethical Advisory Board in its review of any proposed HEW supported research involving human *in vitro* fertilization or embryo transfer. In this 1974 document "fetus" was defined to include "both the product of *in vivo* conception and the product of *in vitro* fertilization which is subsequently implanted in the donor of the ovum" [39 FR 30650 August 23, 1974]. With respect to unimplanted human embryos, the 1974 rules proposed no specific guidelines.

However, the 1974 HEW document recommended that the Ethical Advisory Board take into account certain issues in reviewing research proposals involving *in vitro* fertilization and/or embryo transfer:

> With respect to the fertilization of human ova *in vitro*, it is expected that the Board will consider the extent to which current technology permits the continued development of such ova, as well as the legal and ethical issues surrounding the initiation and disposition of the products of such research.
>
> With respect to implantation of fertilized human ova, it is expected that the Board will consider such factors as the safety of the technique (with respect to offspring) as demonstrated in animal studies, and clarification of the legal responsibilities of the donor and recipient parent(s) as well as the research personnel [39 FR 30650 August 23, 1974].

In August 1975, HEW responded to the National Commission's report and recommendations concerning fetal research. Since the Commission had not specifically addressed the issue of research involving *in vitro* fertilization and/or embryo transfer, HEW chose not to promulgate substantive regulations governing such research. It did, however, clearly reiterate a procedural requirement:

> (e) No application or proposal involving human *in vitro* fertilization may be funded by the Department or any component thereof until the application or proposal has been reviewed by the Ethical Advisory Board and the Board has rendered advice as to its acceptability from an ethical standpoint [40 FR 33529 August 8, 1975].

The effect of this review requirement between August 1975 and September 1977, when the Ethics Advisory Board was appointed by HEW Secretary Califano, was to place a de facto moratorium on all HEW supported human research involving *in vitro* fertilization and/or embryo transfer.

CHAPTER 2

Laboratory Research Involving Human *in vitro* Fertilization and/or the Culture of Early Human Embryos: Technical and Ethical Issues

The technical and ethical issues surrounding *in vitro* fertilization using human gametes depend, to some extent, on whether or not the procedure is performed with the intent of transferring the resulting embryos to women for further development. The discussion in this chapter relates to *in vitro* fertilization of human ova when there is no intention of transferring the product to establish a pregnancy. Chapter 3 deals with human *in vitro* fertilization performed with the specific intent of initiating a pregnancy.

In one of the papers prepared at the request of the Board, LeRoy Walters surveyed the ethical literature on *in vitro* fertilization published through August 1978.[1] This survey noted that most of the ethical discussion on *in vitro* fertilization has concentrated on clinical applications of the technique (the topic of Chapter 3) rather than on laboratory research with early human embryos (the topic of the present chapter). Central issues in the ethical literature on basic research with human embryos included the moral status of the early embryo, the need for such research, and the potential long-term consequences of the research. According to the same survey, commentators on ethical issues in the application of *in vitro* fertilization and/or embryo transfer discussed, among other topics, the need for *in vitro* fertilization as a method for overcoming infertility, the adequacy of prior laboratory and animal research, the risks of *in vitro* fertilization and embryo transfer to the ovum donor as well as to potential offspring, and the appropriateness of allocating scarce health care resources to the clinical application of such techniques. Many of these issues recurred in the papers presented to the Board, which are systematically reviewed in this and the following chapter.

A. The Goals and Potential Benefits of the Research

As noted in the preceding chapter many studies in experimental embryology do not include embryo transfer as a component. Several possible goals of laboratory research with human embryos have been identified:

1. Developing or testing more adequate contraceptives;[2]
2. Determining causes of infertility;[3]
3. Investigating the circumstances leading to the development of hyatidiform moles and their potential transformation into malignant tumors;[4]
4. Evaluating the effect of noxious agents or teratogens on the early embryo by means of an *in vitro* screening system;[5]
5. Studying the mechanisms by which chromosomal abnormalities are produced;[6] and
6. Investigating the totipotential cells of very early embryos to increase understanding of normal and abnormal cell growth and differentiation.[7]

One additional potential goal of human *in vitro* fertilization and embryo culture is more controversial and therefore merits more detailed comment. R.V. Short suggests that a kind of *in vitro* assessment (or "toxicology testing") study might be performed to determine whether *in vitro* fertilization produces a higher incidence of embryonic abnormalities than the conventional *in vivo* method of human reproduction. In Short's view, if *in vitro* fertilization techniques do in fact lead to an excess of embryonic abnormalities, it would be preferable to discover that excess in the laboratory rather than at the time of amniocentesis or birth. Short argues that such a controlled *in vitro* study would also provide information concerning the probable success rate of *in vitro* fertilization.[8]

Several objections can be raised to such a proposal, as Short himself observes. First, there would be little basis for comparison following such a laboratory study since data concerning the incidence of abnormalities, particularly chromosomal abnormalities, in early human embryos following *in vivo* fertilization are quite limited. In fact, the totality of *in vivo* information relating to human preimplantation ova and embryos is "confined to 15 specimens, 9 recovered from the oviduct and 6 from the uterus."[9] At least two replies to this objection can be made. First, James Schlesselman notes that one can extrapolate statistically from three major studies of the incidence of chromosomal abnormalities following *in vivo* fertilization[10] that the natural incidence of such abnormalities in humans is between 396 per 1,000 and 477 per 1,000 at the time of implantation; prior to implantation the incidence of such abnormalities is presumably somewhat higher.[11] Schlesselman concludes that a 40–50% chromosomal abnormality rate in human embryos following *in vivo* fertilization is a reasonable baseline against which to compare the results of *in vitro* fertilization. A second reply is proposed by Short himself, who suggests that one could perform a controlled study of the actual incidence of embryonic defects following *in vivo* fertilization by flushing early embryos from the reproductive tracts of consenting volunteer research subjects. Short concedes that this aspect of the proposed risk-assessment study would present both medical and ethical difficulties of its own.[12]

A second possible objection to Short's proposal for a laboratory risk-assessment study is that it is unnecessary. This objection can take one of two forms. Schlesselman notes that for every 1,000 chromosomal abnormalities which are present in implanted blastocysts, only 5 to 7 survive to the point of live birth. Thus, 99.3% to 99.5% of chromosomally abnormal fetuses are eliminated *in vivo* through spontaneous abortion or fetal death. It follows, therefore, that even a doubling in the incidence of chromosomal abnormalities following *in vitro* fertilization—assuming that the technique or ancillary medical treatment did not facilitate the survival of abnormal embryos—would yield only an additional 6 to 7 chromosomally abnormal fetuses, which could, in Schlesselman's view, be detected by means of prenatal diagnosis and selectively aborted.[13]

An alternative argument against the necessity of Short's proposed risk-assessment study can be based on the essays of Biggers, who asserts that for the investigation of most questions concerning human reproduction a suitable animal model can be found. In his view, women should not be subjected to research risks and valuable human ova and embryos should not be used in research unless there is no reasonable alternative to a study in humans.[14]

Biggers' position suggests a final issue to be considered under the rubric of goals and potential benefits of the research: How stringent a standard should be set with respect to the need for laboratory research on human *in vitro* fertilization and embryo transfer? There are three possible answers to this question. The least stringent standard would be that benefits can be expected from the human research. A somewhat more stringent standard would be that human research should hold out the prospect of more significant or more reliable benefits than research employing animal models.[15] The most stringent standard would require that the promised benefits of human research be achievable only through research using human gametes and early human embryos.

B. The Design of the Research

Biggers emphasizes that research on human *in vitro* fertilization and embryo culture, since it involves human volunteers, "should only be undertaken if efficiently designed experiments of adequate size are possible."[16] In his view, this stipulation may require that collaborative trials be conducted. Schlesselman's discussion of appropriate sample size for answering specific questions regarding human *in vitro* fertilization illustrates both the complexity of the design issue and the essential role of the biostatistician in helping to plan laboratory research with human gametes and embryos.[17]

C. The Consent of Sperm and Ovum Donors

Most discussion of the consent question for laboratory studies of *in vitro* fertilization has focused on the ovum donor. In most cases ova are harvested from women with intact ovaries by means of laparoscopy. The donation of ova may be associated with receiving hormones to induce superovulation and/or to mature the ova *in vivo* prior to harvest. In some cases ova are harvested at the same time that a tubal ligation is performed. There is unanimous agreement that the informed consent of ovum donors must be secured in advance of their participation as research subjects.[18] In addition, the particular vulnerability of infertility patients, who are dependent on the health professions for assistance in achieving pregnancy and who nonetheless may be asked to serve as ovum donors, has been noted in the literature on the consent question.[19]

Less thoroughly discussed are the issues of consent by semen donors and the use of ova excised from ovarian tissue removed for clinical reasons. Consent by semen donors might be particularly difficult to secure if semen were secured from a sperm bank rather than from a prospectively recruited donor. The view expressed in one published assessment of *in vitro* fertilization is that prior consent should be secured from all males whose sperm are to be used for *in vitro* fertilization.[20]

The harvesting of ova from excised ovarian tissue may prove to be inefficient from a purely practical standpoint unless hormone treatments are administered in advance of surgery. Prior consent to such hormone treatment would presumably be secured. However, even if ova were harvested from such tissue, without the previous administration of hormone to the female patient, gradually evolving general standards with respect to the use of human tissues for research purposes[21] would seem to suggest the necessity for securing the patient's consent to the use of her ova in laboratory research.

D. The Status of the Early Human Embryo

Two primary objections to laboratory research with human *in vitro* fertilization and embryo culture have been raised. The first is that such research is incompatible with the respect that is due to early human embryos. The second is that the potential adverse consequences of the research outweigh the potential benefits. These two objections will be discussed in the present and the succeeding section of this chapter.

The shape of the embryonic status question differs somewhat in the laboratory research context and the clinical context. As Leon Kass points out, many human embryos which would be studied in the laboratory would have been created solely for research purposes.[22] The major alternative would be to perform laboratory studies on untransferred embryos remaining after the fertilization of multiple ova and the transfer of only one to the uterus. However, from a research design standpoint, total reliance on the use of untransferred embryos would seem to exclude research on the fertilization process and on the earliest stages of embryonic development.

At least three distinguishable answers to the embryonic-status question in the research context have been proposed. Kass himself, impressed by the continuities in embryonic and fetal development and by the potential viability of the early human embryo if it is transferred at the proper time, argues (1) that embryos ought not be deliberately created for research purposes[23] and (2) that no invasive or manipulative research should be performed on already-existing human embryos.[24] Any other policy would, according to Kass, symbolize the belief that early human embryos are "things or mere stuff."[25]

A second position on the embryonic-status issue is presented by Charles Curran, who argues that

> From my ethical perspective truly human life is present two to three weeks after conception or shortly after the implantation of the embryo. Hence experimentation after that time and attempts to culture embryos *in vitro* beyond this stage raise insurmountable ethical problems.[26]

However, even for research involving the earliest stages of embryonic life Curran asserts that "[t]he nature of the matter involved in the research calls for respect and economy avoiding unnecessary waste."[27]

A similar position is articulated by Clifford Grobstein who suggests that "human cells, tissues and organs that have no reasonable prospect of possessing or developing sentient awareness" are "human materials rather than human beings or persons." Grobstein notes that "there are established practices for dealing with and disposing of human materials, practices that take into account the special status they have, having originated as human."[28] Grobstein's position is characterized as being similar rather than identical to Curran's for two reasons. First, it is not clear that Curran would extend his principle of respect to include non-embryonic human organs, tissues, or cells. Second, the criterion of possessing a potential for sentience seems not to be a part of Curran's position on embryonic status. Indeed, one could construe this criterion broadly to include all preimplantation embryos since, as Kass notes, they could be transferred, implanted, and develop to maturity; or one could interpret the criterion narrowly to exclude all preimplantation embryos since it is infeasible, given the current state of medical technology, to culture human embryos *in vitro* beyond the blastocyst stage.

A third position on embryonic status, represented by Samuel Gorovitz, adopts sentience (rather than the potential for sentience) as the primary criterion for determining the moral status of the human embryo or fetus. In Gorovitz's view:

> The status of the embryo is not equivalent to that of a person, a child, an infant, or a fetus—at least a fetus from the point of development of the capacity for even primitive sentience.[29]

If by "primitive sentience" Gorovitz means the capacity to respond to sensory stimuli, then the transition from embryonic to fetal status (at the eighth week of gestation) or, at the latest, the tenth gestational week of fetal development would seem to mark the transition from nonprotected to protected status.[30] In fact, however, Gorovitz notes that he would draw the line of acceptability somewhat conservatively, that is, "rather close to the point where cell differentiation begins, rather far from the capacity for independent survival."[31]

A possible reason for the multiplicity of viewpoints on the status of the human embryo is suggested by Gorovitz. In his view, questions like embryonic status or the appropriate criteria of death are not matters of fact which can be clarified through appropriate research programs. Rather, these questions provide the occasion for individuals to make decisions and for societies to establish policies.[32] In contrast, while Kass does not directly address the fact/decision distinction, he clearly regards the discontinuity of fertilization and the continuity of the embryonic development which follows as factual considerations which lead ineluctably to certain moral conclusions.[33]

E. Potential Adverse Consequences of the Research

Concerns about adverse consequences of laboratory research with human *in vitro* fertilization and embryo culture have been focused in three areas: (1) the same types of research *procedures* that have been performed with nonhuman mammalian embryos may be performed with human embryos; (2) certain undesirable technological or clinical *applications* may arise from such research; and (3) the research may have a desensitizing or dehumanizing *effect on investigators*.

Kass outlines some of the scientific procedures which in his view are likely to be applied in the future to human embryos:

1. Culture beyond the blastocyst stage;
2. Formation of hybrids or chimeras (intraspecific and inter-specific);
3. Gene, chromosome, and plasmid insertion, excision, or alteration;
4. Nuclear transplantation or cloning; and
5. The freezing of embryos.[34]

Kass ventures this prediction because, in his view, the same arguments which can be advanced to justify, for example, the simpler and earlier procedures proposed by Pierre Soupart can without *logical* contradiction be extended to the more ambitious and later procedures outlined above. Among these justifying principles are the following:

1. It is desirable to learn as much as possible about the process of fertilization, growth, implantation, and differentiation of human embryos and about human gene expression and its control.
2. It would be desirable to acquire improved techniques for *enchancing* conception and implantation, for *preventing* conception and implantation, for the treatment of genetic and chromosomal abnormalities, etc.
3. Finally, only research using human embryos can answer these questions and provide these techniques.
4. There should be no censorship or limitation of scientific inquiry or research.[35]

Without specifically advocating the types of experiments which Kass regards as undesirable, Gorovitz adopts a general position which could in principle allow him to approve such experiments. If one extrapolates from Gorovitz's views on embryonic status, one concludes that he would approve any type of research procedure on the human embryo, provided only that the research terminated prior to the onset of embryonic or fetal sentience and that other canons of research ethics (consent of gamete donors, appropriate research design, etc.) were carefully followed.[36] Gorovitz explicitly accepts Kass's formal point that the justifying arguments for such research should be carefully formulated, in order to avoid the "slippery slope."[37] However, his material principle of drawing the dividing line at the point of sentience rather than fertilization or implantation seems, at least, to lead Gorovitz to approve as potentially beneficial the experiments which Kass regards as negative consequences of laboratory research with preimplantation embryos.

A specific research technique, interspecies fertilization using human sperm or ova, has provoked considerable discussion and therefore merits brief further comment. Cross-fertilization raises both conceptual and ethical questions. Conceptually, is fertilization research involving the use of only human sperm or human ova and the culture of the resultant hybrid embryo human research? Ethically, Kass regards such research as an adverse consequence of intraspecific *in vitro* fertilization. On the other hand, Short, while acknowledging that interspecific fertilization carries with it undertones of a novel type of genetic manipulation,[38] argues that technical and ethical hedges could be constructed to prevent what he regards as the major potential adverse consequence of such research —namely, any effort to transfer the hybrid embryo into the uterus of a human or animal female for further development.

A second type of potential adverse consequence identified by some critics of human *in vitro* fertilization and embryo culture concerns possible applications of the research rather than the research procedures themselves. Kass suggests that the research might lead to the banking of human ova or embryos for commercial purposes.[39] In the literature on this topic several other potential adverse consequences are noted: the cloning of human beings, the creation of human/animal hybrids, and the development of devices which would allow for the extracorporeal gestation, or ectogenesis, of human embryos and fetuses.[40] Without commenting specifically on these potential developments, Gorovitz expresses reservations about the wedge argument in its predictive (as distinguished from its logical) form. He also expresses confidence in the collective capacity of human beings to exercise good judgment, citing as examples public policy on abortion, appropriate treatment of newborn infants, the treatment of irretrievably comatose patients, and the setting of limits on the freedom of scientific inquiry.[41]

In an earlier essay on *in vitro* fertilization and cloning Leon Kass identified a third general type of potential adverse consequence which might result from laboratory research involving human embryos. According to Kass, one should "be concerned about the effects on the attitude toward and respect for human life engendered in persons who are engaged in such practices."[42] No other author has commented on the possibly dehumanizing effects on the researcher of human *in vitro* fertilization and embryo culture. It is probable that authors like Curran and Gorovitz would link the dehumanization question to the issue of embryonic or fetal status, arguing that only research on embryos which have developed beyond the two-to-three-week stage (Curran) or to the point of sentience (Gorovitz) would show disrespect for the human embryo or fetus and that only research which manifested such disrespect would be likely to desensitize the researcher.

CHAPTER 3

Clinical Applications of *In Vitro* Fertilization and/or Embryo Transfer: Technical and Ethical Issues

A. The Need for and Potential Benefits of *In Vitro* Fertilization and Embryo Transfer

The major potential benefit to be derived from clinical applications of *in vitro* fertilization and embryo transfer is that it may enable some otherwise-infertile women to conceive and bear children. Most commentators on the clinical use of *in vitro* fertilization and embryo transfer view the alleviation of infertility, particularly in the context of heterosexual marriage, as a desirable goal.[1] In opposition to this majority position, however, Stanley Hauerwas argues that even within marriage, resort to *in vitro* fertilization as a method to overcome infertility reflects an undue emphasis on the importance of biological parentage.[2]

There are at least two senses in which the *need* for this potential benefit has been discussed. First, how many women who wish to bear children are infertile because of blocked Fallopian tubes? Second, of these infertile women, how many need *in vitro* fertilization and embryo transfer in the sense that they have no alternative means for producing children of their own?

Precise data on the extent of need in these two senses are unavailable. Rough estimates of the upper limits of need in the United States are provided by Biggers:

> There are 60 million women reproductively active in the USA; seven percent of couples are infertile, and a third of these are infertile because of sterility of the wife. Thus, there are 1,400,000 sterile women in the population. Pathology of the oviduct accounts for 40 percent of the cases so that there are about 560,000 women with diseased oviducts.[3]

The major alternative to *in vitro* fertilization and embryo transfer for women is one of several surgical procedures available for repairing blocked oviducts: salpingolysis, resection and reanastomosis, fimbrioplasty, and tubal implantation. According to a recent survey, the rates of term pregnancy following the first three of these procedures are 40–50%, 25–40%, and 10–25% respectively.[4] Thus, at least 280,000 U.S. women with tubal obstruction are not likely to achieve pregnancy by surgical methods alone. Of these women, an unknown number may also suffer from ovarian and/or uterine dysfunction and thus may be incapable of producing offspring even with the aid of *in vitro* fertilization and embryo transfer.[5] An additional adjustment in the estimate of the "need" for *in vitro* fertilization would be required if one were to consider women who had previously elected sterilization by tubal ligation but who later desire to become pregnant.

While the alleviation of infertility among couples is generally regarded as the major potential benefit of clinical *in vitro* fertilization and embryo transfer, some witnesses and some commentators in the literature have identified what they regard as additional benefits. Sid Leiman regards the surrogate-motherhood role as closely analogous to that of a wet nurse and therefore sees no ethical objection to extramarital involvement in gestation in cases in which intramarital reproduction is physically impossible.[6] In his writings on this topic R.G. Edwards mentions sex preselection as an additional potential benefit of clinical *in vitro* fertilization and embryo transfer.[7] Other potential benefits cited by various authors are pre-transfer screening for abnormalities,[8] pre-transfer repair of defects,[9] and extracorporeal gestation.[10] The potential consequences enumerated in this paragraph are not universally judged to be beneficial, however, as Section F below illustrates.

* * *

C. Risks of Procedures

1. *Risks to potential offspring.* The major sources of potential risk to offspring from *in vitro* fertilization and embryo transfer have been briefly outlined in Chapter 1, Section B.[11] In general, the surgical procedure of embryo transfer seems to occasion the least concern, in part perhaps because of the widespread use of embryo transfer following natural fertilization in farm animals.[12] The conditions under which the early embryo is cultured are also not a matter of primary concern, since the early mammalian embryo is known to be highly resistant to damage from environmental insults.[13] The major potential sources of damage to the early embryo are related to either the development of ova, the selection of sperm, the fertilization process, or the freezing of gametes or embryos. Specifically, potential sources of damage are the following:

a. Superovulation, sometimes employed prior to *in vitro* fertilization, may be correlated with an increase in the incidence of a chromosomal abnormality (trisomy) in embryos.[14]
b. The quality of sperm reaching and fertilizing the ovum *in vitro* may differ from the quality of sperm fertilizing the ovum in the Fallopian tube, since the female reproductive tract selects against some types of abnormal sperm.[15]
c. The quantity of sperm reaching the ovum simultaneously *in vitro* may break down the usual block to fertilization by multiple sperm; a polyploid embryo may result.[16]
d. The use of freezing techniques to preserve gametes or embryos may produce mutations.[17]

The precise extent to which each of these theoretical sources of risk is likely to be realized in human clinical applications of *in vitro* fertilization and embryo transfer cannot be estimated with certainty. The data and calculations of Schlesselman suggest that even if an excess of chromosomally abnormal embryos were produced by *in vitro* techniques, only a small proportion (less than 10%) would develop to term because of the natural process by which most such embryos are lost early in gestation. Whether the ancillary medical treatment associated with *in vitro* fertilization and embryo transfer would enhance the survivability of chromosomally abnormal embryos is unknown, as Schlesselman acknowledges.[18] Similarly, if subtler genetic (as distinguished from chromosomal) abnormalities were to result from *in vitro* techniques, the abnormal embryos might not be affected by the natural screening process described by Schlesselman.

Judgments about the *acceptability* of various levels of risk to offspring diverge. Kass would require that such risks be equivalent to or less than those of natural reproduction.[19] Curran adopts a similar (although perhaps slightly less stringent) position, arguing that the risks of the *in vitro* fertilization and transfer procedures to the offspring ought to be "about the same as in the normal process."[20] On the other hand, Biggers notes that there is an estimated three percent additional risk of abnormality in offspring suggested by animal studies, and suggests that such an added risk would be acceptable, particularly in light of the fact that some couples who receive genetic counseling are not deterred from procreation by a twenty-five percent risk of genetically-abnormal offspring.[21]

Schlesselman explicitly raises the question: to what are the risks of human *in vitro* fertilization being compared? His answer is that the women and embryos being used for comparison should have the same medical history relevant to their infertility as those undergoing *in vitro* fertilization and embryo transfer.

2. *Risks to donors.* Most discussion of risks to donors has focused on risks to the women donating ova. The following sources of risk have been identified:

a. Hormonal treatment of the women, sometimes employed to induce superovulation; this treatment can lead to ovarian hyperstimulation or ovarian cysts.[22]

b. Laparoscopy, a surgical procedure generally performed under general anesthesia; this procedure may have to be repeated.[23]
c. Ectopic pregnancy, a potential danger if the embryo fails to implant in the uterus.[24]
d. Careful monitoring of any resulting uterine pregnancy, often including amniocentesis.[25]
e. The possibility of a higher-than-average rate of embryo loss or spontaneous abortion.[26]

These risks are considered to be comparable to the risks faced by female infertility patients, in general, and by women who undergo surgery for the correction of blocked Fallopian tubes, in particular.[27]

D. The Consent of Sperm and Ovum Donors

The issue of informed consent by sperm and oocyte donors was not addressed by the expert witnesses who testified before the Board. In the literature, however, there is unanimous agreement that the informed consent of the would-be mother and presumably of both parents must be secured. Several specific items of information have been identified by various commentators as being material to the decision of the couple and therefore requiring disclosure:

a. The availability of potentially effective alternative therapies, e.g., surgical reconstruction of the Fallopian tubes.[28]
b. The anticipated need for repeated laparoscopies.
c. The low probability of success.
d. The likelihood that the primary beneficiaries of the research will be other couples rather than the research participants themselves.[29]
e. The sources of the gametes to be used in the attempted *in vitro* fertilization (i.e., a guarantee that only the sperm and ova of the couple will be employed).[30]
f. The disposition to be made of sperm, ova, and embryos not used in the transfer attempt.[31]

In the literature on informed consent, several commentators have remarked that infertility patients may be strongly influenced by their desperate desire to have children.[32] On the other hand, R.G. Edwards notes that many candidates for *in vitro* fertilization and embryo transfer are professional persons or their wives. Edwards expresses confidence that the patients seeking this therapy are fully capable of understanding and consenting to its procedures.[33]

E. The Status of the Early Human Embryo

The question of embryonic status in the clinical context differs to some extent from the same question in the laboratory-research context. Perhaps the most obvious difference is that in the clinical context there is at least a possibility that each embryo "created" will be transferred to the uterus, will implant, and will develop to the point of viability. Because of this difference in probabilities, as well as the directly-therapeutic intention present in the clinical context, most expert witnesses on ethical issues surrounding *in vitro* fertilization and embryo transfer viewed the status of the early embryo as less problematic in the clinical situation.

For persons who regard the embryo as deserving of respect or protection from the time of fertilization there are two major concerns: (1) loss of embryos following transfer, and (2) the disposition of untransferred embryos. Kass argues that there is no qualitative difference between embryonic loss following natural reproduction and that which follows *in vitro* fertilization.[34] The second issue is somewhat more complex, however, since, as Kass notes, the "surplus" embryos can be transferred to women other than the donor, used for laboratory research purposes, or allowed to die.[35] A fourth possibility, not mentioned by Kass, would be to freeze the untransferred embryos, perhaps for later transfer to the same donor. Among the first three possibilities, Kass expresses a clear preference for allowing untransferred embryos to die. In his view, this choice is most compatible with concerns about lineage (which would argue against transfer to other women) and about the respect which is owed to early human embryos.[36] Curran's position on the discard of embryos is similar to that of Kass, although Curran adds the note that discards and losses should be minimized insofar as possible.[37]

A potential method for reducing the number of untransferred embryos is suggested by both Kass and Leiman[38]: ova could be fertilized one at a time, and any additional ova could be stored, perhaps by freezing, for future attempts at *in vitro* fertilization and embryo transfer. A possible objection to this one-at-a-time procedure is that if fertilization failed to occur, embryo transfer might be delayed until the next menstrual cycle.

An issue not discussed by the expert witnesses and only hinted at in the literature on *in vitro* fertilization is the disposition of grossly abnormal embryos. Some have argued that to decide that such embryos should not be transferred is the first step toward deciding which fetuses (or persons) are not worthy to live.

Finally, some witnesses such as Gorovitz and Short do not explicitly consider the issue of embryonic status in the clinical context. However, if one extrapolates from their views on embryonic status in general or on laboratory research with early embryos, one can conclude with some confidence that they would regard the embryonic loss following embryo transfer and the discard of untransferred embryos as ethically acceptable.

F. Potential Adverse Consequences of Clinical Applications

Two types of potential adverse consequences of *in vitro* fertilization and embryo transfer have been identified: (1)

adverse consequences for the family; and (2) other adverse consequences. Kass notes that even if the initial aim of clinical applications is to assist married couples to bear children of their own, the techniques employed provide "the *immediate* possibility" of egg donation (egg from donor, sperm from husband), embryo donation (egg and sperm both from outside the marriage), and foster pregnancy (another woman carrying the pregnancy to term).[39] In Kass's view, there will be a strong demand for such extramarital uses of the clinical procedures—a demand which, if fulfilled, will further compromise "the virtues of family, lineage, and heterosexuality" or weaken "the taboos against adultery and even incest."[40]

Responses to the thesis that clinical uses of *in vitro* fertilization and embryo transfer will weaken the family have taken two forms. The first, represented by Gorovitz, is to argue that the demand for laboratory-assisted methods of reproduction in general will be limited and that other technological innovations (e.g., modern contraceptive techniques) will have a much more significant adverse impact on the family.[41] A second kind of response, briefly developed by Leiman, is to deny that surrogate motherhood is necessarily detrimental to the family, if this novel method of becoming a parent is resorted to for good reasons (e.g., if a couple would otherwise be unable to have a child).[42]

Other potential consequences considered adverse by some expert witnesses and commentators include

a. The development of commercial ovum and embryo banks.[43]
b. The genetic selection or manipulation of early embryos.[44]
c. The transfer of nuclei from adult individuals to early embryos, or cloning.[45]
d. Extracorporeal gestation, or bringing an embryo all the way to viability in the laboratory.[46]

As noted above in Section A of the present chapter, the second and fourth consequences in this list are regarded by some commentators as potential benefits of clinical *in vitro* fertilization and embryo transfer. Few have advocated that commercial ovum and embryo banks be created or that human beings be cloned. Some commentators (for example, Gorovitz) have advanced the procedural suggestion that each potential consequence of *in vitro* fertilization and embryo transfer be carefully evaluated from the standpoint of both likelihood and probable impact. . . .[47]

CHAPTER 6

Summary and Conclusions

It is now technically possible to fertilize a human egg outside the body of a woman and then transfer the fertilized egg (sometimes called a blastocyst or preimplantation embryo) back into the woman to establish a pregnancy. For some women, *in vitro* fertilization may be the only way to bear children of their own. It does not appear, however, that the procedure for achieving pregnancy by this means is yet very effective; the best available data indicate that a number of attempts have been necessary before a pregnancy in a particular woman can be established, if at all. In addition, many questions remain as to the safety of the procedure for the offspring. Nevertheless, there is reason to believe that clinics may soon be established, both in this country and abroad, where *in vitro* fertilization and embryo transfer will be offered as "therapy" for infertile couples.

The Board is required by HEW regulations to review research proposals involving human *in vitro* fertilization and advise the Secretary as to their "acceptability from an ethical standpoint" [45 CFR 46.204(d)]. This phrase is broad enough to include at least two interpretations: (1) "clearly ethically right" or (2) "ethically defensible but still legitimately controverted." In finding that research involving human *in vitro* fertilization is "acceptable from an ethical standpoint" the Board is using the phrase in the second sense; the Board wishes to emphasize that it is *not* finding that the ethical considerations against such research are insubstantial. Indeed, concerns regarding the moral status of the embryo and the potential long-range consequences of this research were among the most difficult that confronted the Board.

In its deliberations on human *in vitro* fertilization, the Board confronted many ethical, scientific and legal issues. Among the more difficult were the following: (A) the moral status of the embryo; (B) the safety and efficacy of the procedure [by "efficacy" the Board means not only whether the procedure can be done but also how efficient it is, e.g., the number of procedures required to achieve the desired result]; (C) the potential long-range adverse effects of such research; and (D) the appropriateness of Departmental support.

A. After much analysis and discussion regarding both scientific data and the moral status of the embryo, the Board is in agreement that the human embryo is entitled to profound respect; but this respect does not necessarily encompass the full legal and moral rights attributed to persons. In addition, the Board noted the high rate of embryo loss that occurs in the natural process of reproduction. It concluded that some embryo loss associated with attempts to assist otherwise infertile couples to bear children of their own through *in vitro* fertilization may be regarded as acceptable from an ethical standpoint, under certain conditions, as more fully described below.

B. The Board is concerned about still unanswered questions of safety for both mother and offspring of *in vitro* fertilization and embryo transfer; it is concerned, as well, about the physical and mental health of the children born following such a procedure and about their legal status.

Many women have told the Board that in order to bear a child of their own they will submit to whatever risks are involved. The Board believes that while the Department should not interfere with such reproductive decisions, it has a legitimate interest in developing and disseminating information regarding safety and health so that fully informed choices about reproduction can be made.

C. A number of fears have been expressed with regard to adverse effects of technological intervention in the reproductive process: fears that such intervention might lead to genetic manipulation or encourage casual experimentation with human embryos, or bring with it the use of surrogate mothers, cloning, or the creation of genetic hybrids. Some have suggested that such research might also have a dehumanizing effect on investigators, the families involved, and society generally. (See Chapter 3 of this report.)

Although the Board recognizes that there is an opportunity for abuse in the application of this technology as [with] other technologies, it concluded that a broad prohibition of research involving human *in vitro* fertilization is neither justified nor wise. Among the developments warned against by some who testified before the Board, a few (e.g., the cloning of human beings and the creation of animal/human hybrids) are of uncertain or remote risk. Other possible developments, such as the use of surrogate mothers, may be contained by regulation or legislation. Other abuses may be avoided by the use of good judgment based upon accurate information of the type collected by the Board and now being disseminated in this report. Finally, where reproductive decisions are concerned, it is important to guard against unwarranted governmental intrusion into personal and marital privacy.

D. The question of Federal support of research involving human *in vitro* fertilization and embryo transfer was troublesome for the Board in view of the uncertain risks, the dangers of abuse and because funding the procedure is morally objectionable to many. In weighing these considerations, the Board noted that the procedures may soon be in use in the private sector and that Departmental involvement might help to resolve questions of risk and avoid abuse by encouraging well-designed research by qualified scientists. Such involvement might also help to shape the use of the procedures through regulation and by example. The Board concluded that it should not advise the Department on the level of Federal support, if any, of such research; but it concluded that Federal support, if decided upon after due consideration of all that is at issue, would be acceptable from an ethical standpoint.

Evidence presented to the Board indicates that human *in vitro* fertilization and embryo transfer techniques may, in the near future, be employed throughout the world in both research and clinical practice settings. The Board believes that data from these activities as well as related types of animal research should be collected, analyzed and, when appropriate, given wide public dissemination. Accordingly, the Board recommends in conclusion #4 below, that the Department take the primary initiative in carrying out these functions.

Having carefully weighed diverse ethical points of view and a broad base of scientific considerations regarding human *in vitro* fertilization and embryo transfer, the Board has concluded that: (1) the Department should consider support of more animal research in order to assess the risks to both mother and offspring associated with the procedures; (2) the conduct of research involving human *in vitro* fertilization designed to establish the safety and effectiveness of the procedures is ethically acceptable under certain conditions; (3) Departmental support of such research would be acceptable from an ethical standpoint, although the Board did not address the question of the level of funding, if any, which such research might be given; (4) the Department should take the initiative in collecting, analyzing and disseminating data from both research and clinical practice involving *in vitro* fertilization throughout the world; and (5) model or uniform laws should be developed to define the rights and responsibilities of all parties involved in such activities.

Finally, the Board is aware of the possibility of research that involves the collection and culture of early human embryos in the laboratory which have been fertilized naturally rather than *in vitro*. The ethical aspects of such research, which appears to bear a close resemblance to research involving *in vitro* fertilization, have not been examined by the Board. Therefore it has not reached a conclusion concerning the ethical acceptability of these procedures. However, the Board intends to consider in the near future the need for setting standards for such research.

Conclusion 1

The department should consider support of carefully designed research involving *in vitro* fertilization and embryo transfer in animals, including nonhuman primates, in order to obtain a better understanding of the process of fertilization, implantation and embryo development, to assess the risks to both mother and offspring associated with such procedures, and to improve the efficacy of the procedure.

DISCUSSION

As indicated in Chapter 3 of the Board's report, available scientific data do not indicate clearly either the relative safety or the efficacy of procedures of *in vitro* fertilization and embryo transfer. Some scientists have suggested that *in vitro* fertilization may result in a higher incidence of abnormal embryos than is associated with the normal reproductive process, although there are no animal data that clearly demonstrate such an effect. Neither are there data that demonstrate an absence of increased abnormality in embryos following *in vitro* fertilization. The Board feels that additional data should be gathered that might indicate whether abnormal embryos are more likely to result and, if so, whether there is a significant increase in the risk of abnormal offspring actually being born following such procedures.

Experts appearing before the Board agreed that there has been insufficient controlled animal research designed to determine the long-range effects of *in vitro* fertilization and embryo transfer. The lack of primate work is particularly noteworthy in view of the opportunity provided by primate models for assessing subtle neurological, cognitive and developmental effects of such procedures. The Board has been advised that controlled studies of embryo transfer following *in vitro* fertilization in animals, designed to include developmental assessments, may be feasible and may permit more confident estimates of the risk to human offspring associated with such procedures.

Information regarding the effectiveness of the procedures for *in vitro* fertilization and embryo transfer is also lacking. It does not appear possible to predict with reliability the number of laparoscopies and embryo transfers that might be required, or the likelihood of success of the procedure for any couple, given the fact that, to date, only three successes have been reported in humans, and that very limited information is available concerning this work. Such data as are available suggest that any woman hoping to bear a child through *in vitro* fertilization is likely to face numerous unsuccessful procedures and delays with no assurance of achieving her goal.

Careful research with animal models might provide a more accurate estimate of the chances of achieving a successful pregnancy. It might also reduce the inconvenience and risk to women of undergoing multiple procedures to establish a pregnancy by improving techniques for recovering ova, identifying embryonic abnormalities and achieving implantation. It is often the case in medicine that, even after therapies are already being applied to humans, investigations continue in animals in order to test further or to improve their safety and effectiveness. The Board believes that the Department should consider support of well-designed animal studies whether or not human research or clinical trials are also in progress.

Conclusion 2

The Ethics Advisory Board finds that it is acceptable from an ethical standpoint to undertake research involving human *in vitro* fertilization and embryo transfer provided that

A. If the research involves human *in vitro* fertilization without embryo transfer, the following conditions are satisfied:

1. The research complies with all appropriate provisions of the regulations governing research with human subjects (45 cfr 46);
2. The research is designed primarily: (a) to establish the safety and efficacy of embryo transfer and (b) to obtain important scientific information toward that end not reasonably attainable by other means;
3. Human gametes used in such research will be obtained exclusively from persons who have been informed of the nature and purpose of the research in which such materials will be used and have specifically consented to such use;
4. No embryos will be sustained *in vitro* beyond the stage normally associated with the completion of implantation (14 days after fertilization); and
5. All interested parties and the general public will be advised if evidence begins to show that the procedure entails risks of abnormal offspring higher than those associated with natural human reproduction.

B. In addition, if the research involves embryo transfer following human *in vitro* fertilization, embryo transfer will be attempted only with gametes obtained from lawfully married couples.

DISCUSSION

This conclusion relates to the ethics of conducting research involving *in vitro* fertilization in general; it does not address the question of Departmental support of such research. The purpose of this more general conclusion is to provide guidance to Institutional Review Boards and other groups who are asked to review research that will not be supported by HEW. Whether or not the Department decides to provide funds for such research, the Board wishes to express its views regarding the conduct of human *in vitro* fertilization and embryo transfer, so that review groups may benefit from the deliberations of the Board as they conduct their own review of specific research proposals.

As emphasized above, the Board believes that much remains to be learned about the safety and effectiveness of these procedures before they can be considered standard, accepted medical practice. Research designed to provide reliable data regarding safety and efficacy is acceptable from an ethical standpoint if conducted within the constraints indicated above. In the case of research involving embryo transfer, the Board intends not only that the gametes be obtained from lawfully married couples but also that the embryo be transferred back to the wife whose ova were used for fertilization.

The Board also discussed research designed primarily to establish safety and efficacy but which may, in addition, obtain information of scientific importance unrelated to *in vitro* fertilization and embryo transfer. The Board believes that such research, if performed as a corollary to research designed primarily to establish safety and efficacy of *in vitro* fertilization and embryo transfer, would also be acceptable from an ethical standpoint.

Conclusion 3

The Board finds it acceptable from an ethical standpoint for the department to support or conduct research involving human *in vitro* fertilization and embryo transfer, provided that the applicable conditions set forth in Conclusion 2 are met. However, the board has decided not to address the question of the level of funding, if any, which such research might be given.

DISCUSSION

1. *Departmental support.* The Board consciously adopted the language "acceptable from an ethical standpoint" to indicate the limits of its inquiry. Even though the members are aware that ethical considerations pervade decisions regarding the level, if any, of Departmental support of human *in vitro* fertilization, the Board has concluded that it lacks the resources needed to render meaningful advice with respect to such decisions. The Board, therefore, defers to established political, scientific and administrative procedures for allocating public research funds.

The Board wishes to note that such decisions have significant ethical dimensions. For example, some believe that research involving human *in vitro* fertilization should have a relatively low priority at a time when other health needs, arguably more basic in character and long-term in nature, are unmet. Others find such research objectionable either on grounds related to the moral status of the embryo or because it may lead to undesirable genetic interventions or have a long-range adverse effect. (See Chapter 3 of this report.) Still others believe that research on human *in vitro* fertilization and embryo transfer should have a high priority because it might help parents overcome physical obstacles to having their own children and ensure the mothers' safety and the normality of offspring.

The Board has found that these and other ethical arguments for and against public funding of research involving human *in vitro* fertilization, by themselves, are not conclusive. Instead, the Board believes that the questions of whether to fund and at what level should be made in the larger context where all relevant data and arguments—scientific, political, economic, legal and ethical—can be considered. In that context questions such as health and safety, availability of funds, and alternative research proposals, must be considered along with the very difficult type of ethical issues described above which arise in allocation of resources.

2. *Research without embryo transfer.* As previously noted the risks of producing abnormal offspring are still undetermined; therefore, an important goal would be to gain as much information as possible from well-designed research on *in vitro* fertilization not involving embryo transfer in humans. The Department should conduct a careful scientific evaluation of the possibility, supported by some expert testimony before the Board, that animal research and studies involving human *in vitro* fertilization without embryo transfer, over a relatively short period, might substantially increase our knowledge concerning the possible risk of abnormal offspring as well as lead to the development of safe and more effective techniques.

3. *Research involving embryo transfer.* While initial research efforts designed to gain as much information as possible from animal studies and human research not involving embryo transfer may be desirable, the Board does not wish to discourage planning and preparation that may lead to clinical trials or other forms of research involving embryo transfer. The Department's participation in, or support of, clinical trials is often an effective method to evaluate the safety and efficacy of innovative medical procedures, particularly as the use of the procedures increases.

4. *Research for other purposes.* Potentially valuable information about reproductive biology, the etiology of birth defects, and other subjects may be revealed through research involving human *in vitro* fertilization, without embryo transfer, and unrelated to the safety and efficacy of procedures for overcoming infertility. The Board makes no judgment at this time regarding the ethical acceptability of such research nor does it speculate about what research might be sufficiently compelling to justify the use of human embryos. Instead, it notes that applications for support of such research should be submitted to the Board for ethical review in accordance with 45 CFR 46.204(d).

5. *Pending research application.* Given the criteria specified in Conclusion 2 and incorporated in Conclusion 3 for evaluating research involving human *in vitro* fertilization, and the Board's views about Departmental support of such research, the Board recommends that the Secretary refer the pending application of Vanderbilt University back to the National Institutes of Health for a determination as to whether the proposal meets those criteria and for further review in light of the considerations set forth in this report.

Conclusion 4

The National Institute of Child Health and Human Development (NICHD) and other appropriate agencies should work with professional societies, foreign governments and international organizations to collect, analyze and disseminate information derived from research (in both animals and humans) and clinical experience throughout the world involving *in vitro* fertilization and embryo transfer.

DISCUSSION

The Board is aware that the most valuable information regarding *in vitro* fertilization and embryo transfer is likely to come from well-controlled clinical trials. But it is expected that *in vitro* fertilization and embryo transfer will soon be performed in clinics throughout the world, sometimes without benefit of research design or experimental controls. It would be unfortunate not to have access to the information that might be gained from such clinical experience, notwithstanding the fact that well-designed investigations would be preferable. With that in mind, the Board recommends that every effort be made to collect whatever information may be elicited from practitioners in this country and abroad. NICHD should also consider suggesting to practitioners a basic protocol for collecting vital information, to which each would be encouraged to add their own observations.

The data from such clinical experience and from research conducted throughout the world should be analyzed along with that derived from animal studies so that individuals contemplating *in vitro* fertilization and embryo transfer will have access to the best information available regarding risks to both mother and offspring. Timely dissemination of the information would increase the opportunity for investigators, clinicians and prospective patients to be fully informed.

Conclusion 5

The secretary should encourage the development of a uniform or model law to clarify the legal status of children born as a result of *in vitro* fertilization and embryo transfer. To the extent that funds may be necessary to develop such legislation, the Department should consider providing appropriate support.

DISCUSSION

The Board is concerned about the ambiguity regarding the legal status of children born following artificial insemination and a similar ambiguity that may surround the legal status of children born following *in vitro* fertilization and embryo transfer. The Board is also concerned about lack of clarity regarding the legal responsibilities of those who utilize, support, or permit use of such procedures. Because of the complexity of the legal problems involved in new techniques for human reproduction, the Board recommends that a model or uniform law be drafted that would establish with clarity the rights and responsibilities of donor and recipient "parents," of offspring, and of those who participate in the process of reproduction through new technologies.

The Board urges that such a uniform or model law be drafted by the National Conference of Commissioners on Uniform State Laws, the American Law Institute, or some other qualified body. Because of the complex nature of the subject matter, however, the Board is aware that the task may be a major undertaking and suggests that the Department consider providing funds for drafting the legislation. Since the purpose is to safeguard the health and welfare of children and their families, it appears to be an appropriate project for Departmental support.

NOTES

Notes to Chapter 2

1. Short, R.V., "Human *In Vitro* Fertilization and Embryo Transfer," a paper prepared for the Ethics Advisory Board, 1978, pp. 2–3; Mastroianni, Luigi, Jr., "*In Vitro* Fertilization and Embryo Transfer," a paper prepared for the Ethics Advisory Board, 1978, p. 5.
2. Short, op. cit., pp. 3–5; Mastroianni, op. cit., p. 5.
3. Short, op. cit., pp. 5–6.
4. Mastroianni, op. cit., p. 5.
5. Ibid.
6. Ibid.
7. Short, op. cit., pp. 6–7.
8. Ibid., pp. 8–10.
9. Schlesselman, James J., "How Does One Assess the Risk of Abnormalities from Human *In Vitro* Fertilization?," a paper prepared for the Ethics Advisory Board, 1979, p. 17; cf. Biggers, John D., "*In Vitro* Fertilization, Embryo Culture and Embryo Transfer in the Human," a paper prepared for the Ethics Advisory Board, 1978, p. 6 and Appendix I, Table 3.
10. Schlesselman, op. cit., pp. 7–8, citing, Boue, J.G. and Boue, A., "Chromosomal Anomalies in Early Spontaneous Abortion," *Current Topics in Pathology*, vol. 62, 1976, pp. 193–208; Creasy, M.R., Crolla, J.A., and Alberman, E.D., "A Cytogenetic Study of Human Spontaneous Abortions Using Banding Techniques," *Humangenetik*, vol. 31, 1976, pp. 177–196; Alberman, E.D. and Creasy, M.R., "Frequency of Chromosomal Abnormalities in Miscarriages and Perinatal Deaths," *Journal of Medical Genetics*, vol. 14, 1977, pp. 313–315.
11. Schlesselman, op. cit., p. 19.
12. Short, op. cit., p. 10; cf. Schlesselman, op. cit., pp. 24–25.
13. Schlesselman, op. cit., p. 30.
14. Biggers, op. cit., p. 412; cf. Kass, Leon R., "Ethical Issues in Human *In Vitro* Fertilization, Embryo Culture and Research, and Embryo Transfer," a paper prepared for the Ethics Advisory Board, 1978, p. 27.
15. Walters, LeRoy, "Ethical Issues in Human *In Vitro* Fertilization and Research Involving Early Human Embryos," a paper prepared for the Ethics Advisory Board, 1978, fn. 178, citing Mastroianni, Luigi, Jr., *In Vitro* Fertilization, in: Reich, Warren, ed., *Encyclopedia of Bioethics*, (vol. 4), New York, Free Press-Macmillan, 1978, pp. 1448–1451.

16. Biggers, op. cit., p. 41a.
17. Schlesselman, op. cit., pp. 20–27.
18. Short, op. cit., p. 9; cf. Walters, op. cit., pp. 37–38.
19. Walters, op. cit., fn. 182, citing National Research Council, Assembly of Behavioral and Social Sciences, Committee on the Life Sciences and Social Policy, *Assessing Biomedical Technologies: An Inquiry into the Nature of the Process*, Washington, D.C., National Academy of Sciences, 1975, p. 27.
20. Ibid.
21. Holder, Angela R. and Levine, Robert J., "Informed Consent for Research on Specimens Obtained at Autopsy or Surgery: A Case Study in the Overprotection of Human Subjects," *Clinical Research*, vol. 24, 1976, pp. 68–77.
22. Kass, op. cit., fn. 14, p. 28.
23. Ibid., p. 5.
24. Ibid., pp. 10–11.
25. Ibid., p. 11.
26. Curran, Charles E., "*In Vitro* Fertilization and Embryo Transfer: From a Perspective of Moral Theology," a paper prepared for the Ethics Advisory Board, 1978, p. 22.
27. Ibid., p. 26.
28. Grobstein, Clifford, Statement to the Ethics Advisory Board, Transcript of Meeting III, September 15, 1978, *National Technical Information Service*, PB-288 764, p. 229.
29. Gorovitz, Samuel, "*In Vitro* Fertilization: Sense and Nonsense," a paper prepared for the Ethics Advisory Board, 1979, p. 28.
30. Williams, John W., *Williams Obstetrics*, Pritchard, Jack A. and MacDonald, Paul C., eds., 14th ed., New York, Appleton-Century-Crofts, 1971, p. 223.
31. Gorovitz, op. cit., p. 28.
32. Ibid., pp. 1–4.
33. Kass, op. cit., pp. 5–7.
34. Ibid., pp. 18–19.
35. Ibid., p. 20.
36. Gorovitz, op. cit., pp. 27–28.
37. Ibid., p. 15.
38. Short, op. cit., p. 7.
39. Kass, op. cit., p. 19.
40. Walters, op. cit., pp. 39–40.
41. Gorovitz, op. cit., p. 14.
42. Kass, Leon, "Making Babies—the New Biology and the 'Old' Morality," *Public Interest*, vol. 26, 1972, p. 33.

Notes to Chapter 3

1. Kass, Leon R., "Ethical Issues in Human *In Vitro* Fertilization, Embryo Culture and Research, and Embryo Transfer," a paper prepared for the Ethics Advisory Board, 1978, pp. 13–14; Leiman, Sid Z., Statement to the Ethics Advisory Board, Transcript of Meeting V, November 10, 1978, *National Technical Information Service*, PB-288 405, p. 130.
2. Hauerwas, Stanley, "Theological Reflections on *In Vitro* Fertilization," a paper prepared for the Ethics Advisory Board, 1978, pp. 6–12.
3. Biggers, John D., "*In Vitro* Fertilization, Embryo Culture and Embryo Transfer in the Human," a paper prepared for the Ethics Advisory Board, 1978, p. 35.
4. Biggers, op. cit., p. 36 and Table 4, p. 37, citing Shane, J.M., Schiff, I., and Wilson, E.A., "The Infertile Couple," *Clinical Symposia*, vol. 28, 1976, pp. 1–40.
5. Biggers, op. cit., p. 35; Kass, op. cit., pp. 36–37.
6. Leiman, op. cit., pp. 126–130.
7. Walters, LeRoy, "Ethical Issues in Human *In Vitro* Fertilization and Research Involving Early Human Embryos," a paper prepared for the Ethics Advisory Board, 1978, fn. 112, citing Edwards, R.G., "Fertilization of Human Eggs *In Vitro*: Morals, Ethics, and the Law," *Quarterly Review of Biology*, vol. 49, 1974, p. 12.
8. Walters, op. cit., fn. 113, citing Karp, Laurence E. and Donahue, Roger P., "Preimplantational Ectogenesis: Science and Speculation Concerning *In Vitro* Fertilization and Related Procedures," *Western Journal of Medicine*, vol. 124, 1976, p. 295.
9. Walters, op. cit., fn. 115, citing Sinshiemer, Robert L., "Prospects for Future Scientific Developments: Ambush or Opportunity," in Hilton, Bruce et al., eds., *Ethical Issues in Human Genetics: Genetic Counseling and the Use of Genetic Knowledge*, New York, Plenum Press, 1973, pp. 346–348.
10. Walters, op. cit., fn. 118, citing Fletcher, Joseph, *The Ethics of Genetic Control: Ending Reproductive Roulette*, Garden City, N.Y., Anchor Press/Doubleday, 1974, pp. 163–165.
11. See Chapter 1 of this report, pp. 9–10.
12. Short, op. cit., p. 8; Foote, R.H., "*In Vitro* Fertilization in Perspective, Relative to the Science and Art of Domestic Animal Reproduction," a paper prepared for the Ethics Advisory Board, 1978, p. 17.
13. Biggers, op. cit., p. 34.
14. Biggers, op. cit., p. 34, citing Boue, J.G. and Boue, A., "Increased Frequency of Chromosomal Anomalies in Abortions After Induced Ovulation," *Lancet*, vol. i, 1973, p. 679.
15. Biggers, op. cit., p. 33, citing Ahlgren, M., "Sperm Transport to and Survival in the Human Fallopian Tube," *Gynecologic Investigation*, vol. 6, 1975, pp. 206–214.
16. Biggers, op. cit., p. 33, citing Fraser, L.R., Zenellotti, H.M., Paton, G.R. and Drury, L.M., "Increased Incidence of Triploidy in Embryos Derived from Mouse Eggs Fertilized *In Vitro*," *Nature*, vol. 260, 1976, pp. 39–40; Fraser, L.R., and Maudlin, I., "Relationship Between Sperm Concentration and the Incidence of Polyspermy in Mouse Embryos Fertilized *In Vitro*," *Journal of Reproduction and Fertility*, vol. 52, 1978, pp. 103–106.
17. Biggers, op. cit., p. 34.
18. Schlesselman, op. cit., pp. 29–31.
19. Kass, op. cit., 1978, p. 12.
20. Curran, Charles E., "*In Vitro* Fertilization and Embryo Transfer: From a Perspective of Moral Theology," a paper prepared for the Ethics Advisory Board, 1978, p. 19.
21. Biggers, Statement to the Ethics Advisory Board, op. cit., pp. 261–263; see also Shulman, Joseph, Testimony for the Ethics Advisory Board, 1978, p. 3.
22. Gould, op. cit., p. 17; Mastroianni, op. cit., p. 3.
23. Gould, op. cit., pp. 17–18.
24. Ibid., pp. 18–19.
25. Ibid., p. 19.
26. Schlesselman, op. cit., pp. 29–31.

27. Gould, op. cit., p. 17; Edwards, op. cit., p. 8; Mastroianni, Luigi, Jr., "*In Vitro* Fertilization," in Reich, Warren, ed., *Encyclopedia of Bioethics*, vol. 4, New York, Free Press-Macmillan, 1978, pp. 1448–1451.
28. Kass, Leon, "Making Babies—the New Biology and the 'Old' Morality," *Public Interest*, vol. 26, 1972, p. 31.
29. Items (b) through (d) are enumerated in National Research Council, Assembly of Behavioral and Social Sciences, Committee on the Life Sciences and Social Policy, *Assessing Biomedical Technologies: An Inquiry into the Nature of the Process*, Washington, D.C., National Academy of Sciences, 1975, p. 21.
30. British Medical Association, Board of Science and Education Panel, *Professional Standards*, London, British Medical Association, 1972, p. 10.
31. National Research Council, op. cit., pp. 21, 27.
32. Mastroianni, Luigi, Jr., "*In Vitro* Fertilization of Human Ova and Blastocyst Transfer: An Invitational Symposium," in: Schumacher, Gebhard, F., et al., *Journal of Reproductive Medicine*, vol. 11, 1973, p. 197; National Research Council, op. cit., 1975, p. 21.
33. Edwards, op. cit., p. 11.
34. Kass, op. cit., pp. 9–10.
35. Ibid., p. 10.
36. Ibid., pp. 9–11.
37. Curran, op. cit., pp. 17, 26.
38. Kass, op. cit., 1972, p. 34; Leiman, op. cit., p. 126.
39. Kass, op. cit., 1978, p. 15.
40. Ibid.
41. Gorovitz, op. cit., pp. 20–21.
42. Leiman, op. cit., pp. 128–129.
43. Kass, op. cit., 1978, p. 19.
44. Walters, op. cit., fn. 113 (see fn. 9 above).
45. Ibid.
46. Ibid, fn. 118 (see fn. 10 above).
47. Gorovitz, op. cit., pp. 14–15.

HUMAN FETAL TISSUE TRANSPLANTATION RESEARCH PANEL: NATIONAL INSTITUTES OF HEALTH, 1988

INTRODUCTION. *In the late 1980s, scientific reports began to appear suggesting that (1) the transplantation of tissue taken from the brains of aborted human fetuses might prove therapeutic for Parkinson's Disease, and (2) the transplantation of fetal pancreatic tissue might help persons afflicted with Insulin Dependent Diabetes. Tissue for use in this research—and for research related to the development of new vaccines—derives from fetuses that are deliberatively or spontaneously aborted. However, the Reagan and Bush administrations had banned federal support for transplantation research (though not for other fetal tissue research) if the researchers were using fetal tissue derived from deliberate abortions. Following a 1988 request for federal support of this research, the Assistant Secretary for Health requested the establishment of an outside advisory committee to "consider whether this kind of research should be performed and if so, under what circumstances." A committee called the Human Fetal Tissue Transplantation Research Panel was subsequently appointed as an ad hoc consultation to the Advisory Committee to the Director, National Institutes of Health; and charged to review the "legal, scientific, and ethical issues surrounding the use of fetal tissue derived from induced abortions in transplantation research." The Panel presented its report to the NIH on December 14, 1988. The Advisory Committee to the Director unanimously accepted its report and recommendations. The Director, however, declined to accept its recommendations.*

QUESTION 1. Is an induced abortion of moral relevance to the decision to use human fetal tissue for research? Would the answer to this question provide any insight on whether and how this research should proceed?

Response to Question 1

It is of moral relevance that human fetal tissue for research has been obtained from induced abortions. However, in light of the fact that abortion is legal and that the research in question is intended to achieve significant medical goals, the panel concludes that the use of such tissue is acceptable public policy.

This position must not obscure the profound moral dimensions of the issue of abortion, nor the principled positions that divide scholars, scientists, and the public at large. It is not the charge of this panel to attempt to settle the issue of abortion or to weigh the worthiness of competing principled perspectives on abortion itself. The panel notes that induced abortion creates a set of morally relevant considerations, but notes further that the possibility of relieving suffering and saving life cannot be a matter of moral indifference to those who shape and guide public policy.

Recognizing the moral convictions deeply held in our society, the panel concludes that appropriate guidelines are required even as the research proceeds. Accordingly, the following points are noted:

Reprinted from Human Fetal Tissue Transplantation Research Panel, Report of the Human Fetal Tissue Transplantation Research Panel. 2 vols. (Bethesda, MD: National Institutes of Health, 1988).

1. The decision to terminate a pregnancy and the procedures of abortion should be kept independent from the retrieval and use of fetal tissue.
2. Payments and other forms of remuneration and compensation associated with the procurement of fetal tissue should be prohibited, except payment for reasonable expenses occasioned by the actual retrieval, storage, preparation, and transportation of the tissues.
3. Potential recipients of such tissues, as well as research and health care participants, should be properly informed as to the source of the tissues in question.
4. Procedures must be adopted that accord human fetal tissue the same respect accorded other cadaveric human tissues entitled to respect.

[Panel Vote: 18 Yes, 3 No, 0 Abstain]

Considerations for Question 1

In reaching its answer to the first question, the panel weighed the proposition that the morality of abortion could be separated in principle from the morality of the uses to which fetal tissue from induced abortions might be put. It was noted that fetal tissue would be obtained as a result of lawful, constitutionally protected decisions and actions to terminate unwanted pregnancy, and that use of cadaveric fetal tissue from induced abortions for research or therapy was generally legal. But it was also noted that the lawfulness of decisions and actions can be distinguished from their morality.

On the morality of research use of fetal tissue from induced abortion, three positions were discussed during the panel's deliberations.

1. Abortion is morally acceptable, and thus the research and therapeutic use of fetal tissue derived from induced abortion is also morally acceptable.
2. Abortion is immoral and so is the use of fetal tissue obtained thereby. No amount of good achieved in research or therapy could erase institutional complicity in the immorality of abortion itself or in encouragement of future abortions. No efforts at separating the procurement and use of fetal tissue from the abortion decision and procedure could make the use of fetal tissue from induced abortion morally acceptable.
3. Abortion is immoral or undesirable, but as abortion is a legal procedure in our society and with appropriate safeguards can be separated from the subsequent research use of tissue derived therefrom, the use of fetal tissue in research and therapy is not seen as complicitous with the immorality of abortion.

A decisive majority of the panel found that it was acceptable public policy to support transplant research with fetal tissue either because the source of the tissue posed no moral problem or because the immorality of its source could be ethically isolated from the morality of its use in research. Considerations supporting this decision were the fact that these abortions would occur regardless of their use in research, that neither the researcher nor the recipient would have any role in inducing or performing the abortion, and that a woman's abortion decision would be insulated from inducements to abort to provide tissue for transplant research and therapy. Accordingly, the panel found it essential that abortion decisions and procedures be kept separate from considerations of fetal tissue procurement and use in research and therapy. In keeping with that separation, it is essential that there be no offer of financial incentives or personal gain to encourage abortion or donation of fetal tissue.

Because some persons opposed to abortion would not accept the use of fetal tissue from induced abortions regardless of these insulating measures, the interests of those persons in neither participating in the research nor in receiving fetal tissue transplants should be protected by informing them of the source of such tissue.

The majority's approval of the research use of tissue from elective abortions is not to be construed as a majority vote for the moral acceptability of elective abortion.

QUESTION 2. Does the use of the fetal tissue in research encourage women to have an abortion that they might otherwise not undertake? If so, are there ways to minimize such encouragement?

Response to Question 2

Research using fetal tissue has been conducted and publicized for over 30 years. There is no evidence that this use of fetal tissue for research has had a material effect on the reasons for seeking an abortion in the past. Some panel members were concerned that a more publicized and promising research program might have such an effect in the future. To minimize any encouragement for abortion as might arise from the use of fetal tissue in research, we recommend that the measures outlined above under Question 1 be implemented, as well as the following:

- The decision and consent to abort must precede discussion of the possible use of the fetal tissue and any request for such consent as might be required for that use.
- The pregnant woman should be prohibited from designating the transplant-recipient of the fetal tissue.

The foregoing recommendations are not to be construed as denying or in any way impeding a pregnant woman's access to information regarding the use of fetal tissue in research should she request this information.

[Panel Vote: 19 Yes, 1 No, 1 Abstain]

Considerations for Question 2

The panel noted that the reasons for terminating a pregnancy are complex, varied, and deeply personal. The panel regarded it highly unlikely that a woman would be encouraged to make this decision because of the knowledge that the fetal remains might be used in research.

The panel concluded further that it was sound public policy to separate as much as possible the deliberations and decisions about the abortion from any discussion of the disposition of the fetal remains.

QUESTION 3. As a legal matter, does the very process of obtaining informed consent from the pregnant woman constitute a prohibited "inducement" to terminate the pregnancy for the purposes of the research—thus precluding research of this sort, under HHS regulations?

Response to Question 3

The panel agrees that a pregnant woman should not be induced to terminate pregnancy in order to furnish fetal tissue for transplantation or medical research.

The process for obtaining informed consent from a pregnant woman for fetal tissue research does not by itself constitute a prohibited inducement to terminate the pregnancy for the purposes of research. However, knowledge of the possibility for using fetal tissue in research and transplantation might constitute motivation, reason, or incentive for a pregnant woman to have an abortion. This would not constitute a prohibited "inducement," since it is not a promise of financial reward or personal gain, nor is it coercive.

However, because the panel believes strongly that we should keep transplantation and research on fetal tissue from encouraging abortion, the panel recommends that informed consent for an abortion should precede informed consent or even the provision of preliminary information for tissue donation.

Moreover, anonymity between donor and recipient shall be maintained, so that the donor does not know who will receive the tissue, and the identity of the donor is concealed from the recipient and transplant team.

Further, the timing and method of abortion should not be influenced by the potential uses of fetal tissue for transplantation or medical research.

In the long term, the problem alluded to by this question may be able to be addressed by deferring the discussion of possible tissue donation until after the abortion procedure has been performed. The feasibility of this approach to fetal tissue procurement should be reviewed on a regular basis by the Department.

[Panel Vote: 20 Yes, 0 No, 1 Abstain]

Considerations for Question 3

As a preliminary matter, we assume that the informed consent mentioned in the question refers to the consent sought for the purpose of using the fetal tissue in research—as distinguished from the informed consent for the abortion itself. As we have emphasized in several places, in the consent process for termination of pregnancy, we believe there should be no mention at all of the possibility of fetal tissue use in transplantation and research. The one exception might be if the pregnant woman were to ask a direct question. And even then only general information should be given; there should be no promise that her fetal tissue either could or would be so used. Panel members individually take this stand either because they do not want to do anything that might encourage abortion or as a concession to those who do not want to risk encouraging abortion.

The heart of the question pivots on the meaning of "prohibited 'inducement.'" It is not clear which inducements are in fact prohibited by Department of Health and Human Services (HHS) regulations nor is it clear exactly what an inducement is. Therefore, some clarifications are in order to determine what would be a reasonable and defensible position in the matter.

An inducement could be a coercion, an incentive, or a reason. (1) Coercion is in any case unacceptable and would surely be prohibited. In order for consent to be valid it must at least be free, voluntary, and informed. (2) We would also find incentives to be unacceptable inasmuch as our panel recommends at every turn that we should (for reasons articulated elsewhere) keep fetal tissue transplantation and research from encouraging abortion. Also, incentives to terminate a pregnancy would probably be prohibited under HHS regulations, though it might turn on how strong, i.e., how irresistible, the incentive was. (3) However, with respect to reasons, it would be unrealistic not to consider the possibility that transplantation and research with fetal tissue may enter the balance of considerations of a pregnant woman in deciding whether to have an abortion. It would be unrealistic because transplantation and research with fetal tissue will become general knowledge; it will not be possible to keep the populace from knowing about it.

By no reasonable interpretation can sheer information constitute a "prohibited 'inducement.'" The point of labeling some inducements as prohibited is to avoid manipulation of persons by coercion (a threat of harm) or by incentives (the promise of personal gain) unrelated to the risks, harms, and benefits of the act itself. Thus, that fetal tissue could benefit others might be one of many reasons to be weighed in deciding whether to terminate a pregnancy. We clearly would be unable to keep such knowledge from functioning as a reason, and in any case it does not and should not be construed to constitute a "prohibited 'inducement.'"

QUESTION 4. Is maternal consent a sufficient condition for the use of the tissue, or should additional consent be obtained? If so, what should be the substance and who should be the source(s) of the consent, and what procedures should be implemented to obtain it?

Response to Question 4

Fetal tissue from induced abortions should not be used in medical research without the prior consent of the pregnant woman. Her decision to donate fetal remains is sufficient for the use of tissue, unless the father objects (except in cases of incest or rape).

The consent should be obtained in compliance with State law and with the Uniform Anatomical Gift Act.

Customary review procedures should apply to research involving transplantation of tissue from induced abortions.

[Panel Vote: 17 Yes, 3 No, 1 Abstain]

Considerations for Question 4

There are several possible ways to transfer or acquire any human tissue: donation (express or presumed), abandonment, sales, and expropriation. Although each method of transfer has been used for some human biological materials in some contexts in the United States, our society has largely adopted express donation—by the decedent while alive or by the next of kin after his or her death—as the method of transfer of cadaver organs and tissues. In cases where the decedent while alive could not or did not express his or her wishes about donation, the Uniform Anatomical Gift Act (UAGA) allows express donation by the next of kin. Presumed donation (or presumed consent) is used in 12 States for the removal of corneas; the donation of corneas by the decedent and next of kin is presumed to have been made if there is no express objection. The panel believes that express donation by the pregnant woman after the abortion decision is the most appropriate mode of transfer of fetal tissues because it is the most congruent with our society's traditions, laws, policies, and practices, including the Uniform Anatomical Gift Act and current Federal research regulations.

When a woman chooses a legal abortion for her own reasons, that act does not legally disqualify her—and should not disqualify her—as the primary decisionmaker about the disposition of fetal remains, including the donation of fetal tissue for research. Objections to this conclusion are grounded in the assumption that the decision to abort severs kinship in any but the biological sense. Nonetheless, the panel concludes that disputes about the morality of her decision to have an abortion should not deprive the woman of the legal authority to dispose of fetal remains. She still has a special connection with the fetus, and she has a legitimate interest in its disposition and use. Furthermore, the dead fetus has no interests that the pregnant woman's donation would violate. In the final analysis, any mode of transfer of fetal tissue other than maternal donation appears to raise more serious ethical problems. For all these reasons, the pregnant woman's consent, or decision to donate, should be sufficient (within the limits identified below). The panel heard no compelling reasons why federally funded transplantation research should depart from ordinary and legal practice in the disposition and use of cadaver tissues, including fetal cadaver tissues.

However, questions have been raised about whether additional consent is needed from other parties, such as the father or a hospital ethics committee or an institutional review board. We believe that the structure provided by the UAGA (revised 1987) is generally adequate but that a modification in policy is needed for the donation of fetal tissue. Where the decedent did not express his or her wishes, the UAGA authorizes "either parent of the decedent" to make a donation, unless there is a known objection to such a donation from the other parent (or from the decedent's spouse or adult children). As applied to the donation of fetal tissue, the UAGA provides that either parent may donate unless there is a known objection by the other parent. In the panel's view, the pregnant woman's consent should be *necessary* for donation—that is, the father should not be able to authorize the donation by himself, and the mother should always be asked before the fetal tissue is used. In addition, her consent or donation should be *sufficient*, except where the procurement team knows of the father's objection to such donation. There is no legal or ethical obligation to seek the father's permission, but there is a legal and ethical obligation not to use the tissue if it is known that he objects (unless the pregnancy resulted from rape or incest).

Review procedures have been developed for federally funded research involving human subjects. These review procedures would also apply to fetal tissue transplantation research, which must be reviewed and approved by Institutional Review Boards (IRBs) before it can proceed. Such research would fall under the purview of IRBs because human subjects would receive experimental transplants of fetal tissue in a research protocol. In addition, IRBs will need to consider the adequacy of the information disclosed to the pregnant woman who is considering whether to consent to tests (e.g., for antibody to the human immunodeficiency virus) to determine the acceptability of the fetal tissue for transplantation research. Nevertheless, the pregnant woman's consent to donate the tissue is legally sufficient and should be sufficient in federally funded transplantation research, as long as there is no known objection from the father (except in cases of rape or incest).

QUESTION 5. Should there be and could there be a prohibition on the donation of fetal tissue between family members, or friends and acquaintances? Would a prohibition on donation between family members jeopardize the likelihood of clinical success?

Response to Question 5

There should be no Federal funding of experimental transplants performed with fetal tissue from induced abortions provided by a family member, friend, or acquaintance. Absent such prohibition, the potential benefits to friends and family members might encourage abortion or encourage pregnancy for the purpose of abortion—encouragements that the panel strongly opposed.

Concerns regarding maternal welfare as well as the moral status of the human fetus and, therefore, the morality of abortion itself, militate against Federal practices or policies that could have the effect of in any way encouraging abortions for the purpose of benefiting family members or acquaintances.

There is no evidence now that a prohibition against the intrafamilial use of fetal tissue would affect the attainment of valid clinical objectives. Given the current state of scientific knowledge, the treatment of diabetes with intrafamilial transplants would be contraindicated. For other conditions that are considered to be candidates for fetal tissue transplantation, currently available scientific evidence allows no definitive conclusions to be drawn with respect to this question.

[Panel Vote: 19 Yes, 0 No, 1 Abstain (Note: One panel member was out of the room when this vote was taken.)]

Considerations for Question 5

There was no plea from the scientists for doing intrafamilial transplantation. In fact, the experts gave testimony that there ought to be a prohibition. If circumstances change, however, there may be reasons to modify the prohibition.

The panel did not hear any compelling evidence that suggests that a relationship between the donor and the fetus would improve the likelihood of success. Repeatedly, testimony of the experts emphasized the lack of scientific justification for intrafamilial donation by reason of current state of knowledge of immunology and disease pathophysiology. In fact, some argued that relatedness may induce the potential for disease recurrence, e.g., diabetes mellitus. It was strongly urged that the Secretary for Health and Human Services review these recommendations at regular intervals.

QUESTION 6. If transplantation using fetal tissue from induced abortions becomes more common, what impact is likely to occur on activities and procedures employed by abortion clinics? In particular, is the optimal or safest way to perform an abortion likely to be in conflict with preservation of the fetal tissue? Is there any way to ensure that induced abortions are not intentionally delayed in order to have a second trimester fetus for research and transplantation?

Response to Question 6

If fetal tissue transplants become more common, the impact on the activities and procedures of abortion clinics will depend upon the demand for tissue and the regulations and safeguards that restrict tissue procurement. To minimize this impact, it is essential that requests to donate tissue be separated from consent to the abortion, and that no fees be paid to the woman to donate, or to the clinic for its efforts in procuring fetal tissue (other than expenses incurred in retrieving fetal tissue).

The most certain impact if fetal tissue transplants become more common is that abortion facilities will more frequently—perhaps even routinely—ask women to donate fetal remains for research and therapy after they have decided to abort the fetus. The abortion clinic will also coordinate retrieval and temporary storage of fetal remains with tissue procurement organizations, either retrieving the tissue themselves or permitting procurement agency personnel to do so.

The greatest pressure for change in abortion clinic practices beyond requesting women to donate fetal tissue would occur if abortion clinics and women could profit financially from procuring fetal tissue. Current Federal law and the law of many States prohibit the buying and selling of fetal tissue, though they do permit payment of expenses incurred in procuring tissue for transplantation. Enforcement of these laws, including clear guidelines about what constitutes procurement expenses, is essential to prevent pressure to abort and to donate fetal tissue.

One could contemplate a scenario in which demand outstripped the supply of fetal tissue from abortions to end unwanted pregnancies. More effective contraception, greater acceptance of pharmacologically induced abortions, and great success in treating major diseases (such as Parkinson's and diabetes) could make the demand greater than the supply. To accommodate this scarcity, mechanisms for distributing fetal tissue to the larger number of patients demanding it would have to be devised, such as now exist for distributing the scarce supply of hearts, livers, and kidneys to patients on waiting lists for transplants.

However, this situation alone would not change the activities and practices of abortion clinics. Pressures to conceive and abort for transplantation purposes would arise outside of or apart from the activities of such clinics. Adherence to rules that specify when the request to donate tissue is made and that ban sales of fetal tissue would also limit the impact of such demand on abortion clinics.

The future medical possibilities cannot be foreseen with clarity. If, however, presently unexpected conflicts arise in the future, the choice of the abortion procedure should always be dictated by the health considerations of the woman.

[Panel Vote: 19 Yes, 2 No, 0 Abstain]

Considerations for Question 6

Predicting the impact on abortion clinics of a greater frequency of fetal tissue transplants is difficult and necessarily speculative at this time. The impact will depend upon many factors, including the extent of the demand for tissue, the number of abortions, the time at which viable fetal tissue may be obtained, the rules for obtaining consent, and rules against buying and selling fetal tissue. History, of course, will supply the most accurate answers, for no one can tell just how successful the research under consideration will be.

Ideally, permission to use tissues from the aborted fetus would not even be sought until the abortion itself had been performed. The timing of and the procedures associated with the abortion would be set and the abortion would be performed before the question of tissue donation was even raised. However, post mortem tissue quickly deteriorates, and, in most instances, (e.g., transplantation of neural tissue) cryogenic storage is not a scientifically effective alternative. Thus, the pregnant woman must be consulted before the abortion is actually performed. In such instances, it is always possible for the woman herself to consider procedural options that might render the fetal tissue more useful for research or therapy; possible, but, according to experienced persons, entirely unlikely.

It was the judgment of the panel that the concerns behind Question 6 are best addressed by strict adoption of a number of safeguards; safeguards that would eliminate or at least radically reduce profit motives and tendencies toward commercialization, and safeguards that would ensure the greatest possible separation between abortion procedures, facilities, and personnel on the one hand, and fetal-tissue research procedures, facilities and personnel on the other.

Where the panel was divided was on the question of which "scenario" to adopt in framing recommendations; a so-called "worst-case" situation in which demand so outstrips supply as to exert great financial and altruistic pressures, or a so-called "reasonable-case" situation in which modest medical objectives are met only over a long period. The energetic support of research by the NIH would, of course, affect the rate of progress in this area. The strictest principles of separation would be necessary in the "worst case" and would not be untoward in their effects even under current conditions.

QUESTION 7. What actual ateps are involved in procuring the tissue from the source to the researcher? Are there any payments involved? What types of payments in this situation, if any, would fall inside or outside the scope of the Hyde Amendment?

Response to Question 7

Past experience with fetal tissue research usually has had the medical researcher directly requesting fetal remains for research from physicians performing abortions, usually in the same institution. Occasionally, medical researchers have requested fetal tissue from freestanding abortion clinics in the same city.

In these instances, it is assumed that the woman aborting has consented to donation of fetal remains, though it is possible that in some instances the tissue, which would otherwise be discarded, has been treated as abandoned and used without maternal consent. If consent was obtained, it would ordinarily have been obtained before the abortion occurred but after the decision to abort had been made.

More recently, agencies or organizations have developed to provide tissue, including fetal tissue, to researchers. These have been nonprofit agencies that have solicited fetal tissue from abortion facilities and paid them a small fee for each fetal tissue retrieved to cover the costs of retrieval, including time of staff and rental of space. They have then distributed the tissue to previously identified and approved researchers conducting legitimate medical research. These agencies have usually charged the researchers the cost they have incurred in procuring the tissue.

There sometimes have been payments made to abortion facilities and physicians who have provided fetal tissue for research. These payments are intended to cover the costs to the abortion facility of providing access to the procurement agency, including staff time in requesting consent and retrieving tissue, and use of the clinic space by employees of the procurement agency.

If Federal research funds were used to pay the cost of the abortion procedure that makes fetal tissue available for research, such payment would violate the Hyde Amendment. On the other hand, the use of Federal research funds to pay tissue retrieval agencies for the costs of retrieving fetal tissue after the abortion has occurred would not violate the Amendment. Those funds would not be used "to perform abortions," but to obtain fetal tissue from abortions that would otherwise be occurring. Similarly, Federal support of fetal tissue research activities other than the cost of fetal tissue retrieval would also not violate the Hyde Amendment.

[Panel Vote: 19 Yes, 2 No, 0 Abstain]

Considerations for Question 7

The description of fetal tissue procurement procedures described here is based on information presented to the panel concerning past experience in obtaining fetal tissue and on information about new organizations that have arisen to provide fetal tissue for research and therapy. Some further development along these lines may be expected, with a strong emphasis on nonprofit retrieval agencies and no payments for tissue procurement beyond expenses.

There is no evidence that women who abort are paid money or other consideration to donate fetal tissue. Payments to abortion facilities have purported to cover expenses involved in collecting tissue and making it available. To prevent abortion clinics from making profits from fetal tissue donation, specific rules for what counts as a reasonable payment for retrieval expenses may be required.

The Hyde Amendment prohibits the use of designated Federal funds "to perform abortions except where the life of the pregnant woman would be endangered if the fetus were carried to term." It would appear, therefore, that the Hyde Amendment is not violated by support of research with fetal tissue or payment of costs incurred in retrieving that tissue because those funds would not be paid "to perform abortions."

QUESTION 8. According to HHS regulations, research on dead fetuses must be conducted in compliance with State and local laws. A few States' enacted version of the Uniform Anatomical Gift Act contains restrictions on the research applications of dead fetal tissue after an induced abortion. In those States, do these restrictions apply to therapeutic transplantation of dead fetal tissue after an induced abortion? If so, what are the consequences for NIH-funded researchers in those States?

Response to Question 8

While the Uniform Anatomical Gift Act in every State permits donations of fetal remains with maternal consent (as long as the father does not object), the panel is aware of eight States (Arkansas, Arizona, Illinois, Indiana, Ohio, Louisiana, New Mexico, and Oklahoma) that have statutes that prohibit the experimental use of cadaveric fetal tissue from induced abortions. Provisions of one statute (that in Louisiana) have been struck down on constitutional grounds.

Six of the eight States prohibit experimentation on fetuses from induced abortion. By their terms, these statutes do not apply to *nonexperimental* therapeutic transplants, but arguably would apply only to *experimental* therapeutic transplants. However, if the subject of the research is deemed to be the recipient of the fetal tissue transplant, then it may be that these statutes do not apply to experimental therapeutic transplants because they are experiments on the recipient and not on the aborted fetus.

Two of the six States would ban any use of fetal tissue from induced abortions, whether experimental or not.

Several States also have laws requiring that maternal consent be obtained before fetal tissue may be used, and ban payments for fetal tissue or providing the abortion free as an inducement to obtain fetal tissue for research.

The consequences for NIH researchers in those States depend upon the meaning of the term "experimentation" in the statutes at issue. In at least two of the States no use could be made of aborted fetal tissue. In the other six they could be used for *nonexperimental* therapeutic transplants or for experimental therapeutic transplants that are reasonably viewed as experiments on the recipient of the transplant and not on the fetal tissue itself.

Researchers in States with statutes appearing to ban fetal tissue transplants may seek clarification of the law.

[Panel Vote: 20 Yes, 0 No, 1 Abstain]

Considerations for Question 8

Research using tissue from dead fetuses is permitted in most States, because these States have statutes modeled on the Uniform Anatomical Gift Act, which treats fetal tissue like other cadaveric remains. The panel knows of only two States that prohibit all use of fetal remains from induced abortion. In six other States known to the panel, whether tissue from induced abortions may be used is dependent upon clarification of the statutory meaning of the term "experimental."

QUESTION 9. For those diseases for which transplantation using fetal tissue has been proposed, have enough animal studies been performed to justify proceeding to human transplants? Because induced abortions during the first trimester are less risky to the woman, have there been enough animal studies for each of those diseases to justify the reliance on the equivalent of the second trimester human fetus?

Response to Question 9

There is sufficient evidence from animal experimentation to justify proceeding with human clinical trials in Parkinson's disease and juvenile diabetes. Although fetal tissue of diverse ages may be scientifically and clinically advantageous for transplantation to relieve various pathologies, no abortion should be scheduled or otherwise accommodated to suit the requirements of research.

In terms of Parkinson's disease there is a wealth of positive data on graft efficacy from animal models. Extensive research has been conducted in rodents and in non-human primates. Additional testimony from some scientists suggested that further animal studies would be helpful. It is not known, for example, if there are any long-term adverse immunological effects of the grafts. It was also pointed out that the same disease processes that caused the initial dopamine neuron degeneration could also produce degeneration of grafted neurons. Testimony stressed the need for additional research, especially in terms of developing cell lines, as discussed in Question 10, below.

In terms of diabetes, there was presented a considerable body of data with animal models of diabetes supporting the efficacy of fetal islet transplants in man and suggesting that human clinical trials were timely and appropriate. Such trials are now in progress and are currently being evaluated.

Experts testified that in other disease states, such as Alzheimer's disease, Huntington's disease, spinal cord injury, and neuroendocrine deficiencies, promising results have derived from experiments using allografts in animal disease models. In these latter diseases, experts urged further animal studies before using human fetal tissue. Acceptable preliminary data would then need to be presented to an appropriate Institutional Review Board, NIH Initial Review Group, and National Advisory Council before Public Health Service funds would be obtained.

Research in diabetes, Parkinson's disease, and neural regeneration has found that first trimester fetal tissue is not only more apt, but optimal, for transplantation, since it survives better and contains cells at a stage of differentiation which is more appropriate for the therapeutic goals. Animal studies on other disorders have not revealed a transplantation protocol that would require the use of more mature fetal tissue.

Should that possibility arise and not be restricted by law, then tissue available from abortions that have already occurred during the second trimester may be used. But, to the extent that Federal sponsorship or funding is involved, no abortion should be put off to a later date nor should any abortion be performed by an alternate method entailing greater risk to the pregnant woman in order to supply more useful fetal materials for research.

[Panel Vote: 18 Yes, 2 No, 1 Abstain]

CONSIDERATIONS FOR QUESTION 9

A summary of current literature underlying this response is to be found in the Addendum. The scientific testimony presented to the panel is provided in the appendices.

QUESTION 10. What is the likelihood that transplantation using fetal cell cultures will be successful? Will this obviate the need for fresh fetal tissue? In what time frame might this occur?

Response to Question 10

In terms of alternatives to the use of fetal tissue for transplantation, an option that was presented to the panel was the use of established lines of cells that are maintained in culture. The scientific testimony was optimistic that transplantation using cell cultures may ultimately be successful. This use of cultured cells might obviate the need for tissue directly obtained from the fetus for some purposes of research and therapy. The time frame for use of defined cell lines for transplantation is estimated to be at least 10 years, given the problems of genetic engineering to have the cells synthesize chemical messengers and differentiate after grafting.

[Panel Vote: 21 Yes, 0 No, 0 Abstain]

Considerations for Question 10

The evidence in the field and expert testimony indicate that an established cell line for transplantation in diabetes must be able to synthesize, store, and release appropriate amounts of insulin when the blood sugar exceeds normal limits. At the present time, it is possible to construct cell lines by genetic engineering which synthesize insulin, but the newly formed insulin is released immediately regardless of the level of blood sugar. The genetic information for the storage and controlled release of insulin is not available at the moment and thus cannot be inserted into these cells.

A second problem may occur even if a cell line could be developed which would synthesize, store and release insulin upon demand. A normal insulin-producing cell in the pancreas is surrounded by other cells which secrete hormones that control and modulate the secretion of insulin. Thus, it may require the development of additional cell lines to release these hormones and permit the normal secretion of insulin from an insulin-producing cell line.

In regard to Parkinson's disease, it is unknown whether the transplanted neural cells will be needed only to release a specific chemical messenger or whether the transplanted cells must contact other neural cells. If both properties are required, then these two different types of genetic information would have to be inserted into the cell line.

A final problem for the development of cell lines for transplantation into patients with either diabetes or Parkinson's disease is that genetic information would have to be inserted to permit the multiplication of the cells before transplantation and then stop multiplying after transplantation. If cell multiplication could not be stopped after transplantation, the cell line would form a tumor in the patient.

Part II

THE ETHICS OF DEATH AND DYING

THE ETHICS OF DEATH AND DYING: CHANGING ATTITUDES TOWARD DEATH AND MEDICINE

Robert M. Veatch

ONE OF THE DOMINANT ISSUES in public policy debate during the last part of the twentieth century has been the controversies in bioethics over the care of the dying. By the middle of the century, the professional physician's sense of an imperative to preserve life whenever possible had reached its zenith. New-found technologies—antibiotics, respirators, dialysis machines, and cardiopulmonary resuscitation (CPR)—gave physicians their first real chance to do something to postpone death in a significant way. It became increasingly clear, however, that sometimes this postponement comes with a great price. Cancer patients had their lives prolonged to face a bedridden horrible existence in intractable pain. Heart attack victims, stroke patients, and those suffering other neurological accidents were snatched from the jaws of death only to live lives of severe debilitation sometimes to the point of total, irreversible unconsciousness. In extreme cases, such patients literally had dead brains. The time had come to ask whether such preservation of biological existence was always a morally wise choice.

Death in History

Many living in the twentieth century are surprised to discover that the monomaniacal drive to preserve life is a relatively new phenomenon in the history of medicine. Historian Darrel Amundsen called it "[a] Duty without Classical Roots."[1] Death was a great concern for the Greeks, but much of their attention was devoted to what happened after death.[2] The Greeks were quite open to ending life when it seemed appropriate based on their understanding of the meaning of life. Plato described decisions to terminate life including the purposeful killing of defective infants.

The Hippocratic cult with its school of medicine was somewhat different from other medical traditions in Greek medicine. In the Hippocratic Oath the physician pledges, "I will neither give a deadly drug to anybody if asked for it, nor will I make a suggestion to this effect."[3] The exact meaning of this prohibition is debated. Some see it as merely a condemnation of conspiracy to help a patient's enemies poison a patient, but most see it as a significant censuring of helping patients actively end their lives.[4] It is not, however, a broad mandate to Hippocratic physicians to use their skills, such as they were, to preserve human life whenever possible. In fact, elsewhere in the Hippocratic writings, the physician is advised to avoid taking a terminally ill person as a patient. Doing so was bad for the physician's reputation and apparently not expected by the morality of the day. Nowhere in the Hippocratic literature is there any notion that the physician must do everything possible to preserve life.

The Judeo-Christian tradition is the other major source of the ethics of Western culture. Judaism has long held to the doctrine that all human life is sacred, a precious divine creation. Many interpreters of the Talmudic tradition, especially those identified with the Orthodox readings of the tradition, hold that all human life is to be preserved, at least until the patient is *goses* (moribund).

Christianity has also held that life is sacred, but it has not manifested an ethic requiring all life to be preserved even when the patient is dying and prolonging dying merely burdens the patient. The Roman Catholic tradition, while condemning all euthanasia, has, since the days of Thomas Aquinas, recognized the legitimacy of forgoing extraordinary means of preserving life—and has defined "extraordinary" as all means that are "gravely burdensome to oneself or another."[5] That view has consistently been reflected in U.S. Catholic thought even during the time that secular physicians were compulsively striving for more moments of heart beat and blood flow.

The Twentieth Century to 1970

Certainly, the duty to preserve life can be dated no earlier than the beginning of the modern period. Francis Bacon describes this duty as "new, and deficient; and the most noble of all."[6] More realistically, it became the dominant duty of physicians only in the twentieth century, when medicine really could have an effect on the dying trajectory.

This sense among physicians that it was their duty to preserve life was reinforced during the Nazi era in response to the physicians of national socialism who took the leadership in the German euthanasia movement. Still, no medical professional organization has any language in its code of ethics that would commit its members to the duty to preserve life whenever possible. And no public organization regulating the medical profession has ever expected its licensees to do whatever is possible to preserve life. Public and professional organizations of the middle of the century differentiated active interventions to kill for mercy from the clinician's duty to do everything that will predictably extend life.

In the 1950s and 1960s, new technologies made the prolongation of life a more realistic possibility. First the iron lung, an enormous, engulfing machine that surrounded the entire body except the head, made mechanical ventilation possible in patients without spontaneous control of their lungs. Then more compact ventilators, CPR, dialysis machines, cardiac surgery, and transplants gave clinicians a whole new range of options for preserving life. Often these devices did not succeed, but sometimes they did. Sometimes when they succeeded in preserving life, they did so at an enormous price of pain, suffering, and degradation. Although kidney transplants began on a limited basis in 1954, the first human heart transplant in December 1967 marked a watershed that captured the public's imagination. People began to question for the first time whether these interventions were justified. People questioned whether they were "playing God." When these new high-tech heroics turned out to produce terrible side effects, the stage was set for a movement that would challenge the authority of physicians to make decisions about life preservation.

The challenge to medical authority was bolstered by developments in the broader social culture of the 1960s. The antiwar and civil rights movements led people, particularly in the United States, to question the authority of elites. The rights movements—civil rights, women's rights, and students' rights—thrived on this questioning of authority. The traditional medical ethic was soon caught up in this trend; it saw its authority dismissed as paternalism in what was dubbed the patients' rights movement. The stage was set for a radical reshaping of the public policy on the care of the dying.

The Death and Dying Era

Soon the American denial of death[7] was replaced with what was to become an obsession with death. The previous denial of death was no longer noble but a "pornography."[8] Thousands of college and health professional schools offered courses dealing with death. Led by psychiatrist Elisabeth Kübler-Ross, author of the immensely popular *Death and Dying*,[9] a social movement on death and dying began that changed forever our view of death and the way we care for the dying.

The movement differentiated two questions: the definition of death and the ethics of stopping treatment on the dying. The definition debate was clearly stimulated by the development of organ transplants. The first heart transplant occurred in December 1967, and the interdisciplinary Harvard Ad Hoc Committee on the Definition of Death published its reforming report proposing a brain-based definition in May 1968.[10] The report in effect addressed both issues: the availability of organs for transplant and the controversy over whether it was acceptable to stop medical treatment on certain dying patients by the bold move of claiming that those with total, irreversible loss of brain function were actually already dead. Since it is widely held that organs can only be procured from the deceased and no one believes that we are morally required to continue "life support" on someone who is dead, this redefinition solved both problems at once, at least for those who had truly lost all brain function irreversibly.

The first two states to pass a brain-based definition of death were Kansas (1970) and Maryland (1971). For a time it was believed that eventually all jurisdictions would follow suit, but we encountered an unexpected delay. The philosophical problems were more complex than people had realized, and the question at stake did not lend itself to resolution by scientific data. The issue was this: under what conditions should society treat people as dead—as no longer members of the human community?

The social pronouncement of death triggers important societal responses: it creates widowhood, triggers the payment of life insurance, produces murder charges in the case of assaults, and allows for the procurement of organs, among other social "death" practices. Different social, philosophical, and religious views about when these activities should occur continue to exist. One group continues to hold that death should not be pronounced until the heart and lung systems stop functioning. Another group is pressing for an even more radical redefinition in which individuals could be called dead when "higher-brain" functions are lost irreversibly even if some other brain functions continued.

These issues were all reviewed by the President's Commission for the Study of Ethical Problems in Medicine and Biomedical and Behavioral Research, a national interdisciplinary body established in 1980. Its first report, published in 1981, took on the definition of death debate. A major portion of that report is reproduced here.

As early as 1970, it was realized that even if we completely solved the problem of defining death, we would still have to face, the second, more significant issue of when to stop treatment on the still-living. Some terminally and critically ill patients with cancer, stroke, and neurological impairment are clearly not dead by anyone's definition. Some groups, such as Orthodox Jews, hold that everything possible should be done to preserve life in these patients, but most groups, including Roman Catholic theologians and members of the American Medical Association, deny that it is morally necessary to preserve life in all cases by all means.

Court cases focusing on the right to refuse life-prolonging medical treatments go back well before this time. They often dealt with the convictions of Jehovah's Witnesses or other religious objections to medical life-support. But by about 1970 laypeople's questioning of efforts to preserve life had become a social phenomenon. Court actions increased leading to a 1975 case that captured the public attention.

Karen Ann Quinlan, a twenty-one-year-old New Jersey woman spending an evening with friends at a local bar, lost consciousness from reasons that were never definitively established. Rushed to a hospital, she was resuscitated—her heartbeat was restored and she was placed on a mechanical respirator, but she did not regain consciousness. Months later she became the focus of a court action. Her parents sought to have her father named her guardian so that he could withdraw consent for the ventilator that was believed necessary to maintain her breathing.

Dr. Robert Morse, her physician, believing that he was obligated to maintain her life, was unwilling to stop the ventilator without a court order. A lower court first sided with the physician, but the Supreme Court in New Jersey, in an opinion reproduced in this chapter, reversed the lower court. The case is a watershed: it established public recognition of the right of persons to refuse life-prolonging treatment. Although the role of families and other surrogate decisionmakers remains controversial to this day, cases focused on routine refusals of treatment based on desires that the patient expressed while competent have ceased to be an issue.

While the New Jersey courts were struggling over the Quinlan case, California legislators were debating a statutory approach to a similar problem. California assemblyman Barry Keene introduced a bill, called the California Natural Death Act, that gives certain people the authority to write an advance directive (sometimes referred to as a "living will") whereby they could refuse medical treatment rather than be maintained in a terminal condition. Several states had been considering similar laws since the early 1970s, but the California law (reprinted in this section) was the first to get through the entire legislative process. It passed in 1976.

The result has been a social consensus, at least within the United States, that competent patients have the right to refuse medical treatment provided that the treatment is offered for the patient's own good.[11] The only remaining issues were those involving decisions for incompetent patients whose wishes were not known, and those involving special treatments, such as nutrition and hydration, that were considered so "basic" that they could not be refused.

Limits to the Consensus

One of the ambiguities in the Quinlan opinion is exactly why Mr. Quinlan was given the authority to decide on his daughter's behalf whether to withdraw the ventilator. The court claimed that it could not know Karen's wishes, but it never made clear whether it thought Mr. Quinlan could know them. It may be that the court believed that Mr. Quinlan was in a position to know his daughter so well that he could deduce what she would have chosen based on her own values. That interpretation would have involved a standard now referred to as *substituted judgment*.

On the other hand, some patient's wishes can never be known even by close family members. Infants and the severely retarded presumably have never formulated their own wishes and still someone must decide. It could be that Mr. Quinlan was appointed to make a choice based on his estimate of what would be best for Karen. If so, his decision would have involved a *best interest standard*.

It can also be argued that someone has to make the choice. Consider the case, reprinted here, of Joseph Saikewicz, a severely retarded sixty-seven-year-old man suffering from leukemia for which chemotherapy and blood transfusions were considered. The issue in his case was whether the trauma of the treatment, which Mr. Saikewicz could not understand because of his mental condition, would make the treatment too burdensome. The highest court in Massachusetts confirmed that the treatment should not be provided.

The Saikewicz case involved a patient who had no family available to act as surrogate. Two cases involving dispute over forgoing nutrition and hydration are presented in this section that involve formerly competent adult patients and family who offer to help interpret the patient's wishes. The issue raised is whether some treatments are special, or so basic, that they must be provided to all patients regardless of their wishes and regardless of whether the treatments offer benefits that exceed the benefits of refusal. The case of Claire Conroy involved a woman who had a history of resistance to physicians. She suffered from organic brain syndrome that left her incompetent to decide whether to continue feeding via a nasogastric tube. The New Jersey Supreme Court, in accepting the decision of her nephew (her next of kin) to refuse the treatment on her behalf, articulated three standards for cases in which refusals may be accepted. These standards are described in the record of the case, which is included in this section.

The second case confronting these issues concerned Nancy Cruzan, a Missouri woman who was left persistently vegetative as a result of an automobile accident. She was being fed through a gastrostomy, which her parents insisted she would have refused. After several preliminary state rulings, the case was heard by the United States Supreme Court, the first case of its kind to reach this level. In its ruling, the Supreme Court acknowledged that a state may establish standards, including the requirement of clear and convincing evidence of a patient's wishes. At the same time, the opinion stated a presumption of the patient's constitutional right to refuse any life-prolonging treatment, regardless of its nature.

This ruling appears to provide the basis for exercising a right of refusal for competent and formerly competent patients of any treatment including nutrition and hydration. It leaves open the question of whether parents and other surrogates for never-competent patients have the authority to refuse life-prolonging treatment as a matter of constitutional law. Many states have since acknowledged that right, but not all have. In particular, Missouri and New York still require that refusal decisions be based on the patient's own wishes. Certainly, more debate is needed to establish whether family members have such authority.

One set of federal regulations is important both in understanding the role of family members as surrogates and in deciding the limits on forgoing nutrition and hydration. In response to reports of cases involving parents' attempting to refuse life-supporting interventions for their infant children, the federal government has intervened to establish protections. After an initial effort grounded in the federal prohibition against discrimination against the handicapped,[12] a law was passed mandating protections grounded in the notion of child neglect and abuse.

The regulations growing out of this law ban payments for child welfare protection to states that do not set up mechanisms to protect infants from decisions of surrogates to forgo certain life-prolonging treatments.[13] The regulations, often referred to as the "Baby Doe" regulations, establish three conditions under which surrogates may refuse treatment of infants: when the infant is terminally ill, when it is irreversibly comatose, or when the treatment would be virtually futile for preserving life and would be inhumane. Even in these cases, however, "appropriate nutrition and hydration" must be provided to the infants.

Thus, the federal regulations for infants appear to differ from those governing treatment refusal for adults. The 1985 Federal Regulations (or Baby Doe regulations) are the next to the last document presented in this section.

The role of the family as surrogate decisionmaker has been addressed in federal courts in cases in which the issue was the right of the parent to choose in favor of life-prolonging treatment for a child who was believed by the physicians involved not to be benefiting from the treatment.[14] These cases, often misleadingly called *futile care* cases, involve ventilator support for patients whose lives predictably could be extended with a ventilator, but in ways the clinician considers pointless.

In the case of Baby K, a baby born with anencephaly, it was agreed that the baby could never be made conscious, but the mother nevertheless felt there was value in the baby's life. The federal court, supported by a court of appeals, agreed that the baby must be treated at the request of the mother, at least in this case in which an insurer was willing to pay the bills.

This shift in the public debate — from the right to refuse treatment to the right of access to treatment signals the beginning of a new era in the medical ethical debate over the care of the dying.

NOTES

1. Darrel W. Amundsen, "The Physician's Obligation to Prolong Life: A Medical Duty without Classical Roots," *Hastings Center Report* 8 (August 1978): 23–30.
2. Jacques Choron, *Death and Western Thought* (New York: Collier Books, 1963); Arnold Toynbee, ed., *Man's Concern With Death* (St. Louis: McGraw-Hill, 1968).
3. Ludwig Edelstein, "The Hippocratic Oath: Text, Translation and Interpretation," in Owsei Temkin and C. Lilian Temkin, editors, *Ancient Medicine: Selected Papers of Ludwig Edelstein* (Baltimore, Maryland: The Johns Hopkins Press, 1967), pp. 3–64 (page 6).
4. Ibid., p. 9–14.
5. Pope Pius XII. "The Prolongation of Life: An Address of Pope Pius XII to an International Congress of Anesthesiologists," *The Pope Speaks* 4 (Spring 1958): 393–398.
6. *The Philosophical Works of Francis Bacon*, ed. J. M. Robertson (Ellis and Spedding translation) 1905. Reprinted, Freeport, N.Y.: Books for Libraries Press, 1970,

pp. 485, 489. Cited in Amundsen, "The Physician's Obligation," p. 27.

7. Ernest Becker, *The Denial of Death* (New York: The Free Press, 1973).
8. Geoffrey Gorer, *Death, Grief, and Mourning* (New York: Doubleday, 1965).
9. Elizabeth K. Kübler-Ross, *On Death and Dying* (New York: Macmillan, 1969).
10. Harvard Medical School. "A Definition of Irreversible Coma. Report of the Ad Hoc Committee of the Harvard Medical School to Examine the Definition of Brain Death." *Journal of the American Medical Association* 205 (1968): 337–340.
11. Robert M. Veatch, *Death, Dying, and the Biological Revolution*, Revised Edition (New Haven, Connecticut: Yale University Press, 1989; Alan Meisel, "The Legal Consensus about Forgoing Life-Sustaining Treatment: Its Status and Its Prospects," *Kennedy Institute of Ethics Journal* 2 (1992): 309–45.
12. "Nondiscrimination on the Basis of Handicap, Procedures and Guidelines Relating to Health Care for Handicapped Infants, Final Rule." 49 *Federal Register* No. 8, 1622, January 12, 1984 (Part 84).
13. U.S. Department of Health and Human Services, "Child Abuse and Neglect Prevention and Treatment Program: Final Rule: 45 CFR 1340." *Federal Register: Rules and Regulations 50* (No. 72, April 15, 1985):14878–14892.
14. *In re Jane Doe*, a minor, Civil Action File No. D-93064, Superior Court of Fulton County, State of Georgia, October 1991; In the Matter of Baby "K", United States Court of Appeals for the Fourth Circuit, February 10, 1994.

DEFINING DEATH: MEDICAL, LEGAL, AND ETHICAL ISSUES IN THE DEFINITION OF DEATH

INTRODUCTION. *By 1980, the United States, beginning with Kansas, had been adopting brain-oriented definitions of death for a decade. While there was clearly a shift in the direction of legalizing death pronouncement based on irreversible loss of all brain functions, states were reaching this position through different routes and based on different arguments. Still, a significant minority of the U.S. population was holding to the traditional heart and lung-oriented definition. Others were beginning to advocate what has been called a "higher-brain-oriented" definition. The President's Commission for the Study of Ethical Problems in Medicine and Biomedical and Behavioral Research was established by an Act of Congress in 1980. Its first report analyzed the definition of death and endorsed what is now called the "whole-brain-oriented" definition. It has now been adopted in all U.S. jurisdictions and in almost all countries of the world, Japan being the major exception. Opposition has been found among Orthodox Jews, Native Americans, and some conservative Christians.*

Summary of Conclusions and Recommended Statute

The enabling legislation for the President's Commission directs it to study "the ethical and legal implications of the matter of defining death, including the advisability of developing a uniform definition of death" [142 USC 1802 (1978)]. In performing its mandate, the Commission has reached conclusions on a series of questions which are the subject of this Report. In summary, the central conclusions are

1. That recent developments in medical treatment necessitate a restatement of the standards traditionally recognized for determining that death has occurred.
2. That such a restatement ought preferably to be a matter of statutory law.
3. That such a statute ought to remain a matter for state law, with federal action at this time being limited to areas under current federal jurisdiction.
4. That the statutory law ought to be uniform among the several states.
5. That the "definition" contained in the statute ought to address general physiological standards rather than medical criteria and tests, which will change with advances in biomedical knowledge and refinements in technique.
6. That death is a unitary phenomenon which can be accurately demonstrated either on the traditional grounds of irreversible cessation of heart and lung functions or on the basis of irreversible loss of all functions of the entire brain.
7. That any statutory "definition" should be kept separate and distinct from provisions governing the donation of cadaver organs and from any legal rules on decisions to terminate life-sustaining treatment.

1. WHY "UPDATE" DEATH?

For most of the past several centuries, the medical determination of death was very close to the popular one. If a person fell unconscious or was found so, someone (often but not al-

President's Commission for the Study of Ethical Problems in Medicine and Biomedical and Behavioral Research, *Defining Death: Medical, Legal, and Ethical Issues in the Definition of Death* (Washington, D.C.: U.S. Government Printing Office, 1981, pp. 1, 13–43, 55–61, 72–84, 159–166. To avoid confusion, footnotes in the original report have been renumbered consecutively within each chapter and set as endnotes at the end of the Appendix.

ways a physician) would feel for the pulse, listen for breathing, hold a mirror before the nose to test for condensation, and look to see if the pupils were fixed. Although these criteria have been used to determine death since antiquity, they have not always been universally accepted.

Developing Confidence in the Heart-Lung Criteria

In the eighteenth century, macabre tales of "corpses" reviving during funerals and exhumed skeletons found to have clawed at coffin lids led to widespread fear of premature burial. Coffins were developed with elaborate escape mechanisms and speaking tubes to the world above, mortuaries employed guards to monitor the newly dead for signs of life, and legislatures passed laws requiring a delay before burial.[1]

The medical press also paid a great deal of attention to the matter. In *The Uncertainty of the Signs of Death and the Danger of Precipitate Interments* in 1740, Jean-Jacques Winslow advanced the thesis that putrefaction was the only sure sign of death. In the years following, many physicians published articles agreeing with him. This position had, however, notable logistic and public health disadvantages. It also disparaged, sometimes with unfair vigor, the skills of physicians as diagnosticians of death. In reply, the French surgeon Louis published in 1752 his influential *Letters on the Certainty of the Signs of Death*. The debate dissipated in the nineteenth century because of the gradual improvement in the competence of physicians and a concomitant increase in the public's confidence in them.

Physicians actively sought to develop this competence. They even held contests encouraging the search for a cluster of signs—rather than a single infallible sign—for the diagnosis of death.[2] One sign did, however, achieve prominence. The invention of the stethoscope in the mid-nineteenth century enabled physicians to detect heartbeat with heightened sensitivity. The use of this instrument by a well-trained physician, together with other clinical measures, laid to rest public fears of premature burial. The twentieth century brought even more sophisticated technological means to determine death, particularly the electrocardiograph (EKG), which is more sensitive than the stethoscope in detecting cardiac functioning.

The Interrelationships of Brain, Heart, and Lung Functions

The brain has three general anatomic divisions: the cerebrum, with its outer shell called the cortex; the cerebellum; and the brainstem, composed of the mid-brain, the pons, and the medulla oblongata. Traditionally, the cerebrum has been referred to as the "higher brain" because it has primary control of consciousness, thought, memory and feeling. The brainstem has been called the "lower brain," since it controls spontaneous, vegetative functions such as swallowing, yawning and sleep-wake cycles. It is important to note that these generalizations are not entirely accurate. Neuroscientists generally agree that such "higher brain" functions as cognition or consciousness probably are not mediated strictly by the cerebral cortex; rather, they probably result from complex interrelations between brainstem and cortex.

Respiration is controlled in the brainstem, particularly the medulla. Neural impulses originating in the respiratory centers of the medulla stimulate the diaphragm and intercostal muscles, which cause the lungs to fill with air. Ordinarily, these respiratory centers adjust the rate of breathing to maintain the correct levels of carbon dioxide and oxygen. In certain circumstances, such as heavy exercise, sighing, coughing or sneezing, other areas of the brain modulate the activities of the respiratory centers or even briefly take direct control of respiration.

Destruction of the brain's respiratory center stops respiration, which in turn deprives the heart of needed oxygen, causing it too to cease functioning. The traditional signs of life—respiration and heartbeat—disappear: the person is dead. The "vital signs" traditionally used in diagnosing death thus reflect the direct interdependence of respiration, circulation and the brain.

The artificial respirator and concomitant life-support systems have changed this simple picture. Normally, respiration ceases when the functions of the diaphragm and intercostal muscles are impaired. This results from direct injury to the muscles or (more commonly) because the neural impulses between the brain and these muscles are interrupted. However, an artificial respirator (also called a ventilator) can be used to compensate for the inability of the thoracic muscles to fill the lungs with air. Some of these machines use negative pressure to expand the chest wall (in which case they are called "iron lungs"); others use positive pressure to push air into the lungs. The respirators are equipped with devices to regulate the rate and depth of "breathing," which are normally controlled by the respiratory centers in the medulla. The machines cannot compensate entirely for the defective neural connections since they cannot regulate blood gas levels precisely. But, provided that the lungs themselves have not been extensively damaged, gas exchange can continue and appropriate levels of oxygen and carbon dioxide can be maintained in the circulating blood.

Unlike the respiratory system, which depends on the neural impulses from the brain, the heart can pump blood without external control. Impulses from brain centers modulate the inherent rate and force of the heartbeat but are not required for the heart to contract at a level of function that is ordinarily adequate. Thus, when artificial respiration provides adequate oxygenation and associated medical treatments regulate essential plasma components and blood pressure, an intact heart will continue to beat, despite loss of brain functions. At present, however, no machine can take over the functions of the heart except for a very limited time and in limited circumstances (e.g., a heart-lung machine used during surgery). Therefore, when a severe injury to the heart or major blood vessels prevents the circulation of the crucial blood supply to the brain, the loss of brain functioning is inevitable because no oxygen reaches the brain.

Loss of Various Brain Functions

The most frequent causes of irreversible loss of functions of the whole brain are (1) direct trauma to the head, such as from a motor vehicle accident or a gunshot wound, (2) massive spontaneous hemorrhage into the brain as a result of ruptured aneurysm or complications of high blood pressure, and (3) anoxic damage from cardiac or respiratory arrest or severely reduced blood pressure.[3]

Many of these severe injuries to the brain cause an accumulation of fluid and swelling in the brain tissue, a condition called cerebral edema. In severe cases of edema, the pressure within the closed cavity increases until it exceeds the systolic blood pressure, resulting in a total loss of blood flow to both the upper and lower portions of the brain. If deprived of blood flow for at least 10–15 minutes, the brain, including the brainstem, will completely cease functioning.[4] Other pathophysiologic mechanisms also result in a progressive and, ultimately, complete cessation of intracranial circulation.

Once deprived of adequate supplies of oxygen and glucose, brain neurons will irreversibly lose all activity and ability to function. In adults, oxygen and/or glucose deprivation for more than a few minutes causes some neuron loss.[5] Thus, even in the absence of direct trauma and edema, brain functions can be lost if circulation to the brain is impaired. If blood flow is cut off, brain tissues completely self-digest (autolyze) over the ensuing days.

When the brain lacks all functions, consciousness is, of course, lost. While some spinal reflexes often persist in such bodies (since circulation to the spine is separate from that of the brain), all reflexes controlled by the brainstem as well as cognitive, affective and integrating functions are absent. Respiration and circulation in these bodies may be generated by a ventilator together with intensive medical management. In adults who have experienced irreversible cessation of the functions of the entire brain, this mechanically generated functioning can continue only a limited time because the heart usually stops beating within two to ten days. (An infant or small child who has lost all brain functions will typically suffer cardiac arrest within several weeks, although respiration and heartbeat can sometimes be maintained even longer.[6])

Less severe injury to the brain can cause mild to profound damage to the cortex, lower cerebral structures, cerebellum, brainstem, or some combination thereof. The cerebrum, especially the cerebral cortex, is more easily injured by loss of blood flow or oxygen than is the brainstem. A 4–6 minute loss of blood flow—caused by, for example, cardiac arrest—typically damages the cerebral cortex permanently, while the relatively more resistant brainstem may continue to function.[7]

When brainstem functions remain, but the major components of the cerebrum are irreversibly destroyed, the patient is in what is usually called a "persistent vegetative state" or "persistent noncognitive state."[8] Such persons may exhibit spontaneous, involuntary movements such as yawns or facial grimaces, their eyes may be open and they may be capable of breathing without assistance. Without higher brain functions, however, any apparent wakefulness does not represent awareness of self or environment (thus, the condition is often described as "awake but unaware"). The case of Karen Ann Quinlan has made this condition familiar to the general public. With necessary medical and nursing care—including feeding through intravenous or nasogastric tubes, and antibiotics for recurrent pulmonary infections—such patients can survive months or years, often without a respirator. (The longest survival exceeded 37 years.[9])

Conclusion: The Need for Reliable Policy

Medical interventions can often provide great benefit in avoiding *irreversible* harm to a patient's injured heart, lungs, or brain by carrying a patient through a period of acute need. These techniques have, however, thrown new light on the interrelationship of these crucial organ systems. This has created complex issues for public policy as well.

For medical and legal purposes, partial brain impairment must be distinguished from complete and irreversible loss of brain functions or "whole brain death."[10] The President's Commission, as subsequent chapters explain more fully, regards the cessation of the vital functions of the entire brain—and not merely portions thereof, such as those responsible for cognitive functions—as the only proper neurologic basis for declaring death. This conclusion accords with the overwhelming consensus of medical and legal experts and the public.

Present attention to the "definition" of death is part of a process of development in social attitudes and legal rules stimulated by the unfolding of biomedical knowledge. In the nineteenth century increasing knowledge and practical skill made the public confident that death could be diagnosed reliably using cardiopulmonary criteria. The question now is whether, when medical intervention may be responsible for a patient's respiration and circulation, there are other equally reliable ways to diagnose death.

The Commission recognizes that it is often difficult to determine the severity of a patient's injuries, especially in the first few days of intensive care following a cardiac arrest, head trauma, or other similar event. Responsible public policy in this area requires that physicians be able to distinguish reliably those patients who have died from those whose injuries are less severe or are reversible. In the next chapter, medical evidence on these points is examined. Ascertaining the medical facts is only a part of the process of framing a "definition," however. Therefore, the third chapter examines concepts of death at a more basic, albeit not technical level.

2. THE "STATE OF THE ART" IN MEDICINE

Until the past few decades, comatose patients fairly rapidly either improved or died. If no other complication supervened and the patient did not improve, death followed from starvation and dehydration within days; pneumonia, apnea, or effects of the original disease typically brought on death even more quickly. Before such techniques as intravenous hydration, nasogastric feeding, bladder catheterization and respirators, no patient continued for long in deep coma.

With the aid of modern medicine, some comatose patients can be kept from a rapid death. Many, however, become permanently and totally unresponsive. In other words, their appearance resembles that of the dead as traditionally perceived: they no longer respond to their environment by sensate and intellectual activity. But their appearance also differs from that traditionally associated with the dead because mechanical support generates breathing, heartbeat, and the associated physical characteristics (e.g., warm, moist skin) of life.

The ever more sophisticated capabilities developed by biomedical practitioners during the past quarter century to support or supplant certain vital functions have thus created new problems in diagnosing death. If these diagnostic problems were the only consequence of medicine's new capabilities, those who developed and employed them might well be criticized for having opened a Pandora's Box of troubles for physicians and for society. But, as witnesses told the Commission, in a portion of the cases the armamentarium of resuscitative medicine brings comatose patients back from the brink of death by supporting their breathing and blood flow during a period of acute need.

Since the witnesses and existing medical literature lacked information on the relative proportion of comatose, respirator-assisted patients who survive versus those who die (as determined by either brain-based or heart/lung-based tests), the Commission sponsored a small study. This study was not intended to generate definitive data on the incidence of such outcomes but rather to provide a rough estimate of the extent of the various outcomes. The study examined the experience over a period ranging from two months to one year at seven hospitals serving major metropolitan areas. . . . At the four acute care centers from which such data were available, 2–4 cases of irreversible loss of all brain functions arose each month, a figure consistent with other data.[1] These figures convey a useful, if limited, perspective on the frequency with which the medicolegal dilemma of determining death in comatose, respirator-assisted cases arises at such hospitals.

The social and legal as well as medical consequences attached to a determination of death make it imperative that the diagnosis be incontrovertible. One must be certain that the functions of the entire brain are irreversibly lost and that respiration and circulation are, therefore, solely artifacts of mechanical intervention. Indeed, though suspicious that their interventions may be doing nothing more than masking what would otherwise manifestly be death by the traditional measures, physicians are concerned about doing anything—such as removing a respirator—that would hinder the recovery of a patient whose loss of brain functioning might be only partial or reversible.[2]

Development of the Concept of "Brain Death"

The concept of "brain death" and efforts to refine criteria to identify that condition have been developing during the last two decades, concomitant with the spread of life support systems in clinical medicine. In 1959, several French neurophysiologists published results of research they had conducted on patients in extremely deep coma receiving respirator assistance, a condition they termed "coma dépassé."[3] Multiple tests showed these patients lacked reflexes and electrophysiologic activity. The investigators concluded that the patients had suffered permanent loss of brain functions—they were, in other words, "beyond coma." Postmortem examinations of those patients revealed extensive destruction (necrosis and autolysis) of the brain—a phenomenon that has since been called the "respirator brain."[4]

With the advent of transplant surgery employing cadaver donors—first with kidney transplantation in the 1950s and later, and still more dramatically, with heart transplantation in the 1960s—interest in "brain death" took on a new urgency.[5] For such transplants to be successful, a viable, intact organ is needed. The suitability of organs for transplantation diminishes rapidly once the donor's respiration and circulation stop. The most desirable organ donors are otherwise healthy individuals who have died following traumatic head injuries and whose breathing and blood flow are being artificially maintained. Yet even with proper care, the organs of these potential donors will deteriorate. Thus, it became important for physicians to be able to determine when the brains of mechanically supported patients irretrievably ceased functioning.

Yet, the need for viable organs to transplant does not account fully for the interest in diagnosing irreversible loss of brain functions. The Commission's study illustrates this point; of 36 comatose patients who were declared dead on the basis of irreversible loss of brain functions, only six were organ donors. Other studies also report that organs are procured in only a small percentage of cases in which brain-based criteria might be applied.[6] Thus, medical concern over the determination of death rests much less with any wish to facilitate organ transplantation than with the need both to render appropriate care to patients and to replace artificial support with more fitting and respectful behavior when a patient has become a dead body. Another incentive to update the criteria for determining death stems from the increasing realization that the dedication of scarce and expensive intensive care facilities to bodies without brain functions may not only prolong the uncertainty and suffering of grieving families but also preclude access to the facilities for patients with reversible conditions.[7]

The Emergence of a Medical Consensus

Medical concern over making the proper diagnosis in respirator-supported patients led to the development of criteria which reliably establish permanent loss of brain functions. A landmark in this process was the publication in 1968 of a report by an *ad hoc* committee of the Harvard Medical School which became known as the "Harvard criteria."[8] The Committee's report described the following characteristics of a permanently nonfunctioning brain, a condition it referred to as "irreversible coma":

1. *Unreceptivity and unresponsitivity.* The patient shows a total unawareness to externally applied stimuli and inner need, and complete unresponsiveness, even when intensely painful stimuli are applied.
2. *No movements or breathing.* All spontaneous muscular movement, spontaneous respiration, and response to stimuli such as pain, touch, sound or light are absent.
3. *No reflexes.* Among the indications of absent reflexes are fixed, dilated, pupils; lack of eye movement even when the head is turned or ice water is placed in the ear; lack of response to noxious stimuli; and generally, unelicitable tendon reflexes.

In addition to these three criteria, a flat electroencephalogram (EEG), which shows that there is no discernible electrical activity in the cerebral cortex, was recommended as a confirmatory test, when available. All tests were to be repeated at least 24 hours later without showing change. Drug intoxication (e.g., barbiturates) and hypothermia (body temperature below 90 °F), which can cause a *reversible* loss of brain functions, also had to be excluded before the criteria could be used.

The "Harvard criteria" have been found to be quite reliable. Indeed, no case has yet been found that met these criteria and regained any brain functions despite continuation of respirator support. Criticisms of the criteria have been of five kinds. First, the phrase "irreversible coma" is misleading as applied to the cases at hand. "Coma" is a condition of a living person, and a body without any brain functions is dead and thus *beyond* any coma. Second, the writers of these criteria did not realize that the spinal cord reflexes actually persist or return quite commonly after the brain has completely and permanently ceased functioning. Third, "unreceptivity" is not amenable to testing in an unresponsive body without consciousness. Next, the need adequately to test brainstem reflexes, especially apnea, and to exclude drug and metabolic intoxication as possible causes of the coma, are not made sufficiently explicit and precise. Finally, although all individuals that meet "Harvard criteria" are dead (irreversible cessation of all functions of the entire brain), there are many other individuals who are dead but do not maintain circulation long enough to have a 24-hour observation period. Various other criteria have been proposed since 1968 that attempt to ameliorate these deficiencies.[9]

As the Harvard Committee noted, permanent loss of brain functions can also be confirmed by absence of circulation to the brain. The brain necessarily ceases functioning after a short period without intracranial circulation, unless it is protected by hypothermia or drug induced depression of neuronal metabolism. In recent years, several procedures have been developed to test for absence of intracranial blood flow, including radioisotope cerebral angiography by bolus or static imaging and four vessel intracranial contrast angiography.[10]

Clinical research has emphasized the development of procedures that can be performed reliably at a patient's bedside, so as to interfere as little as possible with treatment and not to risk harming the patient when recovery may still be possible. The aim of the tests is to reduce mistaken diagnoses that a patient is still alive, without incurring risks of erroneous diagnoses that a patient lacks all brain functioning when such functions actually remain or could recur. This is achieved by establishing first that all brain functions have ceased and then ascertaining that the cessation is irreversible. To do this, the cause of coma must be established and this may require, in addition to history and physical examination, such tests as computerized axial tomography, electroencephalography and echoencephalography.[11] The cause of the cessation of functions must be sufficient to explain the individual's clinical status and must be demonstrated to be permanent during a period of observation.[12]

The studies that document the adequacy of criteria have followed one of two general formats. Some define a group of subjects who have met the proposed criteria and demonstrate that in all such cases the heart soon stopped beating despite intensive therapy.[13] Other studies identify a group of subjects who met the proposed criteria and demonstrate widespread brain necrosis at autopsy, providing the body has remained on a respirator for sufficient time for necrosis to occur.[14] All the studies focus on patients with deep coma including absence of spontaneous breathing (apnea); in addition, some require known and sufficient cause for the absence of brain functions, isoelectric electroencephalogram, dilated pupils, or absent circulation shown by angiography. The published criteria for determining cessation of brain functions have been uniformly successful in diagnosing death. The differences among criteria often arise from differing assessments of the technical skill and instrumentation available to the physician. Experts now generally agree that careful clinical assessment (including identification of a cause of the damage to the brain which is sufficient to explain the clinical findings) is the sine qua non of a diagnosis.

The role of confirmatory tests such as electroencephalography or circulation tests beyond such bedside judgments in establishing either the cessation of brain functions or the irreversibility of such cessation has been the subject of considerable discussion.[15] For example, the Conference of Royal Colleges and Faculties in Britain focused on the function of the brainstem alone to diagnose death.[16] Since the brainstem's reticular activating formation is essential to generating consciousness and its transmittal of motor and sensation impulses is essential to these functions, loss of brainstem functions precludes discernable functioning of the cerebral hemispheres. In addition, the brainstem is the locus of homeostatic control, cranial nerve reflexes, and control of respiration. Thus, if the brainstem completely lacks functions, the brain as a whole cannot function. American physicians, however, judge the reliability of brainstem testing to be incomplete. Therefore they endorse the appropriate use of cerebral blood flow testing or electroencephalography in order to confirm the completeness of injury and the irreversibility of conditions that have led to cessation of brain functions.[17] The published data support the reliability of both approaches.

The prevailing British viewpoint on the neurologic diagnosis of death is closer to a *prognostic* approach (that a "point of no return"[18] has been reached in the process of dying), while the American approach is more *diagnostic* in seeking to determine that all functions of the brain have irreversibly ceased at the time of the declaration of death. Also, the British diagnose brain death almost entirely where irremediable structural injury has occurred while the American concept has encompassed all etiologies that may lead to irreversible loss of brain functions in respirator-maintained patients.

The British criteria resemble the American, however, in holding that death has been established when "all functions of the brain have permanently and irreversibly ceased."[19] In measuring *functions*, physicians are not concerned with mere *activity* in cells or groups of cells if such activity (metabolic, electrical, etc.) is not manifested in some way that has significance for the organism as a whole. The same is true of the cells of the heart and lungs; they too may continue to have metabolic and electrical activity after death has been diagnosed by cardiopulmonary standards [note omitted]. Tests that measure cellular activity are thus relevant to the determination of death only when they forecast whether missing functions may reappear.

Translating Medical Knowledge into Policy

Knowledgeable physicians agree that, when used in appropriate combinations, available procedures for diagnosing death by brain criteria are at least as accurate as the customary cardiopulmonary test. Indeed, medical experts testified to the Commission that the risk of mistake in a competently performed examination was infinitesimal. Plainly, the results depend on the personal knowledge, judgment and care of the physicians who apply them. Expert witnesses before the Commission pointed out that many physicians (including some neurologists and neurosurgeons) are not sufficiently familiar with the criteria (much less the detailed tests) by which the cessation of total brain functions is assessed. As one step toward professional education, a group of physicians, working with the encouragement of the Commission, has developed a summary of currently accepted medical practices. (The statement appears as Appendix F to this Report.) Such criteria—particularly as they relate to diagnosing death on neurological grounds will be continually revised by the biomedical community in light of clinical experience and new scientific knowledge.

At present, the accepted norm is that the tests will be employed by a physician who has specialized knowledge of their use. Consultation with another appropriately trained physician is typically undertaken to confirm a brain-based diagnosis in an artificially supported individual before any decisions are made on whether to discontinue support.

Particular care must be exercised to establish the cause of the patient's condition and especially to rule out conditions (such as drug intoxication or treatable brain lesions) that can give the misleading appearance that brain functions have stopped irreversibly. (Research is currently underway to test whether hypothermia and large doses of barbiturates might be used to reduce brain injury after trauma or surgery. This will complicate the diagnosis of death in these patients.)

The Commission concludes that reliable means of diagnosis are essential for determinations of death and that the medical community has developed such means. Insistence that determinations of death accord with "accepted medical standards" would thus, in the opinion of the Commission, bring to bear all the usual stimuli for assuring accuracy in medical diagnosis: the testing of practices through biomedical research and the dissemination of the results of such research; the continuing education of physicians and other health care personnel; the conscientious application of professional skills and knowledge; and the encouragement of due care provided by professional standards and by state civil and criminal laws. In the Commission's view, it is not necessary—indeed, it would be a mistake—to enshrine any particular medical criteria, or any requirements for procedure or review, as part of a statute.

3. UNDERSTANDING THE "MEANING" OF DEATH

It now seems clear that a medical consensus about clinical practices and their scientific basis has emerged: certain states of brain activity and inactivity, together with their neurophysiological consequences, can be reliably detected and used to diagnose death. To the medical community, a sound basis exists for declaring death even in the presence of mechanically assisted "vital signs." Yet before recommending that public policy reflect this medical consensus, the Commission wished to know whether the scientific viewpoint was consistent with the concepts of "being dead" or "death" as they are commonly understood in our society. These questions have been addressed by philosophers and theologians, who have provided several formulations.[1]

The Commission believes that its policy conclusions, including the statute recommended in Chapter 5, must accurately reflect the social meaning of death and not constitute a mere legal fiction. The Commission has not found it necessary to resolve all of the differences among the leading concepts of death because these views all yield interpretations consistent with the recommended statute.

Three major formulations of the meaning of death were presented to the Commission: one focused upon the functions of the whole brain, one upon the functions of the cerebral hemispheres, and one upon non-brain functions. Each of these formulations (and its variants) is presented and evaluated.

The "Whole Brain" Formulations

One characteristic of living things which is absent in the dead is the body's capacity to organize and regulate itself. In animals, the neural apparatus is the dominant locus of these functions. In higher animals and man, regulation of both maintenance of the internal environment (homeostasis) and interaction with the external environment occurs primarily within the cranium.

External threats, such as heat or infection, or internal ones, such as liver failure or endogenous lung disease, can stress the body enough to overwhelm its ability to maintain organization and regulation. If the stress passes a certain level, the organism as a whole is defeated and death occurs.

This process and its denouement are understood in two major ways. Although they are sometimes stated as alternative formulations of a "whole brain definition" of death, they are actually mirror images of each other. The Commission has found them to be complementary; together they enrich one's understanding of the "definition." The first focuses on the integrated functioning of the body's major organ systems, while recognizing the centrality of the whole brain, since it is neither revivable nor replaceable. The other identifies the functioning of the whole brain as the hallmark of life because the brain is the regulator of the body's integration. The two conceptions are subject to similar criticisms and have similar implications for policy.

The Concepts The functioning of many organs—such as the liver, kidneys, and skin—and their integration are "vital" to individual health in the sense that if any one ceases and that function is not restored or artificially replaced, the organism as a whole cannot long survive. All elements in the system are mutually interdependent, so that the loss of any part leads to the breakdown of the whole and, eventually, to the cessation of functions in every part.[2]

Three organs—the heart, lungs and brain—assume special significance, however, because their interrelationship is very close and the irreversible cessation of any one very quickly stops the other two and consequently halts the integrated functioning of the organism as a whole. Because they were easily measured, circulation and respiration were traditionally the basic "vital signs." But breathing and heartbeat are not life itself. They are simply used as signs—as one window for viewing a deeper and more complex reality: a triangle of interrelated systems with the brain at its apex. As the biomedical scientists who appeared before the Commission made clear, the traditional means of diagnosing death actually detected an irreversible cessation of integrated functioning among the interdependent bodily systems. When artificial means of support mask this loss of integration as measured by the old methods, brain-oriented criteria and tests provide a new window on the same phenomenon.

On this view, death is that moment at which the body's physiological system ceases to constitute an integrated whole. Even if life continues in individual cells or organs, life of the organism as a whole requires complex integration, and without the latter, a person cannot properly be regarded as alive.

This distinction between systemic, integrated functioning and physiological activity in cells or individual organs is important for two reasons. First, a person is considered dead under this concept even if oxygenation and metabolism persist in some cells or organs. There would be no need to wait until all metabolism had ceased in every body part before recognizing that death has occurred.

More importantly, this concept would reduce the significance of continued respiration and heartbeat for the definition of death. This view holds that continued breathing and circulation are not in themselves tantamount to life. Since life is a matter of integrating the functioning of major organ systems, breathing and circulation are necessary but not sufficient to establish that an individual is alive. When an individual's breathing and circulation lack neurologic integration, he or she is dead.

The alternative "whole brain" explanation of death differs from the one just described primarily in the vigor of its insistence that the traditional "vital signs" of heartbeat and respiration were merely surrogate signs with no significance in themselves. On this view, the heart and lungs are not important as basic prerequisites to continued life but rather because the irreversible cessation of their functions shows that the brain had ceased functioning. Other signs customarily employed by physicians in diagnosing death, such as unresponsiveness and absence of pupillary light response, are also indicative of loss of the functions of the whole brain.

This view gives the brain primacy not merely as the sponsor of consciousness (since even unconscious persons may be alive), but also as the complex organizer and regulator of bodily functions. (Indeed, the "regulatory" role of the brain in the organism can be understood in terms of thermodynamics and information theory.[3]) Only the brain can direct the entire organism. Artificial support for the heart and lungs, which is required only when the brain can no longer control them, cannot maintain the usual synchronized integration of the body. Now that other traditional indicators of cessation of brain functions (*i.e.*, absence of breathing), can be obscured by medical interventions, one needs, according to this view, new standards for determining death—that is, more reliable tests for the complete cessation of brain functions.

Critique: Both of these "whole brain" formulations—the "integrated functions" and the "primary organ" views—are subject to several criticisms. Since both of these conceptions of death give an important place to the integrating or regulating capacity of the whole brain, it can be asked whether that characteristic is as distinctive as they would suggest. Other organ systems are also required for life to continue—for example, the skin to conserve fluid, the liver to detoxify the blood.

The view that the brain's functions are more central to "life" than those of the skin, the liver, and so on, is admittedly arbitrary in the sense of representing a choice. The view is not, however, arbitrary in the sense of lacking reasons. As discussed previously, the centrality accorded the brain reflects both its overarching role as "regulator" or "integrator" of other bodily systems and the immediate and devastating consequences of its loss for the organism as a whole. Furthermore, the Commission believes that this choice overwhelmingly reflects the views of experts and the lay public alike.

A more significant criticism shares the view that life consists of the coordinated functioning of the various bodily systems, in which process the whole brain plays a crucial role. At the same time, it notes that in some adult patients lacking all brain functions it is possible through intensive support to achieve constant temperature, metabolism, waste disposal, blood pressure, and other conditions typical of living organisms and not found in dead ones. Even with extraordinary medical care, these functions cannot be sustained indefinitely—typically, no longer than several days—but it is argued that this shows only that patients with nonfunctional brains are dying, not that they are dead. In this view, the respirator, drugs, and other resources of the modern intensive-care unit collectively substitutes for the lower brain, just as a pump used in cardiac surgery takes over the heart's function.

This criticism rests, however, on a premise about the role of artificial support vis-à-vis the brainstem which the Commission believes is mistaken or at best incomplete. While the respirator and its associated medical techniques do substitute for the functions of the intercostal muscles and the diaphragm, which without neuronal stimulation from the brain cannot function spontaneously, they cannot replace the myriad functions of the brainstem or of the rest of the brain. The startling contrast between bodies lacking *all* brain functions and patients with intact brainstems (despite severe neocortical damage) manifests this. The former lie with fixed pupils, motionless except for the chest movements produced by their respirators. The latter can not only breathe, metabolize, maintain temperature and blood pressure, and so forth, *on their own* but also sigh, yawn, track light with their eyes, and react to pain or reflex stimulation.

It is not easy to discern precisely what it is about patients in this latter group that makes them alive while those in the other category are not. It is in part that in the case of the first category (*i.e.*, absence of all brain functions) when the mask created by the artificial medical support is stripped away what remains is not an integrated organism but "merely a group of artificially maintained subsystems."[4] Sometimes, of course, an artificial substitute can forge the link that restores the organism as a whole to unified functioning. Heart or kidney transplants, kidney dialysis, or an iron lung used to replace physically-impaired breathing ability in a polio victim, for example, restore the integrated functioning of the organism as they replace the failed function of a part. Contrast such situations, however, with the hypothetical of a decapitated body treated so as to prevent the outpouring of blood and to generate respiration: continuation of bodily functions in that case would not have restored the requisites of human life.

The living differ from the dead in many ways. The dead do not think, interact, autoregulate or maintain organic identity through time, for example. Not all the living can always do *all* of these activities, however; nor is there one single characteristic (e.g., breathing, yawning, etc.) the loss of which signifies death. Rather, what is missing in the dead is a cluster of attributes, all of which form part of an organism's responsiveness to its internal and external environment.

While it is valuable to test public policies against basic conceptions of death, philosophical refinement beyond a certain point may not be necessary. The task undertaken in this Report, as stated at the outset, is to provide and defend a statutory standard for determining that a human being has died. In setting forth the standards recommended in this Report, the Commission has used "whole brain" terms to clarify the understanding of death that enjoys near universal acceptance in our society. The Commission finds that the "whole brain" formulations give resonance and depth to the biomedical and epidemiological data presented in Chapter Two. Further effort to search for a conceptual "definition" of death is not required for the purpose of public policy because, separately or together, the "whole brain" formulations provide a theory that is sufficiently precise, concise and widely acceptable.

Policy Consequences Those holding to the "whole brain" view—and this view seems at least implicit in most of the testimony and writing reviewed by the Commission—believe that when respirators are in use, respiration and circulation lose significance for the diagnosis of death. In a body without a functioning brain these two functions, it is argued, become mere artifacts of the mechanical life supports. The lungs breathe and the heart circulates blood only because the respirator (and attendant medical interventions) cause them to do so, not because of any comprehensive integrated functioning. This is "breathing" and "circulation" only in an analogous sense: the function and its results are similar, but the source, cause, and purpose are different between those individuals with and those without functioning brains.

For patients who are not artificially maintained, breathing and heartbeat were, and are, reliable signs either of systemic integration and/or of continued brain functioning (depending on which approach one takes to the "whole brain" concept). To regard breathing and respiration as having diagnostic significance when the brain of a respirator-supported patient has ceased functioning, however, is to forget the basic reasoning behind their use in individuals who are not artificially maintained.

Although similar in most respects, the two approaches to "whole brain death" could have slightly different policy consequences. The "primary organ" view would be satisfied with a statute that contained only a single standard—the irreversible cessation of all functions of the entire brain. Nevertheless, as a practical matter, the view is also compatible with a statute establishing irreversible cessation of respiration and circulation as an alternative standard, since it is inherent in this view that the loss of spontaneous breathing and heartbeat are surrogates for the loss of brain functions.

The "integrated functions" view would lead one to a "definition" of death recognizing that collapse of the organism as a whole can be diagnosed through the loss of brain functions as well as through loss of cardiopulmonary functions. The latter functions would remain an explicit part of the policy statement because their irreversible loss will continue to provide an independent and wholly reliable basis for determining that death has occurred when respirators and related means of support are not employed.

The two "whole brain" formulations thus differ only modestly. And even conceptual disagreements have a context; the context of the present one is the need to clarify and update the "definition" of death in order to allow principled decisions to be made about the status of comatose respirator-supported patients. The explicit recognition of both standards—cardiopulmonary and whole brain—solves that problem fully. In addition, since it requires only a modest reformulation of the generally-accepted view, it accounts for the importance traditionally accorded to heartbeat and respiration, the "vital signs" which will continue to be the grounds for determining death in the overwhelming majority of cases for the foreseeable future. Hence the Commission, drawing on the aspects that the two formulations share and on the ways in which they each add to an understanding of the "meaning" of death, concludes that public policy should recognize both cardiopulmonary and brain-based standards for declaring death.

The "Higher Brain" Formulations

When all brain processes cease, the patient loses two important sets of functions. One set encompasses the integrating and coordinating functions, carried out principally but not exclusively by the cerebellum and brainstem. The other set includes the psychological functions which make consciousness, thought, and feeling possible. These latter functions are located primarily but not exclusively in the cerebrum, especially the neocortex. The two "higher brain" formulations of brain-oriented definitions of death discussed here are premised on the fact that loss of cerebral functions strips the patient of his psychological capacities and properties.

A patient whose brain has permanently stopped functioning will, by definition, have lost those brain functions which sponsor consciousness, feeling, and thought. Thus the higher brain rationales support classifying as dead bodies which meet "whole brain" standards, as discussed in the preceding section. The converse is not true, however. If there are parts of the brain which have no role in sponsoring consciousness, the higher brain formulation would regard their continued functioning as compatible with death.

The Concepts Philosophers and theologians have attempted to describe the attributes a living being must have to be a person.[5] "Personhood" consists of the complex of activities (or of capacities to engage in them) such as thinking, reasoning, feeling, human intercourse which make the human different from, or superior to, animals or things. One higher brain formulation would define death as the loss of what is essential to a person. Those advocating the personhood definition often relate these characteristics to brain functioning. Without brain activity, people are incapable of these essential activities. A breathing body, the argument goes, is not in itself a person; and, without functioning brains, patients are merely breathing bodies. Hence personhood ends when the brain suffers irreversible loss of function.

For other philosophers, a certain concept of "personal identity" supports a brain-oriented definition of death.[6] According to this argument, a patient literally ceases to exist as an individual when his or her brain ceases functioning, even if the patient's body is biologically alive. Actual decapitation creates a similar situation: the body might continue to function for a short time, but it would no longer be the "same" person. The persistent identity of a person as an individual from one moment to the next is taken to be dependent on the continuation of certain mental processes which arise from brain functioning. When the brain processes cease (whether due to decapitation or to "brain death") the person's identity also lapses. The mere continuation of biological activity in the body is irrelevant to the determination of death, it is argued, because after the brain has ceased functioning the body is no longer identical with the person.

Critique: Theoretical and practical objections to these arguments led the Commission to rely on them only as confirmatory of other views in formulating a definition of death. First, crucial to the personhood argument is acceptance of one particular concept of those things that are essential to being a person, while there is no general agreement on this very fundamental point among philosophers, much less physicians or the general public. Opinions about what is essential to personhood vary greatly from person to person in our society—to say nothing of intercultural variations.

The argument from personal identity does not rely on any particular conception of personhood, but it does require assent to a single solution to the philosophical problem of identity. Again, this problem has persisted for centuries despite the best attempts by philosophers to solve it. Regardless of the scholarly merits of the various philosophical solutions, their abstract technicality makes them less useful to public policy.

Further, applying either of these arguments in practice would give rise to additional important problems. Severely senile patients, for example, might not clearly be persons, let alone ones with continuing personal identities; the same might be true of the severely retarded. Any argument that classified these individuals as dead would not meet with public acceptance.

Equally problematic for the "higher brain" formulations, patients in whom only the neocortex or subcortical areas have been damaged may retain or regain spontaneous respiration and circulation. Karen Quinlan is a well-known example of a person who apparently suffered permanent damage to the higher centers of the brain but whose lower brain continues to function. Five years after being removed from the respirator that supported her breathing for nearly a year, she remains in a persistent vegetative state but with heart and lungs that function without mechanical assistance.[7] Yet the implication of the personhood and personal identity arguments is that Karen Quinlan, who retains brainstem function and breathes spontaneously, is just as dead as a corpse in the traditional sense. The Commission rejects this conclusion and the further implication that such patients could be buried or otherwise treated as dead persons.

Policy Consequences In order to be incorporated in public policy, a conceptual formulation of death has to be amenable to clear articulation. At present, neither basic neurophysiology nor medical technique suffices to translate the "higher brain" formulation into policy. First, as was discussed in Chapter One, it is not known which portions of the brain are responsible for cognition and consciousness; what little is known points to substantial interconnections among the brainstem, subcortical structures and the neocortex. Thus, the "higher brain" may well exist only as a metaphorical concept, not in reality. Second, even when the sites of certain aspects of consciousness can be found, their cessation often cannot be assessed with the certainty that would be required in applying a statutory definition.

Even were these difficulties to be overcome, the adoption of a higher brain "definition" would depart radically from the traditional standards. As already observed, the new standard would assign no significance to spontaneous breathing and heartbeat. Indeed, it would imply that the existing cardiopulmonary definition had been in error all along, even before the advent of respirators and other life-sustaining technology.

In contrast, the position taken by the Commission is deliberately conservative. The statutory proposal presented in Chapter Five offers legal recognition for new diagnostic measures of death, but does not ask for acceptance of a wholly new concept of death. On a matter so fundamental to a society's sense of itself—touching deeply held personal and religious beliefs—and so final for the individuals involved, one would desire much greater consensus than now exists before taking the major step of radically revising the concept of death.

Finally, patients declared dead pursuant to the statute recommended by the Commission would be also considered dead by those who believe that a body without higher brain functions is dead. Thus, all the arguments reviewed thus far are in agreement that irreversible cessation of *all* brain functioning is sufficient to determine death of the organism.

The Non-Brain Formulations

The Concepts The various physiological concepts of death so far discussed rely in some fashion on brain functioning. By contrast, a literal reading of the traditional cardiopulmonary criteria would require cessation of the flow of bodily "fluids," including air and blood, for death to be declared. This standard is meant to apply whether or not these flows coincide with any other bodily processes, neurological or otherwise. Its support derives from interpretations of religious literature and cultural practices of certain religious and ethnic groups, including some Orthodox Jews[8] and Native Americans.[9]

Another theological formulation of death is, by contrast, not necessarily related to any physiologic phenomenon. The view is traditional in many faiths that death occurs the moment the soul leaves the body.[10] Whether this happens when the patient loses psychological capacities, loses all brain functions, or at some other point, varies according to the teachings of each faith and according to particular interpretations of the scriptures recognized as authoritative.

Critique: The conclusions of the "bodily fluids" view lack a physiologic basis in modern biomedicine. While this view accords with the traditional criteria of death, as noted above, it does not necessarily carry over to the new conditions of the intensive care unit—which are what prompts the reexamination of the definition of death. The flow of bodily fluids could conceivably be maintained by machines in the absence of almost all other life processes; the result would be viewed by most as a perfused corpse, totally unresponsive to its environment.

Although the argument concerning the soul could be interpreted as providing a standard for secular action, those who adhere to the concept today apparently acknowledge the need for a more public and verifiable standard of death. Indeed, a statute incorporating a brain-based standard is accepted by theologians of all backgrounds.[11]

Policy Consequences The Commission does not regard itself as a competent or appropriate forum for theological interpretation. Nevertheless, it has sought to propose policies consistent with as many as possible of the diverse religious tenets and practices in our society.

The statute set forth in Chapter Five does not appear to conflict with the view that the soul leaves the body at death. It provides standards by which death can be determined to have occurred, but it does not prevent a person from believing on religious grounds that the soul leaves the body at a point other than that established as marking death for legal and medical purposes.

The concept of death based upon the flow of bodily fluids cannot be completely reconciled with the proposed statute. The statute is partially consistent with the "fluids" formulation in that both would regard as dead a body with no respiration and circulation. As noted previously, the overwhelming majority of patients, now and for the foreseeable future, will be diagnosed on such basis. Under the statute, however, physicians would declare dead those bodies in which respiration and circulation continued *solely* as a result of artificial maintenance, in the absence of all brain functions. Nonetheless, people who believe that the continued flow of fluids in such patients means they are alive would not be forced by the statute to abandon those beliefs nor to change their religious conduct. While the recommended statute may cause changes in medical and legal behavior, the Commission urges those acting under the statute to apply it with sensitivity to the emotional and religious needs of those for whom the new standards mark a departure from traditional practice. Determinations of death must be made in a consistent and evenhanded fashion, but the statute does not preclude flexibility in responding to individual circumstances after determination has been made. . . .

5. WHAT "DEFINITION" OUGHT TO BE ADOPTED?

The Commission has concluded that legislatures ought to set the rules for determining human death and that those rules should recognize brain-oriented techniques of establishing death because traditional standards often cannot be employed with patients whose respiration and circulation are artificially maintained. This chapter asks: by what principles should the drafting of a statute on death be guided, how does the law stand at present, and what would a good statute provide?

The Specificity of Public Policy

A statute on death should guide those who will decide whether (and if so, when) a person has passed from being alive to being dead. Such guidance can be general or specific. An initial question for legislative drafters is what level of detail should be incorporated within a statute and what supporting concepts or details can be drawn from other sources. Four levels of generality for such a "definition" have been suggested:[1]

> The *basic concept* of death is fundamentally a philosophical matter. Examples of possible "definitions" of death at this level include "permanent cessation of the integrated functioning of the organism as a whole," "departure of the animating or vital principle," or "irreversible loss of personhood." These abstract definitions offer little concrete help in the practical task of determining whether a person has died but they may very well influence how one goes about devising standards and criteria.
>
> In setting forth the *general physiological standard(s)* for recognizing death, the definition moves to a level which is more medico-technical, but not wholly so. Philosophical issues persist in the choice to define death in terms of organ systems, physiological functions, or recognizable human activities, capacities, and conditions. Examples of possible general standards include "irreversible cessation of spontaneous respiratory and/or circulatory functions," "irreversible loss of spontaneous brain functions," "irreversible loss of the ability to respond or communicate," or some combination of these.
>
> *Operational criteria* further define what is meant by the general physiological standards. The absence of cardiac contraction and lack of movement of the blood are examples of traditional criteria for "cessation of spontaneous circulatory functions," whereas deep coma, the absence of reflexes, and the lack of spontaneous muscular movements and spontaneous respiration are among criteria proposed for "cessation of spontaneous brain functions" by the Harvard Committee.
>
> Fourth, there are the *specific tests and procedures* to see if the criteria are fulfilled. [Measurement of] pulse, heart beat, and blood pressure, electrocardiogram, and examination of blood flow in the retinal vessels are among the specific tests of cardiac contraction and movement of the blood. Reaction to painful stimuli, appearance of the pupils and their responsiveness to light, and observation of movement and breathing over a specified time period are among specific tests of the "brain function" criteria enumerated above.

The Commission has concluded that legislation should be formulated at the second level, that of general standards. Broader formulations would lead down arcane philosophical paths which are at best somewhat removed from practical application in the formulation of law. To truly redefine the very concepts of life and death, such a course might be necessary; but that is not the Commission's objective. Physicians, applying the traditional procedures that corresponded to societal expectations, were not maintaining that death *is* the irreversible loss of heart and lung functions. They were affirming only that the loss of those functions *indicated* that a person had died. Modern treatments that interfere with these indicators do not necessitate a change in concepts, provided that alternative indicators of the current concept are available. As discussed in Chapters Two and Three, the brain-oriented indicators provide such an alternative. Thus, it seems proper to proceed on the assumption that the widespread agreement in traditional understanding of death (i.e., that it is manifested by cessation of spontaneous cardiopulmonary functioning) would apply equally for alternative procedures congruent with the traditional concept.

The third and fourth levels of specificity have problems opposite to those of the first. Agreement might be reached about the details, but this agreement would be fleeting, since new criteria and tests—unlike new concepts—will be repeatedly generated by changes in biomedical knowledge and clinical abilities. It would seem more realistic to leave the technical details to physicians and other biomedical scientists. Once the public has set its goal, specialists in the field can be delegated the responsibility of elaborating the means toward it.

The distinction between general standards (which a statute ought to articulate) and operational criteria (which are better left to medical bodies to establish) is not always recognized. The term "criteria" reflects the usage of the ad hoc Harvard committee whose 1968 report on "the definition of irreversible coma" brought the issue to the fore.[2] In the years since that group made its recommendations, the criteria by which an irreversible cessation of total brain functioning is detected have been repeatedly revised.[3] Were a statute to incorporate such criteria, its inflexibility might chill the development of more accurate criteria and of faster, more precise, and more economical tests. By remaining at a slightly greater level of generality—e.g.,"irreversible cessation of all functions of the entire brain"—a statute may be able to remain valid indefinitely and not to require repeated amendments.

The Objectives to Be Sought

General principles of drafting—such as clarity and brevity—apply as well to a statute on the standards for death determination as to any legislation. But there are also certain objectives particular to the subject at hand.

Death Is a Single Phenomenon The statute must address the right question. The Commission conceives the question to be, "how, given medical advances in cardiopulmonary support, can the evidence that death has occurred be obtained and recognized?" When the presence of a mechanical ventilator precludes the use of traditional vital signs (i.e., respiration and heartbeat) to ascertain whether a person is alive, the use of brain-based criteria provides another means of making such a determination. Thus, brain-based criteria do not introduce a new "kind of death", but rather reinforce the concept of death as a single phenomenon—the collapse of psycho-physical integrity. The statute merely allows new ways to recognize that this phenomenon has occurred.

Death of the Organism as a Whole The death of a human being—not the "death" of cells, tissues or organs—is the matter at issue. The cessation of vital bodily systems provides the basis for broad standards by which death can be judged to have occurred. But such functional cessation is not of interest in and for itself, but for what it reveals about the status of the person. What was formerly a person is now a dead body and can be socially and legally treated as such. Although absence of breathing and heartbeat may often have been spoken of as "defining" death, review of history and of current medical and popular understanding makes clear that these were merely evidence for the disintegration of the organism as a whole, as discussed in Chapter Three.

Incremental (Not Radical) Change Two advantages of the traditional vital signs were their accessibility to measurement (not only by the medically-trained) and their obvious connection to the reality of death as perceived in everyday life. Although fewer and fewer people actually witness death (how many children, for example, today are gathered with their families around the death bed of an elderly relative?), most Americans still feel they recognize the manifest signs of death, at least through the arts and the communications media, if not first-hand. The "whole brain" signs of life and death are less well comprehended by nonspecialists, and they measure functions that are less clearly manifest. The heart and the lungs move when they work; the brain does not. Thus, since any incorporation of brain-oriented standards into the law necessarily changes the *type* of measures permitted somewhat, a statute will be more acceptable the less it otherwise changes legal rules.

Conservatism seems justified in articulating a rule that will not only be applied within the legal system but will also guide the beliefs and behavior of physicians and the public. People's attitudes toward death evolve, and changes in medical capabilities certainly come to be reflected in public as well as professional circles: heart transplantation, for example, cannot help but alter the romantic notion of the heart as the seat of soul or personality. Change does not occur overnight, however, and there seems to be no reason to force it by statute when wrenching change is not necessary. Any statute on death should, therefore, supplement rather than supplant the existing legal concept.

The conservative nature of the reform here proposed will be more apparent if the statute refers explicitly to the existing cardiopulmonary standard for determination of death. The brain-based standard is, after all, merely supplementary to the older standard, which will continue to be adequate in the overwhelming majority of cases in the foreseeable future. Indeed, of all hospital deaths at four acute hospitals in the Commission's survey, only about 8 percent could have been declared dead by neurologic criteria prior to cardiac arrest. The study clearly illustrates that the use of cardiopulmonary criteria predominates. In the first place, the brain-based criteria are relevant only to a limited patient population (i.e., comatose patients on respirators). Even among this population, only one-fourth of those who died at the four acute care centers in the Commission's study met brain-based criteria before meeting the cardiopulmonary standard. Moreover, among those in that population who are likely to meet the criteria, cardiac standstill sometimes intervenes (i.e., cardiopulmonary criteria are met) prior to completion of the waiting period necessary to confirm the irreversibility of the loss of brain functions. In addition, as the Commission's study illustrates, physicians who conclude that still living patients have no chance for recovery sometimes forego extraordinary treatment; as a result, patients who might have met brain-based criteria if placed on respirators die instead from cardiac standstill or collapse. Thus, although brain-based criteria are needed in those cases where traditional criteria cannot be applied, these instances at present represent, and will in all probability continue to represent, a small percentage of all determinations of death.

Uniformity Among People and Situations Besides moving slowly, the law ought to move evenhandedly. The statute ought not to reinforce the misimpression that there are different "kinds" of death, defined for different purposes, and hence that some people are "more dead" than others.

In many contexts, definitions are handmaidens to other purposes lawmakers are seeking to achieve. Rather than asking "what is death"? one might ask, "what difference does it make whether somebody is dead"?[4] That question has many answers, most of them familiar to everyone. Criminal law (murder v. aggravated assault), tort law (wrongful death), family law (the status of spouse and children), property and estate law, insurance law (payment of life insurance benefits and termination of health insurance payments), and tax law, as well as some actions and culturally determined behaviors of family members, physicians, clerics and undertakers are all initiated by the determination that a death has occurred. Were there good reason for one branch or another of the law or one or another cultural institution to employ a different "definition" of death, logic would not preclude such a step. But in fact, society has found it desirable to employ a single standard for declaring death in all these circumstances and no special-purpose definitions have been seriously advanced. Calling the same person "dead" for one purpose and "alive" for another would engender nothing but confusion.[5] Thus, in setting forth the law in statutory form, the wisest and most cautious course (furthering the principle of incrementalism as well) would be to adopt a rule recognizing the unity of the concept of death. Such a "definition" of death can be applied in all appropriate circumstances; if a special need is identified for acting on a different basis, a separate status—other than that of being "dead"—could be defined for that purpose.[6]

Adaptability to Advances in Technique Some, particularly in the medical community, have voiced a fear of statutory "inflexibility." A statute should apply uniformly at any one time, but it need not fix at the current level of scientific sophistication or biomedical technology the means by which it is to be implemented. In the terms used earlier, a statute should be confined to the standards by which death is to be determined and leave to experts in biomedicine the continuing development of criteria and specific tests that fulfill them.

The Legal Changes That Have Occurred

The gap between the common law definition of death and the skills of modern medicine has not gone unnoticed by lawmakers. Spurred initially by the interest in transplantation,[7] later by the widely publicized tragedy of Karen Ann Quinlan,[8] and finally by a recognition of the perplexities in the civil and criminal law processes, legislators in twenty-seven states[9] have enacted statutes that permit reliance on brain-oriented criteria for determining death. Moreover, in several states where legislators had not yet acted, judges have given some recognition to similar standards. . . .[10]

The Proposal for a Uniform Statute

The Language and Its History The array of "model laws" and state variations reveals two major problems: first, their diversity, and second, the overly complex or inexact wording that characterizes many of them. Diversity is a problem for several reasons. In the case of enacted statutes, diversity means nonuniformity among jurisdictions. In most areas of the law, provisions that diverge from one state to the next create, at worst, inconvenience and the occasional failure of a finely honed business or personal plan to achieve its intended result. But on the subject of death, nonuniformity has a jarring effect. Of course, the diversity is really only superficial; all the enacted statutes appear to have the same intent. Yet even small differences raise the question: if the statutes all mean the same thing, why are they so varied? And it is possible to think of medical situations—and, even more freely, of legal cases that would be unlikely but not bizarre—in which the differences in statutory language *could* lead to different outcomes.[11]

More fundamental is the obstacle that diversity presents for the process of statutory enactment. Legislators, presented with a variety of proposals and no clear explanation of the significance of their differences, are (not surprisingly) wary of *all* the choices. . . .

A uniform proposal that is broadly acceptable would significantly ease the enactment of good law on death throughout the United States. To that end, the Commission's Executive Director met in May 1980 with representatives of the American Bar Association, the American Medical Association and the National Conference of Commissioners on Uniform State Laws. Through a comparison of the then existing "models" with the objectives that a statute ought to serve, they arrived at a proposed Uniform Determination of Death Act:

> §1. [*Determination of Death.*] An individual who has sustained either (1) irreversible cessation of circulatory and respiratory functions, or (2) irreversible cessation of all functions of the entire brain, including the brain stem, is dead. A determination of death must be made in accordance with accepted medical standards.

> §2. [*Uniformity of Construction and Application.*] This act shall be applied and construed to effectuate its general purpose to make uniform the law with respect to the subject of this Act among states enacting it.

This model law has now been approved by the Uniform Law Commissioners, the ABA [American Bar Association] and the AMA [American Medical Association] as a substitute for their previous proposals. It has also been endorsed by the American Academy of Neurology and the American Electroencephalographic Society.

Construction of the Statute As recommended at the outset of this Chapter, the proposed statute addresses the matter of "defining" death at the level of general physiological standards rather than at the level of more abstract concepts or the level of more precise criteria and tests. The proposed statute articulates alternative standards, since in the vast majority of cases irreversible circulatory and respiratory cessation will be the obvious and sufficient basis for diagnosing death. When a patient is not supported on a respirator, the need to evaluate brain functions does not arise. The basic statute in this area should acknowledge that fact by setting forth the basis on which death *is* determined in such cases (namely, that breathing and blood flow have ceased and cannot be restored or replaced).

It would be possible, as in the statute drafted by the Law Reform Commission of Canada, to propound the irreversible cessation of brain functions as *the* "definition" and then to permit that standard to be met not only by direct measures of brain activity but also "by the prolonged absence of spontaneous cardiac and respiratory functions."[12] Although conceptually acceptable (and vastly superior to the adoption of brain cessation as a primary standard conjoined with a nonspecific reference to other, apparently unrelated "usual and customary procedures,")[13] the Canadian proposal breaks with tradition in a manner that appears to be unnecessary. For most lay people—and in all probability for most physicians as well—the permanent loss of heart and lung function (for example, in an elderly person who has died in his or her sleep) clearly manifests death. As previous chapters in this Report recount, biomedical scientists can explain the brain's particularly important—and vulnerable—role in the organism as a whole and show how temporary loss of blood flow (ischemia) becomes a permanent cessation because of the damage it inflicts on the brain. Nonetheless, most of the time people do not, and need not, go through this two-step process. Irreversible loss of circulation is recognized as death because—setting aside any mythical connotations of the heart—a person without blood flow simply cannot live. Thus, the Commission prefers to employ language which would reflect the continuity of the traditional standard and the newer, brain-based standard.

"Individual": Other aspects of the statutory language, as well as several phrases that were intentionally omitted, deserve special mention. First, the word "individual" is employed here to conform to the standard designation of a human being in the language of the uniform acts. The term "person" was not used here because it is sometimes used by the law to include a corporation. Although that particular confusion would be unlikely to arise here, the narrower term "individual" is more precise and thus avoids the possibility of confusion.

"Irreversible Cessation of Functions": Second, the statute emphasizes the degree of damage to the brain required for a determination of death by stating "*all* functions of the *entire* brain, *including the brain stem*" (emphasis added). This may be thought doubly redundant, but at least it should make plain the intent to *exclude* from application under the "definition" any patient who has lost only "higher" brain functions or, conversely, who maintains those functions but has suffered solely a direct injury to the brain stem which interferes with the vegetative functions of the body.

The phrase "cessation of *functions*" reflects an important choice. It stands in contrast to two other terms that have been discussed in this field: (a) "loss of activity" and (b) "destruction of the organ."

Bodily parts, and the subparts that make them up, are important for the functions they perform. Thus, detecting a loss of the ability to function is the central aim of diagnosis in this field. After an organ has lost the ability to *function* within the organism, electrical and metabolic *activity* at the level of individual cells or even groups of cells may continue for a period of time. Unless this cellular activity is organized and directed, however, it cannot contribute to the operation of the organism as a whole. Thus, cellular activity alone is irrelevant in judging whether the organism, as opposed to its components, is "dead."

At the other pole, several commentators have argued that organic *destruction* rather than cessation of functions should be the basis for declaring death.[14] They assert that until an organ has been destroyed there is always the *possibility* that it might resume functioning. The Commission has rejected this position for several reasons. Once brain cells have permanently ceased metabolizing, the body cannot regenerate them. The loss of the brain's functions precedes the destruction of the cells and liquefaction of the tissues.

Theoretically, even *destruction* of an organ does not prevent its functions from being restored. Any decision to recognize "the end" is inevitably restricted by the limits of available medical knowledge and techniques.[15] Since "irreversibility" adjusts to the times, the proposed statute can incorporate new clinical capabilities. Many patients declared dead fifty years ago because of heart failure would have not experienced an "*irreversible* cessation of circulatory and respiratory functions" in the hands of a modern hospital.

Finally, the argument for using "brain destruction" echoes the proposal about "putrefaction" made two centuries ago and overcome by advances in diagnostic techniques. The traditional cardiopulmonary standard relies on the vital signs as a measure of heart-lung function; the declaration of death does not await evidence of destruction. Since the evidence reviewed by the Commission indicates that brain criteria, properly applied, diagnose death as reliably as cardiopulmonary criteria, the Commission sees no reason not to use the same standards of cessation for both. The requirement of "irreversible cessation of functions" should apply to both cardiopulmonary and brain-based determinations.

"Is Dead": Most of the model statutes previously proposed state that a person meeting the statutory standards "will [or shall] be considered dead." This formulation, although probably effective in achieving the desired clarification of the place of "brain death" in the law, is somewhat disconcerting since it might be read to indicate that the law will *consider* someone dead who by some other, perhaps wiser, standard *is not* dead. The President's Commission does not endorse this view. It favors stating more directly (as had the Uniform State Law Commissioners in their 1978 proposal) that a person "is dead" when he or she meets one of the standards set forth in the statute.

In declaring that an individual "is dead," physicians imply that at some moment prior to the diagnosis the individual moved from the status of "being alive" to "being dead." The Commission concurs in the view that "death should be viewed not as a process but as the event that separates the process of dying from the process of disintegration."[16] Although it assumes that each dead person became dead at some moment prior to the time of diagnosis, the statute does not specify that moment. Rather, this calculation is left to "accepted medical practices" and the law of each jurisdiction.

Determining the time of passage from living to dead can be troublesome in certain situations; like all aspects of assessing whether a body is dead, it relies heavily on the clinical skills and judgment of the person making the determination. In most cases, it appears to be the custom simply to record the time when a diagnosis of death is made as the time of death. When precision is important for legal purposes, the scientific basis for determining the time of death may be reexamined and resolved through legal proceedings.

A determination of death immediately changes the attitudes and behavior of the living toward the body that has gone from being a person to being a corpse. Discontinuation of medical care, mourning and burial are examples of customary behavior; people usually provide intimate care for living patients and identify with them, while withdrawing from contact with the dead. In ordinary circumstances, the time at which medical diagnosis causes a change in legal status should be synchronous with the time that social behaviors naturally change.

In some cases of death determined by neurologic criteria, however, it is necessary to allow for repeated testing, observation, or metabolism of drugs. This may interpose hours or even days between the actual time of death and its confirmation. Procedures for certifying time of death, like those for determining the status of being dead, will be a matter for locally "accepted medical standards," hospital rules and custom, community mores and state death certificate law. Present practice in most localities now parallels the determination of death by cardiopulmonary criteria: death by brain criteria is certified at the time that the fact of death is established, that is, after all tests and confirmatory observation periods are complete.

When the time of "brain death" has legal importance, a best medical estimate of the actual time when all brain functions irreversibly ceased will probably be appropriate. Where this is a matter of controversy, it becomes a point to be resolved by the law of the jurisdiction. Typically, judges decide this on the basis of expert testimony—as they do with a contested determination of unwitnessed cessation of cardiopulmonary functions.

"Accepted Medical Standards": The proposed statutes variously describe the basis on which the criteria and tests actually used to diagnose death are to be selected and employed. The variations were:

Capron-Kass (1972): "based on ordinary standards of medical practice"
ABA (1975): "according to usual and customary standards of medical practice"
NCCUSL [National Conference of Commissioners on Uniform State Laws] (1978): "in accordance with reasonable medical standards"
AMA (1979): "in accordance with accepted medical standards"

Despite their linguistic differences, the Capron/Kass, ABA and AMA models apparently intend the same result: to require the use of diagnostic measures and procedures that have passed the normal test of scrutiny and adoption by the biomedical community. In contrast, the 1978 uniform proposal sounded a different note by proposing "reasonableness" as the standard. The problem is: whose reasonableness? Might lay jurors conclude that a medical practice, although generally adopted, was "unreasonable"? It would be unfair to subject a physician (and others acting pursuant to his or her instructions) to liability on the basis of an after-the-fact determination of standards if he or she had been acting in good faith and according to the norms of professional practice and belief. Even the prospect of this liability would unnecessarily disrupt orderly decision making in this field.

The process by which a norm of medical practice becomes "accepted" varies according to the field and the type of procedure at issue. The statutory language should eliminate wholly idiosyncratic standards or the use of experimental means of diagnosis (except in conjunction with adequate customary procedures). On the other hand, the statute does not require a procedure to be universally adopted; it is enough if, like any medical practice which is later challenged, it has been accepted by a substantial and reputable body of medical men and women as safe and efficacious for the purpose for which it is being employed.[17]

The Commission has also concluded that the statute need not elaborate the legal consequences of following accepted practices. The model statute proposed earlier by the AMA contained separate sections precluding criminal and civil prosecution or liability for determinations of death made in accordance with the statute or actions taken "in good faith in reliance on a determination of death."[18] It is not necessary to address this issue in a statute because the existing common law already eliminates such liability.

Scope of Application: The Kansas statute specified that it established when a person is considered "medically and legally dead."[19] Although this unnecessary language was deleted in the 1972 model statute, it partially resurfaced in the 1975 ABA proposal which begins "for all legal purposes."[20] Three years later it was back in full flower in the Uniform Brain Death Act, whose scope includes all "legal and medical purposes."[21]

Besides being unnecessary, the broader provisions are misleading. A law setting a general standard without explicit limitations would be assumed to apply for *all* legal purposes; to say so in the statute, however, only raises needless questions (e.g., what does "all *legal* purposes" leave out? For example, proceedings in equity?).

By mentioning "medical purposes," the Kansas act and 1978 Uniform proposal compounded the confusion. Without this language, a statute would certainly reach the practice of medicine and its consequences for patients. The only additional area that might be encompassed by the phrase "medical purposes" is medical theory, a plane which a statute cannot reach whatever it may proclaim. Society cannot legislate the laws of nature, nor is there any reason to think that in this case it should want to try to do so. Thus, the language proclaiming a "definition" of death "for all medical purposes" is at best unnecessary and at worst foolish.

Finally, since the proposed statute is intended to apply in all situations, it ought not to be incorporated into a state's

Uniform Anatomical Gift Act (UAGA). Placing it there would create the mistaken impression that a special "definition" of death needs to be applied to organ transplantation, which is not the case. (As a matter of fact, most of the respirator-supported cases in which the brain-oriented standard would be applicable are not potential donors, as noted in Chapter 2.) Section 7(b) of the UAGA makes the time of death a matter to be determined by the attending physician; the proposed Uniform Determination of Death Act specifies the grounds on which such a determination are made. Some people have expressed concern that a determination of death in a potential organ donor might be made by a physician with a conflict of interest, but the UAGA specifies that the physician who determines that death has occurred "shall not participate in the procedures for removing or transplanting a part."[22]

Personal Beliefs: Should a statute include a "conscience clause" permitting an individual (or family members, where the individual is incompetent) to specify the standard to be used for determining his or her death based upon personal or religious beliefs?[23] While sympathetic to the concerns and values that prompt this suggestion, the Commission has concluded that such a provision has no place in a statute on the determination of death. Were a non-uniform standard permitted, unfortunate and mischievous results are easily imaginable.[24]

If the question were what actions (e.g., termination of treatment, autopsy, removal of organs, etc.) could be taken, there might be room for such a conscience clause. Yet, as the question is one of legal *status,* on which turn the rights and interests not only of the one individual but also the other people and of the state itself, the subject is not one for personal (or familial) self-determination.[25]

The statute specifies that death has occurred if *either* cardiopulmonary or brain criteria are met. Although, as a legal matter, there is no personal discretion as to the *fact* of death when either criteria is met, room remains for reasonable accommodation of personal beliefs regarding the actions to be taken once a determination of death has been made. Such actions, whether medical (e.g., maintaining a dead body on a respirator until organs are removed for transplantation) or religious (e.g., withholding religious pronouncement of death until the blood has ceased flowing), can vary with the circumstances. Some subjects in the Commission's hospital survey, for example, were maintained on ventilators for several hours after they were dead, in deference to family wishes or in order for the family to decide whether to donate the deceased's organs.

Ethical Aspects of the Proposal

In addition to the issues discussed earlier, particularly in Chapter Three, two further ethical issues deserve mention: (a) concerns about the certainty of diagnosis and (b) concerns about the medical steps that may be taken after death is pronounced.

Certainty of Diagnosis Part of the public concern over employing a brain-based standard to determine death seems to arise from fear that this may cause medical treatment to be withdrawn from some patients who might have "recovered," that is, regained consciousness or at least the ability to breathe without the aid of a respirator. This fear is expressed in anecdotes about patients who have resumed normal lives after long periods of coma or even after having been pronounced dead.[26] The ethical question is whether a new, brain-oriented definition of death would lead to abandonment of patients who might have responded to continued medical care. Those who press this objection to "redefinition" of death insist that death should not be pronounced until it is certain that recovery is impossible.[27]

The moral gravity of the concern over premature cessation of care cannot be questioned. It is important, however, to be clear on the relation of this concern to the proposed brain-oriented standard. Under that standard, death will be pronounced in cases in which there is an irreversible loss of brain functions while respiration is artificially supplied. Such bodies might have been regarded as alive if only heart-lung tests for death were permissible. Yet ethical concern over the accuracy of the criteria used to establish a standard and the certainty of the resulting diagnosis can be expressed about both standards—brain or heart-lung—or indeed about any standard. The certainty issue, then, is not peculiar to a brain-oriented standard.

It is true that public attention has not recently focused on the certainty of the diagnosis of death under the heart-lung formulation. But this has not always been so. From time to time in centuries past, the public questioned the ability of doctors to determine when a person had suffered irreversible cessation of life functions. Writers were able to excite the public imagination with tales of buried people awakening and escaping from coffins.[28] The prospect of premature burial has been eliminated by the practice of embalming. Increased public confidence in the diagnostic ability of physicians has laid the remaining fears largely to rest, although reports of occasional "mistakes" (for example, by paramedics in battle) continue to circulate.

The ethical concern over certainty, then, is addressed to a relatively narrow and technical question: with what assurance can a physician state that the relevant organs will not resume functioning in a person diagnosed to have lost certain vital functions? This question cannot be answered by any moral or philosophical argument; it requires empirical evidence. Since experts testified before the Commission that determinations of death based on the irreversible cessation of total brain functioning are today no more, and perhaps less, subject to error than those based on irreversible cessation of heart and lung functions, this ethical question can be satisfactorily answered: a statute establishing a whole-brain standard for determining death would not lead to an increase in the number of patients declared dead who actually possessed the capacity for recovery. Both standards contained in the proposed statute provide the basis for accurate and reliable determinations, when proper criteria and tests are used with due care by qualified people.

Terminating Medical Interventions on Dead Bodies

A patient correctly diagnosed as having lost brain functions permanently and totally will never regain consciousness. He or she will experience no pleasure or pain, enjoy no social interaction, and be unable to pursue or complete his or her life's projects. Why, then, is there an ethical issue over discontinuing medical interventions? For many, there will be none. As with all dead bodies, it is appropriate to discontinue interventions—indeed, it is usually inappropriate, on both practical and moral grounds, to continue to intervene,[29] except under closely circumscribed conditions (as when a dead person's organs are kept functioning briefly while preparations for organ removal and transplantation are completed).

For some people, however, the withdrawal of treatment from a mechanically respirated patient diagnosed as dead because of loss of all brain functions is difficult and perhaps ethically questionable. Such corpses after all, typically have some appearance of life, such as a moving chest, pulsing blood vessels, and bodily warmth. It is these factors, of course, that make the status of such bodies ambiguous and present the issues for biomedical professionals and the public discussed in this Report.

Ceasing to intervene medically in such cases should be compared with the appropriate behavior in regard to other dead bodies. For example, medical personnel may labor vigorously over a patient with a cardiac arrest. If they are not able to restore spontaneous circulation, they know that the patient is dead and treatment ceases.

The use of the respirator—and the decision to withdraw it from a patient who has been declared dead on the basis of an irreversible cessation of all brain functions—only appears to be different. The superficial difference arises because of differences in the clinical situations. An attempt at cardiac resuscitation is acute and dramatic (typically involving numerous people who labor vigorously, shouting orders and employing ever more Draconian measures). By comparison, an attempt at brain resuscitation is chronic (taking hours or days, not minutes) and typically peaceful (the loudest noise may be the quiet "whoosh" of air from a mechanical respirator and the rhythmic beeping of a cardiac monitor). At the moment of cardiac failure, one can almost see the life pass from a patient, while from the other it has slipped away so stealthily that its image lingers on. Although undeniably disconcerting for many people, the confusion created in personal perception by a determination of "brain death" does not, in the Commission's view, provide a basis for an ethical objection to discontinuing medical measures on these dead bodies any more than on other dead bodies.

Indeed, it is quite important to be clear on this matter because of the attention paid in recent years to the ethical issues in decisions to forego treatment of *dying*—but still living—patients. That is a separate issue, and one which the Commission will address in a subsequent report. Mechanical respirators and associated treatments are applied to two groups of patients: those whom they are helping to keep alive and those who have died despite such treatment. Failure to recognize the distinctness of those two situations will only obscure and exaggerate the difficulties of framing policy. The statute recommended in this Report aids in that process of recognition by providing a legal standard to distinguish the dead from the dying.

APPENDIX F: Guidelines for the Determination of Death

Report of the Medical Consultants on the Diagnosis of Death to the President's Commission for the Study of Ethical Problems in Medicine and Biomedical and Behavioral Research.

FOREWORD

The advent of effective artificial cardiopulmonary support for severely brain-injured persons has created some confusion during the past several decades about the determination of death. Previously, loss of heart and lung functions was an easily observable and sufficient basis for diagnosing death, whether the initial failure occurred in the brain, the heart and lungs, or elsewhere in the body. Irreversible failure of either the heart and lungs or the brain precluded the continued functioning of the other. Now, however, circulation and respiration can be maintained by means of a mechanical respirator and other medical interventions, despite a loss of all brain functions. In these circumstances we recognize as dead an individual whose loss of brain functions is complete and irreversible.

To recognize reliably that death has occurred, accurate criteria must be available for physicians' use. These now fall into two groups, to be applied depending on the clinical situation. When respiration and circulation have irreversibly ceased, there is no need to assess brain functions directly. When cardiopulmonary functions are artificially maintained, neurologic criteria must be used to assess whether brain functions have irreversibly ceased.

More than half of the states now recognize, through statutes or judicial decisions, that death may be determined on the basis of irreversible cessation of all functions of the brain. Law in the remaining states has not yet departed from the older, common law view that death has not occurred until "all vital functions" (whether or not artificially maintained) have ceased. The language of the statutes has not been uniform from state to state, and the diversity of proposed and enacted laws has created substantial confusion. Consequently, the American Bar Association, the American Medical Association, the National Conference of Commissioners on Uniform State Laws, and the President's Commission for the Study of Ethical Problems in Medicine and Biomedical and Behavioral Research have proposed the following model statute, intended for adoption in every jurisdiction:

Uniform Determination of Death Act

An individual who has sustained either (1) irreversible cessation of circulatory and respiratory functions, or (2) irreversible cessation of all functions of the entire brain, including the brain stem, is dead. A determination of death must be made in accordance with accepted medical standards.

This wording has also been endorsed by the American Academy of Neurology and the American Electroencephalographic Society.

The statute relies upon the existence of "accepted medical standards" for determining that death has occurred. The medical profession, based upon carefully conducted research and extensive clinical experience, has found that death can be reliably determined by either cardiopulmonary or neurologic criteria. The tests used for determining cessation of brain functions have changed and will continue to do so with the advent of new research and technologies. The "Harvard criteria" (*Journal of the American Medical Association* 205 [1968]: 337) are widely accepted, but advances in recent years have led to the proposal of other criteria. As an aid to the implementation of the proposed uniform statute, we provide here one statement of currently accepted medical standards.

INTRODUCTION

The criteria that physicians use in determining that death has occurred should:

(1) Eliminate errors in classifying a living individual as dead,
(2) Allow as few errors as possible in classifying a dead body as alive,
(3) Allow a determination to be made without unreasonable delay,
(4) Be adaptable to a variety of clinical situations, and
(5) Be explicit and accessible to verification.

Because it would be undesirable for any guidelines to be mandated by legislation or regulation or to be inflexibly established in case law, the proposed Uniform Determination of Death Act appropriately specifies only "accepted medical standards." Local, state, and national institutions and professional organizations are encouraged to examine and publish their practices.

The following guidelines represent a distillation of current practice in regard to the determination of death. Only the most commonly available and verified tests have been included. The time of death recorded on a death certificate is at present a matter of local practice and is not covered in this document.

These guidelines are advisory. Their successful use requires a competent and judicious physician, experienced in clinical examination and the relevant procedures. All periods of observation listed in these guidelines require the patient to be under the care of a physician. Considering the responsibility entailed in the determination of death, consultation is recommended when appropriate. . . .

THE CRITERIA FOR DETERMINATION OF DEATH

An individual presenting the findings in *either* section A (cardiopulmonary) *or* section B (neurologic) is dead. In either section, a diagnosis of death requires that *both cessation of functions,* as set forth in subsection 1, *and irreversibility,* as set forth in subsection 2, be demonstrated.

A. An individual with irreversible cessation of circulatory and respiratory functions is dead.

1. *Cessation* is recognized by an appropriate clinical examination.

Clinical examination will disclose at least the absence of responsiveness, heartbeat, and respiratory effort. Medical circumstances may require the use of confirmatory tests, such as an ECG.

2. *Irreversibility* is recognized by persistent cessation of functions during an appropriate period of observation and/or trial of therapy.

In clinical situations where death is expected, where the course has been gradual, and where irregular agonal respiration or heartbeat finally ceases, the period of observation following the cessation may be only the few minutes required to complete the examination. Similarly, if resuscitation is not undertaken and ventricular fibrillation and standstill develop in a monitored patient, the required period of observation thereafter may be as short as a few minutes. When a possible death is unobserved, unexpected, or sudden, the examination may need to be more detailed and repeated over a longer period, while appropriate resuscitative effort is maintained as a test of cardiovascular responsiveness. Diagnosis in individuals who are first observed with rigor mortis or putrefaction may require only the observation period necessary to establish that fact.

B. An individual with irreversible cessation of all functions of the entire brain, including the brainstem, is dead.

The "functions of the entire brain" that are relevant to the diagnosis are those that are clinically ascertainable. Where indicated, the clinical diagnosis is subject to confirmation by laboratory tests as described below. Consultation with a physician experienced in this diagnosis is advisable.

1. *Cessation* is recognized when evaluation discloses findings of a *and* b:

a. Cerebral functions are absent, and . . .

There must be deep coma, that is, cerebral unreceptivity and unresponsivity. Medical circumstances may require the use of confirmatory studies such as EEG or blood flow study.

b. Brainstem functions are absent.

Reliable testing of brainstem reflexes requires a perceptive and experienced physician using adequate stimuli. Pupillary light, corneal, oculocephalic, oculovestibular, oropharyngeal, and respiratory (apnea) reflexes should be tested. When these reflexes cannot be adequately assessed, confirmatory tests are recommended.

Adequate testing for apnea is very important. An accepted method is ventilation with pure oxygen or an oxygen and carbon dioxide mixture for ten minutes before withdrawal of the ventilator, followed by passive flow of oxygen. (This procedure allows $PaCO_2$ to rise without hazardous hypoxia.) Hypercarbia adequately stimulates respiratory effort within thirty seconds when $PaCO_2$ is greater than 60 mmHg. A ten minute period of apnea is usually sufficient to attain this level of hypercarbia. Testing of arterial blood gases can be used to confirm this level. Spontaneous breathing efforts indicate that part of the brainstem is functioning.

Peripheral nervous system activity and spinal cord reflexes may persist after death. True decerebrate or decorticate posturing or seizures are inconsistent with the diagnosis of death.

2. *Irreversibility* is recognized when evaluation discloses findings of a *and* b *and* c:

a. The cause of coma is established and is sufficient to account for the loss of brain functions, and . . .

Most difficulties with the determination of death on the basis of neurologic criteria have resulted from inadequate attention to this basic diagnostic prerequisite. In addition to a careful clinical examination and investigation of history, relevant knowledge of causation may be acquired by computed tomographic scan, measurement of core temperature, drug screening, EEG, angiography, or other procedures.

b. The possibility of recovery of any brain functions is excluded, and . . .

The most important reversible conditions are sedation, hypothermia, neuromuscular blockade, and shock. In the unusual circumstance where a sufficient cause cannot be established, irreversibility can be reliably inferred only after extensive evaluation for drug intoxication, extended observation, and other testing. A determination that blood flow to the brain is absent can be used to demonstrate a sufficient and irreversible condition.

c. The cessation of all brain functions persists for an appropriate period of observation and/or trial of therapy.

Even when coma is known to have started at an earlier time, the absence of all brain functions must be established by an experienced physician at the initiation of the observation period. The duration of observation periods is a matter of clinical judgment, and some physicians recommend shorter or longer periods than those given here.

Except for patients with drug intoxication, hypothermia, young age, or shock, medical centers with substantial experience in diagnosing death neurologically report no cases of brain functions returning following a six hour cessation, documented by clinical examination and confirmatory EEG. In the absence of confirmatory tests, a period of observation of at least twelve hours is recommended when an irreversible condition is well established. For anoxic brain damage where the extent of damage is more difficult to ascertain, observation for twenty-four hours is generally desirable. In anoxic injury, the observation period may be reduced if a test shows cessation of cerebral blood flow or if an EEG shows electrocerebral silence in an adult patient without drug intoxication, hypothermia, or shock.

Confirmation of clinical findings by EEG is desirable when objective documentation is needed to substantiate the clinical findings. Electrocerebral silence verifies irreversible loss of cortical functions, except in patients with drug intoxication or hypothermia. (Important technical details are provided in: American Electroencephalographic Society, *Guidelines in EEG 1980*, Section 4: "Minimum Technical Standards for EEG Recording in Suspected Cerebral Death," pp. 19–24, Atlanta, 1980.) When joined with the clinical findings of absent brainstem functions, electrocerebral silence confirms the diagnosis.

Complete cessation of circulation to the normothermic adult brain for more than ten minutes is incompatible with survival of brain tissue. Documentation of this circulatory failure is therefore evidence of death of the entire brain. Four-vessel intracranial angiography is definitive for diagnosing cessation of circulation to the entire brain (both cerebrum and posterior fossa) but entails substantial practical difficulties and risks. Tests are available that assess circulation only in the cerebral hemispheres, namely radioisotope bolus cerebral angiography and gamma camera imaging with radioisotope cerebral angiography. Without complicating conditions, absent cerebral blood flow as measured by these tests, in conjunction with the clinical determination of cessation of all brain functions for at least six hours, is diagnostic of death.

COMPLICATING CONDITIONS

A. Drug and Metabolic Intoxication

Drug intoxication is the most serious problem in the determination of death, especially when multiple drugs are used. Cessation of brain functions caused by the sedative and anesthetic drugs, such as barbiturates, benzodiazepines, meprobamate, methaqualone, and trichloroethylene, may be completely reversible even though they produce clinical cessation of brain functions and electrocerebral silence. In cases where there is any likelihood of sedative presence, toxicology screening for all likely drugs is required. If exogenous intoxication is found, death may not be declared until the intoxicant is metabolized or intracranial circulation is tested and found to have ceased.

Total paralysis may cause unresponsiveness, areflexia, and apnea that closely simulates death. Exposure to drugs such as neuromuscular blocking agents or aminoglycoside antibiotics, and diseases like myasthenia gravis are usually apparent by careful review of the history. Prolonged paralysis after use of succinylcholine chloride and related drugs requires evaluation for pseudo-cholinesterase deficiency. If there is any question, low-dose atropine stimulation, electromyogram, peripheral nerve stimulation, EEG, tests of intracranial circulation, or extended observation, as indicated, will make the diagnosis clear.

In drug-induced coma, EEG activity may return or persist while the patient remains unresponsive, and therefore the EEG may be an important evaluation along with extended observation. If the EEG shows electrocerebral silence, short latency auditory or somatosensory evoked potentials may be used to test brainstem functions, since these potential are unlikely to be affected by drugs.

Some severe illnesses (e.g., hepatic encephalopathy, hyperosmolar coma, and preterminal uremia) can cause deep coma. Before irreversible cessation of brain functions can be determined, metabolic abnormalities should be considered and, if possible, corrected. Confirmatory tests of circulation or EEG may be necessary.

B. Hypothermia

Criteria for reliable recognition of death are not available in the presence of hypothermia (below 32.2 °C core temperature). The variables of cerebral circulation in hypothermic patients are not sufficiently well studied to know whether tests of absent or diminished circulation are confirmatory. Hypothermia can mimic brain death by ordinary clinical criteria and can protect against neurologic damage due to hypoxia. Further complications arise since hypothermia also usually precedes and follows death. If these complicating factors make it unclear whether an individual is alive, the only available measure to resolve the issue is to restore normothermia. Hypothermia is not a common cause of difficulty in the determination of death.

C. Children

The brains of infants and young children have increased resistance to damage and may recover substantial functions even after exhibiting unresponsiveness on neurological examination for longer periods than do adults. Physicians should be particularly cautious in applying neurologic criteria to determine death in children younger than five years.

D. Shock

Physicians should also be particularly cautious in applying neurologic criteria to determine death in patients in shock because the reduction in cerebral circulation can render clinical examination and laboratory tests unreliable.

NOTES

1. Why Update Death?

1. Marc Alexander, "The Rigid Embrace of the Narrow House: Premature Burial and the Signs of Death," 10 *Hastings Center Report* 25 (1980); John D. Arnold, Thomas F. Zimmerman and Daniel C. Martin, "Public Attitudes and the Diagnosis of Death," 206 *Journal of the American Medical Association* 1949 (1968).
2. Alexander, "The Rigid Embrace," at 30, citing, Orifila, *A Popular Treatise on the Remedies to be Employed in Case of Poisoning and Apparent Death; Including Means of Detecting Poisons, of Distinguishing Real From Apparent Death, and of Ascertaining the Adulteration of Wines,* trans. from French, Philadelphia (1818) at 154; G. Tourdes, "Mort (Medicine legate)," *Dictionnaire Encyclopedique des Sciences Medicales* Ser. II, X (1875) at 579–708, 603.
3. Ronald E. Cranford and Harmon L. Smith, "Some Critical Distinctions Between Brain Death and Persistent Vegetative State" 6 *Ethics in Science and Medicine* (1979): 199, 201.
4. H. A. H. van Till-d'Aulnis de Bourouill, "Diagnosis of Death in Comatose Patients under Resuscitation Treatment: A Critical Review of the Harvard Report," 2 *Am. J. L. & Med.* 1 (1976): 21–22.
5. One exception to this general picture requires brief mention. Certain drugs or low body temperature (hypothermia) can place the neurons in "suspended animation." Under these conditions, the neurons may receive virtually no oxygen or glucose for a significant period of time without sustaining irreversible damage. This effect is being used to try to limit brain injury in patients by giving them barbiturates or reducing temperature; the use of such techniques will, of course, make neurological diagnoses slower or more complicated.
6. Julius Korein, "Brain Death," *in* J. Cottrell and H. Turndorf (eds.) *Anesthesia and Neurosurgery*, C.V. Mosby & Co., St. Louis (1980), 282, 284, 292–293.
7. Cranford and Smith, "Some Critical Distinctions," at 203.
8. Bryan Jennett and Fred Plum, "The Persistent Vegetative State: A Syndrome in Search of a Name," 1 *Lancet* 734 (1972); Fred Plum and Jerome B. Posner, *The Diagnosis of Stupor and Coma*, F. A. David Co., Philadelphia (1980 3rd. ed.) at 6–7.
9. See Norris McWhirter (ed.) *The Guinness Book of World Records*, Bantam Books, New York (1981) at 42, citing the case of Elaine Esposito who lapsed into coma following surgery on August 6, 1941, and died on November 25, 1978, 37 years and 111 days later.

2. The "State of the Art" in Medicine

1. Ake Grenvik, David J. Powner, James V. Snyder, Michael S. Jastremski, Ralph A. Babcock and Michael G. Loughhead, "Cessation of Therapy in Terminal Illness and Brain Death," 6 *Critical Care Medicine* 284 (1978).
2. Accordingly, in the procedures for diagnosing death set forth by the Commission's medical consultants in Appendix F (of the original report) . . . the test for apnea involves elevating the level of circulating oxygen before turning off the respirator and allowing the level of carbon dioxide to rise as a stimulus for spontaneous respiration. The high level of oxygen protects the brain cells (if any remain active) from further damage.

3. P. Mollaret and M. Goulon, "Le Coma Dépassé," 101 *Revue Neurologique* 3 (1959).
4. A. Earl Walker, E. L. Diamond and John Moseley, "The Neuropathological Findings in Irreversible Coma; A Critique of the Respirator Brain," 34 *Journal Neuropath Exp Neurol* 295 (1975); John I. Moseley, Gaetano F. Molinari and A. Earl Walker, "Respirator Brain: Report of a Survey and Review of Current Concepts," 100 *Arch. Pathol. Lab. Med.* 61 (1976).
5. See, e.g., Renee C. Fox and Judith P. Swazey, *The Courage to Fail: A Social View of Organ Transplantation and Dialysis*, University of Chicago Press, Chicago, (1978); Francis D. Moore, *Give and Take: The Biology of Tissue Transplantation*, W.B. Sanders, Co., Philadelphia, Pa. (1964).
6. See, e.g., Howard H. Kaufman, John D. Hutchton, Megan M. McBride, Carolyn A. Beardsley and Barry D. Kahan, "Kidney Donation: Needs and Possibilities," 5 *Neurosurg.* 237 (1979); K. J. Bart, "The Prevalence of Cadaveric Organs for Transplantation" in S.W. Sell, U.P. Perry and M.M. Vincent (eds.) *Proceedings of the 1977 Annual Meeting of American Association Tissue Banks*, American Association of Tissue Banks, Rockville, Md. (1977), at 124–130; A. Earl Walker, "The Neurosurgeon's Responsibility for Organ Procurement," 44 *J. Neurosurg.* 1 (1976).
7. B.D. Colen, "Medical Examiner's Solution to Life and Death Problem," January 28, 1978, *Washington Post*, section A, 8, col. 1, describing the attempts of Dr. Ron Wright, deputy chief medical examiner for Dade County Florida, to have medical interventions ceased for bodies declared dead on the basis of brain-oriented criteria. (Florida did not enact a statute on the subject until 1980.) "Wright was able to get a judge to hold a special Sunday morning hearing at the hospital—with reporters and photographers in attendance—at which he successfully argued that the family was being forced to pay $2,000 a day to keep a dead body in the intensive care unit." Patricia H. Butcher, "Management of the Relatives of Patients with Brain Death" in Ronald V. Trubuhovich (ed). *Management of Acute Intracranial Disasters*, Little, Brown and Company, Boston, Mass. (1979) at 327.
8. Ad Hoc Committee of the Harvard Medical School to Examine the Definition of Brain Death, "A Definition of Irreversible Coma," 205 *J.A.M.A.* 337 (1968).
9. David J. Powner, James V. Snyder, and Ake Grenvik, "Brain Death Certification: A Review," 5 *Crit. Care Med.* 230 (1977); Julius Korein, "Brain Death," *in* J. Cottrell and H. Turndorf (eds.) *Anesthesia and Neurosurgery* (1980) at 282; Peter McL. Black, "Brain Death" 299 *New England Journal of Medicine* (1978), 338 and 393.
10. See, e.g., Julius Korein (ed.), *Brain Death: Interrelated Medical and Social Issues* 315 *Annual of the New York Academy of Science* 62–214 (1978); Julius Korein, Phillip Braunstein, Ajax George, Melvin Wichter, Irving Kricheff, Abraham Lieberman and John Pearson, "Brain Death: I. Angiographic Correlation with the Radioisotopic Bolus Technique for Evaluation of Critical Deficit of Cerebral Blood Flow," 2 *Ann. Neurol.* 206 (1977); Andrew J.K. Smith and A. Earl Walker, "Cerebral Blood Flow and Brain Metabolism as Indicators of Cerebral Death: A Review," 133 *Johns Hopkins Medical Journal* 107 (1973); Julius M. Goodman and Larry I. Heck, "Confirmation of Brain Death by Bedside Isotope Angiography," 238 *Journal of the American Medical Association* 966 (1977).
11. See, e.g., Gian Emilio Chatrian, "Electrophysiologic Evaluation of Brain Death: A Critical Appraisal," *in* M. J. Aminoff (ed.) *Electrodiagnosis in Clinical Neurology*, Churchill Livingstone, New York (1980); Donald R. Bennett, Julius Korein, John R. Hughes, Jerome K. Merlis and Cary Suter, *Atlas of Electroencephalography in Coma and Cerebral Death*, Raven Press, New York (1976); Fred Plum and Jerome B. Posner, *The diagnosis of stupor and coma*; Stuart A. Schneck, "Brain Death and Prolonged State of Impaired Responsiveness," 58 *Denver Law Journal* 609, 612–613 (1981).
12. See, e.g., U.S. Department of Health and Human Services, *The NINCDS Collaborative Study of Brain Death*, NIH Publication 81-2286, U.S. Government Printing Office (1980), reported in, "An Appraisal of the Criteria of Cerebral Death. A Summary Statement. A Collaborative Study," 237 *Journal of the American Medical Association* 982 (1977); Peter McL. Black, "Brain Death"; Pamela F. Prior, "Brain Death" 1980(i) *Lancet* 1142.
13. See, e.g., Bryan Jennett, John Gleave and Peter Wilson, "Brain Death in Three Neurosurgical Units" 282 *British Medical Journal* 533 (1981).
14. See, e.g., U.S. Department of Health and Human Services, *The NINCDS Collaborative Study*.
15. Peter McL. Black, "Brain Death."
16. Conference of Royal Colleges and Faculties of the United Kingdom, "Memorandum on the Diagnosis of Death" (January 1979), *in* Working Party of the United Kingdom Health Departments, *The Removal of Cadaveric Organs for Transplantation: A Code of Practice* (1979) at 32–36.
17. See Appendix F; Peter McL. Black, "Brain Death"; Julius Korein, "Brain Death."
18. Conference of Royal Colleges and Faculties, *The Removal of Cadaveric Organs*, at 35. "Medicine and the Media," 281 *British Medical Journal* 1064 (1980). See also A. Mohandas and Shelley Chou, "Brain death: A Clinical and pathological study," 35 *Journal of Neurosurgery* 211, 215 (1971) (authors of so-called "Minnesota criteria" hold that "the state of irreversible damage to the brain-stem . . . is the point of no return"). The more typical contrast between the American and British approaches is illustrated by the criteria employed at the University of Pittsburgh School of Medicine where "brain death" is defined as the "irreversible cessation of all brain function," as demonstrated by coma of established cause, absence of movements and brain stem reflexes, and an isoelectric EEG. David J. Powner and Ake Grenvik, "Triage in Patient Care: From Expected Recovery to Brain Death," 8 *Heart & Lung* 1103 (1979). The British rely instead on another observation, confirmed by the University of Pittsburgh, that "*prognosis* appears to be *similarly hopeless* for those patients who have clinical findings consistent with brain death but who have a nonisoelectric EEG" . . . 1107 (emphasis added) (cited by British neurologist Christopher Pallis in lecture at Conference on Brain Death, Boston, Mass., April 4, 1981).
19. Conference of Royal Colleges and Faculties, *The Removal of Cadaveric Organs* at 36.

3. Understanding the Meaning of Death

1. See, e.g., Robert M. Veatch, *Death, Dying and the Biological Revolution: Our Last Quest for Responsibility,* Yale University Press, New Haven, Conn. (1977) at 21–76; Douglas N. Walton, *Defining Death: An Analytic Study of the Concept of Death in Philosophy and Medical Ethics,* McGill-Queen's University Press, Montreal, Quebec (1979); William C. Charron, "Death: A Philosophical Perspective on the Legal Definitions," 4 *Washington University Law Quarterly* 797 (1975); Dallas M. High, "Death: Its Conceptual Elusiveness," 55 *Soundings* 438 (1972); Paul Ramsey, *The Patient as Person: Explorations in Medical Ethics,* Yale University Press, New Haven, Conn. (1971) at 59–112; Stanley Hauerwas, "Religious Concepts of Brain Death and Associated Problems," 315 *Annals of the New York Academy of Science* 329 (1978).
2. Germain Grisez & Joseph M. Boyle, Jr., *Life and Death with Liberty and Justice: A Contribution to the Euthanasia Debate,* University of Notre Dame Press, Notre Dame, Ind. (1979) at 59–61, and page 77:

   > If death is understood in theoretical terms as the permanent termination of the integrated functioning characteristic of a living body as a whole, then one can see why death of higher animals is usually grasped in factual terms by the cessation of the vital functions of respiration and circulation, which correlates so well with bodily decomposition. Breathing is the minimum in "social interaction." However, considering the role of the brain in the maintenance of the dynamic equilibrium of any system which includes a brain, there is a compelling reason for defining death in factual terms as that state of affairs in which there is complete and irreversible loss of the functioning of the entire brain. To accept this definition is not to make a choice based on one's evaluation of various human characteristics, but is to assent to a theory which fits the facts.

3. Julius Korein, "The Problem of Brain Death: Development and History," 315 *Annals of the New York Academy of Science* 19 (1978).
4. James L. Bernat, Charles M. Culver and Bernard Gert, "On the Definition and Criterion of Death," 94 *Annual of Internal Medicine* 389, 391 (1981); and Grisez & Boyle, *Life and Death with Liberty and Justice* at 77:

   > . . . When the respirator maintains the organism, it is questionable whether there is complete and irreversible loss of the functioning of the entire brain. But this is a question to be settled by empirical inquiry, not by philosophy. Philosophically, we answer the objection by saying that if the functioning of the brain is the factor which principally integrates any organism which has a brain, then if that function is lost, what is left is no longer as a whole an organic unity. If the dynamic equilibrium of the remaining parts of the system is maintained, it nevertheless as a whole is a mechanical, not an organic system.

5. H. Tristram Engelhardt, Jr., "Defining Death: A Philosophical Problem for Medicine and Law," 112 *Annual Review of Respiratory Diseases* 587 (1975); Robert M. Veatch, "The Whole-Brain Oriented Concept of Death: An Out-moded Philosophical Formulation," 3 *Journal of Thanatology* 13 (1975).
6. Michael B. Green and Daniel Wikler, "Brain Death and Personal Identity," 9 *Philosophy and Public Affairs* 105 (1980); Bernard Gert, "Personal Identity and the Body," *Dialogue* 458 (1971); Roland Puccetti, "The Conquest of Death" 59 *The Monist* 252 (1976); Azriel Rosenfeld, "The Heart, the Head and the Halakhah," *New York State Journal of Medicine* 2615 (1970).
7. "Karen Ann Quinlan: A Family's Fate," May 26, 1981, *Washington Post,* A at 1, col. 1.
8. J. David Bleich, "Neurological Criteria of Death and Time of Death Statutes," *in* Fred Rosner and J. David Bleich (eds.), *Jewish Bioethics.* Hebrew Publishing Co., New York (1979) at 303–316.
9. Telephone conversation with Richard E. Grant, Assistant Professor of Nursing, Arizona State University, July 17, 1981.
10. Milton McC. Gatch, "Death: Post-Biblical Christian Thought" in Warren T. Reich (ed.), *Encyclopedia of Bioethics* (v. 1), MacMillan Publishing Co., New York (1976) at 249, 250; Saint Augustine, *The City of God,* Vernon H. Bourke (ed.) Image Books, Garden City, NY (1958) at 269, 277; J. David Bleich, "Establishing Criteria of Death," *in* Fred Rosner and J. David Bleich (eds.), *Jewish Bioethics,* Hebrew Publishing Co., New York (1979) at 285.
11. Bernard Haring, *Medical Ethics,* Fides Publishers, Inc., Notre Dame, Ind. (1973) at 136; Charles J. McFadden, *"The Dignity of Life: Moral Values in a Changing Society,* Our Sunday Visitor, Inc., Huntington, Ind. (1976) at 202; Paul Ramsey, *The Patient as Person,* at 59–112; Seymour Siegel, "Updating the Criteria of Death," 30 *Conservative Judaism* 23 (1976); Moses D. Tendler, "Cessation of Brain Function: Ethical Implications In Terminal Care and Organ Transplant," 315 *Annals of the New York Academy of Science* 394 (1978). . . .

5. What "Definition" Ought to Be Adopted?

1. Alexander M. Capron and Leon R. Kass, "A Statutory Definition of the Standards for Determining Human Death: An Appraisal and a Proposal," 121 *University of Pennsylvania Law Review* 87, 102–104 (1972); see also Robert M. Veatch, *Death, Dying and the Biological Revolution: Our Last Quest for Responsibility,* Yale University Press, New Haven, Conn. (1977) at 68; Task Force on Death and Dying of the Institute of Society, Ethics and the Life Sciences, "Refinements for the Determination of Death: An Appraisal," 221 *Journal of the American Medical Association* 48, 52 (1972).
2. Ad Hoc Committee of the Harvard Medical School to Examine the Definition of Brain Death, "A Definition of Irreversible Coma," 205 *Journal of the American Medical Association* 337 (1968).
3. Black, "Brain Death": Ronald E. Cranford, "Minnesota Medical Association Criteria: Brain Death: Concept and Criteria," 61 *Minn. Med.* 600 (1978).

4. Roger B. Dworkin, "Death in Context," 48 *Indiana Law Journal* 623, 629 (1973).
5. See, e.g., Fred Fabro, "Bacchiochi vs. Johnson Memorial Hospital" 45 *Connecticut Journal of Medicine* 267 (1981) chronicling the troublesome case of Melanie Bacchiochi. On February 11, 1981, after repeated clinical examinations confirmed by electroencephalography, physicians found she had suffered irreversible loss of total brain function. Her physician was unwilling to remove her from the respirator because of legal uncertainty since Connecticut's statute on "brain death" applies only to organ transplantation. "It is ironic that if the patient had been a donor, she could have been pronounced dead on February 11 and the respirator could have been withdrawn. Dead for transplantation, but not dead otherwise!" (p. 268).
6. Alexander M. Capron, "The Purpose of Death: A Reply to Professor Dworkin," 48 *Indiana Law Journal* 640, 643–45 (1973); Capron and Kass, "A Statutory Definition of the Standards for Determining Human Death," at 107–08.
7. David Sanders and Jesse Dukeminier, Jr., "Medical Advance and Legal Lag: Hemodialysis and Kidney Transplantation," 15 *UCLA Law Review* 357, 410 (1968).
8. Although the *Quinlan* case focused public attention on the capabilities of intensive medical care to resuscitate comatose individuals, legislation of the type recommended in this Report and already adopted in some states would not hold Karen Quinlan to be dead. As this Report has repeatedly emphasized, situations like Ms. Quinlan's do not involve determinations of death but rather decisions about whether to cease treatment of patients with no prospect of recovery to consciousness. This is a distinct bioethical and legal issue receiving separate attention from the President's Commission. Joseph Quinlan and Julia Quinlan (with Phyllis Battelle), *Karen Ann: The Quinlans Tell Their Story*, Doubleday and Co., Garden City, N. Y. (1977); *In the Matter of Karen Ann Quinlan: The Complete Briefs, Oral Arguments and the Opinion of the New Jersey Supreme Court, Washington, D.C., University Publications of America*, Inc. (1975) (2 vols.); *In Re Quinlan*, 70 N.J. 10 (1976).
9. See Appendix C, Parts I and III [in the original report].
10. See Appendix D [in the original report].
11. For example, the Kansas statute might be (mis)applied to declare dead a patient who still has some brain functions but who is experiencing repeated and apparently terminal respiratory difficulties, because the first paragraph of Kan. Stat. Ann. §777-02 states that a person is dead when "Attempts at resuscitation [of respiratory and cardiac function] are considered hopeless." Disputes could arise under the Oregon statute over the propriety of a physician declaring a person dead after a severe trauma to the heart and lungs without attempting resuscitation; Or. Rev. Stat. §146.087 treats a person as alive only if "*spontaneous* respiration and circulatory function" can be restored.
12. Law Reform Commission of Canada, *Criteria for the Determination of Death*, Report No. 15), Minister of Supply and Service, Canada (1981) at 7–20.
13. See, e.g., California Health and Safety Code §7180 (West 1975).
14. Paul A. Bryne, Sean O'Reilly and Paul M. Quay, "Brain Death: An Opposing Viewpoint," 242 *Journal of the American Medical Association* 1985 (1979).
15. Already, a hand "destroyed" in an accident can be reconstructed using advanced surgical methods. The functions of the kidney can be artificially restored through extracorporeal devices; an implantable artificial heart has been tested in animals and is now proposed for human trials. It is impossible to predict what other "miracles" biomedical science may some day produce in the restoration of natural functions or their substitution through artificial means.
16. James L. Bernat, Charles M. Culver and Bernard Gert. "On the Definition and Criterion of Death," 94 *Annual of Internal Medicine* 389 (1981):

> If we regard death as a process then either the process starts when the person is still living, which confuses the "process of death" with the process of dying, for we all regard someone who is dying as not yet dead, or the "process of death" starts when the person is no longer alive, which confuses death with the process of disintegration.

17. *Edwards v. United States*, 519 F.2d 1137 (5th Cir. 1975); *Price v. Neyland*, 320 F.2d 674 (D.C. Cir. 1963).
18. 243 *Journal of the American Medical Association* 420 (1980) (editorial).
19. Kan. Stat. Ann. §77–202 (Supp. 1971).
20. 100 *American Bar Association Annual Report*. 231–232 (1978) (February 1975 Midyear Meeting).
21. Uniform Brain Death Act §1, 12 *Uniform Laws Annot.* 15 (Supp. 1980).
22. Uniform Anatomical Gift Act §7(b), 8 *Uniform Laws Annot.* 608 (1972).
23. Veatch, *Death, Dying and the Biological Revolution*, at 72–76; Michael T. Sullivan, "The Dying Person—His Plight and His Right," 8 *New England Law Review* 197, 216 (1973).
24. Capron, "Legal Definition of Death," 356–357.
25. Physicians have recognized the need for sensitivity and good communication on this point. For example, see David J. Powner and Ake Grenvik, "Triage in Patient Care: From Expected Recovery to Brain Death," *Heart and Lung* 8 (1979): 1103, 1107:

> Before and during the diagnostic evaluation of brain death, the patient's family is informed not only of the patient's medical condition but also of the concept of brain death, its diagnosis, and the consequences of death certification in these cases. Because the declaration of death is the legal responsibility of the medical practitioner, the family's permission for this procedure is not sought but their questions and concerns must be answered honestly and with the necessary education and communication regarding the events following discontinuation of cardiopulmonary support. . . . When transplantation is not planned, family members may request to be at the bedside when the ventilator is removed. This is permitted but the family is advised that peripheral muscle movements may be observed during the ensuing anoxia and that these are not dependent on remaining brain function.

26. Bethia S. Currie, "The Redefinition of Death," *in* S.F. Spicker (ed.) *Organism, Medicine, and Metaphysics*, D. Reidel Publishing Co., Dordrecht, Holland (1978) at 177, 184–191. Review of the cases cited established that in none

was a patient who subsequently recovered spontaneous functioning ever dead according to the standard of "irreversible cessation of all functions of the brain" or by the detailed medical guidelines set forth in Appendix F to this Report.

27. Byrne, O'Reilly and Quay, "Brain Death: An Opposing Viewpoint."
28. See pp. 13–15 [in the original report; here: the beginning of Chapter 1]; Edgar Allan Poe, "Fall of the House of Usher," David Galloway (ed.) *Edgar Allan Poe: Selected Writings,* Penguin Books, New York (1979) at 138.
29. Cf. Markku Kaste, Matti Hillbom, and Jorma Palo, "Diagnosis and Management of Brain Death," 1 *British Medical Journal* 525, 527 (1979): "As soon as it is obvious that the patient cannot recover, life-supporting measures should perhaps be withdrawn, since continued support may increase reluctance to embark on resuscitative measures generally."

IN THE MATTER OF KAREN QUINLAN: THE SUPREME COURT, STATE OF NEW JERSEY (1976)

INTRODUCTION. *The terminal illness treatment refusal case that captured the lay public's attention involved a twenty-one-year-old young woman who apparently suffered respiratory arrest following consumption of an overdose of alcohol together with a tranquilizing drug. She would never regain consciousness, but emergency medical intervention stabilized her breathing on a ventilator, leaving her in a persistent vegetative state. Her father, acting on behalf of himself and his wife, sought to be appointed her guardian for the announced purpose of withdrawing the ventilator, even though they believed this action would mean their daughter's death. After a lower court sided with the physician who insisted on continuing the life-support, the Supreme Court gave her father the authority to select his daughter's physician, in effect, giving him the power to decide whether the ventilator would be withdrawn. The court introduced the notion of an ethics committee, which was asked to review the case and confirm the patient's prognosis. The court rejected the physician's claim that the profession of medicine had the authority to resolve such matters.*

The Factual Base

An understanding of the issues in their basic perspective suggests a brief review of the factual base developed in the testimony and documented in greater detail in the opinion of the trial judge. *In re Quinlan*, 137 N.J.Super. 227, 348 A.2d 801 (Ch.Div.1975).

On the night of April 15, 1975, for reasons still unclear, Karen Quinlan ceased breathing for at least two 15 minute periods. She received some ineffectual mouth-to-mouth resuscitation from friends. She was taken by ambulance to Newton Memorial Hospital. There she had a temperature of 100 degrees, her pupils were unreactive and she was unresponsive even to deep pain. The history at the time of her admission to that hospital was essentially incomplete and uninformative.

Three days later, Dr. Morse examined Karen at the request of the Newton admitting physician, Dr. McGee. He found her comatose with evidence of decortication, a condition relating to derangement of the cortex of the brain causing a physical posture in which the upper extremities are flexed and the lower extremities are extended. She required a respirator to assist her breathing. Dr. Morse was unable to obtain an adequate account of the circumstances and events leading up to Karen's admission to the Newton Hospital. Such initial history or etiology is crucial in neurological diagnosis. Relying as he did upon the Newton Memorial records and his own examination, he concluded that prolonged lack of oxygen in the bloodstream, anoxia, was identified with her condition as he saw it upon first observation. When she was later transferred to Saint Clare's Hospital she was still unconscious, still on a respirator and a tracheotomy had been performed. On her arrival Dr. Morse conducted extensive and detailed examinations. An electroencephalogram (EEG) measuring electrical rhythm of the brain was performed and Dr. Morse characterized the result as "abnormal but it showed some activity and was consistent with her clinical state." Other significant neurological tests, including a brain scan, an angiogram, and a lumbar puncture were normal in result. Dr. Morse testified that Karen has been in a state of coma, lack of consciousness, since he began treating her. He explained that there are basically two types of coma, sleep-like unresponsiveness and awake unresponsiveness. Karen was originally in

Condensed from 355 *Atlantic Reporter* 2d Series. Matter of Quinlan. Cite as 355 A.2d 647.

a sleep-like unresponsive condition but soon developed "sleep-wake" cycles, apparently a normal improvement for comatose patients occurring within three to four weeks. In the awake cycle she blinks, cries out and does things of that sort but is still totally unaware of anyone or anything around her.

Dr. Morse and other expert physicians who examined her characterized Karen as being in a "chronic persistent vegetative state." Dr. Fred Plum, one of such expert witnesses, defined this as a "subject who remains with the capacity to maintain the vegetative parts of neurological function but who . . . no longer has any cognitive function."

Dr. Morse, as well as the several other medical and neurological experts who testified in this case, believed with certainty that Karen Quinlan is not "brain dead." They identified the Ad Hoc Committee of Harvard Medical School report (*infra*) as the ordinary medical standard for determining brain death, and all of them were satisfied that Karen met none of the criteria specified in that report and was therefore not "brain dead" within its contemplation.

In this respect it was indicated by Dr. Plum that the brain works in essentially two ways, the vegetative and the sapient. He testified:

> We have an internal vegetative regulation which controls body temperature which controls breathing, which controls to a considerable degree blood pressure, which controls to some degree heart rate, which controls chewing, swallowing and which controls sleeping and waking. We have a more highly developed brain which is uniquely human which controls our relation to the outside world, our capacity to talk, to see, to feel, to sing, to think. Brain death necessarily must mean the death of both of these functions of the brain, vegetative and the sapient. Therefore, the presence of any function which is regulated or governed or controlled by the deeper parts of the brain which in laymen's terms might be considered purely vegetative would mean that the brain is not biologically dead.

Because Karen's neurological condition affects her respiratory ability (the respiratory system being a brain stem function) she requires a respirator to assist her breathing. From the time of her admission to Saint Clare's Hospital Karen has been assisted by an MA-1 respirator, a sophisticated machine which delivers a given volume of air at a certain rate and periodically provides a "sigh" volume, a relatively large measured volume of air designed to purge the lungs of excretions. Attempts to "wean" her from the respirator were unsuccessful and have been abandoned.

The experts believe that Karen cannot now survive without the assistance of the respirator; that exactly how long she would live without it is unknown; that the strong likelihood is that death would follow soon after its removal, and that removal would also risk further brain damage and would curtail the assistance the respirator presently provides in warding off infection.

It seemed to be the consensus not only of the treating physicians but also of the several qualified experts who testified in the case, that removal from the respirator would not conform to medical practices, standards and traditions.

The further medical consensus was that Karen in addition to being comatose is in a chronic and persistent "vegetative" state, having no awareness of anything or anyone around her and existing at a primitive reflex level. Although she does have some brain stem function (ineffective for respiration) and has other reactions one normally associates with being alive, such as moving, reacting to light, sound and noxious stimuli, blinking her eyes, and the like, the quality of her feeling impulses is unknown. She grimaces, makes stereotyped cries and sounds and has chewing motions. Her blood pressure is normal.

Karen remains in the intensive care unit at Saint Clare's Hospital, receiving 24-hour care by a team of four nurses characterized, as was the medical attention, as "excellent." She is nourished by feeding by way of a nasal-gastro tube and is routinely examined for infection, which under these circumstances is a serious life threat. The result is that her condition is considered remarkable under the unhappy circumstances involved.

Karen is described as emaciated, having suffered a weight loss of at least 40 pounds, and undergoing a continuing deteriorative process. Her posture is described as fetal-like and grotesque; there is extreme flexion-rigidity of the arms, legs and related muscles and her joints are severely rigid and deformed.

From all of this evidence, and including the whole testimonial record, several basic findings in the physical area are mandated. Severe brain and associated damage, albeit of uncertain etiology, has left Karen in a chronic and persistent vegetative state. No form of treatment which can cure or improve that condition is known or available. As nearly as may be determined, considering the guarded area of remote uncertainties characteristic of most medical science predictions, she can *never* be restored to cognitive or sapient life. Even with regard to the vegetative level and improvement therein (if such it may be called) the prognosis is extremely poor and the extent unknown if it should in fact occur.

She is debilitated and moribund and although fairly stable at the time of argument before us (no new information having been filed in the meanwhile in expansion of the record), no physician risked the opinion that she could live more than a year and indeed she may die much earlier. Excellent medical and nursing care so far has been able to ward off the constant threat of infection, to which she is peculiarly susceptible because of the respirator, the tracheal tube and other incidents of care in her vulnerable condition. Her life accordingly is sustained by the respirator and tubal feeding, and removal from the respirator would cause her death soon, although the time cannot be stated with more precision.

The determination of the fact and time of death in past years of medical science was keyed to the action of the heart and blood circulation, in turn dependent upon pulmonary activity, and hence cessation of these functions spelled out the reality of death [note omitted].

Developments in medical technology have obfuscated the use of the traditional definition of death. Efforts have been made to define irreversible coma as a new criterion for death, such as by the 1968 report of the Ad Hoc Committee of the Harvard Medical School (the Committee comprising ten physicians, an historian, a lawyer and a theologian), which asserted that:

> From ancient times down to the recent past it was clear that, when the respiration and heart stopped, the brain would die in a few minutes; so the obvious criterion of no heart beat as synonymous with death was sufficiently accurate. In those times the heart was considered to be the central organ of the body; it is not surprising that its failure marked the onset of death. This is no longer valid when modern resuscitative and supportive measures are used. These improved activities can now restore "life" as judged by the ancient standards of persistent respiration and continuing heart beat. This can be the case even when there is not the remotest possibility of an individual recovering consciousness following massive brain damage. ["A Definition of Irreversible Coma," 205 J.A.M.A. 337, 339 (1968)].

The Ad Hoc standards, carefully delineated, included absence of response to pain or other stimuli, pupillary reflexes, corneal, pharyngeal and other reflexes, blood pressure, spontaneous respiration, as well as "flat" or isoelectric electroencephalograms and the like, with all tests repeated "at least 24 hours later with no change." In such circumstances, where all of such criteria have been met as showing "brain death," the Committee recommends with regard to the respirator:

> The patient's condition can be determined only by a physician. When the patient is hopelessly damaged as defined above, the family and all colleagues who have participated in major decisions concerning the patient, and all nurses involved, should be so informed. Death is to be declared and *then* the respirator turned off. The decision to do this and the responsibility for it are to be taken by the physician-in-charge, in consultation with one or more physicians who have been directly involved in the case. It is unsound and undesirable to force the family to make the decision. [205 J.A.M.A., *supra* at 338 [emphasis in original]].

But, as indicated, it was the consensus of medical testimony in the instant case that Karen, for all her disability, met none of these criteria, nor indeed any comparable criteria extant in the medical world and representing, as does the Ad Hoc Committee report, according to the testimony in this case, prevailing and accepted medical standards.

We have adverted to the "brain death" concept and Karen's disassociation with any of its criteria, to emphasize the basis of the medical decision made by Dr. Morse. When plaintiff and his family, finally reconciled to the certainty of Karen's impending death, requested the withdrawal of life support mechanisms, he demurred. His refusal was based upon his conception of medical standards, practice and ethics described in the medical testimony, such as in the evidence given by another neurologist, Dr. Sidney Diamond, a witness for the State. Dr. Diamond asserted that no physician would have failed to provide respirator support at the outset, and none would interrupt its life-saving course thereafter, except in the case of cerebral death. In the latter case, he thought the respirator would in effect be disconnected from one already dead, entitling the physician under medical standards and, he thought, legal concepts, to terminate the supportive measures. We note Dr. Diamond's distinction of major surgical or transfusion procedures in a terminal case not involving cerebral death, such as here:

> The subject has lost human qualities. It would be incredible, and I think unlikely, that any physician would respond to a sudden hemorrhage, massive hemorrhage or a loss of all her defensive blood cells, by giving her large quantities of blood. I think that . . . major surgical procedures would be out of the question even if they were known to be essential for continued physical existence.

This distinction is adverted to also in the testimony of Dr. Julius Korein, a neurologist called by plaintiff. Dr. Korein described a medical practice concept of "judicious neglect" under which the physician will say:

> Don't treat this patient anymore, . . . it does not serve either the patient, the family, or society in any meaningful way to continue treatment with this patient.

Dr. Korein also told of the unwritten and unspoken standard of medical practice implied in the foreboding initials DNR (do not resuscitate), as applied to the extraordinary terminal case:

> Cancer, metastatic cancer, involving the lungs, the liver, the brain, multiple involvements, the physician may or may not write: Do not resuscitate. . . . [I]t could be said to the nurse: if this man stops breathing don't resuscitate him. . . . No physician that I know personally is going to try and resuscitate a man riddled with cancer and in agony and he stops breathing. They are not going to put him on a respirator. . . . I think that would be the height of misuse of technology.

While the thread of logic in such distinctions may be elusive to the non-medical lay mind, in relation to the supposed imperative to sustain life at all costs, they nevertheless relate to medical decisions, such as the decision of Dr. Morse in the present case. We agree with the trial court that that decision was in accord with Dr. Morse's conception of medical standards and practice.

* * *

It is from this factual base that the Court confronts and responds to three basic issues:

1. Was the trial court correct in denying the specific relief requested by plaintiff, *i.e.*, authorization for termination of the life-supporting apparatus, on the case presented to him? Our determination on that question is in the affirmative.
2. Was the court correct in withholding letters of guardianship from the plaintiff and appointing in his stead a stranger? On that issue our determination is in the negative.
3. Should this Court, in the light of the foregoing conclusions, grant declaratory relief to the plaintiff? On that question our Court's determination is in the affirmative.

* * *

Constitutional and Legal Issues . . .

The Right of Privacy. [Note omitted.] It is the issue of the constitutional right of privacy that has given us most concern, in the exceptional circumstances of this case. Here a loving parent, *qua* parent and raising the rights of his incompetent and profoundly damaged daughter, probably irreversibly doomed to no more than a biologically vegetative remnant of life, is before the court. He seeks authorization to abandon specialized technological procedures which can only maintain for a time a body having no potential for resumption or continuance of other than a "vegetative" existence.

We have no doubt, in these unhappy circumstances, that if Karen were herself miraculously lucid for an interval (not altering the existing prognosis of the condition to which she would soon return) and perceptive of her irreversible condition, she could effectively decide upon discontinuance of the life-support apparatus, even if it meant the prospect of natural death. To this extent we may distinguish *Heston, supra,* which concerned a severely injured young woman (Delores Heston), whose life depended on surgery and blood transfusion; and who was in such extreme shock that she was unable to express an informed choice (although the Court apparently considered the case as if the patient's own religious decision to resist transfusion were at stake), but most importantly a patient apparently salvable to long life and vibrant health;—a situation not at all like the present case.

We have no hesitancy in deciding, in the instant diametrically opposite case, that no external compelling interest of the State could compel Karen to endure the unendurable, only to vegetate a few measurable months with no realistic possibility of returning to any semblance of cognitive or sapient life. We perceive no thread of logic distinguishing between such a choice on Karen's part and a similar choice which, under the evidence in this case, could be made by a competent patient terminally ill, riddled by cancer and suffering great pain: such a patient would not be resuscitated or put on a respirator in the example described by Dr. Korein, and *a fortiori* would not be kept *against his will* on a respirator. . . .

* * *

The claimed interests of the State in this case are essentially the preservation and sanctity of human life and defense of the right of the physician to administer medical treatment according to his best judgment. In this case the doctors say that removing Karen from the respirator will conflict with their professional judgment. The plaintiff answers that Karen's present treatment serves only a maintenance function; that the respirator cannot cure or improve her condition but at best can only prolong her inevitable slow deterioration and death; and that the interests of the patient, as seen by her surrogate, the guardian, must be evaluated by the court as predominant, even in the face of an opinion *contra* by the present attending physicians. Plaintiff's distinction is significant. The nature of Karen's care and the realistic chances of her recovery are quite unlike those of the patients discussed in many of the cases where treatments were ordered. In many of those cases the medical procedure required (usually a transfusion) constituted a minimal bodily invasion and the chances of recovery and return to functioning life were very good. We think that the State's interest *contra* weakens and the individual's right to privacy grows as the degree of bodily invasion increases and the prognosis dims. Ultimately there comes a point at which the individual's rights overcome the State interest. It is for that reason that we believe Karen's choice, if she were competent to make it, would be vindicated by the law. Her prognosis is extremely poor,—she will never resume cognitive life. And the bodily invasion is very great,—she requires 24 hour intensive nursing care, antibiotics, the assistance of a respirator, a catheter and feeding tube.

Our affirmation of Karen's independent right of choice, however, would ordinarily be based upon her competency to assert it. The sad truth, however, is that she is grossly incompetent and we cannot discern her supposed choice based on the testimony of her previous conversations with friends, where such testimony is without sufficient probative weight. 137 N.J. Super. at 260, 348 A.2d 801. Nevertheless we have concluded that Karen's right of privacy may be asserted on her behalf by her guardian under the peculiar circumstances here present.

If a putative decision by Karen to permit this non-cognitive, vegetative existence to terminate by natural forces is regarded as a valuable incident of her right of privacy, as we believe it to be, then it should not be discarded solely on the basis that her condition prevents her conscious exercise of the choice. The only practical way to prevent destruction of the right is to permit the guardian and family of Karen to render their best judgment subject to the qualifications hereinafter stated, as to whether she would exercise it in these circumstances. If their conclusion is in the affirmative this decision should be accepted by a society the overwhelming majority of whose members would, we think, in similar circumstances, exercise such a choice in the same way for themselves or for those closest to them. It is for this reason that we determine that Karen's right of privacy may be asserted in her behalf, in this respect, by her guardian and family under the particular circumstances presented by this record.

* * *

The Medical Factor . . .

The medical obligation is related to standards and practice prevailing in the profession. The physicians in charge of the case, as noted above, declined to withdraw the respirator. That decision was consistent with the proofs below as to the then existing medical standards and practices.

Under the law as it then stood, Judge Muir was correct in declining to authorize withdrawal of the respirator.

However, in relation to the matter of the declaratory relief sought by plaintiff as representative of Karen's interests, we are required to reevaluate the applicability of the medical standards projected in the court below. The question is whether there is such internal consistency and rationality in the application of such standards as should warrant their constituting an ineluctable bar to the effectuation of substantive relief for plaintiff at the hands of the court. We have concluded not.

In regard to the foregoing it is pertinent that we consider the impact on the standards both of the civil and criminal law as to medical liability and the new technological means of sustaining life irreversibly damaged.

The modern proliferation of substantial malpractice litigation and the less frequent but even more unnerving possibility of criminal sanctions would seem, for it is beyond human nature to suppose otherwise, to have bearing on the practice and standards as they exist. The brooding presence of such possible liability, it was testified here, had no part in the decision of the treating physicians. As did Judge Muir, we afford this testimony full credence. But we cannot believe that the stated factor has not had a strong influence on the standards, as the literature on the subject plainly reveals. . . . Moreover our attention is drawn not so much to the recognition by Drs. Morse and Javed of the extant practice and standards but to the widening ambiguity of those standards themselves in their application to the medical problems we are discussing.

The agitation of the medical community in the face of modern life prolongation technology and its search for definitive policy are demonstrated in the large volume of relevant professional commentary [note omitted].

The wide debate thus reflected contrasts with the relative paucity of legislative and judicial guides and standards in the same field. The medical profession has sought to devise guidelines such as the "brain death" concept of the Harvard Ad Hoc Committee mentioned above. But it is perfectly apparent from the testimony we have quoted of Dr. Korein, and indeed so clear as almost to be judicially noticeable, that humane decisions against resuscitative or maintenance therapy are frequently a recognized *de facto* response in the medical world to the irreversible, terminal, pain-ridden patient, especially with familial consent. And these cases, of course, are far short of "brain death."

We glean from the record here that physicians distinguish between curing the ill and comforting and easing the dying; that they refuse to treat the curable as if they were dying or ought to die, and that they have sometimes refused to treat the hopeless and dying as if they were curable. In this sense, as we were reminded by the testimony of Drs. Korein and Diamond, many of them have refused to inflict an undesired prolongation of the process of dying on a patient in irreversible condition when it is clear that such "therapy" offers neither human nor humane benefit. We think these attitudes represent a balanced implementation of a profoundly realistic perspective on the meaning of life and death and that they respect the whole Judeo-Christian tradition of regard for human life. No less would they seem consistent with the moral matrix of medicine, "to heal," very much in the sense of the endless mission of the law, "to do justice."

Yet this balance, we feel, is particularly difficult to perceive and apply in the context of the development by advanced technology of sophisticated and artificial life-sustaining devices. For those possibly curable, such devices are of great value, and, as ordinary medical procedures, are essential. Consequently, as pointed out by Dr. Diamond, they are necessary because of the ethic of medical practice. But in light of the situation in the present case (while the record here is somewhat hazy in distinguishing between "ordinary" and "extraordinary" measures), one would have to think that the use of the same respirator or like support could be considered "ordinary" in the context of the possibly curable patient but "extraordinary" in the context of the forced sustaining by cardio-respiratory processes of an irreversibly doomed patient. And this dilemma is sharpened in the face of the malpractice and criminal action threat which we have mentioned.

We would hesitate, in this imperfect world, to propose as to physicians that type of immunity which from the early common law has surrounded judges and grand jurors, *see e.g., Grove v. Van Duyn*, 44 N. J.L. 654, 656–57 (E. & A.1882); *O'Regan v. Schermerhorn*, 25 N.J.Misc. 1, 19–20, 50 A.2d 10 (Sup.Ct.1940), so that they might without fear of personal retaliation perform their judicial duties with independent objectivity. In *Bradley v. Fisher*, 80 U.S. (13 Wall.) 335, 347, 20 L.Ed. 646, 649 (1872), the Supreme Court held:

> [I]t is a general principle of the highest importance to the proper administration of justice that a judicial officer, in exercising the

> authority vested in him, shall be free to act upon his own convictions, without apprehension of personal consequences to himself.

Lord Coke said of judges that "they are only to make an account to God and the King [the State]." 12 Coke Rep. 23, 25, 77 Eng.Rep. 1305, 1307 (S.C.1608).

Nevertheless, there must be a way to free physicians, in the pursuit of their healing vocation, from possible contamination by self-interest or self-protection concerns which would inhibit their independent medical judgments for the well-being of their dying patients. We would hope that this opinion might be serviceable to some degree in ameliorating the professional problems under discussion.

A technique aimed at the underlying difficulty (though in a somewhat broader context) is described by Dr. Karen Teel, a pediatrician and a director of Pediatric Education, who writes in the *Baylor Law Review* under the title "The Physician's Dilemma: A Doctor's View: What The Law Should Be." Dr. Teel recalls:

> Physicians, by virtue of their responsibility for medical judgments are, partly by choice and partly by default, charged with the responsibility of making ethical judgments which we are sometimes ill-equipped to make. We are not always morally and legally authorized to make them. The physician is thereby assuming a civil and criminal liability that, as often as not, he does not even realize as a factor in his decision. There is little or no dialogue in this whole process. The physician assumes that his judgment is called for and, in good faith, he acts. Someone must and it has been the physician who has assumed the responsibility and the risk.
>
> I suggest that it would be more appropriate to provide a regular forum for more input and dialogue in individual situations and to allow the responsibility of these judgments to be shared. Many hospitals have established an Ethics Committee composed of physicians, social workers, attorneys, and theologians, . . . which serves to review the individual circumstances of ethical dilemma and which has provided much in the way of assistance and safeguards for patients and their medical caretakers. Generally, the authority of these committees is primarily restricted to the hospital setting and their official status is more that of an advisory body than of an enforcing body.
>
> The concept of an Ethics Committee which has this kind of organization and is readily accessible to those persons rendering medical care to patients, would be, I think, the most promising direction for further study at this point. . . .
>
> . . . [This would allow] some much needed dialogue regarding these issues and [force] the point of exploring all of the options for a particular patient. It diffuses the responsibility for making these judgments. Many physicians, in many circumstances, would welcome this sharing of responsibility. I believe that such an entity could lend itself well to an assumption of a legal status which would allow courses of action not now undertaken because of the concern for liability. [27 Baylor L.Rev. 6, 8–9 (1975)].

The most appealing factor in the technique suggested by Dr. Teel seems to us to be the diffusion of professional responsibility for decision, comparable in a way to the value of multi-judge courts in finally resolving on appeal difficult questions of law. Moreover, such a system would be protective to the hospital as well as the doctor in screening out, so to speak, a case which might be contaminated by less than worthy motivations of family or physician. In the real world and in relationship to the momentous decision contemplated, the value of additional views and diverse knowledge is apparent.

* * *

Conclusion

We therefore remand this record to the trial court to implement (without further testimonial hearing) the following decisions:

1. To discharge, with the thanks of the Court for his service, the present guardian of the person of Karen Quinlan, Thomas R. Curtin, Esquire, a member of the Bar and an officer of the court.
2. To appoint Joseph Quinlan as guardian of the person of Karen Quinlan with full power to make decisions with regard to the identity of her treating physicians.

We repeat for the sake of emphasis and clarity that upon the concurrence of the guardian and family of Karen, should the responsible attending physicians conclude that there is no reasonable possibility of Karen's ever emerging from her present comatose condition to a cognitive, sapient state and that the life-support apparatus now being administered to Karen should be discontinued, they shall consult with the hospital "Ethics Committee" or like body of the institution in which Karen is then hospitalized. If that consultative body agrees that there is no reasonable possibility of Karen's ever emerging from her present comatose condition to a cognitive, sapient state, the present life-support system may be withdrawn and said action shall be without any civil or criminal liability therefor on the part of any participant, whether guardian, physician, hospital or others.

By the above ruling we do not intend to be understood as implying that a proceeding for judicial declaratory relief is necessarily required for the implementation of comparable decisions in the field of medical practice.

MODIFIED AND REMANDED

For modification and remandment: Chief Justice Hughes, Justices Mountain, Sullivan, Pashman, Clifford and Schreiber and Judge Conford—7.

Opposed: None.

THE CALIFORNIA NATURAL DEATH ACT: STATE OF CALIFORNIA, 1976 (REVISED THROUGH 1992)

INTRODUCTION. *While the State of New Jersey was relying on the courts to establish the rights of patients and their surrogates to forgo life-sustaining treatments, other states were exploring the legislative route to accomplish something similar. California was the first state to pass such a law. Assemblyman Barry Keene led a complex political struggle, complete with many compromises, to establish that Californians had the right to execute a document refusing certain life-sustaining medical treatments. There were many exclusions, limitations, and special provisions, including those affecting pregnant women and nursing home patients. Written documents were legally binding only if they were written after the patient was certified terminally ill. Terminal illness was defined very narrowly, referring only to patients inevitably dying regardless of treatment.*

The People of the State of California Do Enact as Follows:

NATURAL DEATH ACT OF CALIFORNIA

Sec. 7185.

This act shall be known and may be cited as the Natural Death Act.

Sec. 7186.

The Legislature finds that adult persons have the fundamental right to control the decisions relating to the rendering of their own medical care, including the decision to have life-sustaining procedures withheld or withdrawn in instances of a terminal condition.

The Legislature further finds that modern medical technology has made possible the artificial prolongation of human life beyond natural limits.

The Legislature further finds that, in the interest of protecting individual autonomy, such prolongation of life for persons with a terminal condition may cause loss of patient dignity, and unnecessary pain and suffering, while providing nothing medically necessary or beneficial to the patient.

The Legislature further finds that there exists considerable uncertainty in the medical and legal professions as to the legality of terminating the use or application of life-sustaining procedures where the patient has voluntarily and in sound mind evidenced a desire that such procedures be withheld or withdrawn.

In recognition of the dignity and privacy which patients have a right to expect, the Legislature hereby declares that the laws of the State of California shall recognize the right of an adult person to make a written directive instructing his physician to withhold or withdraw life-sustaining procedures in the event of a terminal condition.

Sec. 7187.

The following definitions shall govern the construction of this chapter:

(a) "Attending physician" means the physician selected by, or assigned to, the patient who has primary responsibility for the treatment and care of the patient.

(b) "Directive" means a written document voluntarily executed by the declarant in accordance with the re-

---

California: A.3060 enacted 1976. Introduced by Assemblyman Barry Keene, Passed by Assembly (43–22) and Senate (22–14), and signed by Gov. Edmund G. Brown, Jr.

quirements of Section 7188. The directive, or a copy of the directive, shall be made part of the patient's medical records.

(c) "Life-sustaining procedure" means any medical procedure or intervention which utilizes mechanical or other artificial means to sustain, restore, or supplant a vital function, which, when applied to a qualified patient, would serve only to artificially prolong the moment of death and where, in the judgment of the attending physician, death is imminent whether or not such procedures are utilized. "Life-sustaining procedure" shall not include the administration of medication or the performance of any medical procedure deemed necessary to alleviate pain.

(d) "Physician" means a physician and surgeon licensed by the Board of Medical Quality Assurance or the Board of Osteopathic Examiners.

(e) "Qualified patient" means a patient diagnosed and certified in writing to be afflicted with a terminal condition by two physicians, one of whom shall be the attending physician, who have personally examined the patient.

(f) "Terminal condition" means an incurable condition caused by injury, disease, or illness, which, regardless of the application of life-sustaining procedures, would, within reasonable medical judgment, produce death, and where the application of life-sustaining procedures, serve only to postpone the moment of death of the patient.

Sec. 7188.

Any adult person may execute a directive directing the withholding or withdrawal of life-sustaining procedures in a terminal condition. The directive shall be signed by the declarant in the presence of two witnesses not related to the declarant by blood or marriage and who would not be entitled to any portion of the estate of the declarant upon his decease under any will of the declarant or codicil thereto then existing or, at the time of the directive, by operation of law then existing. In addition, a witness to a directive shall not be the attending physician, an employee of the attending physician or a health facility in which the declarant is a patient, or any person who has a claim against any portion of the estate of the declarant upon his decease at the time of the execution of the directive. The directive shall be in the following form:

Directive to Physicians

Directive made this ____ day of ____ (month, year).

I ______________. being of sound mind, willfully, and voluntarily make known my desire that my life shall not be artificially prolonged under the circumstances set forth below, do hereby declare:

1. If at any time I should have an incurable injury, disease, or illness certified to be a terminal condition by two physicians, and where the application of life-sustaining procedures would serve only to artificially prolong the moment of my death and where my physician determines that my death is imminent whether or not life-sustaining procedures are utilized, I direct that such procedures be withheld or withdrawn, and that I be permitted to die naturally.

2. In the absence of my ability to give directions regarding the use of such life-sustaining procedures, it is my intention that this directive shall be honored by my family and physician(s) as the final expression of my legal right to refuse medical or surgical treatment and accept the consequences from such refusal.

3. If I have been diagnosed as pregnant and that diagnosis is known to my physician, this directive shall have no force or effect during the course of my pregnancy.

4. I have been diagnosed at least 14 days ago as having a terminal condition by ______________, M.D., whose address is ____________ ____________, and whose telephone number is ______________. I understand that if I have not filled in the physician's name and address, it shall be presumed that I did not have a terminal condition when I made out this directive.

5. This directive shall have no force or effect five years from the date filled in above.

6. I understand the full import of this directive and I am emotionally and mentally competent to make this directive.

Signed ______________

City, County and State of Residence

The declarant has been personally known to me and I believe him or her to be of sound mind.

Witness ______________

Witness ______________

Sec. 7188.5

A directive shall have no force or effect if the declarant is a patient in a skilled nursing facility as defined in subdivision (c) of Section 1250 at the time the directive is executed unless one of the two witnesses to the directive is a patient advocate or ombudsman as may be designated by the State Department of Aging for this purpose pursuant to any other applicable provision of law. The patient advocate or ombudsman shall have the same qualifications as a witness under Section 7188.

The intent of this section is to recognize that some patients in skilled nursing facilities may be so insulated from a voluntary decision-making role, by virtue of the custodial nature of their care, as to require special assurance that they are capable of willfully and voluntarily executing a directive.

Sec. 7189.

(a) A directive may be revoked at any time by the declarant, without regard to his mental state or competency, by any of the following methods:

1. By being canceled, defaced, obliterated, or burnt, torn, or otherwise destroyed by the declarant or by some person in his presence and by his direction.

2. By a written revocation of the declarant expressing his intent to revoke, signed and dated by the declarant. Such revocation shall become effective only upon communication to the attending physician by the declarant or by a person acting on behalf of the declarant. The attending physician shall record in the patient's medical record the time and date when he received notification of the written revocation.
3. By a verbal expression by the declarant of his intent to revoke the directive. Such revocation shall become effective only upon communication to the attending physician by the declarant or by a person acting on behalf of the declarant. The attending physician shall record in the patient's medical record the time, date, and place of the revocation and the time, date, and place, if different, of when he received notification of the revocation.

(b) There shall be no criminal or civil liability on the part of any person for failure to act upon a revocation made pursuant to this section unless that person has actual knowledge of the revocation.

Sec. 7189.5

A directive shall be effective for five years from the date of execution thereof unless sooner revoked in a manner prescribed in Sec. 7189. Nothing in this chapter shall be construed to prevent a declarant from reexecuting a directive at any time in accordance with the formalities of Sec. 7188, including reexecution subsequent to a diagnosis of a terminal condition. If the declarant has executed more than one directive, such time shall be determined from the date of execution of the last directive known to the attending physician. If the declarant becomes comatose or is rendered incapable of communicating with the attending physician, the directive shall remain in effect for the duration of the comatose condition or until such time as the declarant's condition renders him or her able to communicate with the attending physician.

Sec. 7190.

No physician or health facility which, acting in accordance with the requirements of this chapter, causes the withholding or withdrawal of life-sustaining procedures from a qualified patient, shall be subject to civil liability therefrom. No licensed health professional, acting under the direction of a physician, who participates in the withholding or withdrawal of life-sustaining procedures, in accordance with the provisions of this chapter shall be subject to any civil liability. No physician, or licensed health professional acting under the direction of a physician, who participates in the withholding or withdrawal of life-sustaining procedures in accordance with the provisions of this chapter shall be guilty of any criminal act or of unprofessional conduct.

Sec. 7191.

(a) Prior to effecting a withholding or withdrawal of life-sustaining procedures from a qualified patient pursuant to the directive, the attending physician shall determine that the directive complies with Sec. 7188, and, if the patient is mentally competent, that the directive and all steps proposed by the attending physician to be undertaken are in accord with the desires of the qualified patient.

(b) If the declarant was a qualified patient at least 14 days prior to executing or reexecuting the directive, the directive shall be conclusively presumed, unless revoked, to be the directions of the patient regarding the withholding or withdrawal of life-sustaining procedures. No physician, and no licensed health professional acting under the direction of a physician, shall be criminally or civilly liable for failing to effectuate the directive of the qualified patient pursuant to this subdivision. A failure by a physician to effectuate the directive of a qualified patient pursuant to this division shall constitute unprofessional conduct if the physician refuses to make the necessary arrangements, or fails to take the necessary steps, to effect the transfer of the qualified patient to another physician who will effectuate the directive of the qualified patient.

(c) If the declarant becomes a qualified patient subsequent to executing the directive, and has not subsequently reexecuted the directive, the attending physician may give weight to the directive as evidence of the patient's directions regarding the withholding or withdrawal of life-sustaining procedures and may consider other factors, such as information from the affected family or the nature of the patient's illness, injury, or disease, in determining whether the totality of circumstances known to the attending physician justify effectuating the directive. No physician, and no licensed health professional acting under the directive of a physician, shall be criminally or civilly liable for failing to effectuate the directive of the qualified patient pursuant to this subdivision.

Sec. 7192.

(a) The withholding or withdrawal of life-sustaining procedures from a qualified patient in accordance with the provisions of this chapter shall not, for any purpose, constitute a suicide.

(b) The making of a directive pursuant to Sec. 7188 shall not restrict, inhibit, or impair in any manner the sale, procurement, or issuance of any policy of life insurance, nor shall it be deemed to modify the terms of an existing policy of life insurance. No policy of life insurance shall be legally impaired or invalidated in any manner by the withholding or withdrawal of life-sustaining procedures from an insured qualified patient, notwithstanding any term of the policy to the contrary.

(c) No physician, health facility, or other health provider, and no health care service plan, insurer issuing disability insurance, self-insured employee welfare benefit plan, or nonprofit hospital service plan, shall require any person to execute a directive as a condition for being insured for, or receiving, health care services.

Sec. 7193.

Nothing in this chapter shall impair or supersede any legal right or legal responsibility which any person may have to effect the withholding or withdrawal of life-sustaining procedures in any lawful manner. In such respect the provisions of this chapter are cumulative.

Sec. 7194.

Any person who willfully conceals, cancels, defaces, obliterates, or damages the directive of another without such declarant's consent shall be guilty of a misdemeanor. Any person who, except where justified or excused by law, falsifies or forges the directive of another, or willfully conceals or withholds personal knowledge of a revocation as provided in Section 7189, with the intent to cause a withholding or withdrawal of life-sustaining procedures contrary to the wishes of the declarant, and thereby, because of any such act, directly causes life-sustaining procedures to be withheld or withdrawn and death to thereby be hastened, shall be subject to prosecution for unlawful homicide as provided in Chapter 1 (commencing with Section 187) of Title 8 of Part 1 of the Penal Code.

Sec. 7195.

Nothing in this chapter shall be construed to condone, authorize, or approve mercy killing, or to permit any affirmative or deliberate act or omission to end life other than to permit the natural process of dying as provided in this chapter.

SECTION 2.

If any provision of this act or the application thereof to any person or circumstances is held invalid, such invalidity shall not affect other provisions or applications of the act which can be given effect without the invalid provision or application, and to this end the provisions of this act are severable.

SECTION 3.

Notwithstanding Section 2231 of the Revenue and Taxation Code, there shall be no reimbursement pursuant to this section nor shall there be any appropriation made by this act because the Legislature recognizes that during any legislative session a variety of changes to laws relating to crimes and infractions may cause both increased and decreased costs to local government entities and school districts which, in the aggregate, do not result in significant identifiable cost changes.

SUPERINTENDENT OF BELCHERTOWN STATE SCHOOL V. SAIKEWICZ

INTRODUCTION. *The New Jersey Quinlan opinion and the California Natural Death Act were limited in their application to patients who had been legally competent, leaving unclear how decisions should be made for those who had never been competent, such as children and the severely retarded who could never develop a plan about their terminal care. Joseph Saikewicz, a 67-year-old severely retarded institutionalized patient suffering from leukemia, led the Massachusetts courts to clarify the problem. In accepting a court-appointed guardian's recommendation, the court ruled that the treatment could be foregone.*

The court found that the patient's mental retardation was relevant: Mr. Saikewicz was unusually burdened by the treatment because he could not understand what was being done to him. The court rejected the view that Mr. Saikewicz's life was less valuable because of his retardation. In the opinion the Massachusetts court uses the term substituted judgment in an atypical manner. It usually refers to judgments based on the patient's own values. Here it is apparently used to refer to the guardian's views on the best interests of the patient. This standard is now usually referred to as the best interest standard. The Massachusetts court insists that it is the "ultimate" or final authority on such decisions. The court seems to believe its opinion differs from the New Jersey Quinlan opinion in rejecting definitive authority for physicians, family, and ethics committee. A careful reading of the Quinlan opinion, however, suggests that the differences may not be real. The New Jersey court clearly did not give the attending physician real authority, and limited the authority of ethics committees to confirming prognoses. The father was given the immediate authority to make the key decisions. In Saikewicz, however, the patient had no family available to make these choices. It seems clear that in New Jersey as in Massachusetts, the court retains "ultimate" authority.

I.

The judge below found that Joseph Saikewicz, at the time the matter arose, was sixty-seven years old, with an I.Q. of ten and a mental age of approximately two years and eight months. He was profoundly mentally retarded. The record discloses that, apart from his leukemic condition, Saikewicz enjoyed generally good health. He was physically strong and well built, nutritionally nourished, and ambulatory. He was not, however, able to communicate verbally—resorting to gestures and grunts to make his wishes known to others and responding only to gestures or physical contact. In the course of treatment for various medical conditions arising during Saikewicz's residency at the school, he had been unable to respond intelligibly to inquiries such as whether he was experiencing pain. It was the opinion of a consulting psychologist, not contested by the other experts relied on by the judge below, that Saikewicz was not aware of dangers and was disoriented outside his immediate environment. As a result of his condition, Saikewicz had lived in State institutions since 1923 and had resided at the Belchertown State School since 1928. Two of his sisters, the only members of his family who could be located, were notified of his condition and of the hearing, but they preferred not to attend or otherwise become involved.

On April 19, 1976, Saikewicz was diagnosed as suffering from acute myeloblastic monocytic leukemia. Leukemia is a disease of the blood. It arises when organs of the body produce an excessive number of white blood cells as well as other abnormal cellular structures, in particular undeveloped and immature white cells. Along with these symp-

Condensed from 370 North Eastern Reporter, 2d series. *Superintendent of Belchertown v. Saikewicz*. Cite as Mass 370 N.E. 2d 417 (1977).

toms in the composition of the blood the disease is accompanied by enlargement of the organs which produce the cells, e.g., the spleen, lymph glands, and bone marrow. The disease tends to cause internal bleeding and weakness, and, in the acute form, severe anemia and high susceptibility to infection. Attorneys' Dictionary of Medicine L-37–38 (1977). The particular form of the disease present in this case, acute myeloblastic monocytic leukemia is so defined because the particular cells which increase are the myeloblasts, the youngest form of a cell which at maturity is known as the granulocytes. *Id.* at M-138. The disease is invariably fatal.

Chemotherapy, as was testified to at the hearing in the Probate Court, involves the administration of drugs over several weeks, the purpose of which is to kill the leukemia cells. This treatment unfortunately affects normal cells as well. One expert testified that the end result, in effect, is to destroy the living vitality of the bone marrow. Because of this effect, the patient becomes very anemic and may bleed or suffer infections—a condition which requires a number of blood transfusions. In this sense, the patient immediately becomes much "sicker" with the commencement of chemotherapy, and there is a possibility that infections during the initial period of severe anemia will prove fatal. Moreover, while most patients survive chemotherapy, remission of the leukemia is achieved in only thirty to fifty per cent of the cases. Remission is meant here as a temporary return to normal as measured by clinical and laboratory means. If remission does occur, it typically lasts for between two and thirteen months although longer periods of remission are possible. Estimates of the effectiveness of chemotherapy are complicated in cases, such as the one presented here, in which the patient's age becomes a factor. According to the medical testimony before the court below, persons over age sixty have more difficulty tolerating chemotherapy and the treatment is likely to be less successful than in younger patients.[1] This prognosis may be compared with the doctors' estimates that, left untreated, a patient in Saikewicz's condition would live for a matter of weeks or, perhaps, several months. According to the testimony, a decision to allow the disease to run its natural course would not result in pain for the patient, and death would probably come without discomfort.

An important facet of the chemotherapy process, to which the judge below directed careful attention, is the problem of serious adverse side effects caused by the treating drugs. Among these side effects are severe nausea, bladder irritation, numbness and tingling of the extremities, and loss of hair. The bladder irritation can be avoided, however, if the patient drinks fluids, and the nausea can be treated by drugs. It was the opinion of the guardian ad litem, as well as the doctors who testified before the probate judge, that most people elect to suffer the side effects of chemotherapy rather than to allow their leukemia to run its natural course.

Drawing on the evidence before him including the testimony of the medical experts, and the report of the guardian ad litem, the probate judge issued detailed findings with regard to the costs and benefits of allowing Saikewicz to undergo chemotherapy. The judge's findings are reproduced in part here because of the importance of clearly delimiting the issues presented in this case. The judge below found:

5. That the majority of persons suffering from leukemia who are faced with a choice of receiving or foregoing such chemotherapy, and who are able to make an informed judgment thereon, choose to receive treatment in spite of its toxic side effects and risks of failure.
6. That such toxic side effects of chemotherapy include pain and discomfort, depressed bone marrow, pronounced anemia, increased chance of infection, possible bladder irritation, and possible loss of hair.
7. That administration of such chemotherapy requires cooperation from the patient over several weeks of time, which cooperation said JOSEPH SAIKEWICZ is unable to give due to his profound retardation.[2]
8. That, considering the age and general state of health of said JOSEPH SAIKEWICZ, there is only a 30–40 percent chance that chemotherapy will produce a remission of said leukemia, which remission would probably be for a period of time of from 2 to 13 months, but that said chemotherapy will certainly not completely cure such leukemia.
9. That if such chemotherapy is to be administered at all it should be administered immediately, inasmuch as the risks involved will increase and the chances of successfully bringing about remission will decrease as time goes by.
10. That, at present, said JOSEPH SAIKEWICZ's leukemia condition is stable and is not deteriorating.
11. That said JOSEPH SAIKEWICZ is not now in pain and will probably die within a matter of weeks or months a relatively painless death due to the leukemia unless other factors should intervene to themselves cause death.
12. That it is impossible to predict how long said JOSEPH SAIKEWICZ will probably live without chemotherapy or how long he will probably live with chemotherapy, but it is to a very high degree medically likely that he will die sooner, without treatment than with it.

Balancing these various factors, the judge concluded that the following considerations weighed *against* administering chemotherapy to Saikewicz: "(1) his age, (2) his inability to cooperate with the treatment, (3) probable adverse side effects of treatment, (4) low chance of producing remission, (5) the certainty that treatment will cause immediate suffering, and (6) the quality of life possible for him even if the treatment does bring about remission."

The following considerations were determined to weigh in *favor* of chemotherapy: "(1) the chance that his life may be lengthened thereby, and (2) the fact that most people in his situation when given a chance to do so elect to take the gamble of treatment."

Concluding that, in this case, the negative factors of treatment exceeded the benefits, the probate judge ordered on May 13, 1976, that no treatment be administered to Saikewicz for his condition of acute myeloblastic monocytic leukemia except by further order of the court. The judge further ordered that all reasonable and necessary supportive measures be taken, medical or otherwise, to safeguard the well-being of Saikewicz in all other respects and to reduce as far as possible any suffering or discomfort which he might experience.

It is within this factual context that we issued our order of July 9, 1976.

Saikewicz died on September 4, 1976, at the Belchertown State School hospital. Death was due to bronchial pneumonia, a complication of the leukemia. Saikewicz died without pain or discomfort.[3]

II.

We recognize at the outset that this case presents novel issues of fundamental importance that should not be resolved by mechanical reliance on legal doctrine. Our task of establishing a framework in the law on which the activities of health care personnel and other persons can find support is furthered by seeking the collective guidance of those in health care, moral ethics, philosophy, and other disciplines. Our attempt to bring such insights to bear in the legal context has been advanced by the diligent efforts of the guardian ad litem and the probate judge, as well as the excellent briefs of the parties and amici curiae.[4] As thus illuminated, the principal areas of determination are:

A. The nature of the right of any person, competent or incompetent, to decline potentially life-prolonging treatment.
B. The legal standards that control the course of decision whether or not potentially life-prolonging, but not life-saving, treatment should be administered to a person who is not competent to make the choice.
C. The procedures that must be followed in arriving at that decision.

For reasons we develop in the body of this opinion, it becomes apparent that the questions to be discussed in the first two areas are closely interrelated. We take the view that the substantive rights of the competent and the incompetent person are the same in regard to the right to decline potentially life-prolonging treatment. The factors which distinguish the two types of persons are found only in the area of how the State should approach the preservation and implementation of the rights of an incompetent person and in the procedures necessary to that process of preservation and implementation. We treat the matter in the sequence above stated because we think it helpful to set forth our views on (A) what the rights of all persons in this area are and (B) the issue of how an incompetent person is to be afforded the status in law of a competent person with respect to such rights. Only then can we proceed to (C) the particular procedures to be followed to ensure the rights of the incompetent person.

* * *

This survey of recent decisions involving the difficult question of the right of an individual to refuse medical intervention or treatment indicates that a relatively concise statement of countervailing State interests may be made. As distilled from the cases, the State has claimed interest in: (1) the preservation of life; (2) the protection of the interests of innocent third parties; (3) the prevention of suicide; and (4) maintaining the ethical integrity of the medical profession.

It is clear that the most significant of the asserted State interests is that of the preservation of human life. Recognition of such an interest, however, does not necessarily resolve the problem where the affliction or disease clearly indicates that life will soon, and inevitably, be extinguished. The interest of the State in prolonging a life must be reconciled with the interest of an individual to reject the traumatic cost of that prolongation. There is a substantial distinction in the State's insistence that human life be saved where the affliction is curable, as opposed to the State interest where, as here, the issue is not whether but when, for how long, and at what cost to the individual that life may be briefly extended. Even if we assume that the State has an additional interest in seeing to it that individual decisions on the prolongation of life do not in any way tend to "cheapen" the value which is placed in the concept of living, see *Roe v. Wade, supra,* we believe it is not inconsistent to recognize a right to decline medical treatment in a situation of incurable illness. The constitutional right to privacy, as we conceive it, is an expression of the sanctity of individual free choice and self-determination as fundamental constituents of life. The value of life as so perceived is lessened not by a decision to refuse treatment, but by the failure to allow a competent human being the right of choice.[5]

A second interest of considerable magnitude, which the State may have some interest in asserting, is that of protecting third parties, particularly minor children, from the emotional and financial damage which may occur as a result of the decision of a competent adult to refuse life-saving or life-prolonging treatment. Thus, in *Holmes v. Silver Cross Hosp. of Joliet, Ill.,* 340 F.Supp. 125 (D.Ill.1972), the court held that, while the State's interest in preserving an individual's life was not sufficient, by itself, to outweigh the individual's interest in the exercise of free choice, the possible impact on miner children would be a factor which might have a critical effect on the outcome of the balancing process. Similarly, in the *Georgetown* case the court held that one of the interests requiring protection was that of the minor child in order to avoid the effect of "abandonment" on that child as a result of the parent's decision to refuse the necessary medical measures. See Byrn, *supra* at 33; *United States v. George, supra.*[6] We need not reach this aspect of claimed State interest as it is not in issue on the facts of this case.

The last State interest requiring discussion[7] is that of the maintenance of the ethical integrity of the medical profession as well as allowing hospitals the full opportunity to care for people under their control. See *Georgetown, supra; United States v. George, supra; John F. Kennedy Memorial Hosp. v. Heston, supra.* The force and impact of this interest is lessened by the prevailing medical ethical standards. see Byrn, *supra* at 31. Prevailing medical ethical practice does not, without exception, demand that all efforts toward life prolongation be made in all circumstances. Rather, as indicated in *Quinlan,* the prevailing ethical practice seems to be to recognize that the dying are more often in need of comfort than treatment. Recognition of the right to refuse necessary treatment in appropriate circumstances is consistent with existing medical mores; such a doctrine does not threaten either the integrity of the medical profession, the proper role of hospitals in caring for such patients or the State's interest in protecting the same. It is not necessary to deny a right of self-determination to a patient in order to recognize the interests of doctors, hospitals, and medical personnel in attendance on the patient. Also, if the doctrines of informed consent and right of privacy have as their foundations the right to bodily integrity, see *Union Pac. Ry. v. Botsford,* 141 U.S. 250, 11 S.Ct. 1000, 35 L.Ed. 734 (1891), and control of one's own fate, then those rights are superior to the institutional considerations.[8]

Applying the considerations discussed in this subsection to the decision made by the probate judge in the circumstances of the case before us, we are satisfied that his decision was consistent with a proper balancing of applicable State and individual interests. Two of the four categories of State interests that we have identified, the protection of third parties and the prevention of suicide, are inapplicable to this case. The third, involving the protection of the ethical integrity of the medical profession was satisfied on two grounds. The probate judge's decision was in accord with the testimony of the attending physicians of the patient. The decision is in accord with the generally accepted views of the medical profession, as set forth in this opinion. The fourth State interest—the preservation of life—has been viewed with proper regard for the heavy physical and emotional burdens on the patient if a vigorous regimen of drug therapy were to be imposed to effect a brief and uncertain delay in the natural process of death. To be balanced against these State interests was the individual's interest in the freedom to choose to reject, or refuse to consent to, intrusions of his bodily integrity and privacy. We cannot say that the facts of this case required a result contrary to that reached by the probate judge with regard to the right of any person, competent or incompetent, to be spared the deleterious consequences of life-prolonging treatment. We therefore turn to consider the unique considerations arising in this case by virtue of the patient's inability to appreciate his predicament and articulate his desires.

* * *

With this historical perspective, we now reiterate the substituted judgment doctrine as we apply it in the instant case. We believe that both the guardian ad litem in his recommendation and the judge in his decision should have attempted (as they did) to ascertain the incompetent person's actual interests and preferences. In short the decision in cases such as this should be that which would be made by the incompetent person, if that person were competent, but taking into account the present and future incompetency of the individual as one of the factors which would necessarily enter into the decision-making process of the competent person. Having recognized the right of a competent person to make for himself the same decision as the court made in this case, the question is, do the facts on the record support the proposition that Saikewicz himself would have made the decision under the standard set forth. We believe they do.

The two factors considered by the probate judge to weigh in favor of administering chemotherapy were: (1) the fact that most people elect chemotherapy and (2) the chance of a longer life. Both are appropriate indicators of what Saikewicz himself would have wanted, provided that due allowance is taken for this individual's present and future incompetency. We have already discussed the perspective this brings to the fact that most people choose to undergo chemotherapy. With regard to the second factor, the chance of a longer life carries the same weight for Saikewicz as for any other person, the value of life under the law having no relation to intelligence or social position. Intertwined with this consideration is the hope that a cure, temporary or permanent, will be discovered during the period of extra weeks or months potentially made available by chemotherapy. The guardian ad litem investigated this possibility and found no reason to hope for a dramatic breakthrough in the time frame relevant to the decision.

The probate judge identified six factors weighing against administration of chemotherapy. Four of these—Saikewicz's age,[9] the probable side effects of treatment, the low chance of producing remission, and the certainty that treatment will cause immediate suffering—were clearly established by the medical testimony to be considerations that any individual would weigh carefully. A fifth factor—Saikewicz's inability to cooperate with the treatment—introduces those considerations that are unique to this individual and which therefore are essential to the proper exercise of substituted judgment. The judge heard testimony that Saikewicz would have no comprehension of the reasons for the severe disruption of his formerly secure and stable environment occasioned by the chemotherapy. He therefore would experience fear without the understanding from which other patients draw strength. The inability to anticipate and prepare for the severe side effects of the drugs leaves room only for confusion and disorientation. The possibility that such a naturally uncooperative patient would have to be physically restrained to allow the slow intravenous administration of drugs could only compound his pain and fear, as well as possibly jeopardize the ability of his body to withstand the toxic effects of the drugs.

The sixth factor identified by the judge as weighing against chemotherapy was "the quality of life possible for him even if the treatment does bring about remission." To the extent that this formulation equates the value of life with any measure of the quality of life, we firmly reject it. A reading of the entire record clearly reveals, however, the judge's concern that special care be taken to respect the dignity and worth of Saikewicz's life precisely because of his vulnerable position. The judge, as well as all the parties, were keenly aware that the supposed ability of Saikewicz, by virtue of his mental retardation, to appreciate or experience life had no place in the decision before them. Rather than reading the judge's formulation in a manner that demeans the value of the life of one who is mentally retarded, the vague, and perhaps ill-chosen, term "quality of life" should be understood as a reference to the continuing state of pain and disorientation precipitated by the chemotherapy treatment. Viewing the term in this manner, together with the other factors properly considered by the judge, we are satisfied that the decision to withhold treatment from Saikewicz was based on a regard for his actual interests and preferences and that the facts supported this decision.

* * *

Commensurate with the powers of the Probate Court already described, the probate judge may, at any step in these proceedings, avail himself or herself of the additional advice or knowledge of any person or group. We note here that many health care institutions have developed medical ethics committees or panels to consider many of the issues touched on here. Consideration of the findings and advice of such groups as well as the testimony of the attending physicians and other medical experts ordinarily would be of great assistance to a probate judge faced with such a difficult decision. We believe it desirable for a judge to consider such views wherever available and useful to the court. We do not believe, however, that this option should be transformed by us into a required procedure. We take a dim view of any attempt to shift the ultimate decision-making responsibility away from the duly established courts of proper jurisdiction to any committee, panel or group, ad hoc or permanent. Thus, we reject the approach adopted by the New Jersey Supreme Court in the *Quinlan* case of entrusting the decision whether to continue artificial life support to the patient's guardian, family, attending doctors, and hospital "ethics committee."[10] 70 N.J. at 55, 355 A.2d 647, 671. One rationale for such a delegation was expressed by the lower court judge in the *Quinlan* case, and quoted by the New Jersey Supreme Court: "The nature, extent and duration of care by societal standards is the responsibility of a physician. The morality and conscience of our society places this responsibility in the hands of the physician. What justification is there to remove it from the control of the medical profession and place it in the hands of the courts?" *Id.* at 44, 355 A.2d at 665. For its part, the New Jersey Supreme Court concluded that "a practice of applying to a court to confirm such decisions would generally be inappropriate, not only because that would be a gratuitous encroachment upon the medical profession's field of competence, but because it would be impossibly cumbersome. Such a requirement is distinguishable from the judicial overview traditionally required in other matters such as the adjudication and commitment of mental incompetents. This is not to say that in the case of an otherwise justiciable controversy access to the courts would be foreclosed; we speak rather of a general practice and procedure." *Id.* at 50, 355 A.2d at 669.

We do not view the judicial resolution of this most difficult and awesome question—whether potentially life-prolonging treatment should be withheld from a person incapable of making his own decision—as constituting a "gratuitous encroachment" on the domain of medical expertise. Rather, such questions of life and death seem to us to require the process of detached but passionate investigation and decision that forms the ideal on which the judicial branch of government was created. Achieving this ideal is our responsibility and that of the lower court, and is not to be entrusted to any other group purporting to represent the "morality and conscience of our society," no matter how highly motivated or impressively constituted.

III.

Finding no State interest sufficient to counterbalance a patient's decision to decline life-prolonging medical treatment in the circumstances of this case, we conclude that the patient's right to privacy and self-determination is entitled to enforcement. Because of this conclusion, and in view of the position of equality of an incompetent person in Joseph Saikewicz's position, we conclude that the probate judge acted appropriately in this case. For these reasons we issued our order of July 9, 1976, and responded as we did to the questions of the probate judge.

NOTES

1. On appeal, the petitioners have collected in their brief a number of recent empirical studies which cast doubt on the view that patients over sixty are less successfully treated by chemotherapy. E.g., Bloomfield & Theologides, Acute Granulocytic Leukemia in Elderly Patients, 226 J.A.M.A. 1190, 1192 (1973); Grann and others. The Therapy of Acute Granulocytic Leukemia in Patients More Than Fifty Years Old. 80 Annals Internal Med. 15, 16 (1974). (Acute myeloblastic monocytic leukemia is a subcategory of acute granulocytic leukemia.) Other experts maintain that older patients have lower remission rates and are more vulnerable to the toxic effects of the administered drugs. E.g., Crosby, Grounds for Optimism in Treating Acute Granulocytic Leukemia. 134 Archives Internal Med. 177 (1974). None of these authorities was brought to the consideration of the probate judge. We accept the judge's conclusion, based on the expert testimony before him and in accordance with substantial medical evidence, that the patient's age weighed against the successful administration of chemotherapy. . .
2. There was testimony as to the importance of having the full cooperation of the patient during the initial weeks of the chemotherapy process as well as during follow-up visits. For example, the evidence was that it would be necessary to administer drugs intravenously for extended periods of time—twelve or twenty-four hours a day for up to five days. The inability of Saikewicz to comprehend the purpose of the treatment, combined with his physical strength, led the doctors to testify that Saikewicz would probably have to be restrained to prevent him from tampering with the intravenous devices. Such forcible restraint could, in addition to increasing the patient's discomfort, lead to complications such as pneumonia.
3. This information comes to us from the supplemental briefs of the parties.
4. Submitting the brief for the defendant was the guardian ad litem, Patrick J. Melnik. The Attorney General submitted the brief for the plaintiffs. The Civil Rights and Liberties Division of the Department of the Attorney General prepared a brief amicus curiae on behalf of the defendant. Briefs amicus curiae were also submitted by the Mental Health Legal Advisers Committee, the Massachusetts Association for Retarded Citizens, Inc., and the Developmental Disabilities Law Project of the University of Maryland Law School.
5. *Commonwealth v. O'Neal*, 367 Mass 440, 327 N.E. 2d 662 (1975), does not compel a different result. That case considered the magnitude of the State interest in preserving life in the context of an intentional State deprivation. It does not apply to a situation where an individual, without State involvement, may make a decision resulting in the shortening of life by natural causes.
6. The nature of the third party interest discussed here is not one where the decision has clear, immediate, and adverse effects on the third party such as in *Raleigh Fitkin-Paul Morgan Memorial Hosp.*, where a blood transfusion was necessary to preserve the life of a child in utero, as well as the mother. Clearly, different considerations are presented in such a case.
7. The interest in protecting against suicide seems to require little if any discussion. In the case of the competent adult's refusing medical treatment such an act does not necessarily constitute suicide since (1) in refusing treatment the patient may not have the specific intent to die, and (2) even if he did, to the extent that the cause of death was from natural causes the patient did not set the death producing agent in motion with the intent of causing his own death. Byrn, *supra* at 17–18. Cantor, *supra* at 255. Furthermore, the underlying State interest in this area lies in the prevention of irrational self-destruction. What we consider here is a competent, rational decision to refuse treatment when death is inevitable and the treatment offers no hope of cure or preservation of life. There is no connection between the conduct here in issue and any State concern to prevent suicide. Cantor, *supra* at 258.
8. Any threats of civil liability may be removed by a valid giving or withholding of consent by an informed patient. See generally Note, Statutory Recognition of the Right to Die: The California Natural Death Act. 57 B.U.L.Rev. 148 (1977), for a comprehensive discussion of the common law foundations of physicians' duties, and patients' rights, one legislative attempt to modernize the law, and an analysis of the ramifications for doctors and patients of recognizing the option of withholding life-sustaining procedures from a patient incapable of indicating his or her wishes.
9. This factor is relevant because of the medical evidence in the record that people of Saikewicz's age do not tolerate the chemotherapy as well as younger people and that the chance of a remission is decreased. Age is irrelevant, of course, to the question of the value or quality of life.
10. "We repeat for the sake of emphasis and clarity that upon the concurrence of the guardian and family of Karen, should the responsible attending physicians conclude that there is no reasonable possibility of Karen's ever emerging from her present comatose condition to a cognitive, sapient state and that the life-support apparatus now being administered to Karen should be discontinued, they shall consult with the hospital "Ethics Committee" or like body of the institution in which Karen is then hospitalized. If that consultative body agrees that there is no reasonable possibility of Karen's ever emerging from her present comatose condition to a cognitive, sapient state, the present life-support system may be withdrawn and said action shall be without any civil or criminal liability therefor on the part of any participant, whether guardian, physician, hospital or others."

    "By the above ruling we do not intend to be understood as implying that a proceeding for judicial declaratory relief is necessarily required for the implementation of comparable decisions in the field of medical practice." See *In re Quinlan*, 70 NJ at 55, 355 Atlantic Reporter 2d. at 672.

DECIDING TO FOREGO LIFE-SUSTAINING TREATMENT: ETHICAL, MEDICAL, AND LEGAL ISSUES IN TREATMENT DECISIONS

INTRODUCTION. *The same Presidential Commission that reviewed the debate swirling around the definition of death turned its attention to the controversy surrounding foregoing of life-sustaining treatment. It reviewed the issues underlying the Quinlan and Saikewicz cases and the legislative activity giving rise to natural death acts.*

The Commission's report, which appeared in March 1983, expresses the broad public consensus that was emerging at the time. It emphasizes the primary importance of the voluntary choice of the competent or formerly competent patient to refuse life-sustaining treatment. Incompetent patients who have not provided a record of the wishes they expressed while competent should have an appropriate surrogate, ordinarily a family member, whose responsibility is to pursue the best interest of the patient. The Commission urges consultation with hospital-based ethics committees, but recognizes that the only body with the legal authority to override a surrogate's decision is a court. The Commission also puts forward the model of durable powers of attorney for individuals to designate their surrogate should they become incompetent.

The Commission's report remains the single most important summary of the consensus that was emerging in the United States during this time. It continued to evolve throughout the 1980s, and remains in place in the United States regarding foregoing treatment.

INTRODUCTION AND SUMMARY

Americans seem to be increasingly concerned with decisions about death and dying. Why is a subject once thought taboo now so frequently aired by the popular media, debated in academic forums and professional societies, and litigated in well-publicized court cases?

Perhaps it is because death is less of a private matter than it once was. Today, dying more often than not occurs under medical supervision, usually in a hospital or nursing home. Actions that take place in such settings involve more people, and the resolution of disagreements among them is more likely to require formal rules and means of adjudication. Moreover, patients dying in health care institutions today typically have fewer of the sources of nonmedical support, such as family and church, that once helped people in their final days.

Also important, no doubt, are the biomedical developments of the past several decades. Without removing the sense of loss, finality, and mystery that have always accompanied death, these new developments have made death more a matter of deliberate decision. For almost any life-threatening condition, some intervention can now delay the moment of death. Frequent dramatic breakthroughs—insulin, antibiotics, resuscitation, chemotherapy, kidney dialysis, and organ transplantation, to name but a few—have made it possible to retard and even to reverse many conditions that were until recently regarded as fatal. Matters once the province of fate have now become a matter of human choice, a development that has profound ethical and legal implications.

Moreover, medical technology often renders patients less able to communicate or to direct the course of treat-

---

President's Commission for the Study of Ethical Problems in Medicine and Biomedical and Behavioral Research. *Deciding to Forego Life-Sustaining Treatment: A Report on the Ethical, Medical, and Legal Issues in Treatment Decisions*. Washington, D.C.: U.S. Government Printing Office, 1993. This excerpt omits Chapters 1, 3, minor parts of 5 through 7 and the Appendixes; the notes have been lightly edited for

ment. Even for mentally competent patients, other people must usually assist in making treatment decisions or at least acquiesce in carrying them out. Consequently, in recent years there has been a continuing clarification of the rights, duties, and liabilities of all concerned, a process in which professionals, ethical and legal commentators, and—with increasing frequency—the courts and legislatures have been involved.

Thus, the Commission found this an appropriate time to reexamine the way decisions are and ought to be made about whether or not to forego life-sustaining treatment.[1] For example, may a patient's withdrawal from treatment ever be forbidden? Should physicians acquiesce in patients' wishes regarding therapy? Should they offer patients the option to forego life-sustaining therapy? Does it make any difference if the treatment has already been started, or involves mechanical systems of life support, or is very costly?

Summary of Conclusions

Building on a central conclusion of its report on informed consent[2]—that decisions about health care ultimately rest with competent patients—the Commission in this Report examines the situations in which a patient's choice to forego life-sustaining therapy may be limited on moral or legal grounds. In addition to providing clarification of the issues, the Report suggests appropriate procedures for decisions regarding both competent and incompetent patients and scrutinizes the role of various public and private bodies in shaping and regulating the process.

These aims are the only ones that this Commission believes to be within the scope of its role. The Report does not judge any particular future case nor provide a guidebook of the morally correct choice for patients and health care providers who are facing such a decision. Rather, the Commission intends to illuminate the strengths and weaknesses of various considerations and various instruments of social policy. Clarifying the relevant considerations and prohibitions may help decisionmakers, but it may also force them to confront painful realities more directly. The Commission hopes that this Report will help improve the process, but recognizes that an improved process will not necessarily make decisions easier.

The Report addresses a broad range of problems and patient situations. Serious questions about whether life should be sustained through a particular treatment usually arise when a patient is suffering from a known disease likely to prove fatal in the near future rather than in an unanticipated emergency (where any decisionmaking would necessarily have to be truncated). Life-sustaining treatment, as used here, encompasses all health care interventions that have the effect of increasing the life span of the patient. Although the term includes respirators, kidney machines, and all the paraphernalia of modern medicine, it also includes home physical therapy, nursing support for activities of daily living, and special feeding procedures, provided that one of the effects of the treatment is to prolong a patient's life.

The issues addressed in this Report are complex and their resolution depends not only on the context of particular decisions but also on their relationship to other values and principles. Thus, it is exceptionally difficult to summarize the Commission's conclusions on this subject. The synopsis provided here should be read in the context of the reasoning, elaboration, and qualifications provided in the chapters that follow.

(1) The voluntary choice of a competent and informed patient should determine whether or not life-sustaining therapy will be undertaken, just as such choices provide the basis for other decisions about medical treatment. Health care institutions and professionals should try to enhance patients' abilities to make decisions on their own behalf and to promote understanding of the available treatment options.

(2) Health care professionals serve patients best by maintaining a presumption in favor of sustaining life, while recognizing that competent patients are entitled to choose to forego any treatments, including those that sustain life.

(3) As in medical decisionmaking generally, some constraints on patients' decisions are justified.

- Health care professionals or institutions may decline to provide a particular option because that choice would violate their conscience or professional judgment, though in doing so they may not abandon a patient.
- Health care institutions may justifiably restrict the availability of certain options in order to use limited resources more effectively or to enhance equity in allocating them.
- Society may decide to limit the availability of certain options for care in order to advance equity or the general welfare, but such policies should not be applied initially nor especially forcefully to medical options that could sustain life.
- Information about the existence and justification of any of these constraints must be available to patients or their surrogates.

(4) Governmental agencies, institutional providers of care, individual practitioners, and the general public should try to improve the medically beneficial options that are available to dying patients. Specific attention should be paid to making respectful, responsive, and competent care available for people who choose to forego life-sustaining therapy or for whom no such therapies are available.

(5) Several distinctions are employed by health care professionals and others in deliberating about whether a choice that leads to an earlier death would be acceptable or unacceptable in a particular case. Unfortunately, people often treat these distinctions—between acts and omissions that cause death, between withholding and withdrawing

care, between an intended death and one that is merely foreseeable, and between ordinary and extraordinary treatment—as though applying them decided the issue, which it does not. Although there is a danger that relying on such labels will take the place of analysis, these distinctions can still be helpful if attention is directed to the reasoning behind them, such as the degree to which a patient is benefited or burdened by a treatment.

(6) Achieving medically and morally appropriate decisions does not require changes in statutes concerning homicide or wrongful death, given appropriate prosecutorial discretion and judicial interpretation.

(7) Primary responsibility for ensuring that morally justified processes of decisionmaking are followed lies with physicians. Health care institutions also have a responsibility to ensure that there are appropriate procedures to enhance patients' competence, to provide for designation of surrogates, to guarantee that patients are adequately informed, to overcome the influence of dominant institutional biases, to provide review of decisionmaking, and to refer cases to the courts appropriately. The Commission is not recommending that hospitals and other institutions take over decisions about patient care; there is no substitute for the dedication, compassion, and professional judgment of physicians. Nevertheless, institutions need to develop policies because their decisions have profound effects on patient outcomes, because society looks to these institutions to ensure the means necessary to preserve both health and the value of self-determination, and because they are conveniently situated to provide efficient, confidential, and rapid supervision and review of decisionmaking.

Incompetent Patients Generally (8) Physicians who make initial assessments of patients' competence and others who review these assessments should be responsible for judging whether a particular patient's decisionmaking abilities are sufficient to meet the demands of the specific decision at hand.

(9) To protect the interests of patients who have insufficient capacity to make particular decisions and to ensure their well-being and self-determination:

- An appropriate surrogate, ordinarily a family member, should be named to make decisions for such patients. The decisions of surrogates should, when possible, attempt to replicate the ones that the patient would make if capable of doing so. When lack of evidence about the patient's wishes precludes this, decisions by surrogates should seek to protect the patient's best interests.[3] Because such decisions are not instances of self-choice by the patient, the range of acceptable decisions by surrogates is sometimes not as broad as it would be for patients making decisions for themselves.
- The medical staff, along with the trustees and administrators of health care institutions, should explore and evaluate various formal and informal administrative arrangements for review and consultation, such as "ethics committees," particularly for decisions that have life-or-death consequences for incompetent patients.
- State courts and legislatures should consider making provision for advance directives through which people designate others to make health care decisions on their behalf and/or give instructions about their care. Such advance directives provide a means of preserving some self-determination for patients who may lose their decisionmaking capacity. Durable powers of attorney are preferable to "living wills" since they are more generally applicable and provide a better vehicle for patients to exercise self-determination, though experience with both is limited.
- Health care professionals and institutions should adopt clear, explicit, and publicly available policies regarding how and by whom decisions are to be made for patients who lack adequate decisionmaking capacity.
- Families, health care institutions, and professionals should work together to make decisions for patients who lack decisionmaking capacity. Recourse to the courts should be reserved for the occasions when adjudication is clearly required by state law or when concerned parties have disagreements that they cannot resolve over matters of substantial import. Courts and legislatures should be cautious about requiring judicial review of routine health care decisions for patients with inadequate decisionmaking capacity.

Patients with Permanent Loss of Consciousness
(10) Current understanding of brain functions allows a reliable diagnosis of permanent loss of consciousness for some patients. Whether or not life-sustaining treatment is given is of much less importance to such patients than to others.

(11) The decisions of patients' families should determine what sort of medical care permanently unconscious patients receive. Other than requiring appropriate decisionmaking procedures for these patients, the law does not and should not require any particular therapies to be applied or continued, with the exception of basic nursing care that is needed to ensure dignified and respectful treatment of the patient.

(12) Access to costly care for patients who have permanently lost consciousness may justifiably be restricted on the basis of resource use in two ways: by a physician or institution that otherwise would have to deny significantly beneficial care to another specific patient, or by legitimate mechanisms of policy formulation and application if and only if the provision of certain kinds of care to these patients were clearly causing serious inequities in the use of community resources.

Seriously Ill Newborns (13) Parents should be the surrogates for a seriously ill newborn unless they are disqualified by decisionmaking incapacity, an unresolvable disagreement between them, or their choice of a course of action that is clearly against the infant's best interests.

(14) Therapies expected to be futile for a seriously ill newborn need not be provided; parents, health care professionals and institutions, and reimbursement sources, however, should ensure the infant's comfort.

(15) Within constraints of equity and availability, infants should receive all therapies that are clearly beneficial to them. For example, an otherwise healthy Down Syndrome child whose life is threatened by a surgically correctable complication should receive the surgery because he or she would clearly benefit from it.

- The concept of benefit necessarily makes reference to the context of the infant's present and future treatment, taking into account such matters as the level of biomedical knowledge and technology and the availability of services necessary for the child's treatment.
- The dependence of benefit upon context underlines society's special obligation to provide necessary services for handicapped children and their families, which rests on the special ethical duties owed to newborns with undeserved disadvantages and on the general ethical duty of the community to ensure equitable access for all persons to an adequate level of health care.[4]

(16) Decisionmakers should have access to the most accurate and up-to-date information as they consider individual cases.

- Physicians should obtain appropriate consultations and referrals.
- The significance of the diagnoses and the prognoses under each treatment option must be conveyed to the parents (or other surrogates).

(17) The medical staff, administrators, and trustees of each institution that provides care to seriously ill newborns should take the responsibility for ensuring good decisionmaking practices. Accrediting bodies may want to require that institutions have appropriate policies in this area.

- An institution should have clear and explicit policies that require prospective or retrospective review of decisions when life-sustaining treatment for an infant might be foregone or when parents and providers disagree about the correct decision for an infant. Certain categories of clearly futile therapies could be explicitly excluded from review.
- The best interests of an infant should be pursued when those interests are clear.
- The policies should allow for the exercise of parental discretion when a child's interests are ambiguous.
- Decisions should be referred to public agencies (including courts) for review when necessary to determine whether parents should be disqualified as decisionmakers and, if so, who should decide the course of treatment that would be in the best interests of their child.

(18) The legal system has various—though limited—roles in ensuring that seriously ill infants receive the correct care.

- Civil courts are ultimately the appropriate decisionmakers concerning the disqualification of parents as surrogates and the designation of surrogates to serve in their stead.
- Special statutes requiring providers to bring such cases to the attention of civil authorities do not seem warranted, since state laws already require providers to report cases of child abuse or neglect to social service agencies; nevertheless, educating providers about their responsibilities is important.
- Although criminal penalties should be available to punish serious errors, the ability of the criminal law to ensure good decisionmaking in individual cases is limited.
- Governmental agencies that reimburse for health care may insist that institutions have policies and procedures regarding decisionmaking, but using financial sanctions against institutions to punish an "incorrect" decision in a particular case is likely to be ineffective and to lead to excessively detailed regulations that would involve government reimbursement officials in bedside decisionmaking. Furthermore, such sanctions could actually penalize other patients and providers in an unjust way.

Cardiopulmonary Resuscitation (19) A presumption favoring resuscitation of hospitalized patients in the event of unexpected cardiac arrest is justified.

(20) A competent and informed patient or an incompetent patient's surrogate is entitled to decide with the attending physician that an order against resuscitation should be written in the chart. When cardiac arrest is likely, a patient (or a surrogate) should usually be informed and offered the chance specifically to decide for or against resuscitation.

(21) Physicians have a duty to assess for each hospitalized patient whether resuscitation is likely, on balance, to benefit the patient, to fail to benefit, or to have uncertain effect.

- When a patient will not benefit from resuscitation, a decision not to resuscitate, with the consent of the patient or surrogate, is justified.
- When a physician's assessment conflicts with a competent patient's decision, further discussion and consultation are appropriate; ultimately the physician must follow the patient's decision or transfer responsibility for that patient to another physician.
- When a physician's assessment conflicts with that of an incompetent patient's surrogate, further discussion, con-

sultation, review by an institutional committee, and, if necessary, judicial review should be sought.

(22) To protect the interests of patients and their families, health care institutions should have explicit policies and procedures governing orders not to resuscitate, and accrediting bodies should require such policies.

- Such policies should require that orders not to resuscitate be in written form and that they delineate who has the authority both to write such orders and to stop a resuscitation effort in progress.
- Federal agencies responsible for the direct provision of patient care (such as the Veterans Administration, the Public Health Service, and the Department of Defense) should ensure that their health care facilities adopt appropriate policies.

(23) The entry of an order not to resuscitate holds no necessary implications for any other therapeutic decisions, and the level or extent of health care that will be reimbursed under public or private insurance programs should never be linked to such orders.

(24) The education of health care professionals should ensure that they know how to help patients and family make ethically justified decisions for or against resuscitation; those responsible for professional licensure and certification may want to assess knowledge in these areas.

The Commission's Inquiry

When the Commission convened in January 1980, it decided to take up first its Congressional mandate to report on "the matter of defining death, including the advisability of developing a uniform definition of death."[5] In July 1981 the Commission reported its conclusions in *Defining Death*[6] and recommended the adoption of the Uniform Determination of Death Act (UDDA), which was developed in collaboration with the American Bar Association, the American Medical Association, and the National Conference of Commissioners on Uniform State Laws.[7]

During hearings on this subject, the Commission learned that many people were troubled by the uncertainties about the correct care to provide for patients with serious deficits in "higher brain" functions—such as those required for thinking, communicating, and consciously responding to others or to the environment. Decisions about the care of such patients were seen to be at least as troubling as decisions about those who have permanently lost all brain functions. The most pointed example brought to the attention of the Commission is the group of patients who are so damaged as to be permanently devoid of any consciousness—the most severe brain damage compatible with life.[8] The Commission concluded that the situation of such patients—like Karen Quinlan—merited its attention. In *Defining Death*, the Commission stated an intention to report subsequently on the treatment of patients who are dying but not dead.[9]

The present study was undertaken not merely because of the study on the determination of death but also because of its broader relationship to work done by the Commission in several areas over the past three years. Under its mandate, the Commission is authorized to undertake investigation "of any other appropriate matter . . . consistent with the purposes of [its authorizing statute] on its own initiative."[10] Decisions about life-sustaining therapy involve the direct and concrete application of the principles of decisionmaking in medicine, which was the subject of the Commission's mandated study on informed consent.[11] Such decisions also illustrate the ways questions of equity in the allocation of often scarce and expensive resources are resolved, a subject addressed by the Commission in another mandated study.[12] The present Report thus represents an effort to apply the conclusions of two previous studies to a particular area of current concern, while also responding to some particularly difficult clinical and ethical problems noted in *Defining Death.*

The Commission received testimony and public comment on the subject of this Report at four public hearings in as many cities; witnesses from medicine, nursing, hospital administration, the social sciences, philosophy, theology, and law, as well as patients and family members, testified.[13] It also deliberated on partial drafts of the Report at eight Commission meetings. On December 15, 1982, a final draft was discussed and approved unanimously, subject to editorial corrections.

Overview of the Report

Part One of the Report examines the considerations common to all decisionmaking about life-sustaining therapy. Chapter One presents historical, cultural, and psychological information to illuminate the social context of the Report. Chapter Two first considers the importance of shared decisionmaking between provider and patient (in which the voluntary decisions of competent patients are ordinarily binding) and the considerations that arise when patients are inadequate decisionmakers, and then discusses constraints imposed by the community's need to ensure that life is protected and that wrongful death is deterred and punished. Traditional distinctions made between acceptable and unacceptable actions to forego treatment are critically scrutinized and their usefulness in sound decisionmaking is evaluated. Chapter Three analyzes additional constraints on patients' choices that arise from the actions of family and care-giving professionals, from society's pursuit of equitable allocation of resources, and from the policies and practices of health care institutions, which are often where these many forces come together.

In Part Two of the Report, several groups of patients whose situations currently raise special public policy concerns are considered. Chapter Four examines decisionmaking for incompetent patients generally, including "living wills" and other advance directives, intrainstitutional review (such as "ethics committees"), and court proceedings. Chapters Five and Six look at the issues involved in treating two particular categories of incompetent patients—those who have permanently lost all consciousness and seriously ill newborns. Finally, Chapter Seven considers orders not to resuscitate hospitalized patients whose hearts stop beating and recommends institutional policies on such orders.

Extensive appendices follow the Report itself, beginning with a detailed account of the process followed by the Commission in its study. Appendix B reviews some of the medical aspects of caring for dying patients in a format intended to be helpful to clinicians, though it will also be of interest to people concerned with ethics and policy. The remainder of the Appendices consist of various documents that are cited in the text and that might otherwise be difficult for a reader to obtain, including the report of a national survey of hospital ethics committees undertaken for the Commission.

* * *

2. THE ELEMENTS OF GOOD DECISIONMAKING

Patients whose medical conditions require treatment to sustain life usually want the treatment and benefit from it. Sometimes, however, a treatment is so undesirable in itself or the life it sustains is so brief and burdened that a patient—or a surrogate acting on the patient's behalf—decides that it would be better to forego the treatment. This chapter considers how life-sustaining treatment decisions should be made and the ethical and legal constraints on such decisions that might be warranted.

Shared Decisionmaking

In considering the issue of informed consent,[1] the Commission recommended that patient and provider collaborate in a continuing process intended to make decisions that will advance the patient's interests both in health (and well-being generally) and in self-determination.[2] The Commission argued that decisions about the treatments that best promote a patient's health and well-being must be based on the particular patient's values and goals; no uniform, objective determination can be adequate—whether defined by society or by health professionals.

Respect for the self-determination of competent patients is of special importance in decisions to forego life-sustaining treatment because different people will have markedly different needs and concerns during the final period of their lives; living a little longer will be of distinctly different value to them. Decisions about life-sustaining treatment, which commonly affect more than one goal of a patient (for example, prolongation of life and relief of suffering) create special tensions. Nonetheless, a process of collaborating and sharing information and responsibility between care givers and patients generally results in mutually satisfactory decisions.[3] Even when it does not, the primacy of a patient's interests in self-determination and in honoring the patient's own view of well-being warrant leaving with the patient the final authority to decide.

Although competent patients thus have the legal and ethical authority to forego some or all care,[4] this does not mean that patients may insist on particular treatments. The care available from health care professionals is generally limited to what is consistent with role-related professional standards and conscientiously held personal beliefs. A health care professional has an obligation to allow a patient to choose from among medically acceptable treatment options (whether provided by the professional or by appropriate colleagues to whom the patient is referred) or to reject all options. No one, however, has an obligation to provide interventions that would, in his or her judgment, be countertherapeutic.

In most circumstances, patients are presumed to be capable of making decisions about their own care. When a patient's capability to make final decisions is seriously limited, he or she needs to be protected against the adverse consequences of a flawed choice. Yet any mechanism that offers such protection also risks abuse: the individual's ability to direct his or her own life might be frustrated in an unwarranted manner. In its report on informed consent, the Commission recommended that a surrogate—typically a close relative or friend—be named when a patient lacks the capacity to make particular medical decisions.[5] As much as possible, surrogates and providers of care should then make decisions as the particular patient would have.

Decisionmaking Capacity Determining whether a patient has sufficient decisionmaking capacity to make choices about health care treatment is based on three considerations: the abilities of the patient, the requirements of the task at hand, and the consequences to the patient that are likely to flow from the decision. The individual must have sufficiently stable and developed personal values and goals, an ability to communicate and understand information adequately, and an ability to reason and deliberate sufficiently well about the choices.[6]

Just as for medical treatment generally, deciding about a patient's decisionmaking abilities when the patient is facing a complex and confusing situation or making a decision of great consequence requires both the wise judgment of others and procedures that regularly yield morally and legally acceptable decisions. The Commission has found no reason for decisions about life-sustaining therapy to be considered differently from other treatment decisions. A decision to forego such treatment is awesome because it hastens death, but that does not change the elements of decisionmaking capacity and need not require greater abilities on the part of a patient. Decisions about the length of life are not necessarily more demanding of a patient's capabilities than other important decisions. And decisions that might shorten life are not always regarded by patients as difficult ones: a patient who even with treatment has a very short time to live may find a few additional hours rather unimportant, especially if the person has had a chance to take leave of loved ones and is reconciled to his or her situation.

Thus, determining whether or not a patient lacks the capacity to make a decision to forego life-sustaining treatment will rest on generally applicable principles for making assessments of decisional incapacity in medical care. Of course, when a patient who could have a substantial time to live rejects life-sustaining treatment, close inquiry into the components of that person's decisionmaking capacity is warranted in order to protect the individual from harms that arise from incapacities that themselves diminish the value of self-determination.[7]

Voluntariness A patient's choice is binding when it is selected freely—that is, when the patient can decide in accord with his or her own values and goals.[8] Selection among options must not be so influenced by others that free choice is precluded, and relevant treatment options must therefore be made available to the patient. Furthermore, the patient must be situated so as to feel that he or she is expected to have the final word in the treatment decision. Of course, patients do not make decisions in isolation from others. Complex networks of relationships and roles make the responses of other parties very important to patients and to their decisionmaking.

One of the things that patients rightly expect from professionals, and that professionals usually expect to provide, is advice rather than neutral information about treatment options and their risks and benefits. However, the way advice is provided can vary substantially. Individual personality styles, both of the professional and of the patient, range from authoritarian through nondirective to dependent.

Drawing the line between influence that is legitimate and that which is not is difficult both conceptually and in practice.[9] Often distinctions are suggested between "coercion," "fraud," "duress," "deceit," and "manipulation"—all of which are said to be unacceptable—and "influence," "persuasion," and "advice"—which are expected, and perhaps even desired. The use of these labels conveys a judgment as to whether an action would interfere with voluntary choice or not, but the categories are too poorly defined to provide a generally accepted basis for judging the difficult cases. It is important, therefore, to develop a fuller understanding of acceptable conduct in the interaction of health care professionals and others with patients.

Professional care givers and a patient's close friends and family[10] have two major roles to play when someone faces a decision about life-sustaining treatment. First, their actions, words, and presence help shape the patient's assessment of the best course of treatment. Second, their ability and willingness to carry out various decisions often define the range of options available to the patient.[11]

Shaping the patient's deliberations. How information is communicated and continuing care is provided can forcefully induce a patient to make certain choices. In many medical care situations patients are dependent and professionals are relatively powerful.[12] This disparity creates an obligation for professionals to reduce the understandable tendency of some patients to receive and act upon either a distorted understanding of their medical situation or a feeling of powerlessness, so that individuals can truly decide in accord with their own values and goals.[13]

Helping to shape the deliberations of a patient who must decide about the course and duration of his or her life is a complex and weighty obligation. For example, letting a patient know that his or her death is now seen by others to be appropriate—or at least not unexpected—may be "giving permission to die" to a patient who no longer wishes to struggle against overwhelming odds. On the other hand, it may encourage overly rapid acceptance of death by a patient who feels rejected and unimportant.[14]

Deciding on the best response and role is especially difficult for families and often inescapably uncertain. Clearly, family members do best by sustaining the patient's courage and hope, and by advancing the person's interests (and limiting self-serving actions) as much as possible. But family members usually cannot be dispassionate and emotionally uninvolved, nor should they try to be. In addition to any practical effects of the illness, they suffer from fear, anxiety, and grief—often as much or more than the patient. Thus, their ability to respond to the patient's needs is determined by their own capabilities under the circumstances.[15]

Generally, part of the experience of dying involves withdrawing from some goals and relationships that have become unachievable or unimportant, pursuing other goals that are important to accomplish, providing directions for the future disposition of property and body, and giving advice to friends and families. Each of these practical steps entails reciprocal activities by others in a person's social network—acceptance of disengagement, support in revising priorities, legal counsel in writing a will, gathering for farewells, and so forth.[16]

The roles of health care professionals are different from those of family members. Their personal concerns and predispositions are not supposed to interfere with providing patients with competent care[17]; they are expected to develop ways to protect themselves from emotional exhaustion without becoming too distant or impersonal to help patients cope with emotional problems.[18]

The individual health care provider is likely to help dying patients most by maintaining a predisposition for sustaining life (while accepting that prolongation of dying may serve no worthwhile purpose for a particular patient). Indeed, this favoring of life is part of society's expectation regarding health care professionals.[19] Commonly, it is supported by a personal belief or value commitment and by a recognition of the needs of dying patients for reassurance about the worth of their own lives. Until it is quite clear that a patient is making an informed, deliberate, and voluntary decision to forego specific life-sustaining interventions, health care providers should look for and enhance any feelings the patient has about not yet acquiescing in death. As death comes closer, such sentiments generally recede; until then, there need be no haste to encourage a patient's acceptance of death.[20]

Enhancing the experience of those whose lives are drawing to a close is a worthwhile goal, one that requires skill, compassion, honesty, and humility. Here, various individuals can serve different and valued functions: clergy can attend especially to religious questions and rituals that affirm spiritual and temporal meaning; family members can resolve problems in relationships and reaffirm the importance of the patient's life; and health care professionals can focus on relieving immediate sources of distress and on enhancing the self-respect and courage of the patient.

The complex nature of provider-patient relations—each person influencing the attitudes of the other in ways that neither may fully understand—is illustrated by the case of "David G.," a young man who pleaded articulately with his physicians to cease the painful treatments they were providing for the extensive burns he had suffered.

> His sudden and unaccustomed total dependence on others insistently calls into question the psychological basis for commonsense perception that he has an identity separate from other people and from the external world.
>
> The critical ambiguity . . . goes . . . to Mr. G.'s conception of himself as a choice maker; that is, it is not clear whether he sees himself as separate from others in exercising choice regarding his future or whether he chooses death because he believes others want that result for him and he feels incapable of extricating himself from their choice-making for him. Either perspective could lead to the deepest despair; his affliction itself could rob life of all possible meaning for him: his belief that others . . . wished him dead could do the same. If, however, others were deferring to his wish to die because they conceived that they were honoring his self-determination, it would be critical to establish which of these two perspectives led him to this choice.[21]

Making choices available. Providers and others have an obligation to see that patients can choose among a range of available and potentially beneficial treatments.[22] Sometimes the range is limited wrongly because a practitioner is unwilling to make available an option or is ignorant of a possible treatment that is especially pertinent to a particular decision about life-sustaining therapy. Since competent and informed patients ought to be made aware that they can forego medical interventions, the option of no effort at curative therapy should generally be explored with dying patients. Some patients may associate this course with isolation, abandonment, and unmitigated suffering, however, unless supportive care is clearly also made available.

Good medical and nursing care can greatly improve the lives of patients who are dying.[23] Much comfort can be gained by careful attention to such details as proper positioning, vigorous skin care, oral hygiene, disguising of disfigurement, on-demand feeding of preferred foods, and so on. Medical management of symptoms has recently demonstrated that no patient should have to be terrified of physical pain; in fact, presently available drugs and techniques allow pain to be reduced to a level acceptable to virtually every patient, usually without unacceptable sedation.[24] Other symptoms, such as nausea, anxiety, constipation, and shortness of breath, usually respond reasonably well to drugs or other procedures.[25] Providers of care have an obligation to ensure that these supportive measures are available to everyone, whether or not a patient has chosen to pursue life-sustaining treatment. To allow such a decision to result in an avoidably harsh existence, or to let the patient believe that it will, is unjustifiable and may render the patient's decision involuntary.

Nonvoluntary decisionmaking. Nonvoluntary foregoing of life-sustaining therapy takes place when a patient gives neither effective consent nor refusal. Often this arises because a patient's decisionmaking capacity is inadequate, and then a surrogate will have to decide on behalf of the patient.[26] Sometimes, however, a patient, though competent, is excluded from the decisionmaking process. This is unjustifiable since it demeans the patient by barring self-determination and allows others to shorten the patient's life or establish the burdens under which it will be lived without the assurance (which could be obtained) that the patient concurs in the judgment. Although there may be times when a competent patient would prefer not to be involved in these choices, it is impossible to know in advance which patients would come to this conclusion.[27] And the risk of wrongly abrogating decisionmaking for many patients seems generally more grievous than the pain of confronting some seriously ill patients with choices that they would rather not face. The only time that the Commission finds it justified for a patient who could be informed and involved to be excluded is when that patient freely and knowingly transfers some decisionmaking authority to another.[28]

Informing and Communicating

Disclosure. The extent of the obligation of providers to inform patients so that they can make sound choices is no different for life-sustaining treatment than for any other. In the Commission's view, health professionals should ensure that patients understand (1) their current medical status, including its likely course if no treatment is pursued; (2) the interventions that might be helpful to the patient, including a description of the procedures involved and the likelihood and effect of associated risks and benefits; and (3) in most cases, a professional opinion as to the best alternative.[29] Each of these elements must be discussed in light of associated uncertainties.[30]

The purpose of such discussions is not to inundate patients with medical facts but rather to give them the information they need in order to assess options realistically and to choose the treatments most consonant with their own values and goals. Inaccurate or incomplete information limits patients' understanding of what is at stake. For any medical intervention to be warranted, a patient must stand to gain more from having the treatment than from not having it. Since the benefit to be gained must be assessed in terms of the patient's own values and goals, practitioners should be cautious not to rule out prematurely a seemingly undesirable or less-than-optimal alternative that might offer what a particular patient would perceive as a benefit.

Physician attitudes toward communication with terminally ill patients have changed dramatically in recent years. Whereas 20 years ago the majority of physicians did not disclose a fatal diagnosis to their patients, most physicians now do so routinely.[31] Yet both behaviors—generally withholding in the 1960s and generally disclosing today—seem to be based on physicians' judgments of what is best for patients rather than on recognition of the value of self-determination per se.

Three surveys between 1953 and 1961,[32] for example, found that 69–90% of physicians routinely failed to inform cancer patients of their diagnosis, claiming that the unvarnished truth would be too much for their patients—"a death sentence," "torture," or "hitting the patients with a baseball bat."[33] Those surveyed expressed concern about the psychological damage that could ensue from such revelations[34] and gave that as a reason for a "therapeutic privilege" to exempt them from the requirements of informed consent when caring for terminally ill patients.[35] Yet one researcher found "on closer examination, most of the instances in which unhappy results were reported to follow [disclosure] turned out to be vague accounts from which no reliable inference could be drawn."[36] Fearful of the effects of telling the truth, many physicians relied upon incomplete information and euphemisms, resorting to vague terms such as "lesion" or "mass" or using language only suggestive of malignancy, such as a "suspicious" or "degenerated" tumor.[37]

In a 1978 replication of the 1961 survey, 97% of physicians said they preferred to tell cancer patients of their diagnosis, compared with only 10% of those polled earlier.[38] Physician attitudes thus now seem to be more attuned to current desires of patients, the overwhelming majority of whom want to know the whole truth. Indeed, in the Commission's survey of patient-provider relationships, "the public displayed an unflinching desire for facts about their condition, even dismal facts"; 96% of the public stated specifically that they would want to know of a diagnosis of cancer, and 86% said they would want a realistic prognosis.[39]

There are a number of hypotheses about why physicians' attitudes shifted. When physicians avoided telling patients their prognoses explicitly, they may still have found that patients arrived at quite reliable conclusions about the nearness of death from how sick they were and from the behavior of others. In one study, three-fourths of the patients who had not been fully informed nevertheless knew that they were expected to die soon.[40] When this is the case, the issue of whether the doctor should tell the patient loses much of its force. Moreover, most of the surveys have dealt with cancer,[41] which may indeed have been very nearly a death sentence as recently as two decades ago. Today remission and even cure is often possible; the disease is not as ominous or stigmatizing as it once was.[42] Since the medical information is more complex, diagnoses today may actually need much more explanation in order for patients to understand the relevant facts.

Physicians may also be giving more information as a function of the increasingly broad and enforced legal duties of disclosure.[43] And many dying patients are part of clinical research in which the obligation to disclose a diagnosis before consent is obtained is carefully enforced by each hospital's institutional review board.[44] Finally, physicians have doubtless been affected by the desire of terminally ill patients for more information, one manifestation of an era marked by consumerism, "patients' rights," and a wariness of the professions generally.

Some physicians are more willing to talk about dying because they have seen the detrimental effects of not doing so. Failure to disclose information to patients who seek it takes a toll in the erosion of trust—the basic bond between physician and patient. This mistrust is likely to be exacerbated and extended to family members if they conspire in keeping silent.[45] For patients whose intuitions tell them they are seriously ill, unlikely fabrications or euphemisms may result in fear that the doctor does not know the real diagnosis or that the family cannot cope with it. For many, the worry, conjecture, and degradation that can result from misinformation may be more tormenting than the knowledge of the illness itself.[46] Nondisclosure may inhibit further questions from patients, which would limit their capacity to participate in medical care decisions as well as those on other personal and financial affairs.

The issue of whether to tell patients about a terminal diagnosis is less a choice of "to tell or not to tell" than it is a question of how to gauge how much each patient wants to know at a particular time. As one experienced physician has noted, "The real question is not 'what do you tell your patients?' but rather 'what do you let your patients tell you?'"[47] In other words, "Now that we tell our patients more, are we also listening more?"[48]

Clearly, doses of truth must be administered with sensitivity, lest they inflict undue psychic trauma upon patients. The dialectic of provider-patient communication is a sensitive one that varies from case to case.[49] Commonly, communication and cues take nonverbal forms, and verbal expressions sometimes are misleading. Meaningful dialogue does not come easily or cheaply:

> You have to be prepared to spend an enormous amount of time with that person, exploring and talking and being quiet for periods of time and letting conversation go and coming back to conversation. . . . Expenditure of time is something that is a quite precious commodity in medical care generally, and is in fact ladled out rather sparingly . . . particularly with dying patients.[50]

A nurse who has worked with parents of seriously ill newborns in a neonatal intensive care unit told the Commission:

> Very often parents are not ready to talk a great deal initially about the worst and most horrible possibilities for the future of their child. And so a good deal of time is often spent in early weeks . . . on what sounds like casual chitchat. I talked a lot about baseball and TV and other things with this family . . . which really was contributory to building the relationship to use when we needed it.[51]

Learning to communicate. For professionals who work with the dying, as well as for families and loved ones, being with patients who are dying can be painful and emotionally exhausting; in truth, it means facing one's own death.

> It extracts a cost that is usually overlooked in the training of the professional. In fact, it would be more accurate to say that the cost is known but the student is usually warned against paying it. The price of compassion is conveyed by the meaning of the two words, *com* and *passio*, which mean to "suffer *with*" another person. One must be touched by the tragedy of the patient in a literal way, a process that occurs through experiential identification with the dying person. This process, empathy, when evoked by a person facing death or tragic disability, ordinarily meets strong . . . resistance. Who can bear the thought of dying at 20?[52]

For some, avoidance is a way to deal with disconcerting aspects of being with dying patients. Such avoidance can be an impersonal or scientific attitude as much as a failing to be physically present.[53] Patients often express concern about loneliness in their final days, and studies have showed that many professionals tend to avoid dying patients.[54] When this occurs, the patient can end up in a netherworld of neglect, feeling lonely and abandoned; possibly foregoing opportunities to receive palliative, comforting measures; perhaps even missing the chance that a mistaken diagnosis will be corrected.[55]

Of course, dying patients may be difficult to work with and their mental and physical state may be such that communication takes longer than with other patients. Also, avoiding such patients on occasion might be respecting their wish not to be disturbed. Yet if health care professionals recognize that the tendency toward avoidance exists, they can then seek to mitigate its impact themselves and to involve other care givers, including clergy. The importance of teamwork and mutual support among those who work with the dying has been demonstrated in hospices and neonatal intensive care units.[56] Having colleagues who are willing to listen and a forum in which to express one's feelings can help deal with the emotional toll of working with the dying. A tendency to "burnout" after extended periods of such work has been noted, though there are strategies to help cope with this.[57]

Some medical and nursing schools never deal with dying as a subject, and some do so all too shallowly. One professor of psychiatry and family practice reported:

> In the School of Nursing I encountered, . . . the junior nurses were given a half-hour lecture on the Kubler-Ross five, and were then sent to the bedsides of terminally ill patients with the instructions to "get them through to acceptance" in an hour.[58]

The notion that a bit of brief classroom work can transform providers into sensitive humanitarians and effective communicators is, of course, simplistic and dangerous. The training of health care professionals should include serious and systematic attention to the requisite skills for working with dying patients. Whereas only 50 years ago it was the rare household that had not been touched by death, today many students in professional training have not previously been exposed to a dying person. Even medical students and residents are likely during their years of clinical training to miss the chance to attend for any length of time a patient in the shadow of impending death. Indeed, many physicians and nurses have never stayed with a dying patient through the final few hours and have never actually seen a patient die except in an unsuccessful resuscitation effort.

Empirical evidence has shown that many of the skills needed to work with the dying can be learned, while undesirable responses and reactions such as avoidance can be "unlearned" or mitigated.[59] Some health care professionals have cited their lack of such training as an impediment in caring for dying patients.[60]

Educating providers to become better communicators is a process that is both explicit and implicit.[61] Work in formal courses is unlikely to have any impact unless it is validated by behaviors at the bedside. Young physicians and nurses need to see their mentors doing the hard work of attending the dying; they are unlikely to learn if all their role models are people only a few years their senior professionally, especially since, as the Commission found, younger physicians are less likely to be comfortable discussing "dismal" news with their patients.[62]

Educational reform must entail greater change than adding a dash of the humanities to already overburdened health care curricula. What is needed instead is systematic attention to the social, ethical, psychological, and organizational aspects of caring for dying patients. Students should also be encouraged to develop an appreciation for different patterns and styles of dying, especially as they arise from different cultures, medical care settings, or religious views.

Reexamining the Role of Traditional Moral Distinctions

Most patients make their decisions about the alternative courses available to them in light of such factors as how many days or months the treatment might add to their lives, the nature of that life (for example, whether treatment will allow or interfere with their pursuit of important goals, such as completing projects and taking leave of loved ones), the degree of suffering involved, and the costs (financial and otherwise) to themselves and others. The relative weight, if any, to be given to each consideration must ultimately be determined by the competent patient.

Other bases are sometimes suggested for judging whether life-and-death decisions about medical care are acceptable or unacceptable beyond making sure that the results of the decisions are justified in the patient's view by their expected good. These bases are traditionally presented in the form of opposing categories. Although the categories—causing death by acting versus by omitting to act; withholding versus withdrawing treatment; the intended versus the unintended but foreseeable consequences of a choice; and ordinary versus extraordinary treatment—do reflect factors that can be important in assessing the moral and legal acceptability of decisions to forego life-sustaining treatment, they are inherently unclear. Worse, their invocation is often so mechanical that it neither illuminates an actual case nor provides an ethically persuasive argument.[63]

In considering these distinctions, which are discussed in detail in the remainder of this chapter, the Commission reached the following conclusions, which are particularly relevant to assessing the role of such distinctions in public policies that preclude patients and providers from choosing certain options.

- The distinction between acting and omitting to act provides a useful rule-of-thumb by separating cases that probably deserve more scrutiny from those that are likely not to need it. Although not all decisions to omit treatment and allow death to occur are acceptable, such a choice, when made by a patient or surrogate, is usually morally acceptable and in compliance with the law on homicide; conversely, active steps to end life, such as by administering a poison, are likely to be serious moral and legal wrongs. Nonetheless, the mere difference between acts and omissions—which is often hard to draw in any case—never by itself determines what is morally acceptable. Rather, the acceptability of particular actions or omissions turns on other morally significant considerations, such as the balance of harms and benefits likely to be achieved, the duties owed by others to a dying person, the risks imposed on others in acting or refraining, and the certainty of outcome.
- The distinction between failing to initiate and stopping therapy—that is, withholding versus withdrawing treatment—is not itself of moral importance. A justification that is adequate for not commencing a treatment is also sufficient for ceasing it. Moreover, erecting a higher requirement for cessation might unjustifiably discourage vigorous initial attempts to treat seriously ill patients that sometimes succeed.
- A distinction is sometimes drawn between giving a pain-relieving medication that will probably have the unintended consequence of hastening a patient's death and giving a poison in order to relieve a patient's suffering by killing the patient. The first is generally acceptable while the latter is against the law. Actions that lead to death must be justified by benefits to the patient that are expected to exceed the negative consequences and ordinarily must be within the person's socially accepted authority. In the case of physicians and nurses, this authority encompasses the use of means, such as pain-relieving medication, that can cure illnesses or relieve suffering but not the use of means, such as weapons or poisons, whose sole effect is viewed as killing a patient.
- Whether care is "ordinary" or "extraordinary" should not determine whether a patient must accept or may decline it. The terms have come to be used in conflicting and confusing ways, reflecting variously such aspects as the usualness, complexity, invasiveness, artificiality, expense, or availability of care. If used in their historic sense, however—to signify whether the burdens a treatment imposes on a patient are or are not disproportionate to its benefits—the terms denote useful concepts. To avoid misunderstanding, public discussion should focus on the underlying reasons for or against a therapy rather than on a simple categorization as "ordinary" or "extraordinary."

The analysis of these four distinctions in this chapter need not be repeated in decisionmaking for each individual patient. Rather, the Commission intends to point to the underlying factors that may be germane and helpful in making decisions about treatment or nontreatment and, conversely, to free individual decisionmaking and public policy from the mistaken limitations imposed when slogans and labels are substituted for the careful reasoning that is required.

Acting Versus Omitting to Act For many dying patients who decide to forego further life-prolonging treatment when its benefits no longer seem to them worth the burdens it creates, cessation of treatment leads rapidly to an end of life and, with that, to a release from their suffering. Others, however, suffer from conditions that would not be immediately fatal were treatment withdrawn. Some of these patients wish that they (or someone acting at their request) could administer a poison to end their suffering more quickly. The Commission does not believe that society ought to condone that deliberate use of poisons or similar lethal agents in this setting. To do so would certainly risk serious abuse.

Lawyers, health care professionals, and policymakers today are in general accord that treatment refusals by dying patients should be honored.[64] Physicians commonly acquiesce in the wishes of competent patients not to receive specified treatments, even when failure to provide those treatments will increase the chance—or make certain—that the patient will die soon.[65] When some patients are dying of a disease process that cannot be arrested, physicians may, for example, write orders not to provide resuscitation if the heart should stop,[66] forego antibiotic treatment of pneumonia and other infections,[67] cease use of respirators,[68] or withhold aggressive therapy from overwhelmingly burned patients.[69] Courts have sanctioned such decisions by guardians for incompetent patients,[70] as well as by competent patients who might have lived for an indefinite period if treated.[71] Although declining to start or continue life-sustaining treatment is often acceptable, health care providers properly refuse to honor a patient's request to be directly killed. Not only would killing, as by violence or strychnine, be outside the bounds of accepted medical practice, but as murder it would be subject to a range of criminal sanctions, regardless of the provider's motives.[72]

In both scholarly and policy discussions, "killing" is often equated with an action causing death, and "allowing to die" with an omission causing death.[73] Killing and allowing to die are then used as merely descriptive terms, leaving open which actual actions that cause death (that is, killings) are morally wrong. Certainly some actions that cause death, such as self-defense, are morally justified. However, particularly in medicine, "killing" is often understood to mean actions that *wrongfully* cause death, and so is never justifiably done by health care providers. Likewise, "allowing to die" is often used to communicate *approval* of accepting that death will occur rather than simply to describe the behavior.[74] In an attempt to avoid confusion that stems from these conflicting usages and to present the important issues clearly, the Commission's discussion employs the descriptive terms—actions that lead to death and omissions that lead to death—rather than mixing the normative and descriptive connotations of the terms killing and allowing to die.

Although the Commission believes that most omissions that lead to death in medical practice are acceptable, it does not believe that the moral distinction between that practice and wrongful killing lies in the difference between actions and omissions per se. Not only is this distinction often difficult to draw in actual practice, it fails to provide an adequate foundation for the moral and legal evaluation of events leading to death. Rather, the acceptability or unacceptability of conduct turns upon other morally significant factors, such as the duties owed to patients, the patients' prospects and wishes, and the risks created for someone who acts or who refrains from acting.

The difference between actions and omissions that lead to death. The distinction between acts and omissions is often easy to draw. A person acts in a way that results in another's death, for example, by fatally poisoning an otherwise healthy person. On the other hand, a person's omission leads to the death of another if the first person knows he or she has the ability and opportunity to act so as to prevent the other dying (at a particular time and in a particular way)[75] but refrains from doing so. For example, an omission leads to death when a person could, but does not, rescue a nearby child who is drowning. The difference, then, is that when A acts to cause B to die, the course of events into which A's action intervenes is otherwise one in which B is not likely to die, whereas when A omits to act and thus causes B to die, the course of events already under way (into which A fails to intervene) includes B's imminent death. Thus, the distinction between a fatal act and a fatal omission depends both upon the difference between a person physically acting and refraining from acting and upon what might be called the background course of events.

If a patient's death is imminent (for example, death is expected within a matter of days) failing to treat and thus hastening death is seen by some not even to be a case of an omission that leads to death—failing to treat is said to be merely "avoiding prolonging the dying process."[76] To hold that such a failure to treat is neither a fatal act nor an omission is wrong and misleading. No one can prevent a person's ever dying; death can only be postponed by preventing it at the moment. Usually, though not always, to postpone death for only a very short time is less important, but that is relevant to whether an omission is wrong and how serious the wrong is, not to whether it is an omission that leads to a patient's death.

Sometimes deciding whether a particular course involves an act or an omission is less clear. Stopping a respirator at the request of a competent patient who could have lived with it for a few years but who will die without it in just a few hours is such an ambiguous case. Does the physician omit continuing the treatment or act to disconnect it? Discontinuing essential dialysis treatments or choosing not to give the next in a sequence of antibiotic doses are other events that could be described either as acts or omissions.

The moral significance of the difference. Actual instances of actions leading to death, especially outside the medical context, are more likely to be seriously morally wrong than are omissions that lead to death, which, in the medical context, are most often morally justified. Usually, one or more of several factors make fatal actions worse than fatal omissions:

(1) The motives of an agent who acts to cause death are usually worse (for example, self-interest or malice) than those of someone who omits to act and lets another die.
(2) A person who is barred from acting to cause another's death is usually thereby placed at no personal risk of harm; whereas, especially outside the medical context, if a person were forced to intercede to save another's life (instead of standing by and omitting to act), he or she would often be put at substantial risk.
(3) The nature and duration of future life denied to a person whose life is ended by another's act is usually much greater than that denied to a dying person whose death comes slightly more quickly due to an omission of treatment.
(4) A person, especially a patient, may still have some possibility of surviving if one omits to act, while survival is more often foreclosed by actions that lead to death.

Each of these factors—or several in combination—can make a significant moral difference in the evaluation of any particular instance of acting and omitting to act. Together they help explain why most actions leading to death are correctly considered morally worse than most omissions leading to death. Moreover, the greater stringency of the legal duties to refrain from killing than to intervene to save life reinforces people's view of which conduct is worse morally.[77]

However, the distinction between omissions leading to death and acts leading to death is not a reliable guide to their moral evaluation. In the case of medical treatment, the first and third factors are not likely to provide grounds for a distinction: family members and health professionals could be equally merciful in their intention—either in acting or omitting—and life may end immediately for some patients after treatment is withdrawn. Likewise, the second factor—based on the usual rule that people have fairly limited duties to save others with whom they stand in no special relation—does not apply in the medical context.[78] Health professionals have a special role-related duty to use their skills, insofar as possible, on behalf of their patients, and this duty removes any distinction between acts and omissions.

Only the final factor—turning the possibility of death into a certainty—can apply as much in medical settings as elsewhere. Indeed, this factor has particular relevance here since the element of uncertainty—whether a patient really will die if treatment is ceased—is sometimes unavoidable in the medical setting. A valid distinction may therefore arise between an act causing certain death (for example, a poisoning) and an omission that hastens or risks death (such as not amputating a gangrenous limb). But sometimes death is as certain following withdrawal of a treatment as following a particular action that is reliably expected to lead to death.

Consequently, merely determining whether what was done involved a fatal act or omission does not establish whether it was morally acceptable. Some actions that lead to death can be acceptable: very dangerous but potentially beneficial surgery or the use of hazardous doses of morphine for severe pain are examples. Some omissions that lead to death are very serious wrongs: deliberately failing to treat an ordinary patient's bacterial pneumonia or ignoring a bleeding patient's pleas for help would be totally unacceptable conduct for that patient's physician.

Not only are there difficult cases to classify as acts or omissions and difficulties in placing moral significance on the distinction, but making the distinction also presupposes an unsound conception of responsibility, namely (1) that human action is an intervention in the existing course of nature, (2) that not acting is not intervening, and (3) that people are responsible only for their interventions (or, at least, are much more responsible for deliberate interventions than for deliberate omissions). The weaknesses of this position include the ambiguous meaning of "intervention" when someone takes an action as part of a plan of nonintervention (such as writing orders not to resuscitate), the inability to define clearly the "course of nature," and the indefensibility of not holding someone responsible for states of affairs that the person could have prevented.

In sum, then, actions that lead to death are likely to be serious wrongs, while many omissions in the medical context are quite acceptable. Yet this is not a fixed moral assessment based on the mere descriptive difference between acts and omissions, but a generalization from experience that rests on such factors as whether the decision reflects the pursuit of the patient's ends and values, whether the health care providers have fulfilled their duties, and whether the risk of death has been appropriately considered.

The cause of death. Sometimes acts that lead to death seem to be more seriously wrong than omissions that likewise lead to death because the cause of death in the first instance is seen to be the act while the cause of death in an omission is regarded as the underlying disease. For example, were a physician deliberately to inject a patient with a lethal poison, the physician's action would be the cause of the patient's death. On the other hand, if an otherwise dying patient is not resuscitated in the event of cardiac arrest, or if a pneumonia or kidney failure goes untreated, the underlying disease process is said to be the cause of death. Since people ordinarily feel responsible for their own acts but not for another person's disease, this is a very comforting formulation.

The difference in this common account of causation does not actually explain the different moral assessment—rather, the account of causation *reflects* an underlying assessment of what is right or wrong under the circumstances.[79] Commonly, many factors play some causal role in a person's death. When "the cause" of a patient's death is singled out—for example, to be entered on a death certificate—the decision to designate one or more factors as "the cause(s)" depends upon the normative question at issue. Although the process begins with an empirical inquiry to identify the factors that were actually connected with a particular patient's death, both the process of narrowing to those factors that were "substantial" causes[80] and that of deciding which ones should be held legally or morally responsible for the death involve value judgments.[81] In some situations, although one person's action is unquestionably a factual cause of another's death, holding the person responsible for the death is unfair because the death could not reasonably have been foreseen or because the person was under no obligation to prevent the death.[82]

Beyond selecting "the cause" of death from among the many factors empirically determined to have causally contributed to a patient's death, both the legal and the moral inquiry presuppose that some kinds of causal roles in a death are wrong, and then ask whether any person played any of those roles. Therefore, a determination of causation ordinarily must presuppose, and cannot itself justify, the sorts of decisions that ought to be permissible. For example, in a death following nontreatment, designating the disease as the cause not only asserts that a fatal disease process was present but also communicates acceptance of the physician's behavior in foregoing treatment. Conversely, if an otherwise healthy patient who desired treatment died from untreated pneumonia, the physician's failure to treat would be considered to have caused the patient's death. Although pneumonia is among the factual causes of death, one way of stating the physician's responsibility for the death is to identify the physician's omission of his or her duty to treat as the cause of death. As this example shows, the action/omission distinction does not always correspond to the usual understanding of whether the physician or the disease is the cause of death, and so the attribution of what caused a death cannot make acts morally different from omissions.

In addition, the physician's behavior is among the factual causes of a patient's death both in acting and in omitting to act. This is clear enough if a physician were to give a lethal injection—the patient would not have died at that time and in that way if the physician had not given the injection. But exactly the same is true of a physician's omission of treatment: had a physician not refrained from resuscitating or from treating a pneumonia or a kidney failure, a patient would not have died at that time and in that way. In either case, a different choice by the physician would have led to the patient living longer. To refrain from treating is justifiable in some cases—for example, if the patient does not want the treatment, is suffering, and will die very soon whatever is done. But the justification rests on these other reasons, rather than on not classifying a physician's omission as a cause of the patient's death. Thus, calling the disease the cause of death can be misleading but does reflect a sound point: that a physician who omits treatment in such a case is not morally or legally blameworthy.

The role of the distinction in public policy. The moral and legal prohibition against acting to take the life of another human being is deeply rooted in Western society and serves the laudable and extremely important value of protecting and preserving human life. Although health care professionals and families want to do the best they can for patients, both in respecting patients' self-determination and promoting their well-being, they face troubling conflicts when doing so would involve them in conduct that might be considered as the taking of another's life.

Yet in health care, and especially with critically or terminally ill patients, it is common to make decisions that one knows risk shortening patients' lives and that sometimes turn out to do so. As a result, there is a strong motivation to interpret the actions decided upon and carried out, especially if by people other than the patient, as something other than acts of killing. Thus, the concerned parties very much want these to be regarded as cases of "allowing to die" (rather than "killing"), of "not prolonging the dying process" (instead of "hastening death"), or of "failing to stop a disease from causing death" (rather than "someone's action was the cause of death").[83] Consequently, these distinctions, while often conceptually unclear and of dubious moral importance in themselves, are useful in facilitating acceptance of sound decisions that would otherwise meet unwarranted resistance. They help people involved to understand, in ways acceptable to them, their proper roles in implementing decisions to forego life-sustaining treatment.

Law, as a principal instrument of public policy in this area, has sought an accommodation that adequately protects human life while not resulting in officious overtreatment of dying patients.[84] The present general legal prohibition against deliberate, active killing, reinforced by a strong social and professional presumption in favor of sustaining life, serves as a public affirmation of the high value accorded to each human life. The law, and public policy in general, has not interpreted the termination of life-sustaining treatment, even when it requires active steps such as turning off a respirator, as falling under this general prohibition. For competent patients, the principle of self-determination is understood to include a right to refuse life-sustaining treatment, and to place a duty on providers and others to respect that right. Providers, in turn, are protected from liability when they act to aid a patient in carrying out that right. Active steps to terminate life-sustaining interventions may be permitted, indeed required, by the patient's authority to forego therapy even when such steps lead to death.[85] With adequate procedural safeguards, this right can be extended to incompetent patients through surrogates.[86]

Although there are some cases in which the acting-omitting distinction is difficult to make and although its moral importance originates in other considerations, the commonly accepted prohibition of active killing helps to produce the correct decision in the great majority of cases. Furthermore, weakening the legal prohibition to allow a deliberate taking of life in extreme circumstances would risk allowing wholly unjustified taking of life in less extreme circumstances. Such a risk would be warranted only if there were substantial evidence of serious harms to be relieved by a weakened legal protection of life, which the Commission does not find to be the case. Thus the Commission concludes that the current interpretation of the legal prohibition of active killing should be sustained.[87]

One serious consequence of maintaining the legal prohibition against direct killing of terminally ill patients could be the prolongation of suffering. In the final stages of some diseases, such as cancer, patients may undergo unbearable suffering that only ends with death. Some have claimed that sometimes the only way to improve such patients' lot is to actively and intentionally end their lives.[88] If such steps are forbidden, physicians and family might be forced to deny these patients the relief they seek and to prolong their agony pointlessly.

If this were a common consequence of a policy prohibiting all active termination of human life, it should force a reevaluation of maintaining the prohibition. Rarely, however, does such suffering persist when there is adequate use of pain-relieving drugs and procedures.[89] Health care professionals ought to realize that they are already authorized and obligated to use such means with a patient's or surrogate's consent, even if an earlier death is likely to result. The Commission endorses allowing physicians and patients to select treatments known to risk death in order to relieve suffering as well as to pursue a return to health.

Policies prohibiting direct killing may also conflict with the important value of patient self-determination. This conflict will arise when deliberate actions intended to cause death have been freely chosen by an informed and competent patient as the necessary or preferred means of carrying out his or her wishes, but the patient is unable to kill him or herself unaided, or others prevent the patient from doing so. The frequency with which this conflict occurs is not known, although it is probably rare. The Commission finds this limitation on individual self-determination to be an acceptable cost of securing the general protection of human life afforded by the prohibition of direct killing.

Withholding Versus Withdrawing Treatment A variation on the action/omission distinction sometimes troubles physicians who allow competent patients to refuse a life-sustaining treatment but who are uncomfortable about stopping a treatment that has already been started because doing so seems to them to constitute killing the patient. By contrast, not starting a therapy seems acceptable, supposedly because it involves an omission rather than an action.[90]

Although the nature of the distinction between withholding and withdrawing seems clear enough initially, cases that obscure it abound. If a patient is on a respirator, disconnecting would count as stopping. But if the patient is on a respirator and the power fails, does failing to use a manual bellows mechanism count as "stopping" a therapy (artificial respiration) or "not starting" a therapy (manually generated respiration)?[91] Many therapies in medicine require repeated applications of an intervention. Does failing to continue to reapply the intervention count as "stopping" (the series of treatments) or as "not starting" (the next element in the series)? Even when a clear distinction can be drawn between withdrawing and withholding, insofar as the distinction is merely an instance of the acting-omitting distinction it lacks moral significance.[92]

Other considerations may be involved here, however. Even though health care professionals may not be obligated to initiate a therapy with a particular patient, its initiation may create expectations on the part of the patient and others. In some instances these expectations may lead the health care provider to feel obliged not to stop a therapy that initially could have been foregone.[93] (Similarly, a physician, who is under no obligation to accept any particular person as a patient, may not abandon a patient once a physician-patient relationship has been established.[94])

This observation does not actually argue that stopping a treatment is in itself any more serious than not starting it. What it claims is that *if* additional obligations to treat have arisen from any expectations created once a treatment has been initiated, then stopping, because it breaches those obligations, is worse than not starting. The expectations, and the resultant obligation to continue, create whatever moral difference arises. The definition of the professional-patient relationship and the creation of expectations that care will be continued occur in complex ways—from professional codes, patterns of practice, legal decisions, and physician-patient communications. A particular physician faced with stopping or not starting therapy with a particular patient may have to accept a relationship and expectations that are at least partly givens.

Discussions between a physician and competent patient, however, allow redefinition of their relationship and alteration of their expectations and thus of any resulting obligations. For example, a physician and patient could agree to a time-limited trial of a particular intervention, with an understanding that unless the therapy achieved certain goals it should be stopped. Moreover, these relationships and expectations, with their resultant obligations, need not be treated as fixed when public policy is being made but can be redefined where appropriate. Of course, most withdrawals of treatment involve explicit decisions while withholdings are commonly implicit and not clearly discussed (although, in conformity with the Commission's recommendations, they should be discussed, except in emergency situations).[95] Although this may make the withdrawal of treatment more anguishing, or even more likely to precipitate external review, it does not make it morally different.

Adopting the opposite view—that treatment, once started, cannot be stopped, or that stopping requires much greater justification than not starting—is likely to have serious adverse consequences. Treatment might be continued for longer than is optimal for the patient, even to the point where it is causing positive harm with little or no compensating benefit.[96] An even more troubling wrong occurs when a treatment that might save life or improve health is not started because the health care personnel are afraid that they will find it very difficult to stop the treatment if, as is fairly likely, it proves to be of little benefit and greatly burdens the patient.[97] The Commission received testimony, for example, that sometimes the view that a therapy that has been started could not be stopped had unduly raised the threshold for initiating some forms of vigorous therapy for newborns.[98] In cases of extremely low birth weight or severe spina bifida, for example, highly aggressive treatment may significantly benefit a small proportion of the infants treated while it prolongs the survival of a great number of newborns for whom treatment turns out to be futile. Fear of being unable to stop treatment in the latter cases—no matter how compelling the reason to stop—can lead to failure to treat the entire group, including the few infants who would have benefited.

Ironically, if there is any call to draw a moral distinction between withholding and withdrawing, it generally cuts the opposite way from the usual formulation: greater justification ought to be required to withhold than to withdraw treatment. Whether a particular treatment will have positive effects is often highly uncertain before the therapy has been tried. If a trial of therapy makes clear that it is not helpful to the patient, this is actual evidence (rather than mere surmise) to support stopping because the therapeutic benefit that earlier was a possibility has been found to be clearly unobtainable.[99]

Behind the withholding/withdrawing distinction lies the more general acting/omitting distinction in one of its least defensible forms. Given that the Commission considers as unwarranted the view that steps leading to death are always more serious when they involve an act rather than an omission, it also rejects the view that stopping a treatment ("an act") is morally more serious than not starting it ("an omission") could be.

Little if any legal significance attaches to the distinction between withholding and withdrawing. Nothing in law—certainly not in the context of the doctor-patient relationship—makes stopping treatment a more serious legal issue than not starting treatment. In fact, not starting treatment that *might* be in a patient's interests is more likely to be held a civil or criminal wrong than stopping the same treatment when it has proved unavailing.

As is the case with the distinction between acting and omitting, many other factors of moral importance may differentiate the appropriateness of a particular decision not to start from one to stop. Yet whatever considerations justify not starting should justify stopping as well. Thus the Commission concludes that neither law nor public policy should mark a difference in moral seriousness between stopping and not starting treatment.

Intended Versus Unintended But Foreseeable Consequences Since there are sound moral and policy reasons to prohibit such active steps as administering strychnine or using a gun to kill a terminally ill patient, the question arises as to whether physicians should be able to administer a symptom-relieving drug—such as a pain-killer—knowing that the drug may cause or accelerate the patient's death, even though death is not an outcome the physician seeks. The usual answer to this question—that the prohibition against active killing does not bar the use of appropriate medical treatment, such as morphine for pain[100]—is often said to rest on a distinction between the goals physicians seek to achieve or the means they use, on the one hand, and the unintended but foreseeable[101] consequences of their actions on the other.[102]

One problem with assigning moral significance to the traditional distinction is that it is sometimes difficult to determine whether a particular aspect of a course of action ought to be considered to be intended, because it is an inseparable part of the "means" by which the course of action is achieved, or whether it is merely an unintended but foreseeable consequence. In medicine, and especially in the treatment of the critically or terminally ill, many of the courses that might be followed entail a significant risk, sometimes approaching a certainty, of shortening a patient's life. For example, in order to avoid additional suffering or disability, or perhaps to spare loved ones extreme financial or emotional costs, a patient may elect not to have a potentially life-extending operation. Risking earlier death might plausibly be construed as the intended means to these other ends, or as an unintended and "merely foreseeable" consequence. Since there seems to be no generally accepted, principled basis for making the distinction, there is substantial potential for unclear or contested determinations.

Even in cases in which the distinction is clear, however, health care professionals cannot use it to justify a failure to consider all the consequences of their choices.[103] By choosing a course of action, a person knowingly brings about certain effects; other effects could have been caused by deciding differently. The law reflects this moral view and holds people to be equally responsible for all the reasonably foreseeable results of their actions and not just for those results that they acknowledge having intended to achieve.[104] Nevertheless, although medication is commonly used to relieve the suffering of dying patients (even when it causes or risks causing death), physicians are not held to have violated the law. How can this failure to prosecute be explained, since it does not rest on an explicit waiver of the usual legal rule?

The explanation lies in the importance of defining physicians' responsibilities regarding these choices and of developing an accepted and well-regulated social role that allows the choices to be made with due care. The search for medical treatments that will benefit a patient often involves risk, sometimes great risk, for the patient: for example, some surgery still carries a sizable risk of mortality, as does much of cancer therapy. Furthermore, seeking to cure disease and to prolong life is only a part of the physician's traditional role in caring for patients; another important part is to comfort patients and relieve their suffering.[105] Sometimes these goals conflict, and a physician and patient (or patient's surrogate) have the authority to decide which goal has priority. Medicine's role in relieving suffering is especially important when a patient is going to die soon, since the suffering of such a patient is not an unavoidable aspect of treatment that might restore health, as it might be for a patient with a curable condition.

Consequently, the use of pain-relieving medications is distinguished from the use of poisons, though both may result in death, and society places the former into the category of acceptable treatment while continuing the traditional prohibition against the latter.[106] Indeed, in the Commission's view it is not only possible but desirable to draw this distinction. If physicians (and other health professionals) became the dispensers of "treatments" that could only be understood as deliberate killing of patients, patients' trust in them might be seriously undermined.[107] And irreparable damage could be done to health care professionals' self-image and to their ability to devote themselves wholeheartedly to the often arduous task of treating gravely ill patients. Moreover, whether or not one believes there are some instances in which giving a poison might be morally permissible, the Commission considers that the obvious potential for abuse of a public, legal policy condoning such action argues strongly against it.[108]

For the use of morphine or other pain-relieving medication that can lead to death to be socially and legally acceptable, physicians must act within the socially defined bounds of their role.[109] This means that they are not only proceeding with the necessary agreement of the patient (or surrogate) and in a professionally skillful fashion (for example, by not taking a step that is riskier than necessary), but that there are sufficiently weighty reasons to run the risk of the patient dying.[110] For example, were a person experiencing great pain from a condition that will be cured in a few days, use of morphine at doses that would probably lead to death by inducing respiratory depression would usually be unacceptable. On the other hand, for a patient in great pain—especially from a condition that has proved to be untreatable and that is expected to be rapidly fatal—morphine can be both morally and legally acceptable if pain relief cannot be achieved by less risky means.

This analysis rests on the special role of physicians and on particular professional norms of acceptability that have gained social sanction (such as the difference between morphine, which can relieve pain, and strychnine, which can only cause death).[111] Part of acceptable behavior—from the medical as well as the ethical and legal standpoints—is for the physician to take into account all the foreseeable effects, not just the intended goals, in making recommendations and in administering treatment.[112] The degree of care and judgment exercised by the physician should therefore be guided not only by the technical question of whether pain can be relieved but also by the broader question of whether care providers are certain enough of the facts in this case, including the patient's priorities and subjective experience, to risk death in order to relieve suffering. If this can be answered affirmatively, there is no moral or legal objection to using the kinds and amounts of drugs necessary to relieve the patient's pain.

The Commission concludes that the distinction between the decisionmakers' "intending" a patient's death and their "merely foreseeing" that death will occur does not help in separating unacceptable from acceptable actions that lead to death. But, as proved true of the distinctions already discussed, this does point to ethically and legally significant factors—here, the real and symbolic role traditionally assigned to physicians and other practitioners of the healing arts, who can be expected to have developed special sensitivity and skills regarding the judgments to be made, and who are an identifiable group that can be readily held accountable for serious error.[113] Furthermore, the acceptable treatment options that carry a risk of death are limited to those within the special expertise of health care professionals.

The highly valued traditional professional role is not undermined when a physician, with due care, employs a measure—whether radical surgery or medication to relieve pain—that could lead to the patient's death but that is reasonably likely to cure or relieve pain. The relevant distinction, then, is not really that death is forbidden as a means to relieve suffering but is sometimes acceptable if it is merely a foreseeable consequence. Rather, the moral issue is whether or not the decisionmakers have considered the full range of foreseeable effects, have knowingly accepted whatever risk of death is entailed, and have found the risk to be justified in light of the paucity and undesirability of other options.

Ordinary Versus Extraordinary Treatment In many discussions and decisions about life-sustaining treatment, the distinction between ordinary and extraordinary (also termed "heroic" or "artificial") treatment plays an important role. In its origins within moral theology, the distinction was used to mark the difference between obligatory and nonobligatory care—ordinary care being obligatory for the patient to accept and others to provide, and extraordinary care being optional.[114] It has also played a role in professional policy statements[115] and recent judicial decisions about life-sustaining treatment for incompetent patients.[116] As with the other terms discussed, defining and applying a distinction between ordinary and extraordinary treatment is both difficult and controversial and can lead to inconsistent results, which makes the terms of questionable value in the formulation of public policy in this area.

The meaning of the distinction. "Extraordinary" treatment has an unfortunate array of alternative meanings, as became obvious in an exchange that took place at a Commission hearing concerning a Florida case[117] involving the cessation of life-sustaining treatment at the request of a 76-year-old man dying of amyotrophic lateral sclerosis. The attending physician testified:

> I deal with respirators every day of my life. To me, this is not heroic. This is standard procedure. . . . I have other patients who have run large corporations who have been on portable respirators. Other people who have been on them and have done quite well for as long as possible.[118]

By contrast, the trial judge who had decided that the respirator could be withdrawn told the Commission:

> Certainly there is no question legally that putting a hole in a man's trachea and inserting a mechanical respirator is extraordinary life-preserving means.
>
> I do not think that the doctor would in candor allow that that is not an extraordinary means of preserving life.
>
> I understand that he deals with them every day, but in the sense of ordinary as against extraordinary, I believe it to be extraordinary.
>
> There was no question in this case, nobody ever raised the question that this mechanical respirator was not an extraordinary means of preserving life.[119]

The most natural understanding of the ordinary/extraordinary distinction is as the difference between common and unusual care, with those terms understood as applying to a patient in a particular condition. This interprets the distinction in a literal, statistical sense and, no doubt, is what some of its users intend. Related, though different, is the idea that ordinary care is simple and that extraordinary care is complex, elaborate, or artificial, or that it employs elaborate technology and/or great efforts or expense.[120] With either of these interpretations, for example, the use of antibiotics to fight a life-threatening infection would be considered ordinary treatment. On the statistical interpretation, a complex of resuscitation measures (including physical, chemical, and electrical means) might well be ordinary for a hospital patient, whereas on the technological interpretation, resuscitation would probably be considered extraordinary. Since both common/unusual and simple/complex exist on continuums with no precise dividing line, on either interpretation there will be borderline cases engendering disagreement about whether a particular treatment is ordinary or extraordinary.[121]

A different understanding of the distinction, one that has its origins in moral theology, inquires into the usefulness and burdensomeness of a treatment.[122] Here, too, disagreement persists about which outcomes are considered useful or burdensome.[123] Without entering into the complexity of these debates, the Commission notes that any interpretation of the ordinary/extraordinary distinction in terms of usefulness and burdensomeness to an individual patient has an important advantage over the common/unusual or simple/complex interpretations in that judgments about usefulness and burdensomeness rest on morally important differences.

Despite the fact that the distinction between what is ordinary and what is extraordinary is hazy and variably defined, several courts have employed the terms in discussing cases involving the cessation of life-sustaining treatment of incompetent patients. In some cases, the courts used these terms because they were part of the patient's religious tradition.[124] In other cases, the terms have been used to characterize treatments as being required or permissibly foregone. For example, the New Jersey Supreme Court in the *Quinlan* case recognized a distinction based on the possible benefit to the individual patient:

> One would have to think that the use of the same respirator or life support could be considered "ordinary" in the context of the possibly curable patient but "extraordinary" in the context of the forced sustaining by cardio-respiratory processes of an irreversibly doomed patient.[125]

Likewise, the Massachusetts Supreme Judicial Court quoted an article in a medical journal concerning the proposition that ordinary treatment could become extraordinary when applied in the context of a patient for whom there is no hope:

> We should not use *extraordinary* means of prolonging life or its semblance when, after careful consideration, consultation and application of the most well conceived therapy it becomes appar-

> ent that there is no hope for the recovery of the patient. Recovery should not be defined simply as the ability to remain alive; it should mean life without intolerable suffering.[126]

Even if the patient or a designated surrogate is held to be under no obligation to accept "extraordinary" care, there still remains the perplexing issue about what constitutes the dividing line between the two. The courts have most often faced the question of what constitutes "ordinary" care in cases when the respirator was the medical intervention at issue. Generally the courts have recognized, in the words of one judge, that "the act of turning off the respirator is the termination of an optional, extraordinary medical procedure which will allow nature to take its course."[127]

For many, the harder questions lie in less dramatic interventions, including the use of artificial feeding and antibiotics. In one criminal case involving whether the defendant's robbery and assault killed his victim or whether she died because life-supporting treatments were later withdrawn after severe brain injury was confirmed, the court held that "heroic" (and unnecessary) measures included "infusion of drugs in order to reduce the pressure in the head when there was no obvious response to those measures of therapy."[128] In another case, in which a patient's refusal of an amputation to prevent death from gangrene was overridden, antibiotics were described by the physician "as heroic measures, meaning quantities in highly unusual amounts risking iatrogenic disease in treating gangrene."[129] Here the assessment, in addition to relying on "benefits," also seems to rely to some degree upon the risk and invasiveness of the intervention. One court did begin to get at the scope of the questions underlying the ordinary/extraordinary distinction. Faced with the question of treatment withdrawal for a permanently unconscious automobile accident victim, the Delaware Supreme Court asked what might constitute life-sustaining measures for a person who has been comatose for many months:

> Are "medicines" a part of such life-sustaining systems? If so, which medicines? Is food or nourishment a part of such life-sustaining systems? If so, to what extent? What extraordinary measures (or equipment) are a part of such systems? What measures (or equipment) are regarded by the medical profession as not extraordinary under the circumstances? What ordinary equipment is used? How is a respirator regarded in this context?[130]

The moral significance of the distinction. Because of the varied meanings of the distinction, whether or not it has moral significance depends upon the specific meaning assigned to it. The Commission believes there is no basis for holding that whether a treatment is common or unusual, or whether it is simple or complex, is in itself significant to a moral analysis of whether the treatment is warranted or obligatory. An unusual treatment may have a lower success rate than a common one; if so, it is the lower success rate rather than the unusualness of the procedure that is relevant to evaluating the therapy. Likewise, a complex, technological treatment may be costlier than a simple one, and this difference may be relevant to the desirability of the therapy. A patient may choose a complex therapy and shun a simple one, and the patient's choice is always relevant to the moral obligation to provide the therapy.

If the ordinary/extraordinary distinction is understood in terms of the usefulness and burdensomeness of a particular therapy, however, the distinction does have moral significance. When a treatment is deemed extraordinary because it is too burdensome for a particular patient, the individual (or a surrogate) may appropriately decide not to undertake it. The reasonableness of this is evident—a patient should not have to undergo life-prolonging treatment without consideration of the burdens that the treatment would impose. Of course, whether a treatment is warranted depends on its usefulness or benefits as well. Whether serious burdens of treatment (for example, the side effects of chemotherapy treatments for cancer) are worth enduring obviously depends on the expected benefits—how long the treatment will extend life, and under what conditions. Usefulness might be understood as mere extension of life, no matter what the conditions of that life. But so long as mere biological existence is not considered the *only* value, patients may want to take the nature of that additional life into account as well.[131]

This line of reasoning suggests that extraordinary treatment is that which, in the patient's view, entails significantly greater burdens than benefits and is therefore undesirable and not obligatory, while ordinary treatment is that which, in the patient's view, produces greater benefits than burdens and is therefore reasonably desirable and undertaken. The claim, then, that the treatment is extraordinary is more of an expression of the conclusion than a justification for it.

The role of the distinction in public policy. Despite its long history of frequent use, the distinction between ordinary and extraordinary treatments has now become so confused that its continued use in the formulation of public policy is no longer desirable.[132] Although those who share a common understanding of its meaning may still find it helpful in counseling situations, the Commission believes that it is better for those involved in the difficult task of establishing policies and guidelines in the area of treatment decisions to avoid employing these phrases. Clarity and understanding in this area will be enhanced if laws, judicial opinions, regulations, and medical policies speak instead in terms of the proportionate benefit and burdens of treatment as viewed by particular patients. With the reasoning thus clearly articulated, patients will be better able to understand the moral significance of the options and to choose accordingly.

Conclusions

Good decisionmaking about life-sustaining treatments depends upon the same processes of shared decisionmaking that should be a part of health care in general. The hallmark of an ethically sound process is always that it enables competent and informed patients to reach voluntary decisions about care. With patients who may die, care givers need special skills and sensitivities if the process is to succeed.

A number of constraints on the range of acceptable decisions about life-sustaining treatment have been suggested. They are often presented in the form of dichotomies: an omission of treatment that causes death is acceptable whereas an action that causes death is not; withholding treatment is acceptable whereas withdrawing existing treatment is not; extraordinary treatment may be foregone but ordinary treatment may not; a person is permitted to do something knowing that it will cause death but may not aim to kill. The Commission has concluded that none of these dichotomies should be used to prohibit choosing a course of conduct that falls within the societally defined scope of ethical medical practice. Instead, the Commission has found that a decision to forego treatment is ethically acceptable when it has been made by suitably qualified decisionmakers who have found the risk of death to be justified in light of all the circumstances. Furthermore, the Commission has found that nothing in current law precludes ethically sound decisionmaking. Neither criminal nor civil law—if properly interpreted and applied by lawyers, judges, health care providers, and the general public—forces patients to undergo procedures that will increase their suffering when they wish to avoid this by foregoing life-sustaining treatment.

Since these conclusions recognize the importance of societally defined roles, health care professionals, individually and through their professional associations, will need to become more active in creating, explaining, and justifying their standards regarding appropriate professional roles. Within presently accepted definitions, it is already apparent that health care professionals may provide treatment to relieve the symptoms of dying patients even when that treatment entails substantial risks of causing an earlier death. The Commission has also found no particular treatments—including such "ordinary" hospital interventions as parenteral nutrition or hydration, antibiotics, and transfusions—to be universally warranted and thus obligatory for a patient to accept. Nevertheless, a decision to forego particular life-sustaining treatments is not a ground to withdraw all care—nor should care givers treat it in this way, especially when care is needed to ensure the patient's comfort, dignity, and self-determination.

* * *

4. PATIENTS WHO LACK DECISIONMAKING CAPACITY

Determination of Incapacity

In general, a person's choices regarding care ought to override the assessments of others about what best serves that person. Certain people, however, are incapable of making choices that reflect and promote their personal goals and values. Some patients—on account of age, incapacity, or inexperience—have an insufficiently developed set of goals and values. Some lack sufficient capabilities for understanding, communication, and reasoning; among patients facing life-threatening decisions, these faculties are frequently compromised. The principles for determining incapacity[1] and for making decisions on behalf of incapacitated patients that were developed by the Commission in its report on informed consent[2] therefore have special relevance to decisions to forego life-sustaining therapy.

Elements of the Determination Determining whether a patient lacks capacity to make a particular health care decision requires assessing the patient's capability to understand information relevant to the decision, to communicate with care givers about it, and to reason about relevant alternatives against a background of reasonably stable personal values and life goals.[3] The ultimate objective of such an assessment is to diminish two types of errors: mistakenly preventing persons who ought to be considered competent from directing the course of their own treatment, and failing to protect incapacitated persons from the harmful effects of their decisions. Health care professionals usually play a substantial role in making these assessments; their conclusions are often not reviewed by officials outside health care institutions.[4]

Each determination of decisional incapacity focuses on a patient's actual functioning in a particular decisionmaking situation rather than simply on an individual's age or diagnosis. This approach is particularly germane for fairly mature children[5] and for mildly retarded or demented persons. What is relevant is whether a person is in fact capable of making a particular decision despite his or her youth, retardation, or dementia. Even when ultimate decisional authority is not left with a patient, reasonable efforts often should be made to give the person relevant information about the situation and the available options and to solicit and accommodate his or her preferences.

The Commission recommends that determinations of incapacity be made only when people lack the ability to make decisions that promote their well-being in conformity with their own values and preferences.[6] Rarely—infants and unconscious patients are the main exceptions—is incapacity absolute. Even people with impaired capacity usually still possess some ability to comprehend, to communicate, and to form and express a preference. The fact that a patient makes a highly idiosyncratic decision or has a medical or mental condition[7] similar to others who have been unable to make decisions that advance their own well-being may alert health care professionals to the possibility of decisional incapacity, but does not conclusively resolve the matter. "Decisionmaking incapacity" is not a medical or a psychiatric diagnostic category; it rests on a judgment of the type that an informed layperson might make—that a patient lacks sufficient ability to understand a situation and to make a choice in light of that understanding.[8] Indeed, when judges are called upon to make legal determinations of patients' competence, they consider the situation not as medical experts but as laypeople examining the data provided by health care personnel[9] and by others who know the individual well, and possibly from personal observation of the patient.

Finally, in any assessment of capacity, due care should be paid to the reasons for a particular patient's impaired capacity—not because the reasons are the determinant of whether the patient's judgment is to be honored, but because identification of the causes of incapacity may assist in their remedy or removal.[10] The Commission urges that those responsible for assessing capacity not be content with providing an answer to the question of whether or not a particular patient is incapacitated. Rather they should, to the extent feasible, attempt to remove barriers to decisional capacity.

Procedural Policies A decision that a patient is incapacitated can be of great importance, both in the Commission's ethical analysis and in the function of law. Courts have generally held that, whereas competent patients may forego any treatment, incompetent patients' wishes can be overridden in order to protect their lives and well-being.[11] Since the threshold issue of capacity is not only so weighty but often so complex,[12] it is of prime importance that assessments of incapacity be made carefully and adequately.

Health care professionals should therefore be familiar with the reason that a careful determination is important as well as with the procedures necessary to achieve it. Furthermore, health care institutions need to have clear policies as to who is responsible for assessing incapacity and by what standards. Institutions should ensure that those who assess capacity know the kinds of inquiries to make, the data to collect, and the records to keep. Finally, provisions also need to be made for reviewing determinations of incapacity both within the institution and, when necessary, through a judicial proceeding.

The first questions about a patient's decisionmaking capacity will usually be raised by attending health care personnel or by family members. Although formal legal procedures exist for adjudicating incompetency, a determination that a patient lacks the capacity to make some or all medical decisions independently is customarily made extra-judicially; only rarely is it reviewed in court. The legal status of such nonjudicial determinations is therefore uncertain, though this common practice is endorsed in the routine admonition to physicians to secure informed consent from the patient's next-of-kin,[13] in institutional regulations,[14] and even in court cases.[15] Some commentators, however, advocate requiring formal, judicial proceedings for all treatment decisions and especially for decisions to forego life-sustaining treatment on an incompetent patient.[16] Ideally, the courts are better equipped to protect the interests of incompetent patients; unfortunately, judicial proceedings, besides consuming time and resources, seem frequently to diffuse responsibility rather than increasing the acuity with which patients' interests are scrutinized.[17]

The Commission therefore believes that determinations of incapacity are best made without routine recourse to the courts. The Commission recommends that—except where state law clearly requires judicial intervention or where a real dispute persists after intrainstitutional review—determinations of decisional incapacity be made by the attending physician and regulated and reviewed at the institutional level, and that those who make and apply the law be encouraged to recognize the validity of such determinations. This recognition will require institutions to adopt procedures that merit such deference; in turn, it should reinforce for all participants in the decisionmaking process the importance of reaching a sound determination in each case.

Surrogate Decisionmaking

Identification of a Surrogate When a patient lacks the capacity to make a decision, a surrogate decisionmaker should be designated. Ordinarily this will be the patient's next of kin,[18] although it may be a close friend or another relative if the responsible health care professional judges that this other person is in fact the best advocate for the patient's interests.[19]

The Commission's broad use of the term "family" reflects a recognition of the fact that often those with most knowledge and concern for a patient are not relatives by blood or marriage.[20] Although more than one person may fall within this category, it will be necessary to designate one person as the principal decisionmaker for the incapacitated patient. One possibility is to define presumptive priority[21]—for example, that a person living with his or her spouse will speak for that spouse, that adult children will speak for elderly, widowed parents, etc. Although such presumptions may be helpful in some cases, the Commission believes that the health care practitioner is responsible for determining who should act as the patient's surrogate. No neat formulas will capture the complexities involved in determining who among a patient's friends and relatives knows the patient best and is most capable of making decisions in the patient's place. The responsibility is therefore on the practitioner either to assign this role of spokesperson (subject to appropriate institutional review) or to seek judicial appointment of a guardian.

The Commission believes that, for several reasons, a family member ought usually to be designated as surrogate to make health care decisions for an incapacitated patient in consultation with the physician and other health care professionals[22]:

(1) The family is generally most concerned about the good of the patient.
(2) The family will also usually be most knowledgeable about the patient's goals, preferences, and values.
(3) The family deserves recognition as an important social unit that ought to be treated, within limits, as a responsible decisionmaker in matters that intimately affect its members.
(4) Especially in a society in which many other traditional forms of community have eroded, participation in a family is often an important dimension of personal fulfillment.
(5) Since a protected sphere of privacy and autonomy is required for the flourishing of this interpersonal union, institutions and the state should be reluctant to intrude, particularly regarding matters that are personal and on which there is a wide range of opinion in society.

The presumption that a family spokesperson is the appropriate surrogate may be challenged for any of a number of reasons: decisional incapacity of family members, unresolvable disagreement among competent adult members of the family about the correct decision, evidence of physical or psychological abuse or neglect of the patient by the family, an indication that the family's interests conflict substantially with the patient's, or evidence that the family intends to disregard the patient's stable values, preferences, or specific earlier instructions about treatment.[23] Even if all family members are disqualified from being the principal decisionmaker, for one or more of these reasons, it may still be appropriate to consult with the family in the decisionmaking process.

When an incapacitated patient has no family but does have a court-appointed guardian, special issues arise. Although the reasons for having an existing guardian act as the surrogate for medical decisions are weaker when the guardian is a stranger,[24] such a guardian should be the surrogate in the absence of disqualifying factors.[25] Since the guardian is likely to have been making a number of other decisions for the patient, he or she may have acquired a knowledge of the patient's beliefs, concerns, and values. In addition, the guardian has the sanction of court authority, which may ameliorate practitioners' concerns about civil liability. The decisions of court-appointed guardians about matters of importance to an incompetent person are usually subject to review and prior approval or disapproval by the court. Even when such oversight is not required, physicians should have greater leeway to seek to have the decisions of nonfamily guardians overridden than they do for the decisions of family surrogates, whose judgment should be accorded greater discretion.

If no family or legal guardian is initially available, a suitable surrogate decisionmaker should be designated to ensure a clear assignment of authority for decisionmaking and of responsibility for the exercise of this authority. Unless a suitable surrogate decisionmaker is identified, treatment decisions may lack continuity or may rest on an unclear foundation, making it difficult if not impossible to ensure that the process by which decisions are made is ethically and legally sound.

Although the concept of designating a surrogate for an individual who has no family is clearly sound, in practice there often are no appropriate individuals or agencies available to serve as surrogates. In the context of making decisions about life-sustaining treatment, this is likely to be an especially prevalent problem because of the large number of elderly patients with no family or friends available. One attorney, testifying before the Commission, commented that

> the undeniable tragic fact of the matter is that many, many people, into the thousands, do not have a brother or sister, a mother, a parent, a daughter, or son who can be appointed guardian. There isn't anybody. A lot of them are in institutions, and with the deinstitutionalization process, a lot are now in the community. And there isn't a person to appoint. And we have run out of volunteers.[26]

In some states, public guardianship agencies have been established, but they are underfunded and understaffed and quickly become overburdened with responsibility.[27] Proposals have also been made to establish private, nonprofit social service corporations to provide guardianship services, though they would ordinarily have to rely on public funding unless limited to patients with substantial estates.[28] Regardless of the source of payment, the estimated cost is very high.[29]

In addition, the logistics of having a guardian appointed are quite cumbersome. The head of a corporate guardianship endeavor described the legal process by which guardians have traditionally been appointed as "woefully medieval and oftentimes not worthy of the description of a legal hearing."[30] Another witness stated that in one large American city, it can often take up to eight months to have a guardian appointed, other than for emergency treatment.[31]

Whether or not the selection of a surrogate decisionmaker requires judicial proceedings is an issue that has not been faced squarely by many courts. The New Jersey Supreme Court upheld the appointment of Karen Quinlan's father as her guardian, thus confirming the notion that a close relative is an appropriate surrogate, but it did not explicitly pass on the issue of whether or not the surrogate must be court-designated.[32] By contrast, the Massachusetts Supreme Judicial Court, in a series of cases, has insisted that a court-appointed guardian generally be named as surrogate for a patient who lacks decisional capacity (subject to direct judicial oversight on appropriate matters), at least when the patient has no family members who are willing and available to participate in the decisionmaking process.[33]

Although all states have statutory provisions allowing the appointment of guardians, none of the statutes deal with whether a person who makes a decision to forego life-sustaining treatment on behalf of another must first obtain sanction from a court to act as decisionmaker. When family members are available and the patient is terminally ill, no court has required judicial appointment of a family member to act as surrogate, although the issue has not yet been presented in this way. In *Dinnerstein*,[34] the Appeals Court of Massachusetts held that the court need not review an order against resuscitation for a "hopeless" patient with loving family. Other judicial cases involving life-sustaining treatment have usually been brought to court on an application for the appointment of a guardian, or on an application of an individual to be appointed guardian for the express purpose of making a decision to forego treatment.[35] In other words, the question of whether a judicially appointed guardian is necessary in all such cases has been sidestepped, and courts have instead considered whether a particular individual is suited to be a guardian and/or whether treatment can be discontinued.

In the Commission's view, the cumbersomeness and costs of legal guardianship strongly militate against its use and ought to be taken into account by lawmakers before they require that decisions about life-sustaining treatment be made by judicially appointed guardians. Yet where the law or the patient's situation clearly requires a judicially appointed guardian, the Commission recommends that provision be made for the establishment of adequate guardianship services. In light of the gap in the law as to when and whether guardians are necessary, the Commission recommends that health care institutions should have policies for the designation of a surrogate and should be responsible both for providing surrogates for patients who have no close family and for appropriate referral of disputed cases to court.

Substantive Principles of Surrogate Decisionmaking

The procedures for decisionmaking on behalf of incapacitated patients—whether they are established by common practice, courts, or legislatures and whether they require formal adjudication or defer to physician judgment—do nothing more than designate the centers for responsibility and the processes to be followed. Knowing what issues to take into account or what weight to give potentially conflicting interests is still necessary for the surrogate who is trying to make morally justified decisions.

The two values that guide decisionmaking for competent patients—promoting patient welfare and respecting patient self-determination—should also guide decisionmaking for incapacitated patients, though their implementation must differ. These values are reflected, roughly speaking, in the two standards that have traditionally guided decisionmaking for the incapacitated: "substituted judgment" and "best interests." Although these standards are now used in health care situations, they have their origins in a different context—namely, the resolution of family disputes and decisions about the control of the property of legal incompetents. These doctrines were developed to instruct guardians about the boundaries of their powers and to provide a standard for guidance of courts that must review decisions proposed or made by a guardian.[36]

Despite the long legal history of both these standards, they provide only hazy guidance for decisionmaking even in their original contexts, not to mention in the often far more complex, urgent, and personal setting of health care. Although a number of recent cases involving decisions about health care for incapacitated patients have given courts the opportunity to clarify their meanings, increased confusion has actually resulted from some of these attempts to add precision to the doctrines.

Substituted judgment. The substituted judgment standard requires that a surrogate attempt to reach the decision that the incapacitated person would make if he or she were able to choose.[37] As a result, the patient's own definition of "well-being" is respected; indeed, the patient's interest in "self-determination" is preserved to a certain extent, given the fundamental reality that the patient is incapable of making a valid contemporaneous choice.

A surrogate's decision is limited, however, by two general external constraints. First, the surrogate is circumscribed by the same limitations that society legitimately imposes on patients who are capable of deciding for themselves, such as not compromising public health (as in refusing a mandatory vaccination) or not taking steps contrary to the criminal law (for example, through intentional maiming). Second, there are certain decisions that a patient might be permitted to make because of the strong protection afforded self-determination but that are outside the discretion of a substitute decisionmaker. The line is drawn at actions whose potential adverse effects on well-being, as that concept is commonly understood, are so great that they can be permitted only when sufficiently directly chosen by a competent patient. For example, people may choose for themselves not to have a life-sustaining blood transfusion, but a similar decision by a surrogate would require more direct confirmation of the patient's goals and values than a generally expressed disinclination to receive transfusions. Thus even the substituted judgment standard—which is considered "subjective"—is constrained by limitations arising from the inescapable uncertainty of the evidence as to patients' competent preferences and from the significance and irreversibility of the particular medical decisions.

The substituted judgment standard can be used only if a patient was once capable of developing views relevant to the matter at hand; further, there must be reliable evidence of those views. From an ethical perspective—and probably from the perspective of evidentiary adequacy in court as well—the best proof is the patient's prior expression of views about the current medical situation, particularly when abstract statements have been substantiated by choices by the person in similar situations.[38] For example, a person who has repeatedly been willing to undergo painful treatments in order to live long enough to see his or her children grow up is likely to want to do so again as long as that goal might be realized. While decisions may be based on a patient's general values, goals, and desires, courts are more likely to honor written statements (such as a "living will") than oral ones because they make it plainer that the person actually expressed the views in question and that the statements were specifically intended to direct what should be done for the individual in certain situations.

In some cases, although a patient lacks the capacity to make a contemporaneous decision about foregoing treatment and may even have been declared legally incompetent, he or she may still express a view about treatment, and surrogates should evaluate the relevance of such statements when making a substituted judgment.[39]

Best interests. Because many people have not given serious thought to how they would want to be treated under particular circumstances, or at least have failed to tell others their thoughts, surrogates often lack guidance for making a substituted judgment. Furthermore, some patients have never been competent; thus, their subjective wishes, real or hypothetical, are impossible to discern with any certainty.[40] In these situations, surrogate decisionmakers will be unable to make a valid substituted judgment; instead, they must try to make a choice for the patient that seeks to implement what is in that person's best interests by reference to more objective, societally shared criteria.[41] Thus the best interests standard does not rest on the value of self-determination but solely on protection of patients' welfare.[42]

In assessing whether a procedure or course of treatment would be in a patient's best interests, the surrogate must take into account such factors as the relief of suffering, the preservation or restoration of functioning, and the quality as well as the extent of life sustained.[43] An accurate assessment will encompass consideration of the satisfaction of present desires, the opportunities for future satisfactions, and the possibility of developing or regaining the capacity for self-determination.

The impact of a decision on an incapacitated patient's loved ones may be taken into account in determining someone's best interests, for most people do have an important interest in the well-being of their families or close associates.[44] To avoid abuse, however, especially stringent standards of evidence should be required to support a claim that the average, reasonable person in the patient's position would disregard personal interests (for example, in prolonging life or avoiding suffering) in order to avoid creating emotional or financial burdens for their family or other people to whom they were close.[45]

The recommended standard. The Commission believes that, when possible, decisionmaking for incapacitated patients should be guided by the principle of substituted judgment, which promotes the underlying values of self-determination and well-being better than the best interests standard does. When a patient's likely decision is unknown, however, a surrogate decisionmaker should use the best interests standard and choose a course that will promote the patient's well-being as it would probably be conceived by a reasonable person in the patient's circumstances. On certain points, of course, no consensus may exist about what most people would prefer, and surrogates retain discretion to choose among a range of acceptable choices.

Advance Directives

An "advance directive" lets people anticipate that they may be unable to participate in future decisions about their own health care—an "instruction directive" specifies the types of care a person wants (or does not want) to receive; a "proxy directive" specifies the surrogate a person wants to make such decisions if the person is ever unable to do so[46]; and the two forms may be combined. Honoring such a directive shows respect for self-determination in that it fulfills two of the three values that underlie self-determination. First, following a directive, particularly one that gives specific instructions about types of acceptable and unacceptable interventions, fulfills the instrumental role of self-determination by promoting the patient's subjective, individual evaluation of well-being. Second, honoring the directive shows respect for the patient as a person.

An advance directive does not, however, provide self-determination in the sense of active moral agency by the patient on his or her own behalf. The discussion between patient and health care professional leading up to a directive would involve active participation and shared decisionmaking, but at the point of actual decision the patient is incapable of participating. Consequently, although self-determination is involved when a patient establishes a way to project his or her wishes into a time of anticipated incapacity, it is a sense of self-determination lacking in one important attribute: active, contemporaneous personal choice. Hence a decision not to follow an advance directive may sometimes be justified even when it would not be acceptable to disregard a competent patient's contemporaneous choice. Such a decision would most often rest on a finding that the patient did not adequately envision and consider the particular situation within which the actual medical decision must be made.

Advance directives are not confined to decisions to forego life-sustaining treatment but may be drafted for use in any health care situation in which people anticipate they will lack capacity to make decisions for themselves. However, the best known type of directive—formulated pursuant to a "natural death" act—does deal with decisions to forego life-sustaining treatment. Beginning with the passage in 1976 of the California Natural Death Act, 14 states and the District of Columbia have enacted statutory authorization for the formulation of advance directives to forego life-sustaining treatment.[47] In addition, 42 states have enacted "durable power of attorney" statutes; though developed in the context of law concerning property, these statutes may be used to provide a legal authority for an advance directive. . . .[48]

Despite a number of unresolved issues about how advance directives should be drafted, given legal effect, and used in clinical practice, the Commission recommends that advance directives should expressly be endowed with legal effect under state law. For such documents to assist decisionmaking, however, people must be encouraged to develop them for their individual use, and health care professionals should be encouraged to respect and abide by advance directives whenever reasonably possible, even without specific legislative authority.

Existing Alternative Documents Several forms of advance directives are currently used. "Living wills" were initially developed as documents without any binding legal effects; they are ordinarily instruction directives. The intent behind the original "natural death" act was simply to give legal recognition to living wills drafted according to certain established requirements. They are primarily instruction directives, although their terms are poorly enough defined that the physician and surrogate who will carry them out will have to make substantial interpretations. "Durable power of attorney" statutes are primarily proxy directives, although by limiting or describing the circumstances in which they are to operate they also contain elements of instruction directives. Furthermore, durable powers of attorney may incorporate extensive personal instructions.

Living wills. People's concerns about the loss of ability to direct care at the end of their lives have lead a number of commentators as well as religious, educational, and professional groups to promulgate documents, usually referred to as living wills,[49] by which individuals can indicate their preference not to be given "heroic" or "extraordinary" treatments. There have been many versions proposed, varying widely in their specificity. Some explicitly detailed directives have been drafted by physicians—outlining a litany of treatments to be foregone or disabilities they would not wish to suffer in their final days.[50] The model living wills proposed by educational groups have somewhat more general language[51]; they typically mention "life-sustaining procedures which would serve only to artificially prolong the dying process." One New York group has distributed millions of living wills.[52] The columnist who writes "Dear Abby" reports receiving tens of thousands of requests for copies each time she deals with the subject.[53] Despite their popularity, their legal force and effect is uncertain.[54] The absence of explicit statutory authorization in most jurisdictions raises a number of important issues that patients and their lawyers or other advisors should keep in mind when drafting living wills.

First, it is uncertain whether health care personnel are required to carry out the terms of a living will; conversely, those who, in good faith, act in accordance with living wills are not assured immunity from civil or criminal prosecution. No penalties are provided for the destruction, concealment, forgery or other misuse of living wills, which leaves them somewhat vulnerable to abuse. The question of whether a refusal of life-sustaining therapy constitutes suicide is unresolved, as are the insurance implications of a patient's having died as a result of a physician's withholding treatment pursuant to a living will.

Yet even in states that have not enacted legislation to recognize and implement advance directives, living wills may still have some legal effect.[55] For example, should a practitioner be threatened with civil liability or criminal prosecution for having acted in accord with such a document, it should at least serve as evidence of a patient's wishes and assessment of benefit when he or she was competent.[56] Indeed, no practitioner has been successfully subjected to civil liability or criminal prosecution for having followed the provisions in a living will, nor do there appear to be any cases brought for having acted against one.[57]

Natural death acts. To overcome the uncertain legal status of living wills,[58] 13 states and the District of Columbia have followed the lead set by California in 1976 and enacted statutes that formally establish the requirements for a "directive to physicians."[59] The California statute was labeled a "natural death" act and this term is now used generically to refer to other state statutes. Although well-intended, these acts raise a great many new problems without solving many of the old ones.

No natural death act yet deals with all the issues raised when living wills are used without specific statutory sanction. For instance, the acts differ considerably in their treatment of penalties for failing to act in accord with a properly executed directive or to transfer the patient to a physician who will follow the directive.[60] In some jurisdictions, the statutes consider these failures to be unprofessional conduct and therefore grounds for professional discipline, including the suspension of a license to practice medicine.[61] Other statutes fail to address the issue; presumably, however, existing remedies such as injunctions or suits for breach of contract or for battery are available to patients or their heirs,[62] although there do not appear to be any instances of such penalties being sought.

Some of the statutes attempt to provide patients with adequate opportunity to reconsider their decision by imposing a waiting period between the time when a patient decides that further treatment is unwanted and the time when the directive becomes effective. Under the California statute, for example, a directive is binding only if it is signed by a "qualified patient," technically defined as someone who has been diagnosed as having a "terminal condition." This is defined as an incurable condition that means death is "imminent" regardless of the "life-sustaining procedures" used.[63] A patient must wait 14 days after being told of the diagnosis before he or she can sign a directive, which would require a miraculous cure, a misdiagnosis, or a very loose interpretation of the word "imminent" in order for the directive to be of any use to a patient. The statute requires that when a directive is signed, the patient must be fully competent and not overwhelmed by disease or by the effects of treatment, but a study of California physicians one year after the new law was enacted found that only about half the patients diagnosed as terminally ill even remain conscious for 14 days.[64] There is an inherent tension between ensuring that dying patients have a means of expressing their wishes about treatment termination before they are overcome by incompetence and ensuring that people do not make binding choices about treatment on the basis of hypothetical rather than real facts about their illness and dying process. If a waiting period is deemed necessary to resolve this tension the time should be defined in a way that does not substantially undercut the objective of encouraging advance directives by people who are at risk of becoming incapacitated.

Although the California statute was inspired in part by the situation of Karen Quinlan, whose father had to pursue judicial relief for a year in order to authorize the removal of her respirator, it would not apply in a case like hers.

> The only patients covered by this statute are those who are on the edge of death *despite the doctors' efforts.* The very people for whom the greatest concern is expressed about a prolonged and undignified dying process are unaffected by the statute because their deaths are not imminent.[65]

The class of persons thus defined by many of the statutes,[66] if it indeed contains any members, at most constitutes a small percentage of those incapacitated individuals for whom decisions about life-sustaining treatment must be made. Although some statutes have not explicitly adopted the requirement that treatments may be withheld or withdrawn only if death is imminent whether or not they are used,[67] this requirement is still found in one of the most recently passed natural death acts.[68] Such a limitation greatly reduces an act's potential.

Some of the patients for whom decisions to forego life-sustaining treatment need to be made are residents of nursing homes rather than hospitals. Concerned that they might be under undue pressure to sign a directive, the California legislature provided additional safeguards for the voluntariness of their directives by requiring that a patient advocate or ombudsman serve as a witness.[69] The Commission believes that health care providers should make reasonable efforts to involve disinterested parties, not only as witnesses to the signing of a directive under a natural death act, but also as counselors to patients who request such a directive to ensure that they are acting as voluntarily and competently as possible. Yet statutory requirements of this sort may have the effect of precluding use of advance directives by long-term care residents, even though some residents of these facilities might be as capable as any other persons of using the procedure in a free and knowing fashion.

Paradoxically, natural death acts may restrict patients' ability to have their wishes about life-sustaining treatment respected. If health care providers view these as the exclusive means for making and implementing a decision to forego treatment and, worse, if they believe that such a decision cannot be made by a surrogate on behalf of another but only in accordance with an advance directive properly executed by a patient, some dying patients may be subject to treatment that is neither desired nor beneficial. In fact, although 6.5% of the physicians surveyed in California reported that during the first year after passage of the act there they withheld or withdrew procedures they previously would have administered, 10% of the physicians reported that they provided treatment they formerly would have withheld.[70]

In addition, there is the danger that people will infer that a patient who has not executed a directive in accordance with the natural death act does not desire life-sustaining treatment to be ended under any circumstances.[71] Yet the person may fail to sign a directive because of ignorance of its existence, inattention to its significance, uncertainty about how to execute one, or failure to foresee the kind of medical circumstances that in fact develop.[72] Unfortunately, even the explicit disclaimer contained in many of these laws—that the act is not intended to impair or supersede any preexisting common-law legal rights or responsibilities that patients and practitioners may have with respect to the withholding or withdrawing of life-sustaining procedures—does not in itself correct this difficulty.

First, the declarations about the right of competent patients to refuse "life-sustaining procedures" take on a rather pale appearance since such procedures are defined by the statutes as those that cannot stop an imminent death. (In other words, competent patients may refuse futile treatments.) Second, it is hard to place great reliance on preexisting common law rights, since had the common law established such rights there would have been no real need for the statutes. Thus, if health care providers are to treat patients appropriately in states that have adopted natural death acts, they will need the encouragement of their attorneys—backed by sensible judicial interpretation of the statutes—to read the acts as authorizing a new, additional means for patients to exercise "informed consent" regarding life-saving treatment, but not as a means that limits decisionmaking of patients who have not executed binding directives pursuant to the act.

The greatest value of the natural death acts is the impetus they provide for discussions between patients and practitioners about decisions to forego life-sustaining treatment.[73] This educational effect might be obtained, however, without making the documents binding by statute and without enforcement and punishment provisions.

Durable power of attorney statutes. Of the existing natural death acts, only Delaware's explicitly provides for the appointment of an agent for medical decisionmaking if the patient becomes incapacitated.[74] In view of the Commission's conclusion that both instruction and proxy directives are important for medical decisionmaking that respects patients' wishes, this deficiency in the other statutes constitutes a serious shortcoming. Proxy directives allow patients to control decisionmaking in a far broader range of cases than the instruction directives authorized by most existing natural death acts.

Nonetheless, authority to appoint a proxy to act after a person becomes incompetent does exist in the 42 states that have laws authorizing durable powers of attorney.[75] A "power of attorney" is a document by which one person (the "principal") confers upon another person (the "agent") the legally recognized authority to perform certain acts on the principal's behalf. For instance, a person who moves to a new city and who leaves behind an automobile for someone else to sell can execute a power of attorney to permit an agent to complete the necessary legal documents in connection with the sale. In this case the power of attorney is a limited one; it gives the agent authority to perform only a specific act—the transfer of title to a particular piece of property. Powers of attorney may also be general, conferring authority on the agent to act on behalf of the principal in all matters. Such actions by agents are as legally binding on principals as if the latter had performed the acts themselves.

A power of attorney—general or limited—may be employed in making decisions not only about property but about personal matters as well, and in this role powers of attorney might be used to delegate authority to others to make health care decisions. A power of attorney, therefore, can be an advance proxy directive. Using it, a person can nominate another to make health care decisions if he or she becomes unable to make those decisions.

One barrier to this use of a power of attorney, however, is that the usual power of attorney becomes inoperative at precisely the point it is needed; a common-law power of attorney automatically terminates when the principal becomes incapacitated.[76] To circumvent this barrier, many states have enacted statutes creating a power of attorney that is "durable"—which means that an agent's authority to act continues after his or her principal is incapacitated. As a result, durable power of attorney acts offer a simple, flexible, and powerful device for making health care decisions on behalf of incapacitated patients.[77]

Although not expressly enacted for the problems of incompetent patients' health care decisionmaking, the language of these statutes can accommodate the appointment of a surrogate for that purpose and nothing in the statutes explicitly precludes such a use.[78] The flexibility of the statutes allows directives to be drafted that are sensitive both to the different needs of patients in appointing proxy decisionmakers and to the range of situations in which decisions may have to be made.

The Commission therefore encourages the use of existing durable power of attorney statutes to facilitate decisionmaking for incapacitated persons, but it also recognizes the possibility for abuse inherent in the statutes. These statutes do not have rigorous procedures because they were enacted primarily to avoid the expense of full guardianship or conservatorship proceedings when dealing with small property interests.[79] Adapting them to the context of health care may require that greater procedural safeguards be provided: precisely which safeguards are needed might best be determined after more experience has been acquired. Existing durable power of attorney statutes need to be studied, therefore, as they are applied to decisionmaking for incapacitated patients facing health care decisions.

Proposed Statutes Various concerned groups have proposed statutes that might improve upon natural death acts, by being more generally applicable and authorizing proxy designation, as well as upon durable power of attorney statutes, by providing protections and procedures appropriate to health care decisionmaking.

The Society for the Right to Die has proposed a "Medical Treatment Decision Act," which is similar to the existing natural death acts.[80] The proposal shares the narrowness of application of most such acts and makes no explicit provision for designating a proxy for medical decisionmaking.

The National Conference of Commissioners on Uniform State Laws has drafted a "Model Health Care Consent Act."[81] Despite its comprehensive title, this act does not have consent as a central concern; more correctly it is a "substitute authority to decide" act. It provides for the appointment of a health care representative to make decisions should a patient be incompetent. Although its intent to provide for proxy directives is laudable, the proposal does not resolve certain central issues. In particular, it does not specify which standard should guide a health care representative (best interests or substituted judgment). The act is also imprecise in the determination of capacity to consent. Procedures governing revocation of the appointment of a health care representative and redelegation of authority are uncertain and liable to abuse.

A national educational group called Concern for Dying has had its Legal Advisory Committee draft a "Uniform Right to Refuse Treatment Act."[82] The Act enunciates competent adults' right to refuse treatment and provides a mechanism by which competent people can both state how they wish to be treated in the event of incompetence and name another person to enforce those wishes. In terms of its treatment of such central issues as the capacity to consent and standard by which a proxy decisionmaker is to act, the Uniform Right to Refuse Treatment Act is carefully crafted and in conformity with the Commission's conclusions. Greater opportunity for review of determinations of incompetency and of proxy's decisions may be needed, however, to protect patients' self-determination and welfare.

Another proposed statute was developed by a committee of concerned citizens in Michigan. First submitted to the state legislature in 1979, their bill would have established the authority of a competent person to designate a proxy specifically for health care decisionmaking.[83] Although Michigan had a durable power of attorney statute, it was not used for health care, perhaps because many people did not know of its availability and it seemed to require a lawyer's drafting services. The proposed proxy decisionmaking bill is simple and direct, yet includes significant procedural safeguards.

General Considerations in Formulating Legislation

The Commission believes that advance directives are, in general, useful as a means of appropriate decisionmaking about life-sustaining treatment for incapacitated patients. The education of the general public and of health care professionals should be a concern to legislators, as the statutes are ineffective if unknown or misunderstood. Many of the natural death and durable power of attorney statutes are less helpful than they might be. In the drafting or the amending of legislation to authorize advance directives, a number of issues need attention.[84]

Requisites for a valid directive. Some way should be established to verify that the person writing a directive was legally competent to do so at the time. A statute might require evidence that the person has the capacity to understand the choice embodied in the directive when it is executed. The statute should clearly state whether the witnesses that are required attest to the principal's capacity or merely ensure that signatures are not fraudulent. Since such witnesses are likely to be laypeople, the standard of decisionmaking capacity they apply will rest on common sense, not psychological expertise. Furthermore, the standard they are asked to attest to may be as low as that used in wills, unless specified differently.

The principal and the prospective proxy should recognize the seriousness of the step being taken, but this will be difficult to guarantee by statute. One way to increase the likelihood that due regard is given to the subject matter would be to provide that before a directive is executed, the principal (and proxy, where one is involved) must have had a discussion with a health care professional about a directive's potential consequences, in light of the principal's values and goals. This would also help ensure that any instructions reflect a process of active self-determination on the part of the patient.

Legal effect of directives. A statute should ensure that people acting pursuant to a valid directive are not subject to civil or criminal liability for any action that would be acceptable if performed on the valid consent of a competent patient. Since directives—particularly those including instructions—may contain unavoidable ambiguities, some recognition of the need for interpretation will be needed to provide adequate reassurance for health care professionals and proxies. Some of the existing statutes speak of protection for actions taken in "good faith,"[85] which provides sensible protection. Some standard of reasonable interpretation of the directive may need to be imposed, however, on an attending physician's reading of the document, lest "good faith" offer too wide a scope for discretion. Such a standard might best be developed in case law and scholarly commentary rather than in the statute itself.

The wisdom or necessity of penalties for noncompliance (fines, for example, or suspension or revocation of professional licenses[86]) depends upon the problem a statute is attempting to remedy. If health care professionals are unwilling to share responsibility with patients and, in particular, tend to overtreat patients whose physical or mental condition leaves them unable to resist, then—unless they are made legally binding-advance directives are unlikely to protect patients who want to limit their treatment. On the other hand, if health care professionals are simply unsure of what patients want, or if they are willing to share decisionmaking responsibility but are apprehensive about their legal liability if they follow the instructions of a person whose decisionmaking capacity is in doubt, then the threat of penalties would be unnecessary and potentially counterproductive by fostering an adversarial relationship between patient and provider. The evidence available at present does not clearly support substantial penalties.[87]

Proxy's characteristics and authority. Several special questions arise in the context of health care concerning who may act as a proxy and what the proxy may do. A proxy should have the decisionmaking capacity needed for a particular health care situation. The criteria for determining presence of adequate capacity in a proxy are the same as for patients themselves.[88]

Statutes might limit who may serve as proxy so as to avoid the appointment of anyone likely to act upon interests that are adverse to a patient's. In some natural death statutes, the criteria for witnesses explicitly exclude anyone financially involved (as debtor, creditor, or heir) with the patient.[89] If a similar restriction were applied to proxies, this might eliminate virtually everyone who cares about the patient, however. Special restrictions on who may be a proxy may be warranted for patients in long-term care and psychiatric institutions, though the appropriate form of such conditions is uncertain.

In certain circumstances a proxy may be temporarily or permanently unable or unwilling to serve as a substitute decisionmaker. When that occurs, alternate proxies could be limited to people who were named by the principal in an original or amended directive; or, alternately, a proxy could be allowed to delegate his or her authority to another person of the proxy's choosing.[90] This issue might be affected by whether either the original or a substitute proxy was a close relative of the patient, as opposed to a stranger.

Since the proxy stands in the shoes of the patient and is expected to engage in a comparable decisionmaking process, logically the proxy should have access to the patient's medical record. Yet it may sometimes be advisable to allow the proxy's access to be limited to the information needed for the health care decision at hand, in order to respect the patient's privacy.

Any directive issued by a competent person, and especially an instruction directive, can use the Commission's preferred standard for surrogate decisionmaking—substituted judgment.[91] The interpretation of such a directive should ordinarily lie with the surrogate decisionmaker, particularly in the case of a proxy designated by the patient. Provision may have to be made for an administrative mechanism to decide situations in which a health care professional challenges a proxy's decision on the ground that it is based on neither a reasonable interpretation of the patient's instructions nor on the patient's best interests.

Administrative aspects. Several procedural concerns probably need to be addressed in any statute for advance health care directives. A statute needs to specify how a directive becomes effective. Some of the natural death acts, as already mentioned, require that a directive be executed after the patient has been informed of a diagnosis, so that the person's instructions are arrived at in the context of the actual, rather than the hypothetical, choices to be made.[92] Some statutes also provide that the directive be renewed every few years so that the signatory can reconsider the instructions or designation in light of changed circumstances or opinions.[93]

The trigger for a valid directive becoming operative also needs to be specified. A statute may leave that question to the document itself, to be specified by the person executing the directive, or it may provide that a particular event or condition brings the document into play. In either case, the triggering event will require both a standard for action and a specification of who will determine that the standard is met. For example, a directive may become operative when a physician makes a particular prognosis ("terminal illness") or determines that a patient lacks decisional capacity regarding a particular health care choice.

Provision must be made for the process and standard by which a document can be revoked. The value of self-determination suggests that as long as the principal remains competent, he or she should unquestionably have the power to revoke a directive. But what about an incompetent (incapacitated) person? The natural death acts have uniformly provided that *any* revocation by a principal negates a directive.[94] In the context of foregoing life-sustaining treatment, that result may be sensible, since it would generally seem wrong to cease such treatment based upon a proxy's orders when a patient, no matter how confused, asks that treatment be continued.[95] In other circumstances, however, allowing revocations by an incompetent patient could seriously disrupt a course of treatment authorized by a proxy. When the proxy intends to override the principal's contemporaneous instructions because the incompetent principal is contradicting earlier competent instructions and/or acting contrary to his or her best interests, the question of whether to follow the proxy or the principal may have to be resolved by an independent review.

In general, when disputes arise about such things as the choice made by a proxy or an attempted revocation by an apparently incapacitated principal, a review process will be an important safeguard for the patient's interests. In some circumstances the review mechanism need only judge whether the decisionmaking process was adequate. In other circumstances it may be advisable to review the health care decision itself and the application of the appropriate decisionmaking standard. In the absence of a special provision in the statute, questions of this sort should lead to intrainstitutional review and, as needed, to judicial proceedings.[96]

CONCLUSIONS

The Commission commends the use of advance directives. Health care professionals should be familiar with their state's legal mechanisms for implementing advance directives on life-sustaining treatment and encourage patients to use these resources. In particular, practitioners can alert patients to the existence of durable power of attorney devices (in states where they exist) and urge them to discuss their desires about treatment with a proxy decisionmaker. In states without applicable legislation, practitioners can still inform their patients of the value of making their wishes known, whether through a living will or more individual instructions regarding the use of life-sustaining procedures under various circumstances.

Institutions concerned with patient and practitioner education have an important role to play in encouraging patients to become familiar with and use advance directives, and in familiarizing practitioners with the ethical and practical desirability of their patients using these mechanisms. Finally, legislators should be encouraged to draft flexible and clear statutes that give appropriate legal authority to those who write and rely upon advance directives. Such legislation needs to balance the provisions aimed at restricting likely abuses and those intended to allow flexibility and individuality for patients and proxies.

5. PATIENTS WITH PERMANENT LOSS OF CONSCIOUSNESS

The general public probably first became aware of the issues addressed in this chapter following the tragedy that began for a New Jersey family on April 15, 1975. On that day, Karen Ann, the 21-year-old daughter of Joseph and Julia Quinlan, lapsed into a coma from which she has never recovered.[1] In the years since, as her situation ceased being solely a private, family concern and—because of legal proceedings[2]—became front-page news, people across the country have confronted such difficult questions as:

- what is the relationship of permanent unconsciousness to life and death?
- how reliable is the medical prognosis of permanence of unconsciousness?
- what life-extending care should be considered unnecessary in the context of patients with little or no chance of regaining cognitive functions?

Uncertainties regarding the care of long-term unconscious patients have been raised with increasing frequency,[3] though the number of such patients whose care has become the subject of judicial scrutiny still represents only a fraction of the total number of permanently unconscious patients.

The Commission's involvement with the issues raised by this group of patients began with its Congressionally mandated study of the "definition" of death.[4] In an empirical investigation conducted as part of that study, the Commission found that although two-thirds of the patients who are supported by an artificial respirator during a coma of at least six hours duration are dead within a month, about 6% remained indefinitely in a "persistent vegetative state."[5] The Commission was especially interested in this group for two reasons. First, for many years the leading set of clinical criteria for the determination of "brain death" were those published in 1968 under the title "A Definition of Irreversible Coma."[6] Using this term as synonymous with death unfortunately served to perpetuate a confusion in the medical field between the state of being permanently unconscious, as are patients in a persistent vegetative state, and that of being dead.[7] Second, and more importantly, once it is acknowledged that permanently unconscious patients are not dead, difficult questions are raised about the type and extent of care that should be provided for them.

Since permanently unconscious patients raise issues at least as difficult as those considered in *Defining Death*, the Commission resolved to give this group special attention in the present study. Two major issues are presented: Who are these patients exactly? And what issues arise during their care that are different from those of other incompetent patients? The first section of this chapter addresses the theoretical concerns in making a diagnosis of permanent loss of consciousness and identifies the major groups of patients in this state, though the Commission leaves to the appropriate biomedical experts the task of providing working guidelines for making the medical diagnosis. After establishing that some patients' unconsciousness can be reliably predicted to be permanent, the chapter attempts to clarify what should be considered permissible care of these patients. The second section evaluates the considerations that would justify continued treatment of these patients. Next, current treatment practices are described and the Commission's analysis is used to distinguish unacceptable practices from desirable ones. The final section presents the Commission's recommendations for decisionmaking processes that encourage both justifiable assignment of authority to decide and ethically defensible decisions.

Identifying Patients

Unconsciousness No one can ever have more than inferential evidence of consciousness in another person. A detailed analysis of the nature of consciousness is not needed, however, when considering the class of patients in whom *all* possible components of mental life are absent—all thought, feeling, sensation, desire, emotion, and awareness of self or environment.[8] Retaining even a slight ability to experience the environment (such as from an ordinary dose of sedative drugs, severe retardation, or the destruction of most of the cerebral cortex) is different from having no such ability, and the discussion in this chapter is limited to the latter group of patients.

Most of what makes someone a distinctive individual is lost when the person is unconscious,[9] especially if he or she will always remain so. Personality, memory, purposive action, social interaction, sentience, thought, and even emotional states are gone.[10] Only vegetative functions and reflexes persist. If food is supplied, the digestive system functions and uncontrolled evacuation occurs; the kidneys produce urine; the heart, lungs, and blood vessels continue to move air and blood; and nutrients are distributed in the body.

Exceedingly careful neurologic examination is essential in order for a diagnosis of complete unconsciousness to be made. Application of noxious stimuli to the nerve endings of an unconscious patient leads to simple, unregulated reflex responses at both the spinal and the brain stem levels. Reflexes may allow some eye movement, grimacing, swallowing, and pupillary adjustment to light. If the reticular activating system in the brain stem is intact, the eyes can open and close in regular daily cycles. The reflex activity can be unsettling to family and other observers, but the components of behavior that produce this appearance are "accompanied by an apparent total lack of cognitive function."[11] In order to have awareness, a person must have an integrated functioning of the brain stem's activating system with the higher "thinking" functions from the thalamus and cerebral hemispheres.[12] Many patients whose brain dysfunctions cause unconsciousness nevertheless have a fairly intact brain stem and, if provided extensive nursing care, are able to remain alive without respirator support for many years.

Permanence The other essential property of this category of patients is that their unconsciousness is permanent,[13] which means "lasting . . . indefinitely without change; opposed to temporary."[14] Three sources of uncertainty should be acknowledged about any judgment that a particular patient's unconscious state is permanent.

The first uncertainty affects any scientific proposition about as-yet-unobserved cases. No matter how extensive the past evidence is for an empirical generalization, it may yet be falsified by future experience. Certainty in prognosis is always a matter of degree, typically based upon the quantity and quality of the evidence from which a prediction is made.

Second, this empirical qualification is especially serious in predictions about unconsciousness because the evidence relevant to a prognosis of permanence is still quite limited. The overall number of such patients is small,[15] and most cases have not been carefully studied or adequately reported. Furthermore, the number of variables affecting prognosis (for example, the cause of unconsciousness, the patient's age and other diseases, the length of time the patient has been unconscious, and the kinds of therapy applied) is large and imperfectly understood.

Finally, any prediction that a patient will not regain consciousness before dying, regardless of the treatment undertaken, contains an implicit assumption about future medical breakthroughs. Since some such patients can be maintained alive for extended periods of time (often years rather than days, weeks, or months),[16] this assumption about treatment innovations can be a long-range one. At the moment, however, it introduces only a very small uncertainty, since the possibility of repairing the neurologic injuries that destroy consciousness is exceedingly remote.

Given these three qualifications on the meaning and basis of any judgment regarding permanence, such a judgment is always a matter of probability about whether a particular patient will remain unconscious until he or she dies despite any treatment that might be undertaken. Nevertheless, the Commission was assured that physicians with experience in this area can reliably determine that some patients' loss of consciousness is permanent.[17]

Disease Categories Only a few fairly uncommon diseases cause permanent loss of consciousness. The pathophysiology of an unconscious state that becomes permanent entails severe disruption of the coordinated functioning of the cerebral hemispheres and the midbrain but with retention of sufficient brain-stem activity to sustain vegetative functions. Most commonly, this occurs when the cerebral hemispheres are profoundly injured but the brain stem is nearly entirely spared. Diagnosis in these cases typically involves extensive physical examination, special radiographic and other imaging procedures, and circulation studies of the brain.

Although many individuals with such an injury survive only briefly, some stay alive for an indefinite period and die of some other illness, often contracted while they are unconscious. Nearly all such long-term survivors are in the diagnostic category of "persistent vegetative state" (PVS).[18] This syndrome usually arises from head injury (as from fights, gunshots, or automobile accidents), intracranial hypoxia (as from cardiac arrest, asphyxiation, or hypotensive shock), or intracranial hypoglycemia (as from insulin overdose). If a patient who is initially comatose from a head injury fails to become responsive and aware within a few weeks, the prognosis for any recovery becomes extremely remote. The absence of all responsiveness, vocalization, or purposive action one month after the trauma makes a lack of recovery virtually certain, despite vigorous therapy.[19] The incidence of head injuries leading to permanent coma or vegetative state is unclear, as there is no central registry, but preliminary evidence seems to point to at least a few cases each year at each large referral hospital.[20]

As with head injury, hypoxic and hypoglycemic damage to the brain often initially causes loss of function in areas of the brain that might recover with time and treatment. However, probably 12% of patients with nontraumatic coma develop reliably diagnosed PVS.[21] Two patients recovered consciousness after a year of PVS from hypoxia.[22] Recovery of consciousness is very unlikely, however, for patients with hypoxia who remain comatose or in PVS for more than one month.[23] Certainly, extended observation is appropriate before making a diagnosis of permanent unconsciousness, at least for hypoxic injuries in otherwise healthy young people.[24]

In addition to those with PVS, four other groups of patients might be diagnosed to be permanently unconscious. First are those who are unresponsive after brain injury or hypoxia and who do not recover sufficient brain-stem function to stabilize in a vegetative state before dying. Most of these die within a few weeks after the brain damage. Although the number of patients in this category is uncertain, it is probably large; more than half the individuals for whom cardiac resuscitation is initially successful die without recovering consciousness, mostly in the first few days.[25]

Second, the end-stage victims of such degenerative neurologic conditions as Jakob-Creutzfeldt disease and severe Alzheimer's disease are permanently unconscious. Only in their final stages do these illnesses become so severe as to bring on complete unconsciousness, and the life span thereafter is only a few weeks or months, depending in part on the extensiveness of support given. Again, the incidence of this source of irreversible unconsciousness is unknown.

A third group of permanently unconscious patients who are in a coma rather than in persistent vegetative state are those who have intracranial mass lesions from neoplasms or vascular masses. If the lesion is correctable, some of these unconscious patients might have restoration of some consciousness. However those for whom there is no effective therapy will be unconscious until they die. Such states usually last only for a few days or weeks, and their frequency is unknown.

The fourth source of permanent unconsciousness is congenital hypoplasia of the central nervous system (anencephaly). Various degrees of hypoplasia and dysplasia are possible and some engender brief vegetative life without development of any mentation or cognition. Usually such conditions are apparent because of abnormalities of the cranium at birth. Sometimes the infant is fairly normal, however, and only the failure to achieve the usual developmental landmarks or the appearance of other medical complications leads to detection. Most babies whose anencephaly precludes development of any consciousness die within a few days of birth, and none survive for more than a few months. This condition afflicts one of every 850 births, for an annual incidence of 4000 in the United States.[26]

Reasons for Continued Treatment

Physicians arrive at prognoses of permanent unconsciousness only after patients have received vigorous medical attention, careful observation, and complete diagnostic studies, usually over a prolonged period. During this time when improvement is thought to be possible, it is appropriate for therapies to be intensive and aggressive, both to reverse unconsciousness and to overcome any other problems. Once it is clear that the loss of consciousness is permanent, however, the goals of continued therapy need to be examined.

The Interests of the Patient The primary basis for medical treatment of patients is the prospect that each individual's interests (specifically, the interest in well-being) will be promoted. Thus, treatment ordinarily aims to benefit a patient through preserving life, relieving pain and suffering, protecting against disability, and returning maximally effective functioning. If a prognosis of permanent unconsciousness is correct, however, continued treatment cannot confer such benefits. Pain and suffering are absent, as are joy, satisfaction, and pleasure. Disability is total and no return to an even minimal level of social or human functioning is possible.[27]

Any value to the patient from continued care and maintenance under such circumstances would seem to reside in the very small probability that the prognosis of permanence is incorrect.[28] Although therapy might appear to be in the patient's interest because it preserves the remote chance of recovery of consciousness, there are two substantial objections to providing vigorous therapy for permanently unconscious patients.

First, the few patients who have recovered consciousness after a prolonged period of unconsciousness were severely disabled.[29] The degree of permanent damage varied but commonly included inability to speak or see, permanent distortion of the limbs, and paralysis. Being returned to such a state would be regarded as of very limited benefit by most patients; it may even be considered harmful if a particular patient would have refused treatments expected to produce this outcome. Thus, even the extremely small likelihood of "recovery" cannot be equated with returning to a normal or relatively well functioning state. Second, long-term treatment commonly imposes severe financial and emotional burdens on a patient's family, people whose welfare most patients, before they lost consciousness, placed a high value on. For both these reasons, then, continued treatment beyond a minimal level will often not serve the interests of permanently unconscious patients optimally.

The Interests of Others The other possible sources of an interest in continued care for a permanently unconscious patient are the patient's family, health care professionals, and the public. A family possessing hope, however slim, for a patient's recovery shares that individual's interest in the continuation of treatment, namely, the possibility that the prognosis of permanent unconsciousness will prove wrong. Also, families may find personal meaning in attending to an unconscious patient, and they have a substantial interest in that patient's being treated respectfully.[30]

Health care professionals undertake specific and often explicit obligations to render care. People trust these professionals to act in patients' best interests. This expectation plays a complex and crucial part in the professionals' ability to provide care. Failure to provide some minimal level of care, even to a permanently unconscious patient, might undermine that trust and with it the health care professions' general capacity to provide effective care. Furthermore, the self-identity of physicians, nurses, and other personnel is bound in significant ways to the life-saving efforts they make; to fail to do so is felt by some to violate their professional creed.[31] Consequently, health care providers may have an interest in continued treatment of these patients.[32]

Finally, society has a significant interest in protecting and promoting the high value of human life.[33] Although continued life may be of little value to the permanently unconscious patient, the provision of care is one way of symbolizing and reinforcing the value of human life so long as any chance of recovery remains.[34] Moreover, the public may want permanently unconscious patients to receive treatment lest reduced levels of care have deleterious effects on the vigor with which other, less seriously compromised patients are treated. Furthermore the public has reason to support appropriate research on the pathophysiology and treatment of this condition so that decisions always rely upon the most complete and recent data possible.

There are, on the other hand, considerations for each of these parties—the family, health care professionals, and society—that argue against continued treatment of permanently unconscious patients. As mentioned, long-term treatment commonly imposes substantial financial burdens on a patient's family and on society[35] and often creates substantial psychological stresses for family members and providers.[36] Health care professionals must devote scarce time and resources to treatment that is nearly certain to be futile. Any alternate useful allocation of the resources and personnel is likely to benefit other patients much more substantially.

In sum, the interests of the permanently unconscious patient in continued treatment are very limited compared with other patients. These attenuated interests in continuing treatment must be weighed against the reasons to choose nontreatment in order to arrive at sound public policy on the care of the permanently unconscious.

6. SERIOUSLY ILL NEWBORNS

* * *

An Ethical Basis for Decisionmaking

Since newborns are unable to make decisions, they will always need a surrogate to decide for them.[1] In nearly all cases, parents are best situated to collaborate with practitioners in making decisions about an infant's care,[2] and the range of choices practitioners offer should normally reflect the parents' preferences regarding treatment (see Table 1, p. 192). Parents are usually present, concerned, willing to become informed, and cognizant of the values of the culture in which the child will be raised. They can be expected to try to make decisions that advance the newborn's best interests. Health care professionals and institutions, and society generally, bear responsibility to ensure that decisionmaking practices are adequate.

Parental Autonomy and Countervailing Considerations Families are very important units in society. Not only do they provide the setting in which children are raised, but the interdependence of family members is an important support and means of expression for adults as well. Americans have traditionally been reluctant to intrude upon the functioning of families, both because doing so would be difficult and because it would destroy some of the value of the family, which seems to need privacy and discretion to maintain its significance.[3] Parents and a child's physician may choose, for example, to correct a disfiguring birthmark or not, to have a generalist or a specialist attend to an injury, or to accept or reject hospitalization for many illnesses. Public policy should resist state intrusion into family decisionmaking unless serious issues are at stake and the intrusion is likely to achieve better outcomes without undue liabilities.

When parental decisionmaking seems not to take account of a child's best interest, however, the stage is set for public intervention. This issue has usually arisen in cases in which the parent's values differ from those common in society. For example, parents are free to inculcate in their children a religious belief that precludes the acceptance of transfused blood. But when a transfusion is necessary for the success of surgery that would be life-saving or without which a child would suffer substantial, irreversible harm, parents' prerogatives must yield to the child's interest in life or in leading a reasonably healthy life.[4] Parents are not, as the Supreme Court has stated, entitled to make martyrs of their children.[5]

The growth of neonatal intensive care has posed problems for parental decisionmaking in addition to those arising from unusual beliefs. Parents may be reeling emotionally from the shock of having a seriously ill child instead of the normal, healthy infant they had imagined. Assuming they have had no previous experience with the condition in question, they are likely to be poorly informed about long-term prospects for the child, be subject to pressing financial exigencies, and be worried about effects on siblings and the family as a whole. Furthermore, the infant's condition may require rather urgent response, often while the mother is still recovering from delivery.

Yet, with suitable assistance, most parents can overcome these difficulties and make decisions on the child's behalf in an appropriate fashion. In order to make good decisions, parents must be told the relevant information, including as accurate an appraisal of prognosis as possible. The medical information they receive, including its uncertainties, should be up-to-date.[6] Their consideration of the situation may be helped by the opportunity to talk with other parents who have faced such decisions, with consultant medical specialists, and perhaps with religious advisors.[7] When reasonably possible, procedures should be used to sustain the infant's life long enough to avoid undue haste in decisionmaking.[8]

If parents continue to insist on a course of action that presents a substantial risk of seriously jeopardizing the infant's best interests, prompt intrainstitutional review should occur. When a decision consistent with the child's interests is still not reached, the health care provider should seek to have a court appoint a surrogate in place of the parents, on the grounds that the parents are incapacitated to make the decision, unable to agree, unconcerned for the infant's well-being, or acting out of an interest that conflicts with the child's.[9]

Besides information, parents need empathy and understanding; health care professionals face the difficult task of keeping lines of communication open with parents who are often unsure of their own feelings and abilities to cope with this tragedy, uncomfortable in the hospital environment, and burdened by other practical barriers to participating in their child's care. Yet these difficulties should not lead to a hasty judgment that parents are uninterested in a child's welfare or incapable of good decisionmaking.[10] Great efforts must be made to understand parents' values and improve their ability to decide on a course of action. In cases when parents are not present, a suitable surrogate from within the family might well be available (for example, the grandmother of the baby of an adolescent mother), but an infant without family surrogates will always need to have another guardian named.

Best Interests of the Infant In most circumstances, people agree on whether a proposed course of therapy is in a patient's best interests. Even with seriously ill newborns, quite often there is no issue—either a particular therapy plainly offers net benefits or no effective therapy is available. Sometimes, however, the right outcome will be unclear because the child's "best interests" are difficult to assess.

The Commission believes that decisionmaking will be improved if an attempt is made to decide which of three situations applies in a particular case—(1) a treatment is available that would clearly benefit the infant, (2) all treatment is expected to be futile, or (3) the probable benefits to an infant from different choices are quite uncertain (see Table 1). The three situations need to be considered separately, since they demand differing responses.

Clearly beneficial therapies. The Commission's inquiries indicate that treatments are rarely withheld when there is a medical consensus that they would provide a net benefit to a child. Parents naturally want to provide necessary medical care in most circumstances, and parents who are hesitant at first about having treatment administered usually come to recognize the desirability of providing treatment after discussions with physicians, nurses, and others. Parents should be able to choose among alternative treatments with similarly beneficial results and among providers, but not to reject treatment that is reliably expected to benefit a seriously ill newborn substantially, as is usually true if life can be saved.

Many therapies undertaken to save the lives of seriously ill newborns will leave the survivors with permanent handicaps, either from the underlying defect (such as heart surgery not affecting the retardation of a Down Syndrome infant) or from the therapy itself (as when mechanical ventilation for a premature baby results in blindness or a scarred trachea). One of the most troubling and persistent issues in this entire area is whether, or to what extent, the expectation of such handicaps should be considered in deciding to treat or not to treat a seriously ill newborn. The Commission has concluded that a very restrictive standard is appropriate: such permanent handicaps justify a decision not to provide life-sustaining treatment only when they are so severe that continued existence would not be a net benefit to the infant. Though inevitably somewhat subjec-

TABLE 1. Treatment Options for Seriously Ill Newborns—Physician's Assessment in Relation to Parent's Preference

*Physician's Assessment of Treatment Options**	*Parents Prefer to Accept Treatment***	*Parents Prefer to Forego Treatment***
Clearly beneficial	Provide treatment	Provide treatment during review process††
Ambiguous or uncertain	Provide treatment	Forego treatment
Futile	Provide treatment unless provider declines to do so†	Forego treatment

* The assessment of the value to the infant of the treatments available will initially be by the attending physician. Both when this assessment is unclear and when the joint decision between parents and physicians is to forego treatment, this assessment would be reviewed by intra-institutional mechanisms and possibly thereafter by court.

** The choice made by the infant's parents or other duly authorized surrogate who has adequate decisionmaking capacity and has been adequately informed, based on their assessment of the infant's best interests.

† See p. 193 *infra.*

†† See pp. 192–93.

tive and imprecise in actual application, the concept of "benefit" excludes honoring idiosyncratic views that might be allowed if a person were deciding about his or her own treatment. Rather, net benefit is absent only if the burdens imposed on the patient by the disability or its treatment would lead a competent decisionmaker to choose to forego the treatment. As in all surrogate decisionmaking, the surrogate is obligated to try to evaluate benefits and burdens from the infant's own perspective.[11] The Commission believes that the handicaps of Down Syndrome, for example, are not in themselves of this magnitude and do not justify failing to provide medically proven treatment, such as surgical correction of a blocked intestinal tract.

This is a very strict standard in that it excludes consideration of the negative effects of an impaired child's life on other persons, including parents, siblings, and society. Although abiding by this standard may be difficult in specific cases, it is all too easy to undervalue the lives of handicapped infants[12]; the Commission finds it imperative to counteract this by treating them no less vigorously than their healthy peers or than older children with similar handicaps would be treated.

Clearly futile therapies. When there is no therapy that can benefit an infant, as in anencephaly or certain severe cardiac deformities, a decision by surrogates and providers not to try predictably futile endeavors is ethically and legally justifiable. Such therapies do not help the child, are sometimes painful for the infant (and probably distressing to the parents), and offer no reasonable probability of saving life for a substantial period. The moment of death for these infants might be delayed for a short time—perhaps as long as a few weeks—by vigorous therapy.[13] Of course, the prolongation of life—and hope against hope—may be enough to lead some parents to want to try a therapy believed by physicians to be futile. As long as this choice does not cause substantial suffering for the child, providers should accept it, although individual health care professionals who find it personally offensive to engage in futile treatment may arrange to withdraw from the case.[14]

Just as with older patients, even when cure or saving of life are out of reach, obligations to comfort and respect a dying person remain. Thus infants whose lives are destined to be brief are owed whatever relief from suffering and enhancement of life can be provided, including feeding, medication for pain, and sedation, as appropriate. Moreover, it may be possible for parents to hold and comfort the child once the elaborate means of life-support are withdrawn, which can be very important to all concerned in symbolic and existential as well as physical terms.

Ambiguous cases. Although for most seriously ill infants there will be either a clearly beneficial option or no beneficial therapeutic options at all, hard questions are raised by the smaller number for whom it is very difficult to assess whether the treatments available offer prospects of benefit—for example, a child with a debilitating and painful disease who might live with therapy, but only for a year or so, or a respirator-dependent premature infant whose long-term prognosis becomes bleaker with each passing day.

Much of the difficulty in these cases arises from factual uncertainty. For the many infants born prematurely, and sometimes for those with serious congenital defects, the only certainty is that without intensive care they are unlikely to survive; very little is known about how each individual will fare with treatment. Neonatology is too new a field to allow accurate predictions of which babies will survive and of the complications, handicaps, and potentials that the survivors might have.[15]

The longer some of these babies survive, the more reliable the prognosis for the infant becomes and the clearer parents and professionals can be on whether further treatment is warranted or futile. Frequently, however, the prospect of long-term survival and the quality of that survival remain unclear for days, weeks, and months, during which time the infants may have an unpredictable and fluctuating course of advances and setbacks.

One way to avoid confronting anew the difficulties involved in evaluating each case is to adopt objective criteria to distinguish newborns who will receive life-sustaining treatment from those who will not. Such criteria would be justified if there were evidence that their adoption would lead to decisions more often being made correctly.

Strict treatment criteria proposed in the 1970s by a British physician for deciding which newborns with spina bifida[16] should receive treatment rested upon the location of the lesion (which influences degree of paralysis), the presence of hydrocephalus (fluid in the brain, which influences degree of retardation), and the likelihood of an infection. Some critics of this proposal argued with it on scientific grounds, such as objecting that long-term effects of spina bifida cannot be predicted with sufficient accuracy at birth.[17] Other critics, however, claimed this whole approach to ambiguous cases exhibited the "technical criteria fallacy."[18] They contended that an infant's future life—and hence the treatment decisions based on it—involves value considerations that are ignored when physicians focus solely on medical prognosis.[19]

> The decision [to treat or not] must also include evaluation of the meaning of existence with varying impairments. Great variation exists about these essentially evaluative elements among parents, physicians, and policy makers. It must be an open question whether these variations in evaluation are among the relevant factors to consider in making a treatment decision. When Lorber uses the phrase "contraindications to active therapy," he is medicalizing what are really value choices.[20]

The Commission agrees that such criteria necessarily include value considerations. Supposedly objective criteria such as birth weight limits or checklists for severity of spina bifida have not been shown to improve the quality of decisionmaking in ambiguous and complex cases. Instead, their use seems to remove the weight of responsibility too readily from those who should have to face the value questions—parents and health care providers.[21]

Furthermore, any set of standards, when honestly applied, leaves some difficult or uncertain cases. When a child's best interests are ambiguous, a decision based upon them will require prudent and discerning judgment. Defining the category of cases in a way that appropriately protects and encourages the exercise of parental judgment will sometimes be difficult. The procedures the Commission puts forward in the remainder of this chapter are intended to assist in differentiating between the infants whose interests are in fact uncertain and for whom surrogates' decisions (whether for or against therapy) should be honored, and those infants who would clearly benefit from a certain course of action, which, if not chosen by the parents and providers, ought to be authorized by persons acting for the state as *parens patriae*.

7. RESUSCITATION DECISIONS

* * *

Ethical Considerations

The Presumption Favoring Resuscitation Resuscitation must be instituted immediately after cardiac arrest to have the best chance of success. Because its omission or delayed application is a grievous error when it should to have been used to attempt to save a life, most hospitals now provide for the rapid assembling of a team of skilled resuscitation professionals at the bedside of any patient whose heart stops.

When there has been no advance deliberation, this presumption in favor of resuscitation is justified. Although the concern a few years ago was about overtreatment, some health care professionals are now worried about unwarranted undertreatment—a weakening of the presumption in favor of resuscitation.[1] Very different presuppositions are involved when a physician feels a need to justify resuscitating as opposed to not resuscitating someone. In either case, however, the risks of an inappropriate decision with grave consequences for a patient are great if the issues are not properly addressed according to well-developed criteria. In order to avoid using resuscitation in circumstances when it would be appropriate to omit it, advance deliberation on the subject is indicated in most cases. As in all decisions in medicine, the basic issue should be what medical interventions, if any, serve a particular patient's interests and preferences best. When a person's interests or preferences cannot be known under the circumstances, a presumption to sustain the patient's life is warranted.

The Values at Stake In considering the relative merits of a decision to resuscitate a patient, concerns arise from each of three value considerations—self-determination, well-being, and equity.[2]

Self-determination. Patient self-determination is especially important in decisions for or against resuscitation. Such decisions require that the value of extending life—usually for brief periods and commonly under conditions of substantial disability and suffering—be weighed against that of an earlier death. Different patients will have markedly different needs and concerns at the end of their lives; having a few more hours, days, or even weeks of life under constrained conditions can be much less important to some people than to others. In decisions concerning competent patients, therefore, first importance should be accorded to patient self-determination, and the patient's own decision should be accepted.

This great weight accorded to competent patients' self-determination means that attending physicians have a duty to ascertain patients' preferences,[3] which involves informing each patient of the possible need for CPR and of the likely consequences (both beneficial and harmful) of either employing or foregoing it if the need arises.[4] When cardiac arrest is considered a significant possibility for a competent patient, a DNR order should be entered in the patient's hospital chart only after the patient has decided that is what he or she wants. When resuscitation is a remote prospect, however, the physician need not raise the issue unless CPR is known to be a subject of particular concern to the patient or to be against the patient's wishes. Some patients in the final stages of a terminal illness would experience needless harm in a detailed discussion of resuscitation procedures and consequences.[5] In such cases, the physician might discuss the situation in more general terms, seeking to elicit the individual's general preferences concerning "vigorous" or "extraordinary" efforts and inviting any further questions he or she may have.[6]

Well-being. A second important ethical consideration is whether resuscitation will promote a patient's welfare. A physician's assessment of "benefit" to a patient incorporates both objective facts, based on the physician's evaluation of the patient's physical status before and following resuscitation, and subjective values, in considering whether resuscitation or non-resuscitation best serves the patient's own values and goals. In virtually all cases the attending physician is in a better position to evaluate the former, while a competent patient is best able to determine the relative value of alternative outcomes.

Even though decisions about resuscitation should recognize the importance of patients' self-determination it may sometimes be necessary to question patients' choices on the grounds of protecting well-being. First, a patient may be mistaken about the course of treatment that will actually achieve the end he or she desires. Even a competent patient may initially misunderstand the nature of alternative outcomes or their relationship to his or her values because of the complexity of the alternatives, the psychological barriers to understanding information, and so forth. Dissonance between the physician's and the patient's assessments of benefit point to the need for such steps as further discussion, reexamination of the patient's decisionmaking capacity, and reassessment of the physician's understanding of patient's goals and values; indeed, in some cases patients may even wish to evaluate their values and goals.

Second, decisions may have to be based on "well-being" because "self-determination" is not possible under the circumstances. Many patients for whom a decision not to resuscitate is indicated have inadequate decisional capacity, often due to their underlying illnesses. In these cases, providers and surrogates must assess whether resuscitation—like any other medical intervention—is or is not likely to benefit the patient. Of course, physicians face many of the same difficulties in deciding that patients do, and their attempts to assess "benefit" will not always lead to clear conclusions.

Equity. The Commission has concluded previously that "society has an ethical obligation to ensure equitable access to . . . an adequate level of care without excessive burdens."[7] Should resuscitation always be considered part of the "adequate level"? Resuscitation decisions are currently made with little regard to the costs incurred or to the manner in which costs are distributed, except when competent patients decide to include such considerations as a reflection of their own concern for family well-being or for distributional justice. The Commission heard from a number of people, however, who wondered if providers and others should consider whether the costs of resuscitation are warranted for those patients for whom survival is very unlikely and who would, in any case, suffer overwhelming disabilities and diseases.[8]

To determine whether cardiac resuscitation is a component of care that all hospitalized patients should have access to, the predicted value of this procedure would have to be compared with other medical procedures that generate comparable expenses and burdens. It is the Commission's sense that, at the moment, resuscitation efforts usually provide benefits that justify their cost, and thus resuscitation services generally should continue to be provided when desired by a patient or an appropriate surrogate. When, in a particular case, an attempt to resuscitate would clearly be against the patient's stated wishes or best interests, then the reason for not resuscitating does not arise from concerns for equitable use of societal resources, though it may incidentally help conserve them.

Of course, a more refined analysis of whether particular cases or categories of cases should be excluded under the definition of "adequate care" might be attempted. A controversial step would be to attempt to eliminate resuscitations that, while advancing a patient's interests or in accord with a patient's preferences, sustained a very marginal existence at a very high cost.[9]

However, the negative consequences of trying to discern such categories in a workable way provide strong arguments against adopting such policies. Explicitly precluding resuscitation for some categories of patients would almost certainly be insensitive to their values, denigrating to their self-esteem, and distressing to health care professionals.[10] Also, the uncertainties over prognosis with resuscitation for each individual patient would make it very difficult to write clear and workable categories. It is unlikely that the costs incurred by marginally beneficial resuscitation are so substantial that their reduction should be a higher priority than the reduction of other well-documented kinds of wasteful or expensive and marginally beneficial care.[11]

Guidance for Decisionmaking

Competent Patients When a competent patient's preference about resuscitation and a physician's assessment of its probable benefits coincide, the decision should simply be in accord with that agreement (see Table 2). When a physician is unclear whether resuscitation would benefit a patient but a competent patient has a clear preference on the subject, the moral claim of autonomy supports acting in accord with the patient's preference. Self-determination also supports honoring a previously competent patient's instructions.[12]

Some patients, although apparently competent, do not express a preference for one course over another. Such patients may not have reached a judgment in their own minds (saying, for example, merely, "whatever you think, Doc") or they may simply be unwilling to articulate a view one way or the other. Provided that the patient's unwillingness to declare a view at the moment does not reflect incompetence, the physician should not immediately ask family members to substitute their views for those of the patient, but should instead seek to involve family members in other useful ways (assuming that the patient does not object to their participation), comparable to the roles sometimes played by clergy, nurses, and other professionals. First, the family may be able to facilitate communication between the hospital staff and the patient, making sure that the issues to be addressed have been understood and helping to overcome any barriers to understanding. Second, they may be able to help the patient to make his or her preferences known to the care giving professionals. Ideally, these efforts will lead the patient to express a preference for or against resuscitation.

Of course, it is necessary to have some operative policy while a patient is being encouraged to make a choice, and patients should be informed about what that will be. Until the person expresses a clear preference, the policy in effect should be based on the physician's assessment of benefit to the patient; when it is unclear whether an attempt at CPR

Table 2. Resuscitation (CPR) of Competent Patients—Physician's Assessment in Relation to Patient's Preference

Physician's Assessment	*Patient Favors CPR**	*No Preference*	*Patient Opposes CPR**
CPR would benefit patient	Try CPR	Try CPR	Do not try CPR; review decision**
Benefit of CPR unclear	Try CPR	Try CPR	Do not try CPR
CPR would not benefit patient	Try CPR; review decision**	Do not try CPR	Do not try CPR

* Based on an adequate understanding of the relevant information.

** Such a conflict calls for careful reexamination by both patient and physician. If neither the physician's assessment nor the patient's preference changes, then the competent patient's decision should be honored.

would be beneficial, there should be a presumption in favor of trying resuscitation.

When physicians and patients disagree about resuscitation, further discussion is warranted. Each can explain the basis of his or her position and why the other person's judgment seems unwarranted or mistaken. In some cases, consultation with experts may be helpful to resolve doubts about the facts of the case. Together, such steps often produce agreement.

Although disagreement in no way implies that a patient is incompetent, it will often be appropriate for the physician, and perhaps consultants or an advisory committee, to reexamine this issue if discussion does not lead to agreement between patient and physician—and also for the physician to reexamine his or her own thinking and to talk with advisors about it. The serious consequences of the patient's choice—which may include severe disability if resuscitation is tried or death if it is foregone—demand that this process be carried out with care. Once the adequacy of the patient's decisionmaking capacity is confirmed, then the patient's preference should be honored on grounds of self-determination, especially since the choice touches such important subjective values.

If a physician finds the course of action preferred by a competent patient to be medically or morally unacceptable and is unwilling to participate in carrying out the choice, he or she should help the patient find another physician. Indeed, such a change should be explored even when the physician is prepared to carry out the patient's wishes despite an initial disagreement if the difference of opinion created barriers to a good relationship.

Incompetent Patients Decisionmaking for incompetent patients parallels that for competent ones except that when a physician or surrogate decisionmaker believes that resuscitation is not likely to benefit the patient, there are some additional constraints[13] (see Table 3). Whenever a surrogate and physician disagree, as when only one thinks that resuscitation is warranted, the case should receive careful review, initially through intrainstitutional consultation or ethics committees.[14] Urgent situations, however, or disagreements that are not resolved in this way should go to court. During such proceedings, resuscitation should be attempted if cardiac arrest occurs.

The review entailed will vary. When a physician feels that there is no benefit, a surrogate may either concur after additional consultations or may find another physician, especially if a consulting physician disagrees with the doctor who initially attended the patient. When a surrogate opposes resuscitation that a physician feels is beneficial, discussing the reasons in an impartial setting may uncover erroneous presuppositions, misunderstandings, or self-interested motives and allow for a resolution that is in the patient's best interests. When a surrogate is ambivalent,

Table 3. Resuscitation (CPR) of Incompetent Patients—Physician's Assessment in Relation to Surrogate's Preference

Physician's Assessment	*Surrogate Favors CPR**	*No Preference*	*Surrogate Opposes CPR**
CPR would benefit patient	Try CPR	Try CPR	Try CPR until review of decision**
Benefit of CPR unclear	Try CPR	Try CPR	Try CPR until review of decision**
CPR would not benefit patient	Try CPR until review of decision**	Try CPR until review of decision**	Do not try CPR

* Based on an adequate understanding of the relevant information.

** See pp. 246–48 *infra*.

confirmation of the expected value of resuscitation by a consultant may be persuasive; continued ambivalence may signal the need for a new surrogate. The hospital will have to be able to ensure that helpful and effective responses are provided for these various situations.

If a patient has no surrogate and orders against resuscitation are contemplated, at least a *de facto* surrogate should be designated. When the physician feels that the decision against resuscitation is quite uncontroversial, a consultation with another physician, professional staff consensus, or agreement from an institutionally designated patient advocate can provide suitable confirmation of the initial judgment. Decisions like these are made commonly and should be within the scope of medical practice rather than requiring judicial proceedings. Decisions that are more complex or uncertain should occasion more formal intrainstitutional review and sometimes judicial appointment of a guardian.

Judicial Oversight As made clear throughout this Report, the Commission believes that decisionmaking about life-sustaining care is rarely improved by resort to courts. Although physicians might want court adjudication when they believe that a patient's decision against resuscitation is clearly and substantially against his or her interests, courts are unlikely to require people to submit to such an intrusive and painful therapy unless they conclude that the patient is incompetent.[15] Some form of review mechanism within a hospital is generally more appropriate and desirable for such disagreements. The courts are sometimes the appropriate forum for serious, intractable disagreements between a patient's surrogate and physician, however. When intrainstitutional procedures have not led to agreement in such cases, judges may well have to decide between two differing accounts of a patient's interests.

Institutional Policies

If DNR decisions always took place when there was time for deliberation and data gathering and only a few people were involved, little more would need to be said. However, potential rescuers often have limited personal knowledge of the patient and, once cardiac arrest occurs, there is no time for deliberation. Furthermore, too many people are involved to permit everyone to be brought into the decisionmaking process. In response to the special problems that attend resuscitation attempts,[16] formal and informal policies have been developed to govern decisionmaking and communication of decisions within institutions.[17] The Commission believes that institutional policymakers need to address three basic concerns.

The Need for Explicit Policies Hospitals should have an explicit policy[18] on the practice of writing and implementing DNR orders.[19] In the absence of an established mechanism, decisionmaking might fail to meet the requirements of informed consent or the responsibility for making and carrying out the decision might be assigned to an inappropriate person.[20] Physicians should be allowed to decide to stop a resuscitation effort in progress, although the authority of inexperienced or untrained individuals to make such a decision should be limited. Moreover, without a deliberate process for reaching decisions about resuscitation, legitimate options may never receive the full consideration of patients, physicians, and other involved parties. Consultations with the nursing staff might well be required.[21]

Hospital policies should require appropriate communication with patients about the resuscitation decision. DNR policies should require that any such order be written in a patient's chart with sufficient documentation of the supporting reasons. Physicians may also need to review the order periodically, though changing a DNR order due to a revised assessment of its likelihood to benefit the patient will probably be rare.

The Need for Balanced Protection of Patients
Hospital policies should recognize that DNR orders can be justified by being in accord with a patient's competent choice or by serving the incompetent patient's well-being. Such policies can serve to remind staff that reflex resuscitation efforts applied to all patients not only denies people the ability to control the course of their own lives (a legal wrong) but also sometimes inflicts actual harm on individuals. At the same time, hospital policies on resuscitation should aim to protect the interests of incompetent patients (who are least likely to be able to protect themselves), by favoring resuscitation, for example, when the deliberations about a particular patient have not yet been completed. Indeed, for incompetent patients, the policy should make it clear that the presumption in favor of resuscitation can only be overcome by a finding that resuscitation offers a patient no significant overall benefit or that the patient would clearly not have wished to be resuscitated under the circumstances. Especially in treatment areas such as intensive and cardiac care units, where many patients are at risk for cardiac arrest, policies should try to reduce the number who are resuscitated without appropriate prior deliberation.

By encouraging prior deliberation, the policies can also reduce the need some now see for "partial resuscitation," in which less than a full effort to resuscitate the patient is made because the attending physician never made a clear decision or because it was thought important to placate or comfort family members or hospital staff.[22] Success at resuscitation is rare enough when all efforts are expended, so such limited efforts are usually doomed from the start. Thus, "partial codes" become a kind of dishonest effort that needs to be justified by reasons stronger than merely the providers' discomfort in discussing DNR decisions.[23]

Any DNR policy should ensure that the order not to resuscitate has no implications for any other treatment decision. Patients with DNR orders on their charts may still be quite appropriate candidates for all other vigorous care, including intensive care.[24] Thus, orders regarding supportive care that is to be provided should be written separately.

Finally, to respond to the conflict that professional staff feel and yet to protect patients' interests in preserving both personal choice and well-being, institutions may wish to provide guidelines for situations in which a patient with a DNR order suffers cardiac arrest as a result of a medical intervention.[25] Although the subject has not been well studied, patients whose cardiac arrest occurs under such circumstances may well have a better chance of successful resuscitation, since the arrest is more likely to have occurred in closely monitored settings and from fairly reversible causes.[26] Policies might require specific discussion of this issue in certain settings or acknowledge that sometimes the DNR order is justifiably overridden.

The Need for Internal Advice and Review Hospital policy should provide for appropriate resolution of disagreements on resuscitation decisions. Intrainstitutional review of decisions that raise persistent disagreements has been shown to be very effective in some institutions, both for clarifying the issues in a case and for achieving compassionate and responsive resolution of the issues.[27]

Hospital staff should not be forced to undertake an action they regard as unethical. All staff should have access to the review mechanism for advice and for clarifying the issues. If that proves unsatisfactory, every effort should be made to have other staff from within the institution care for the patient. Barring that, if the person's medical condition allows it, transfer to another institution may be appropriate. Hospital staff should try, however, to avoid becoming so inflexible that they are unable to respond comfortably to appropriate orders, whether for or against resuscitation. Hospitals have a responsibility in staff education and recruitment to provide sufficient staff resources and flexibility.

Cases should be brought to court when it is necessary to decide whether a patient is competent to make a decision not to be resuscitated or, if not competent, which decision serves the patient's interests. Very few, if any, cases should be brought to court solely to protect the hospital from the unlikely prospect of liability.

NOTES

Introduction and Summary

1. "To forego life-sustaining treatment" means to do without a medical intervention that would be expected to extend the length of the patient's life. "Foregoing" includes both the non-initiation of a treatment and the discontinuation of an ongoing treatment. The terms "therapy" and "medical intervention" are used interchangeably with "treatment" in this Report. When a patient's underlying condition is incurable and will probably soon be fatal, "therapy" or "treatment" may not seem entirely apt, because these terms usually imply a curative intervention. Nevertheless, the terms are used here both because no better ones are available and because they are commonly used.
2. President's Commission for the Study of Ethical Problems in Medicine and Biomedical and Behavioral Research. *Making Health Care Decisions*, U.S. Government Printing Office, Washington, (1982).
3. "Decisionmaking guided by the best interests standard requires a surrogate to do what, from an objective standpoint, appears to promote a patient's good without reference to the patient's actual or supposed preferences." *Making Health Care Decisions*, at 179. . . .
4. "A determination of this [adequate] level will take into account the value of various types of health care in relation to each other as well as the value of health care in relation to other important goods for which societal resources are needed." President's Commission for the Study of Ethical Problems in Medicine and Biomedical and Behavioral Research, *Securing Access to Health Care*, U.S. Government Printing Office, Washington (1983) at 4–5.
5. 42 U.S.C. 300v-1(a)(1)(B) (Supp. 1981).
6. President's Commission for the Study of Ethical Problems in Medicine and Biomedical and Behavioral Research, *Defining Death*, U.S. Government Printing Office, Washington (1981).
7. The UDDA [Uniform Determination of Death] states:

   > An individual who has sustained either (1) irreversible cessation of circulatory and respiratory functions, or (2) irreversible cessation of all functions of the entire brain, including the brain stem, is dead. A determination of death must be made in accordance with accepted medical standards.

   Ten states and the District of Columbia have enacted the Uniform Determination of Death Act by statute . . . [and it] has been "adopted" through case law by the highest court of two other states. See Swafford v. State, 421 N.E.2d 596, 602 (Ind. 1981) (for homicide law); *In re* Bowman, 94 Wash. 2d 407, 421, 617 P.2d 731, 738 (1982). This brings to 37 the number of jurisdictions that have recognized the determination of death through neurological criteria. For a listing of those states with other statutes, see *Defining Death*, *supra* note 6 at 65, 12034.
8. See, e.g., testimony of Dr. Ronald Cranford, transcript of the 3rd meeting of the President's Commission (July 11, 1980) at 20, 23: "The persistent vegetative state . . . seems to me an even more complex and important issue. . . . These cases of persistent vegetative state are going to become more frequent and they will continue to exist in that state for longer periods of time."
9. *Defining Death*, *supra* note 6 at 4–5.
10. 42 U.S.C. § 300v-1(a)(2) (Supp. 1981).

11. *Making Heath Care Decisions*, supra note 2.
12. *Securing Access to Health Care*, supra note 4.
13. A detailed description of the Commission's inquiry appears in Appendix A [in the original report].

2. The Elements of Good Decisionmaking

1. President's Commission for the Study of Ethical Problems in Medicine and Biomedical and Behavioral Research, *Making Health Care Decisions*, U.S. Government Printing Office, Washington (1982). Arguments for the recommendations given here and further elaborations of the consequences can be found in that Report and its two volumes of Appendices.
2. Self-determination, sometimes called "autonomy," involves a person forming, revising over time, and pursuing his or her own particular plan of life. See John Rawls, "Rational and Full Autonomy," 77 *J. Phil.* 524 (1980)
3. See generally Ned H. Cassem, "Procedural Protocol When Illness Is Judged Irreversible," in Edward Rubenstein and Daniel D. Federman, eds., *Scientific American Medicine*, Scientific American, Inc., New York (1980) at 13-V-1; Bernard Lo and Albert Jonsen, "Clinical Decisions to Limit Treatment," 98 *Annals Int. Med.* 764 (1982).
4. A. M. Capron, "Right to Refuse Medical Care," in 4 *Encyclopedia of Bioethics*, The Free Press, New York (1978) at 1498; Norman L. Cantor, "A Patient's Decision to Refuse Life-Saving Medical Treatment: Bodily Integrity versus the Preservation of Life," 26 *Rutgers LL. Rev.* 228 (1973).
5. *Making Health Care Decisions*, supra note 1, at 181–88. The considerations that enter into a decision to turn to a surrogate (including the steps that are appropriate to overcome the causes of a patient's incapacity) and the procedures and standards for surrogate decisionmaking are also treated in pp. 121–36 infra.
6. *Making Health Care Decisions*, supra note 1, at 169–75.
7. Ibid. at 44–51.
8. Ibid. at 63–68.
9. Ibid.
10. "Family" is defined broadly in this Report to include closest relatives and intimate friends, since under some circumstances, particularly when immediate kin are absent, those most concerned for and knowledgeable about the patient may not be actual relatives. See also notes 18, 19, and 20, Chapter Four infra.
11. This second aspect is discussed in [chapter 3] pp. 91–94 [not reprinted here].
12. Talcott Parsons, *The Social System*, The Free Press, New York (1951) at 445; Charles J. Dougherty and Sandra L. Dougherty, "Moral Reconstruction in the Hospital: A Legal and Philosophical Perspective on Patient Rights," 14 *Creighton L. Rev.* 1409, 1423–24 (1981).
13. This feeling of powerlessness led 27-year-old Ted Vergith, a paralyzed nursing home resident, to resist the recommended appointment of a guardian to consent to treatment for life-threatening infections: "I was not in control and I felt almost like I was being stripped of my dignity. Just because you can't walk anymore doesn't mean you can't think and make decisions for yourself." Although Vergith was successful in resisting the appointment of a guardian, he did accept treatment. *Bioethics Letter* 3 (Dec. 1982).
14. James F. Childress, *Priorities in Biomedical Ethics*, Westminster Press, Philadelphia (1981) at 32:

> Antipaternalistic policies may be construed in ways other than their proponents and practitioners intend. For example, if we do not intervene to prevent suicides out of respect for patient autonomy, our nonintervention may be seen as expressing the conviction that these deaths do not matter. A policy that affirms "you should care for yourself" may be interpreted as "we don't care for you."

15. Austin H. Kutscher, "Practical Aspects of Bereavement," in Bernard Schoenberg et al., eds., *Loss and Grief: Psychological Management in Medical Practice*, Columbia Univ. Press, New York (1970) at 280; Henry J. Heimlich and Austin H. Kutscher, "The Family's Reaction to Terminal Illness," Ibid. at 270.
16. Barton E. Bernstein, "Lawyer and Therapist as an Interdisciplinary Team: Serving the Survivors," 4 *Death Education* 179 (1980); Ann S. Kliman, "The Non-Legal Needs of a Dying Client," *Nat'l L.J.*, Nov. 24, 1980, at § 1-15.
17. Different physicians often see the same situation quite differently, a fact that physicians ought to try to remedy as otherwise it severely biases patients' ability to choose. Robert A. Pearlman, Thomas S. Inui, and William B. Carter, "Variability in Physician Bioethical Decisionmaking: A Case Study of Euthanasia," 97 *Annals Int. Med.* 420 (1982).
18. See note 57 infra.
19. See, e.g., Donald G. McCarthy, "The Responsibilities of Physicians," in Donald G. McCarthy and Albert S. Moraczewski, eds., *Moral Responsibility in Prolonging Life Decisions*, Pope John Center, St. Louis, Mo. (1981) at 255; John Ladd, "Physicians and Society: Tribulations of Power and Responsibility," in Stuart F. Spicker, Joseph M. Healey. Jr., and H. Tristram Engelhardt, Jr., eds., *The Law-Medicine Relationship: A Philosophical Explanation*, D. Reidel Pub., Boston (1981) at 33.
20. Ned H. Cassem, "Treatment Decisions in Irreversible Illness," in Thomas P. Hackett and Ned H. Cassem, eds., Massachusetts General Hospital Handbook of General Hospital Psychiatry, C.V. Mosby Co., St. Louis, Mo. (1978) at 572–73.
21. Robert A. Burt, *Taking Care of Strangers*, The Free Press, New York (1979) at 11. See also Robert B. White and H. Tristram Engelhardt, Jr., "A Demand to Die," 5 *Hastings Ctr. Rep.* 9 (June 1975); Michael Platt, *Commentary: On Asking to Die*, 5 *Hastings Ctr. Rep.* 9 (Dec. 1975).
22. For a discussion of external sources of unavailability, such as financial limitations on access to care, see Chapter Three [of this report, which is not reprinted here].
23. See, e.g., Cicely Saunders, ed., *The Management of Terminal Disease*, Edward Arnold Publishers, Ltd., London (1978); E. Mansell Pattison, ed., *The Experience of Dying*, Prentice-Hall, Inc., Englewood Cliffs, N.J. (1977). . . . [And see also, Jacob Bigelow, "Care in the Absence of Cure-1835," reprinted in 85 *Annals Int. Med.* 825 (1976):

> We may do much good by a palliative course, by alleviating pain, procuring sleep, guarding the diet, regulating the ali-

> mentary canal—in fine, by obviating such sufferings as admit of mitigation . . . Lastly, by a just prognosis . . . we may sustain the patient and his friends during the inevitable course of the disease.

24. Robert G. Twycross, "Relief of Pain," in Saunders, supra note 23, at 65; Ivan K. Goldberg, Sidney Malitz, and Austin H. Kutscher, eds., *Psychopharmacologic Agents for the Terminally Ill and Bereaved*, Columbia Univ. Press, New York (1973).
25. See, e.g., Mary J. Baines, "Control of Other Symptoms," in Saunders, supra note 23, at 99. . . .
26. See [chapter 3; not reprinted here].
27. *Making Health Care Decisions*, supra note 1, at 94–102. One regular exception to this is that most people willingly let professionals make decisions for them when life-sustaining treatment is needed on an emergency basis (Ibid. at 93).
28. Ibid. at 50–51.
29. See also *Making Health Care Decisions*, supra note 1, at 76–79. [and] Franz J. Ingelfinger, "Arrogance," 303 *New Eng. J. Med.* 1507, 1509 (1980):

> A physician who merely spreads an array of vendibles in front of the patient and then says, "Go ahead and choose, it's your life," is guilty of shirking his duty, if not of malpractice. The physician, to be sure, should list the alternatives and describe their pros and cons but then, instead of asking the patient to make the choice, the physician should recommend a specific course of action. He must take the responsibility, not shift it onto the shoulders of the patient. The patient may then refuse the recommendation, which is perfectly acceptable, but the physician who would not use his training and experience to recommend the specific action to a patient—or in some cases frankly admit "I don't know"—does not warrant the somewhat tarnished but still distinguished title of doctor.

30. *Making Health Care Decisions*, supra note 1, at 85–89. See also Parsons, supra note 12, at 449; Renee C. Fox, "The Evolution of Medical Uncertainty," 58 *Milbank Mem. Fund Q./Health & Society* 1, 49 (1980).
31. Dennis H. Novack et al., "Changes in Physicians' Attitudes toward Telling the Cancer Patient," 241 *J.A.M.A.* 897 (1979).
32. William T. Fitts, Jr. and I.S. Ravdin, "What Philadelphia Physicians Tell Patients with Cancer," 153 *J.A.M.A.* 903 (1953); Dan Rennick, "What Should Physicians Tell Cancer Patients?" *New Med. Materia* 51 (March 1960); Donald Oken, "What to Tell Cancer Patients: A Study of Medical Attitudes," 175 *J.A.M.A.* 1120 (1961).
33. Oken, supra note 32, at 1125.
34. The reluctance to disclose information shown by the early surveys seemed ironic in the face of the desire expressed by the overwhelming majority of physicians to be told when they themselves confront serious illness. Herman Feifel, "The Function of Attitudes toward Death," in *Death and Dying: Attitudes of Patient and Doctor*, Symposium #11, Group for the Advancement of Psychiatry, New York 632, 635 (1965). Interestingly, however, they still would not disclose such information to their physician brethren. Jay Katz and A. M. Capron, *Catastrophic Diseases: Who Decides What?* Russell Sage Foundation, New York (1975) at 101 n. 56.
35. Hubert W. Smith, "Therapeutic Privilege to Withhold Specific Diagnosis from Patient Sick with Serious or Fatal Illness," 19 *Tenn. L. Rev.* 349 (1946).
36. Oken, supra note 32, at 1124.
37. Ibid. at 1125. The practice of using misleading euphemistic language has apparently long existed, as can be seen in [the following excerpts from] a well-known nineteenth-century work, [namely] Oliver Wendell Holmes, "The Young Practitioner," in *Medical Essays: 1842–1892*, Houghton Mifflin and Co., Boston (1891):

> The face of a physician, like that of a diplomatist should be impenetrable. Nature is a benevolent old hypocrite; she cheats the sick and dying with illusions better than any anodynes. . . .
>
> Some shrewd old doctors have a few phrases always on hand for patients that will insist on knowing the pathology of their complaints without the slightest capacity of understanding the scientific explanation. I have known the term "spinal irritation" [to] serve well on such occasions, but I think nothing on the whole has covered so much ground, and meant so little, and given such profound satisfaction to all parties, as the magnificent phrase "congestion of the portal system" (at 370, 388–89).

38. Physicians in the 1978 survey cited the patient's age, intelligence, and emotional stability, in addition to the patient's or relatives' expressed wishes to be told, as factors in deciding whether to disclose. Obviously, reliance on these qualifiers as hurdles patients must overcome to receive information could lead to objectionable paternalism. Novack, supra note 31.

    Regarding intelligence as a prerequisite, one physician, writing in a popular magazine, had this observation: "To some highly intelligent people—like John Foster Dulles or Robert A. Taft—you can tell the simple truth and know that it is not going to destroy them as human beings. Their minds . . . are capable of . . . adjusting to it rationally" ("Discussion, Should Doctors Tell the Truth to a Cancer Patient?" 78 *Ladies Home J.* 65, 108 [May 1961]). The wiser view would seem to be that "It is very probable that a doctor feels better able to tell an intelligent patient, but this does not necessarily mean that the less intelligent may not cope with this knowledge as well." John M. Hinton, "The Physical and Mental Distress of the Dying," 32 *Q.J. Med.* 1, 19 (1963). For a critique of paternalistic justifications for withholding information from patients, see Allen E. Buchanan, "Medical Paternalism," in Marshall Cohen et al., eds., *Medicine and Moral Philosophy*, Princeton Univ. Press, Princeton, N.J. (1982) at 214.
39. Louis Harris and Associates, "Views of Informed Consent and Decisionmaking: Parallel Surveys of Physicians and the Public," in President's Commission for the Study of Ethical Problems in Medicine and Biomedical and Behavioral Research, *Making Health Care Decisions, Volume two: Appendices (Empirical Studies of Informed Consent)*, U.S. Government Printing Office, Washington (1982) at 17.
40. Hinton, supra note 38, at 19.

41. See, e.g., notes 21 and 32 supra; William D. Kelly and Stanley R. Frisen, "Do Cancer Patients Want to Be Told?" 27 S *Surgery* 822 (1950); E.M. Litin, "Should the Cancer Patient be Told?" 28 *Postgraduate Med.* 470 (1960); Robert J. Saup and Anthony R. Curreric, "A Questionnaire Survey on Public Cancer Education Obtained from Cancer Patients and Their Families," 10 *Cancer* 382 (1957); Lesley A. Slavin, "Communication of the Cancer Diagnosis to Pediatric Patients: Impact on Long-term Adjustment," 139 *Am. J. Psychiatry* 179 (1982).
42. For an elucidation of some of the myth, metaphor, and imagery surrounding cancer, see Susan Sontag, *Illness as Metaphor*, Farrar, Straus & Giroux, New York (1978).
43. Note, "Informed Consent and the Dying Patient," 83 *Yale L. J.* 1632 (1974); Arnold J. Rosoff, *Informed Consent: A Guide for Health Care Providers*, Aspen Systems Corporation, Rockville, Md. (1981). One example of a statutory duty to disclose a terminal diagnosis is the District of Columbia's Natural Death Act, which requires a physician to inform the patient of his or her terminal condition verbally or in writing so that the Act's provisions have legal force. D.C. Code Ann. 16 § 6-2425(b) (1981). . . .
44. Emil J. Freireich, "Should the Patient Know?" (Editorial), 241 *J.A.M.A.* 928 (1979); President's Commission for the Study of Ethical Problems in Medicine and Biomedical and Behavioral Research, *The Official IRB Guidebook*, U.S. Government Printing Office, Washington (1983).
45. This danger is revealed movingly in the case of Jo Ann Mortenson, a 37-year old woman from whom a diagnosis of brain tumor was withheld. Her family was told the truth; Jo Ann was told she had an "encephalitic scar." She later said:

> Imagine taking the parents of a thirty-seven-year-old woman and a man who is the father of five children into a room, hitting them over the head with the truth and then expecting them to take the responsibility for what should be told to the patient. That's not fair. When the doctor takes on the patient in the first place, he is taking the patient on whether that patient lives or dies; and when something unpleasant comes up, it is the doctor's job to tell the patient.
>
> Perhaps he might start off before he knows the results of any tests and ask if the patient wants to know the truth. He can remind the patient that whatever the diagnosis, he is prepared to be available as long as the patient requires, to supply whatever physical and psychological comfort he can.

Gerald Astor, "What's Really Wrong with Me?," 100 *McCall's* 52, 138 (June 1973). See also Peter Maguire, "The Personal Impact of Dying," in Eric Wilkes, ed., *The Dying Patient*, George A. Bogden & Son, Inc., Ridgewood, N.J. (1982) at 233, 252; W.P.L. Myers, "The Care of the Patient with Terminal Illness," in Paul B. Beeson, Walsh McDermott, and James B. Wyngaarden, eds., *Cecil Textbook of Medicine*, W.B. Saunders Co., Philadelphia (1979) at 1941, 1944.
46. Leo Tolstoy, "The Death of Ivan Ilych," in *The Death of Ivan Ilych and Other Stories*, New American Library, New York (Aylmer Maude trans., 1960):

> What tormented Ivan Ilych most was the deception, the lie, which for some reason they all accepted, that he was not dying but was simply ill, and that he only need keep quiet and undergo a treatment and then something very good would result. He however knew that do what they would nothing would come of it, only still more agonizing suffering and death. This deception tortured him—their not wishing to admit what they all knew and what he knew, but wanting to lie to him concerning his terrible condition, and wishing and forcing him to participate in that lie. Those lies—lies enacted over him on the eve of his death and destined to degrade this awful, solemn act to the level of their visitings, their curtains, their sturgeon for dinner—were a terrible agony for Ivan Ilych (at 95, 137).

See also William F. May, "On Not Facing Death Alone," 1 *Hastings Ctr.Rep.* 8 (June 1971).
47. Cicely Saunders, "The Moment of Truth: Care of the Dying Person," in L. Pearson, ed., *Death and Dying*, Case Western Reserve Univ. Press, Cleveland. Ohio (1969) at 49, 59.
48. Novack, supra note 31, at 899. See also, E.R. Hillier, "Communication Between Doctor and Patient," in Robert G. Twycross and Vittorio Ventafridda, eds., *The Continuing Care of Terminal Cancer Patients*. Pergamon Press, New York (1980) at 37.
49. See Ned H. Cassem, *The Dying Patient*, in Hackett and Cassem, supra note 20, at 300.
50. Testimony of Robert Burt, transcript of 21st meeting of the President's Commission (June 10, 1982) at 169.
51. Testimony of Carole Kennon, transcript of 16th meeting of the President's Commission (Jan. 9, 1982) at 21–22.
52. Ned H. Cassem and Rege S. Stewart, "Management and Care of the Dying Patient," 6 *Int'l. J. Psychiatry in Med.* 293, 298 (1975).
53. Tolstoy, supra note 46, at 121.

> To Ivan Ilych only one question was important: was his case serious or not? But the doctor ignored that inappropriate question. From his point of view it was not the one under consideration, the real question was to decide between a floating kidney, chronic catarrh, or appendicitis. It was not a question of Ivan Ilych's life or death.

54. One dying patient stated: "I feel like a railway station that's been closed down—the ward round doesn't stop here any more." Michael A. Simpson, "Therapeutic Uses of Truth," in Wilkes, supra note 45, at 255, 259. See also Barney G. Glaser and Anselm L. Strauss, "Dying on Time," in Anselm L. Strauss, ed., *Where Medicine Fails*, Aldine Pub. Co., Hawthorne, N.Y. (1970) at 131, 139; Donald G. Gallup, Marco Labudovich, and Paul R. Zambito, "The Gynecologist and the Dying Cancer Patient," 144 *Am. J. Obstet. Gynecol.* 154 (1982); "Physicians Found to Spend Little Time with Oldsters," 22 *Med. World News* 48 (Aug. 17, 1981); David Rabin, Pauline L. Rabin, and Roni Rabin, "Compounding the Ordeal of A.L.S.: Isolation from My Fellow Physicians," 307 *New Eng. J. Med.* 506 (1982).
55. Charles D. Aring, "Intimations of Immortality," 69 *Annals Int. Med.* 137 (1968):

> After the flurry of attention to the diagnosis [carcinoma], ward personnel lost interest. The patient began to be moved further and further from the nursing station at the front of the ward. The withdrawal that our patient experienced was

not so much physical absence as uninterest. . . . [An autopsy revealed] a tumor that should have readily yielded to the correct neurosurgical attack (at 140).

56. Thelma D. Bates, "At Home and in the Ward: The Establishment of a Support Team in an Acute Care General Hospital," in Wilkes, supra note 45, at 263; Kennon, supra note 51, at 31; see also note 89, Chapter Six infra.
57. See Stephen B. Shanfield, "The Mourning of the Health Care Professional: An Important Element in Education about Death and Loss," 4 *Death Education* 385 (1981); Louis E. LaGrand, "Reducing Burnout in the Hospice and the Death Education Movement," 4 *Death Education* 61 (1980); Glaser and Strauss, supra note 54, at 34; Richard A. Kolotkin, "Preventing Burn-Out and Reducing Stress in Terminal Care: The Role of Assertive Training," in Harry J. Sobel, ed., *Behavior Therapy in Terminal Care: A Humanistic Approach*, Ballinger Pub. Co., Cambridge, Mass. (1981) at 229; Cassem, supra note 49.
58. Simpson, supra note 54, at 259.
59. Margaret Shandor Miles, "The Effect of a Course on Death and Grief on Nurses' Attitudes Toward Dying Patients and Death," 4 *Death Education* 245 (1980); George E. Dickinson, "Death Education in U.S. Medical Schools: 1975–1980," 56 *J. Med. Educ.* 111 (1981).
60. See, e.g., Loretta Hoggatt and Bernard Spilka, "The Nurse and the Terminally Ill Patient: Some Perspectives and Projected Actions," 9 *Omega* 255 (1978).
61. *Making Health Care Decisions*, supra note 1, at 135.
62. Ibid. at 96.
63. Such terms are also used in varying ways. In particular, some people may use a term (such as "allowing to die" or "artificial means") descriptively while others attach a normative connotation to the same phrase.
64. See, e.g., John A. Robertson, *The Rights of the Critically Ill*, Bantam Books, New York (1983) at 23; William J. Monahan, "Contemporary American Opinion on Euthanasia," in McCarthy and Moraczewski, supra note 19, at 180.
65. See, e.g., Testimony of Dr. Anne Fletcher, transcript of 16th meeting of the President's Commission (Jan. 9, 1982) at 8, 26; Testimony of Dr. Ned Cassem, S.J., transcript of 10th meeting of the President's Commission (June 4, 1981) at 74; Testimony of Dr. Richard Scott, transcript of 12th meeting of the President's Commission (Sept. 12, 1981) at 398.
66. [See the discussion on resuscitation and patient preferences in chapter 7's "Guidance for Decisionmakers" (included in this volume.]
67. See Appendix B [in the original report]; [and] Norman K. Brown and Donovan J. Thompson, "Nontreatment of Fever in Extended-Care Facilities," 300 *New Eng. J. Med.* 1246 (1979).
68. See, e.g., Ake Grenvik, "Terminal Weaning: Discontinuance of Life-Supporting Therapy in the Terminally Ill Patient," 11 *Crit. Care Med* (May 1983). See also, *In re Quinlan*, 70 N.J. 10, 355 A.2d 647, *cert. denied*, 429 U.S. 922 (1976).
69. Sharon H. Imbus and Bruce E. Zawacki, "Autonomy for Burn Patients When Survival Is Unprecedented," 297 *New Eng. J. Med.* 308 (1977).
70. See, e.g., *In re Quinlan*, 70 N.J. 10, 355 A.2d 647, *cert. denied*, 429 U.S. 922 (1976); *In re Dinnerstein*, 380 N.E.2d 134 (Mass. App. Ct. 1978); *Superintendent of Belchertown State School v. Saikewicz*, 370 N.E.2d 417 (1977). See also David W. Meyers, *Medico-legal Implications of Death and Dying*, The Lawyers Co-operative Pub. Co., Rochester, N.Y. (1981) at 211–62; pp. 121–31 infra.
71. See, e.g., *Satz v. Perlmutter*, 379 So.2d 359 (Fla. 1980); *Lane v. Candura*, 376 N.E.2d 1232 (Mass. App. 1978); *In re Quackenbush*, 383 A.2d 785 (N.J., Morris County Ct. 1978).
72. [See chapter 3 in the original report.]
73. See, e.g., James Rachels, "Active and Passive Euthanasia," 292 *New Eng. J. Med.* 78 (1975); Tom Beauchamp, "A Reply to Rachels on Active and Passive Euthanasia," in Tom Beauchamp and Seymour Perlin, eds., *Ethical Issues in Death and Dying*, Prentice-Hall, Inc., Englewood Cliffs, N.J. (1978) at 246; Sisella Bok, "Death and Dying: Euthanasia and Sustaining Life: Ethical Views," in 1 *Encyclopedia of Bioethics*, at 268; Harold F. Moore, "Acting and Refraining," ibid. at 38. The philosophical and moral issues concerning the nature and significance of the killing-letting die distinction are extensively explored in Bonnie Steinbock, ed., *Killing and Letting Die*, Prentice-Hall, Inc., Englewood Cliffs, N.J. (1980); P. J. Fitzgerald, "Acting and Refraining," in Samuel Gorovitz et al., eds., *Moral Problems in Medicine*, Prentice-Hall, Inc., Englewood Cliffs, N. J. (1976) at 284. See also Jonathan Glover, *Causing Death and Saving Lives*, Penguin Books, New York (1977) at 92.
74. George Fletcher, "Prolonging Life," 42 *Wash. L. Rev.* 999 (1967); Edward J. Gurney, "Is There a Right to Die? A Study of the Law of Euthanasia," 3 *Cum.-Sam. L. Rev.* 235 (1972); Robert S. Morrison, "Alternatives to Striving Too Officiously," in Franz J. Ingelfinger et al., eds., *Controversy in Internal Medicine II*, W.B. Saunders, Philadelphia (1974) at 113.
75. More formally, it can be said that the deceased would not have died as and when he or she did had the person responsible not acted in the way he or she did. For death to be a killing by another, that other's action must have changed the cause of the person's death, or have hastened the moment of death, or both.
76. See, e.g., Glover, supra note 73, at 197; James B. Nelson, Human Medicine: Ethical Perspectives on New Medical Issues, Augsburg Pub. House, Minneapolis, Minn. (1973) at 125. . . .
77. See A. D. Woozley, "Law and the Legislation of Morality," in Arthur L. Caplan and Daniel Callahan, eds., *Ethics in Hard Times*, Plenum Press, New York (1981) at 143.
78. Ernest J. Weinrib, "The Case for a Duty to Rescue," 90 YALE L. J. 247 (1980); Judith Jarvis Thomson, "Killing, Letting Die, and the Trolley Problem," 59 *Monist* 204 (1976). See also [chapter 3 of this original report] for a discussion of role-related obligations to intercede.
79. H.L.A. Hart and A.M. Honore, *Causation in the Law*, Oxford Univ. Press, Oxford, England (1959).
80. The empirical component of causation is referred to as "actual" cause (or "cause-in-fact"). For A to be the cause of X, one might have to be able to say that "but for" (or, without the existence of) A, X would not have occurred.

Where there is more than one causative agent or factor, a different test of "actual" cause must be applied, one called a "substantial factor" or "material factor" test. For instance, if Drs. A and B simultaneously give Patient C a lethal injection, neither A nor B is the "but for" cause of C's death because if A had not given the injection, C would have died anyway (from B's injection), and if B had not given the injection, C still would have died (from A's injection). Since it would be unfair for either A or B to escape liability, which would occur if the "but-for" test were applied, these other tests inquire instead whether A's conduct was a substantial (or material) factor in bringing about C's death. If it was, A is legally culpable—and the same test is applied to B's conduct to establish B's culpability.

81. William L. Prosser, *Handbook of the Law of Torts*, West Publishing Co., St. Paul, Minn. (4th ed. 1971):

> Once it is established that the defendant's conduct has in fact been one of the causes of the plaintiff's injury, there remains the question whether the defendant should be legally responsible for what he has caused. Unlike the fact of causation, with which it is often hopelessly confused, this is essentially a problem of law. . . . This becomes essentially a question of whether the policy of the law will extend the responsibility for the conduct to the consequences which have in fact occurred. . . . The term "proximate cause" is applied by the courts to those more or less undefined considerations which limit liability even where the fact of causation is clearly established (at 244).

82. For instance, if in parking an automobile, a driver carelessly hits the car in front, he or she will be liable for any damage to the other car. But if the other car explodes because there was a concealed bomb in the trunk that required only a small tap to set it off, the driver may not be liable for the destruction of the car even though "but for" the driver's carelessness, the harm would not have occurred; the harm nevertheless was more substantially caused by the bomb than by the car accident and the explosion could hardly have been foreseen. And further, if several blocks away, a nurse holding a baby is startled by the explosion and drops the infant, who dies, the driver most certainly will not be liable for the infant's death despite the fact that, in the absence of the driver's carelessness, the infant would have lived. See *Palsgraf v. Long Island R.R.*, 248 N.Y. 339, 162 N.E. 99 (1928) (Andrews, J., dissenting).

83. "He Forgets Silence Is Golden" (Editorial), *N.Y. Times*, July 26, 1917 (supporting a physician's decision not to treat a microcephalic child):

> There would be, indeed, no defense for a doctor who went so far as to take life because in his opinion it was worthless or worse, that is an exercise of power permitted only to Juries and Judges acting through their agent the Sheriff. But to kill is one thing, and to let die is another, with a difference which, though small, is none the less real (at A10).

And see also Robert and Peggy Stinson, *The Long Dying of Baby Andrew*, Little, Brown, Boston (1983). [These] parents of a severely compromised premature newborn have written of the kinds of reasoning that resulted from the desire of their son's doctors to be seen only as "allowing to die":

> [His doctor] spoke as if this were the moment he had been waiting for, when he could make a decision on Andrew that found its way past *commission* into *omission*. . . . They found their loophole. Because of course I shouldn't say they "took him off" [the respirator]—they couldn't do that, since that would be immoral and illegal. They had to hope for an appropriate accident; once Andrew became accidentally detached from the respirator, and had breathed for a couple of minutes, they could declare him "off" and *omit* to put him back on while they wait for his inadequate breathing to kill him. This is the moral, legal, and "dignified" way (at 343, 345).

84. Helen Beynon, "Doctors as Murderers," 1982 *Crim. L. Rev.* 17:

> The practice of medicine raises a peculiar problem of policy for the law of homicide. It is the doctor's job to take decisions which may affect the span of human life. Therefore, it is especially important that law be neither too strict nor too lenient. If it is too strict, it will begin to make doctors criminally responsible for man's mortality; if it is too lenient it will give doctors a "license to kill." But whether the law does steer a middle course between these two extremes, or, indeed, is capable of doing so without greatly distorting the general principles of the criminal law, is a different matter (at 17–18).

85. See, e.g., *State v. Perlmutter*, 379 So.2d 359 (Fla. 1980); *In re* Quinlan, 70 N.J. 10, 355 A.2d 647, 671, *cert. denied*, 429 U.S. 922 (1976).
86. See Chapter Four infra.
87. Evaluating the policy role of the acting/omitting distinction in regulating behavior requires balancing its positive value as a safeguard that protects human life against its negative consequences of contributing to some undesirable decisions. The law has used conceptually unclear reinterpretations to remove most foregoings of life-sustaining treatment from the behaviors that count as "acting" or "wrongful killing." These are important in reducing the frequency of morally undesirable decisions that might otherwise arise.
88. George Fletcher, "Prolonging Life," 42 *Wash. L. Rev.* 999 (1967); Robertson, supra note 64, at 20–22; Christian Barnard, *Good Life/Good Death*, Prentice-Hall, Inc., Englewood Cliffs, N.J. (1980) at 110–17.
89. [See discussions on this point in chapter 1 and Appendix B; neither is reprinted here.]
90. Louis Shattluck Baer, "Nontreatment of Some Severe Strokes," 4 *Annals Neurol.* 381, 382 (Oct. 1978):

> By not starting a "routine IV" I am not committed to that modality of therapy. It is easier *not* to start daily intravenous parenteral fluids than to stop them, once begun—just as it is easier not to turn on the respiratory assistance machine than to turn the switch off, once started.

91. See, e.g., Alan J. Weisbard, "On the Bioethics of Jewish Law: The Case of Karen Quinlan," 14 *Israel L. Rev.* 337, 346 (1979).

92. See [in this chapter, "The moral significance of the Difference].
93. See, e.g., George J. Annas, *The Rights of Hospital Patients*, Avon Books, New York (1975) at 92, 95–96; Albert R. Jonsen, Mark Siegler, and William J. Winslade, *Clinical Ethics*, Macmillan Pub. Co., New York (1982) at 100.
94. See Jon R. Waltz and Fred E. Inbau, *Medical Jurisprudence*, Macmillan Pub. Co., New York (1971) at 142–51; Angela R. Holder, *Medical Malpractice Law*, John Wiley & Sons, New York (1975) at 375.
95. [See the earlier section in this chapter on "Informing and Communicating."]
96. Such "overtreatment" has resulted in the filing of a lawsuit by a deceased patient's family. *Leach v. Shapiro*, Civ. Action C-81-2559A, Summit County, Oh. (1982); *Leach v. Akron General Medical Center*, 426 N.E.2d 809 (Ohio Com. Pl. 1980).
97. "Comment: Medico-Legal Implications of Orders Not to Resuscitate," 31 *Cath. U.L. Rev.* 515, 519 n.12 (1982) (citation omitted):

> Another problem is whether a distinction should be made between causing someone to die by commission of a positive act and allowing someone to die through inaction, i.e., withholding treatment. Whether one physician would be held criminally liable for "pulling the plug" when another would not be liable for failing to start the initial treatment is unclear. Certainly, however, to maintain that there is a difference in the degree of culpability may have the undesirable effect of promoting nontreatment over treatment.

98. Testimony of Dr. John Freeman, transcript of 16th meeting of the President's Commission (Jan. 9, 1982) at 124–25.
99. Paul Ramsey, *The Patient as Person*, Yale Univ. Press, New Haven, Conn. (1970):

> A decision to stop "extraordinary" life-sustaining treatments requires no greater and in fact the same moral warrant as a decision not to begin to use them. . . . Since a trial treatment is often a part of diagnosis of a patient's condition, one might expect there to be greater reluctance on the part of physicians in not starting than in stopping extraordinary efforts to save life. As I understand them, physicians often have the contrary difficulty. . . . The reasons for these variations are probably psychological rather than rational (at 121–22).

See also James F. Childress, *Priorities in Biomedical Ethics*, Westminster Press, Philadelphia (1981) at 123, n.10.

Commenting on Judge Robert Meade's ruling in the Brother Fox case that "it is important that the law not create a disincentive to the fullest treatment of patients by making it impossible for them in at least some extreme circumstances to choose to end treatment which has proven unsuccessful," John Paris noted: "With that legal support for the standard that once the patient has been given the benefit of all known procedures and these prove unsuccessful in restoring health, they need not be uselessly continued. It is to be hoped that the legal recognition of that moral reality will help overcome physician timidity in similar cases." John J. Paris, "Brother Fox: The Courts and Death with Dignity," 143 *America* 282, 284 (1980).

100. In this situation, death occurs because patients in the terminal stages of diseases like cancer sometimes undergo suffering so great that it can only be relieved by doses of morphine that are so large as to induce respiratory depression or to predispose the patient to pneumonia, which may result in an earlier death. The Commission notes that such an occurrence should not be termed an "overdose," with its implications of excessive dosage, since the use of the correct dose of morphine to relieve suffering is really an acceptable practice. On the other hand, relief of pain can extend life: "the relief and comfort given an aged patient often affects the prolongation of life if only by restoring the willingness to live." Alfred Worcester, *The Care of the Aged, the Dying and the Dead*, Charles C. Thomas, Springfield, Ill. (1935) reprinted by Arno Press, Inc., New York (1977) at 6.
101. The customary use of "foreseeable" is for those things that would be predicted as possible outcomes by a person exercising reasonable foresight; it is not limited to consequences that are certain or nearly certain to occur.
102. The moral importance of this distinction is defended in Charles Fried, *Right and Wrong*, Harvard Univ. Press, Cambridge, Mass. (1978) at 7–53. But see Alan Donagan, *The Theory of Morality*, Univ. of Chicago Press, Chicago (1977) at 112–71.
103. Donagan, supra note 102, at 164; R.G. Frey, "Some Aspects to the Doctrine of Double Effect," 5 *Canadian J. Phil.* 259 (1975); Philippa Foot, "The Problem of Abortion and the Doctrine of the Double Effect," 5 *Oxford Rev.* 5 (1967).
104. *Restatement (Second) of Torts*, American Law Institute Publishers, St. Paul, Minn. (1965) at §§ 289–91.
105. Judicial Council, *Current Opinions of the Judicial Council of the American Medical Association*, American Medical Association, Chicago (1982) at 9. . . .
106. "Neither will I administer a poison to anybody when asked to do so, nor will I suggest such a course": "Selections from the Hippocratic Corpus: Oath," in Stanley Joel Reiser, Arthur J. Dyck, and William J. Curran, eds., *Ethics in Medicine*, MIT Press, Cambridge, Mass. (1977) at 5.
107. "Euthanasia would threaten the patient-physician relationship; confidence might give way to suspicion. . . . Can the physician, historic battler for life, become an affirmative agent of death without jeopardizing the trust of his dependents?" From David W. Louisell, "Euthanasia and Biathanasia: On Dying and Killing," 40 *Linacre Q.* 234, 243 (1973).
108. Yale Kamisar, "Some Non-Religious Views Against Proposed *Mercy-Killing* Legislation," 42 *Minn. L. Rev.* 969 (1958); Beauchamp, supra note 73; John C. Fletcher, "Is Euthanasia Ever Justifiable?" in Peter H. Wiernik, ed., *Controversies in Oncology*, John Wiley & Sons, Inc., New York (1982) at 297.
109. See Dennis Horan, "Euthanasia and Brain Death," 35 *Annals N.Y. Acad. Sci.* 363, 374 (1978). Cf. Tamar Lewin,

"Execution by Injection: A Dilemma for Prison Doctors," *N.Y. Times*, Dec. 12, 1982, at E20; Norman St. John-Stevas, *Life, Death and the Law*, World Publishing Co., New York (1961) at 276–77.

110. This consideration plays a prominent part in what is known in Catholic medical ethics as the "doctrine of double effect." This doctrine, which is designed to provide moral guidance for an action that could have at least one bad and one good effect, holds that such an action is permissible if it satisfies these four conditions: (1) the act itself must be morally good or neutral (for example, administering a pain-killer); (2) only the good consequences of the action must be intended (relief of the patient's suffering); (3) the good effect must not be produced by means of the evil effect (the relief of suffering must not be produced by the patient's death); and (4) there must be some weighty reason for permitting the evil (the relief of great suffering, which can only be achieved through a high risk of death). The Commission makes use of many of the moral considerations found in this doctrine, but endorses the conclusion that people are equally responsible for all of the foreseeable effects of their actions, thereby having no need for a policy that separates "means" from "merely foreseen consequences." See, e.g., William E. May, "Double Effect," in 1 *Encyclopedia of Bioethics*, supra note 73, at 316; Joseph T. Mangan, S.J., "An Historical Analysis of the Principle of Double Effect, 10 *Theological Stud.* 4 (1949); Donagan, supra note 102; Richard A. McCormick, S.J., *Ambiguity in Moral Choice*, Marquette Univ. Press, Milwaukee, Wisc. (1973); J.M. Boyle, "Toward Understanding the Principle of Double Effect" 90 *Ethics* 527 (1980).

111. These issues were addressed in a national survey conducted for the Commission by Louis Harris and Associates. Physicians, especially, distinguished between administering drugs to relieve pain, knowing that the dose might be lethal, and complying with a patient's wish to have his or her life ended. In the case of a patient in severe pain who had no hope of recovery and who asked to have the pain eased, knowing it might shorten life, 79 percent of the public and 82 percent of the physicians said it would be ethically permissible to administer drugs to relieve the pain even at the risk of shortening life. Furthermore, 84 percent of physicians said they would be likely to administer such drugs under these circumstances. When asked whether the law should allow such treatment, assuming the patient has requested the drug and understands the consequences, 71 percent of the public and 53 percent of the physicians said yes. When asked whether a physician would be right or wrong to comply with the wishes of a dying patient in severe pain who directly asks to have his or her life ended, 45 percent of the public said it would be right. Among physicians, however just 5 percent thought such compliance was ethically permissible, and a mere 2 percent said they would comply with such a request. 52 percent of the public thought the law should allow physicians to comply with a request for mercy killing, but only 26 percent of physicians thought so. Harris, supra note 39, at 217–62. See also, John M. Ostheimer, "The Polls: Changing Attitudes toward Euthanasia, 44 *Pub. Opinion Q.* 123 (1980).

112. This is a weighty responsibility, and one that correctly entails serious liabilities for the physician if wrongly carried out. Society does want risky treatments to be offered and suffering to be relieved but wants to circumscribe the authority to risk life or to relieve suffering in ways expected to shorten life. One way to do so is to impose penalties for negligent or otherwise unjustified actions that lead to death, and this is the role of legal proceedings for homicide and wrongful death.

113. Part of this endeavor is the development by professional groups of standards of practice that can be publicly discussed and modified. See, e.g., the policies of various institutions and professional societies. . . . [and]; George P. Fletcher, "Prolonging Life: Some Legal Considerations," in Edwin S. Shneidman ed., *Death: Current Perspectives*, Mayfield Pub. Co., Palo Alto, Calif. (1976) at 484.

114. James J. McCartney, "The Development of the Doctrine of Ordinary and Extraordinary Means of Preserving Life in Catholic Moral Theology before the Karen Quinlan Case," 47 *Linacre Q.* 215 (1980). The first treatment of the topic was Soto's in 1582 when he pointed out that superiors could oblige their subjects under religious obedience to use medicine that could be taken without too much difficulty, but they could not oblige them to undergo excruciating pain because nobody is held to preserve life by such means. It was Banez who in 1595 introduced the terms "ordinary" and "extraordinary" into the discussion of the preservation of life. He stated that while it is reasonable to hold that a human being must conserve his or her life, one is not bound to employ extraordinary means, but only to preserve life by nourishment and clothing common to all, by medicine common to all, and even through some ordinary and common pain or anguish (*dolorem*), but not through any extraordinary or horrible pain or anguish, nor by any undertakings (*sumptos*) extraordinarily disproportionate to one's state in life. Jose Janini, "La operation quirurgica, remedio ordinario," 18 *Revista Espanola de Teologia* 335 (1958). For the current Catholic view, see note 132 infra.

115. For example, a statement of the House of Delegates of the American Medical Association (December 1973) employs the ordinary/extraordinary language: "The cessation of the employment of extraordinary means to prolong life of the body when there is irrefutable evidence that biological death is imminent is the decision of the patient and/or his immediate family." Quoted in Benedict M. Ashley and Kevin D. O'Rourke, *Health Care Ethics: A Theological Analysis*, The Catholic Hospital Association, St. Louis, Missouri (1978) at 390.

116. *In re* Quinlan, 70 N.J. 10, 355 A.2d 647, 667, *cert. denied*, 429 U.S. 922 (1976); *Superintendent of Belchertown State School v. Saikewicz*, 370 N.E.2d 417, 424 (1977).

117. *Satz v. Perlmutter*, 379 So.2d 359 (Fla. 1980).

118. Testimony of Dr. Marshall J. Brumer, transcript of 8th meeting of the President's Commission (April 9, 1981) at 60–61.

119. Testimony of Judge John G. Ferris, transcript of 8th meeting of the President's Commission (April 9, 1981) at 124.
120. See Leslie Steven Rothenberg, "Down's Syndrome Babies: Decisions Not to Feed and the Letter from Washington," 2 J. Calif. Perinatal Assoc. 73, 77–78 (Fall 1982).
121. There are some even less understandable uses of the term "extraordinary." In defining the term "extraordinary life support systems or procedures," the formal response to a question directed by a county's attorney to the Attorney General of California states:

> We further understand the word "extraordinary" to distinguish those systems or procedures which are utilized on a continuing basis as necessary to the person's health. Thus we are not here concerned with those treatment measures employed to replace or assist a vital function on a continuing basis such as a heart transplant, a pacemaker, kidney dialysis, and the like (65 Ops. Cal. Att'y Gen. 417, 418 (1982)). . . .

122. The ordinary-extraordinary distinction has had special importance and a special meaning within Catholic moral theology. The distinction dates back several centuries, but much of its prominence stems from its use by Pope Pius XII in a 1957 address in which he stated: "But normally one is held to use only ordinary means—according to circumstances of persons, places, times, and culture—means that do not involve any grave burden for oneself or another"("The Prolongation of Life," 4 *The Pope Speaks*, Vatican City [1958] at 393, 395–96).

    The distinction is here employed within a general theological view of human life as a gift from God that should not be deliberately destroyed by man. As such, it serves to clarify and qualify the absolute obligation to refrain from deliberately taking innocent human life, in light of medical treatments capable of extending a patient's life only by imposing grave burdens on the patient or others. The obligation to sustain life was extended to accepting ordinary, beneficial medical therapies, but not to require extraordinary therapies. For interpretations of the distinction within the Catholic tradition, see Richard A. McCormick, "To Save or Let Die: The Dilemma of Modern Medicine," 229 *J.A.M.A.* 172 (1974); Edwin F. Healy, *Medical Ethics*, Loyola Univ. Press, Chicago (1956); The Linacre Centre, "Ordinary and Extraordinary Means of Prolonging Life," Paper 3 in *Prolongation of Life*. Linacre Centre, London (1979).
123. Disagreement persists about which outcomes should count as being useful or burdensome (for example, whether the life that is sustained can itself be burdensome or only the treatment; whether financial costs are relevant burdens; whether evaluations can be specified independent of, or only in light of, a particular patient's circumstances and values; and especially whether benefits and burdens only to the patient or also to others such as the patient's family are relevant). See, e.g., McCartney, supra note 114.
124. For example, in *Quinlan*, the New Jersey Supreme Court dealt with the "Catholic view" only insofar as it related to the "conscience, motivation, and purpose of the intended guardian . . . and not as a precedent in terms of civil law." *In re* Quinlan, 70 N.J. 10, 355 A.2d 647, 660, *cert. denied*, 429 U.S. 922 (1976). Likewise the Eichner court admitted evidence as to Catholic teachings as "probative of the basis for Brother Fox's state in mind concerning this question" (*Eichner v. Dillon*, 426 N.Y.S.2d 517, 547 (App. Div. 1980), *modified in*, *In re* Storar, 52 N.Y.2d 363, 420 N.E.2d 64 (1981). The Cruse case also admitted expert testimony on Catholic teaching as evidence of the parents' "good faith" in seeking removal of a respirator. *In re* Benjamin Cruse Nos. J9 14419 and P6 45318, slip op. at 4 (Los Angeles Sup. Ct., Feb. 15, 1979).
125. *In re* Quinlan, 70 N.J. 10, 355 A.2d 647, 668, *cert. denied*, 429 U.S. 922 (1976).
126. *Superintendent of Belchertown State School v. Saikewicz*, 370 N.E.2d 417, 424 (1977) (citing Howard P. Lewis, "Machine Medicine and Its Relation to the Fatally Ill," 206 *J.A.M.A.* 387 (1968), citations omitted). The Dinnerstein court (*In re* Dinnerstein, 380 N.E.2d 134, 137 n.7 [Mass. App. Ct. 1978]) cited the same source and also relied upon fatal illness as a distinguishing factor:

> The essence of this distinction in defining the medical role is to draw the sometimes subtle distinction between those situations in which the withholding of extraordinary measures may be viewed as allowing the disease to take its natural course and those in which the same actions may be deemed to have been the cause of death.

127. *In re* Benjamin Cruse, Nos. J9 14419 and P6 45318, slip op. at 6–7 (Los Angeles Sup. Court, Feb. 15, 1979).
128. *Parker v. U.S.*, 406 A.2d 1275, 1279 n.1 (D.C. Ct. App., 1979).
129. *State Department of Human Services v. Northern*, 563 S.W.2d 197 (Tenn. Ct. App. 1978).
130. *Severns v. Wilmington Medical Center, Inc.*, 421 A.2d 1334, 1349 (Del. 1980).
131. Pope Pius XII acknowledged this in his statement that "Life, health, all temporal activities are in fact subordinate to spiritual ends" (*The Prolongation of Life*, supra note 122). See also Richard McCormick, "The Quality of Life, the Sanctity of Life," 8 *Hastings Ctr. Rep.* 30 (Feb. 1978); Robert M. Veatch, *Death, Dying and the Biological Revolution*, Yale Univ. Press, New Haven, Conn. (1976) at 77.
132. The Commission is not the first to have come to this conclusion. See, e.g.: "You do not need to puzzle for very long over the categorical distinction between 'ordinary' and 'extraordinary' means of saving life. By that I mean those terms as classes or categories of treatment are no longer useful" (Paul Ramsey, *Ethics at the Edge of Life*, Yale Univ. Press, New Haven, Conn. [1978] at 153). The overuse and misuse of the term has led the Vatican to question the usefulness of the terminology. The *Declaration on Euthanasia* proposes substituting "proportionate" and "disproportionate" for the more traditional, but perhaps outmoded, "ordinary/extraordinary." Sacred Congregation for the Doctrine of the Faith, *Declaration on Euthanasia* (June 26, 1980).

4. Patients Who Lack Decisionmaking Capacity

1. The term "incapacitated" is used in this Report to refer to patients who lack decisional capacity, rather than referring to general illness or disability. "Incapacity" as used here is roughly equivalent to the conventional legal usage of the term "incompetent."
2. President's Commission for the Study of Ethical Problems in Medicine and Biomedical and Behavioral Research, *Making Health Care Decisions*, U.S. Government Printing Office, Washington (1982) at 16988.
3. Ibid. at 56–68.
4. Determining the patient's incapacity, designating and informing a surrogate, and helping the surrogate to decide may require time that is not available in an emergency. In general, because of its grave nature and consequences, a decision to forego life-saving treatment should be made under conditions that permit consultation, reflection, and reasoned decision. In an emergency, ordinarily treatment ought to be given if no decision has previously been made to forego treatment. See generally Alan Meisel, "The 'Exceptions' to the Informed Consent Doctrine: Striking a Balance Between Competing Values in Medical Decisionmaking," 1979 *Wis. L. Rev.* 413, 436, 476.
5. Lois A. Weithorn and Susan B. Campbell, "The Competency of Children and Adolescents to Make Informed Treatment Decisions," 53 *Child Dev.* 1589 (1982). See also Thomas Grisso, *Juveniles' Waiver of Rights—Legal and Psychological Competence*, Plenum Press, New York (1981); Gary B. Melton, Gerald P. Koocher, and Michael J. Saks, eds., *Children's Competence to Consent*, Plenum Press, New York (1983). Law has traditionally viewed people under a specified age—long set at 21 years and more recently at 18—as incompetent to make decisions about any contractual matters, including their own health care; this reverses the usual presumption of competency accorded adults. Some exceptions have been created for "emancipated" or "mature" minors, in recognition that sometimes children have adequate capacity to make decisions and social policy ought to find such decisions sufficient. The ever-expanding scope of these exceptions calls into question the underlying presumption; it may be more reasonable to ask—of any person at any age—"is *this* person capable of making *this* decision?" See A. M. Capron, "The Competence of Children as Self-Deciders in Biomedical Interventions," in Willard Gaylin and Ruth Macklin, eds., *Who Speaks for the Child*, Plenum Press, New York (1982) at 57.

   The Commission endorses this general trend, recognizing that there is an age, below about 14 years old, at which the traditional presumption of incompetence remains sensible. The presumption, however, is merely a starting point for inquiry. See *Making Health Care Decisions*, supra note 2, at 170, n.6, and Sanford L. Leikin, "Minors' Assent or Dissent to Medical Treatment," ibid., vol. 3: Appendices (studies on the foundations of informed consent), at 175.
6. *Making Health Care Decisions*, supra note 2, at 172–73.
7. In fact, a diagnosis of a major psychiatric illness only rarely in itself decides the question of the patient's capacity to make a particular treatment decision. There is no necessary correspondence between mental illness and the presence or absence of decisional capacity either in fact or in law. See Rogers v. Okin, 634 F.2d 650, 657–59 (1st Cir. 1980).
8. See also Mark Perl and Earl E. Shelp, "Psychiatric Consultation Making Moral Dilemmas in Medicine," 307 *New Eng. J. Med.* 618 (1982).
9. The "mental status examination" is perhaps the best example of how professional expertise can be enlisted in making assessments of incapacity. Such an evaluation is intended, among other things, to elicit the patient's orientation to person, place, time, and situation, the patient's mood and affect, and the content of thought and perception, with an eye to any delusions and hallucinations; to assess intellectual capacity, that is, the patient's ability to comprehend abstract ideas and to make a reasoned judgment based on that ability; to review past history for evidence of any psychiatric disturbance that might affect the patient's current judgment; and to test the patient's recent and remote memory and logical sequencing.

   In testimony before the Commission, Dr. Paul Hardy, a neurologist, cited the Earle Spring case as an example of need for careful attention to underlying medical conditions bearing on determinations of competence. (Earle Spring's son petitioned a Massachusetts probate court for permission to stop dialysis treatments for his 79-year-old father who had been adjudged incompetent.)

   > If there is a . . . major travesty about the Earle Spring case, it lies in the utter confusion on the part of the judicial community and the medical community on how to go about determining competency . . . There was some conflicting testimony as to whether he was indeed competent or not, and there was even confusion over the exact medical condition and diagnosis. . . . [one psychiatrist] never once recognized that Mr. Spring was clearly aphasic and made certain determinations about Mr. Spring's competency based upon Mr. Spring's speech patterns. . . . I think the field of neuropsychiatry and behavioral neurology will be able to help considerably in the months and years ahead to characterize and define whether an individual is competent or not (Testimony of Paul Hardy, transcript of 10th meeting of the President's Commission [June 4, 1981] at 137–38; *In re* Spring, 405 N.E.2d 115 [Mass. 1980]).

10. See Paul S. Appelbaum and Loren H. Roth, "Clinical Issues in the Assessment of Competency," 138 *Am. J. Psychiatry* 1462 (1981); Loren H. Roth et al., "The Dilemma of Denial in the Assessment of Competency to Refuse Treatment," 139 *Am. J. Psychiatry* 910 (1982); Albert R. Jonsen, Mark Siegler, and William J. Winslade, *Clinical Ethics*, Macmillan Pub. Co., New York (1982) at 56–66.
11. Compare *Satz v. Perlmutter*, 379 So.2d 359 (Fla. 1980); *In re* Quackenbush, 156 N.J. Super. 282, 383 A.2d 785 (1978); *In re* Osborne 294 A.2d 372 (D.C. App. 1972), Lane v. Candura, 376 N.E.2d 1232 (Mass. App. 1978); *with* John F. Kennedy Hosp. v. Heston, 279 A.2d 670 (N.J. 1971); and Application of President and Directors of Georgetown College, Inc., 331 F.2d 1000, *rehearing denied*, 331 F.2d 1010 (D.C. 1964). The court's authority to intervene arises largely from the common-law doctrine of *parens patriae*, which recognizes that the state, through probate, juvenile, chancery, and other courts, must act as guardian for those people whose interests cannot otherwise be defended.

12. See, e.g., *State Dept. of Human Services v. Northern*, 563 S.W.2d 197 (Tenn. 1978); Lane v. Candura, 376 N.E.2d 1232 (Mass. App. 1978).
13. See, e.g., "Consents," 2 *Hospital Law Manual*, Aspen Systems, Rockville, Md. (1975) paragraph 4–12, at 58; Joseph H. King, Jr., *The Law of Medical Malpractice in a Nutshell*, West Publishing Co., St. Paul, Minn. (1977) at 140; "Note," 14 *Cin. L. Rev.* 161, 170–72 (1940). The practice of obtaining consent from family members "is so well known in society at large that any individual who finds the prospect particularly odious has ample warning to make other arrangements better suited to protecting his own ends or interests." A. M. Capron, "Informed Consent in Catastrophic Disease Treatment and Research," 123 *U. Pa. L. Rev.* 340, 424–25 (1974).
14. Joint Commission on Accreditation of Hospitals, *Accreditation Manual for Long Term Care Facilities*, Chicago (1980) at 54.
15. See, e.g., *In re* Dinnerstein 380 N.E.2d 134 (Mass. App. Ct. 1978); *In re* Nemser, 51 Misc.2d 616, 273 N.Y.S.2d 624 (Sup. Ct. 1966).
16. John R. Robertson, *The Rights of the Critically Ill*, Bantam Books, New York (1983) at 33; Charles H. Baron, "Assuring 'Detached but Passionate Investigation and Decision': The Role of Guardians Ad Litem in Saikewicz type Cases," 4 *Am. J. L. & Med.* 111 (1978); see also Testimony of Jonathan Brant, transcript of 10th meeting of the President's Commission (June 4, 1981) at 27–35.
17. Robert A. Burt, *Taking Care of Strangers*, The Free Press, New York (1979).
18. In some cases when a guardian is needed, courts have gone to remarkable lengths to identify and appoint even distant family members. See, e.g., *Application of Long Island Jewish-Hillside Medical Center*, 342 N.Y.S.2d 356 (Sup. Ct. 1973).
19. On occasion courts have substituted friends as decisionmakers for incompetent patients, even over the protest of available family members. See, e.g., George F. Will, "A Trip Toward Death," *Newsweek* 72 (Aug. 31, 1982) (an account of a California couple's attempt to gain custody, instead of the natural parents, of an institutionalized teenager with Down Syndrome). . . .
20. See, e.g., Testimony of David Spackman, J.D., transcript of 10th meeting of the President's Commission (June 4, 1981):

> We have had situations where the only family member was a daughter on the West Coast who had not seen her father for the last 20 years.
>
> He had lived with a drinking buddy of his for the last 20 years. Do we ignore this friend of his whose actions show that he cared also about him? Do we rely on the daughter who has no relationship in terms of interest in this patient? Often there are no family members at all, yet there may be friends and associates who knew the patient well. Do we ignore them because they do not constitute the traditional concept of family? (at 83).

21. See, e.g., Uniform Probate Code § 5–410.
22. See Richard A. McCormick and Robert M. Veatch, "The Preservation of Life and Self-Determination," 41 *Theological Studies* 390 (June 1980).
23. Although the majority of court cases brought on behalf of incompetent patients have involved closely related family members, one court noted the problems that might arise when defining the "family" for such purposes. In the combined appeal of *Storar* and *Eichner*, the majority criticized the "dissent which has abstractly endorsed the right of third parties, at least family members, to adopt a course of 'passive euthanasia' with respect to fatally ill incompetents. . . . Presumably this right could only be exercised by family members, thus imposing a 'restriction' which itself is open-ended, reaching to the limits of the family tree." *In re* Storar, 420 N.E.2d 64, 67 n.2 (N.Y. 1981), rev'g *In re* Storar, 433 N.Y.S.2d 388 (App. Div. 1980) and *modifying* Eichner v. Dillon, 426 N.Y.S.2d 527 (App. Div. 1980). Usually families appearing before courts have been unanimous in their agreement that treatment should be foregone. But see, *In re* Nemser, 51 Misc.2d 616, 273 N.Y.S.2d 624 (Sup. Ct. 1966) (disagreement over amputation for 80-year-old mother, with physician son opposing treatment and lawyer son in favor). See also Rhonda J.V. Montgomery, "Impact of Institutional Care Policies on Family Integration," 22 *The Gerontologist* 54 (1982).
24. If the guardian had been nominated by the patient prior to his or her incapacitation, he or she would almost always be included in the definition of family used here.
25. Allen E. Buchanan, "Medical Paternalism or Legal Imperialism: Not the Only Alternatives for Handling Saikewicz-type Cases," 5 *Am. J. L. & Med.* 97, 111 (1979). If an incapacitated patient has both a competent family and a legal guardian, they should function together as principal decisionmakers to the extent permitted by local law, and family members should know that they can challenge the guardian in court.
26. Testimony of Paul Rogers, transcript of 10th meeting of the President's Commission (June 4, 1981) at 106.
27. John J. Regan, "Protective Services for the Elderly: Commitment, Guardianship, and Alternatives," 13 *Wm. & Mary L. Rev.* 569, 609–12 (1972); Rogers, supra note 26, at 107; Maureen Morrisey, "Guardians Ad Litem: An Educational Program in Virginia," 22 *The Gerontologist* 301 (1982).
28. Testimony of Frank Repenseck, Director, Dade County Guardianship Program, transcript of 8th meeting of the President's Commission (April 9, 1981) at 187–204; Rogers, supra note 26, at 107.
29. The estimated cost given to the Commission for a proposed "corporate" guardianship service in Massachusetts was $3100 per patient per year at 1981 prices. Rogers, supra note 26, at 109.
30. Ibid., at 104. See also George J. Alexander, "Premature Probate: A Different Perspective on Guardianship for the Elderly," 31 *Stan. L. Rev.* 1003 (1979).
31. Testimony of Dr. Marianne Prout, transcript of 10th meeting of the President's Commission (June 4, 1981) at 12. This witness testified that a temporary guardian can be appointed in an emergency within a few hours, though even that delay is often detrimental to patient care.
32. *In re* Quinlan, 70 N.J. 10, 355 A.2d 647, *cert. denied*, 429 U.S. 922 (1976).
33. See *Custody of a Minor*, 385 Mass. 697, 434 N.E.2d 601, 607–09 (1982); *Superintendent of Belchertown State*

School v. Saikewicz, 370 N.E.2d 417 (Mass. 1977). See also pp. 153–57 infra.

34. *In re* Dinnerstein, 380 N.E.2d 134 (Mass. App. Ct. 1978).
35. See, e.g., *In re* Quinlan, 70 N.J. 10, 355 A.2d 647, *cert. denied*, 429 U.S. 922 (1976); *State Department of Human Services v. Northern*, 563 S.W.2d 197 (Tenn. Ct. App. 1978).
36. See generally A.M. Capron, "The Authority of Others to Decide about Biomedical Interventions with Incompetents," in Gaylin and Macklin, supra note 5, at 115, 119–133; Lawrence A. Frolik, "Plenary Guardianship: An Analysis, a Critique, and a Proposal for Reform," 23 *Ariz. L. Rev.* 599 (1981).
37. For example, the substituted judgment doctrine permits a surrogate to make a gift of some of an incompetent's assets to a relative to whom the incompetent person had previously made gifts. The court will approve such a gift to the extent that it does not endanger funds needed for the incompetent's support—even if the incompetent person would have been willing to be more generous.
38. For example, the New Jersey Supreme Court refused to give weight to statements Karen Ann Quinlan was reported to have made about her "distaste for continuance of life by extraordinary medical procedures, under circumstances not unlike those of the present case." Despite the fact that "she was said to have firmly evinced her wish," the court would not consider them because "they were remote and impersonal, [and] lacked significant probative weight." *In re* Quinlan, 70 N.J. 10, 355 A.2d 647, 653, *cert. denied*, 429 U.S. 922 (1976). In contrast, the New York Court of Appeals accepted the prior competent statements, made in the context of a discussion of the moral implications of the *Quinlan* case and in associated classroom teaching, of a religious brother whose medical condition paralleled Quinlan's. Brother Fox had said that "he would not want any of this 'extraordinary business' done for him under those circumstances." *In re* Storar, 52 N.Y.2d 363, 420 N.E.2d 64, 68 (1981).
39. This endeavor is especially difficult when the person expresses inconsistent or contradictory views or holds views that fluctuate over time. See *State Dept. of Human Services v. Northern*, 563 S.W.2d 197 (Tenn. Ct. App. 1978), involving an elderly woman suffering from gangrene who refused to consent to the amputation of her gangrenous feet, a procedure her physicians believed necessary to save her life. Despite the fact that she was, as described by the court, "an intelligent, lucid, communicative and articulate individual," she did not "accept the fact of the serious condition of her feet and [was] unwilling to discuss the seriousness of such condition or its fatal potentiality." Furthermore, the woman "had no wish to die" (ibid. at 205). Thus, the inconsistency of her views was that she both wanted to continue to live and to retain her feet, a position that was most untenable in light of the medical evidence. The court determined that this evidenced incapacity regarding the treatment decision and ordered the amputation.
40. Allen E. Buchanan, "The Limits of Proxy Decision Making for Incompetents," 29 U.C.L.A. L. REV. 393 (1981); John A. Robertson, "Legal Criteria for Orders Not to Resuscitate: A Response to Justice Liacos," in A. Edward Doudera and J. Douglas Peters, eds., *Legal and Ethical Aspects of Treating Critically and Terminally Ill Patients*, Aupha Press, Ann Arbor, Mich. (1982) at 159–63. See also, *In re* Storar, 52 N.Y.2d 363, 420 N.E.2d 64 (1981).
41. The best interests doctrine has received most attention in law in cases involving questions of the custody and care of children, see generally 2 C.J.S., Adoption of Persons §§ 90–91 (1972), and in cases involving the expenditure of trust funds, see generally 76 *Am. Jur.* 2D, Trusts § 288 (1975), neither of which are likely to be accurate guides to understanding how the standard ought to operate in instances of surrogate health care decisionmaking for adults who lack decisionmaking capacity.

    For a discussion of the best interests standard, see Joel Feinberg, *Rights, Justice, and the Bounds of Liberty*, Princeton Univ. Press, Princeton, N.J. (1980); Ruth Macklin, "Return to the Best Interests of the Child," in Gaylin and Macklin, supra note 5, at 265; Capron, supra note 36; Joseph Goldstein, Anna Freud, and Albert J. Solnit, *Beyond the Best Interests of the Child*, The Free Press, New York (1979).
42. This does not mean the surrogate must choose the means that an individual physician believes is most likely to benefit the patient maximally but only that the surrogate must have reason to believe that the patient will be maximally benefited. When multiple therapies have different risks, collateral effects, and degrees of success, the surrogate should try to weigh these reasonably and the surrogate's decision should be honored as long as a significant proportion of physicians would agree, whether or not this particular physician does. However, the best interests standard would preclude the surrogate from choosing a therapy that is professionally unacceptable, even if the surrogate might choose that treatment for him or herself.
43. The phrase "quality of life" has been used in differing ways; sometimes it refers to the value that the continuation of life has for the patient, and other times to the value that others find in the continuation of the patient's life, perhaps in terms of their estimates of the patient's actual or potential productivity or social contribution. In applying the best interest principle, the Commission is concerned with the value of the patient's life for the patient.
44. In the context of a decision about the forcible administration of antipsychotic medication, the Massachusetts Supreme Court counted the "impact upon the ward's family" as one of six factors to be considered in reaching a substituted judgment. See *In re* Richard Roe III, 421 N.E.2d 40, 58 (Mass. 1981):

    > An individual who is part of a closely knit family would doubtless take into account the impact his acceptance or refusal of treatment would likely have on his family. Such a factor is likewise to be considered in determining the probable wishes of one who is incapable of formulating or expressing them himself. In any choice between proposed treatments which entail grossly different expenditures of time or money by the incompetent's family, it would be appropriate to consider whether a factor in the incompetent's decision would have been the desire to minimize the burden on his family.
45. *Leach v. Akron General Medical Center*, 426 N.E.2d 809 (Ohio Com. Pl. 1980).

46. This Report uses "proxy" to mean a surrogate whose appointment rests on the designation of the patient while competent.
47. [Before this note and again before note 48, references to Appendixes (to this Report) and to Figure 1, a map showing state distribution of natural death acts and durable powers of attorney have been omitted.] See also Michael Garland, "Politics, Legislation and Natural Death," 6 *Hastings Ctr. Rep.* 5 (Oct. 1976); Richard A. McCormick and Andre Hellegers, "Legislation and the Living Will," 136 *America* 210 (1977); Barry Keene, "The Natural Death Act: A Well-Baby Check-up on Its First Birthday," 315 *Annals N.Y. Acad. Sci.* 376 (1978).
48. In one additional state, Louisiana, all powers of attorney are durable unless otherwise specified.
49. *Questions and Answers About the Living Wills* (pamphlet), [published by] Concern for Dying, New York (n.d.).
50. Walter Modell, "A 'Will' to Live" (Sounding Board), 290 *New Eng. J. Med.* 907 (1974); "Last Rights" (Letters), 295 *New Eng. J. Med.* 1139 (1976); See also Sissela Bok, "Personal Directions for Care at the End of Life," 295 *New Eng. J. Med.* 367 (1976).
51. Among the groups that have promulgated living wills are the Society or the Right to Die, the Euthanasia Education Council, the American Protestant Hospital Association, the American Catholic Hospital Association, and the American Public Health Association.
52. See note 49 supra.
53. Letter from Abigail van Buren to Joanne Lynn (Sept. 10, 1981). Ann Landers reports similar public enthusiasm. Letter from Ann Landers to Joanne Lynn (Sept. 16, 1981).
54. For a discussion of the legal effects of living wills, see Luis Kutner, "Due Process of Euthanasia: The Living Will, A Proposal," 44 *Ind. L. J.* 539, 552 (1969); Michael T. Sullivan, "The Dying Person—His Plight and His Right," 8 *New Eng. J. Med.* 197, 215 (1973); Comment, "Antidysthanasia Contracts: A Proposal for Legalizing Death with Dignity," 5 *Pac. L.J.* 738, 739–40 (1974); Note, "The 'Living Will': The Right to Death with Dignity?," 26 *Case W. Res. L. Rev.* 485, 509–526 (1976); Note, "Informed Consent and the Dying Patient," 83 *Yale L.J.* 1632, 1663–64 (1974); Note, "The Right to Die," 10 *Cal. W.L. Rev.* 613, 625 (1974).
55. See Note, "Living Wills—Need for Legal Recognition," 78 *W. Va. L. Rev.* 370 (1976); See also, *In re* Storar, 52 N.Y.2d 363, 420 N.E.2d 64 (1981) (on reliance on oral advance directives with burden of proof being clear and convincing evidence).
56. See Kutner, supra note 54; Note, "The 'Living Will': The Right to Death with Dignity?, "supra note 54; David J. Sharpe and Robert F. Hargest, "Lifesaving Treatment for Unwilling Patients," 36 *Fordham L. Rev.* 695, 702 (1968).
57. A UPI study, reported in "The Right to Die," 12 *Trial* (Jan. 1976), stated that no living will had been tested in the courts. None since has come to the Commission's attention.
58. See Note, "Living Wills—Need for Legal Recognition," 78 *W. Va. L. Rev.* 370, 377 (1976); Note, "The 'Living Will': The Right to Death With Dignity?," supra note 54, at 525–26.
59. See note 47 supra.
60. Like most provisions of the statutes, the requirement that the physician who refuses to comply must effectuate a transfer to another physician has not been tested. Such a transfer might at times be very difficult and a "good faith" effort might be the appropriate standard rather than the actual transfer.
61. The California statute stipulates that a physician's failure to effectuate a binding, though not a merely advisory, directive, or to transfer the patient to another physician who will effectuate the directive of the qualified patient, shall constitute unprofessional conduct. . . . The Texas statute weakens this penalty by stipulating that such a failure *may* constitute unprofessional conduct. . . . The statutes of Kansas and the District of Columbia, which do not contain the binding/advisory distinction, provide that the failure to properly transfer a patient when the physician cannot comply with a valid advance directive shall constitute unprofessional conduct. . . . The statutes of the remaining states make no explicit provision for penalties for physicians who do not comply with valid advance directives or transfer patients to physicians who will effectuate the directives. . . .
62. See Michigan House Bill No. 4492 (March 26, 1981), Appendix E, pp. 431–37 infra, which provides for the appointment of an agent for medical decisionmaking and presents an approach to physician penalties that is worth considering. Section 12(2) states:

> A physician or other health care professional acting under the direction of a physician who fails to observe a refusal of medical treatment or a request for continued medical treatment by an agent shall be legally liable in the same manner and degree as would have been the case if the appointor had been capable of making the decision and had refused or requested the treatment in his or her own right under similar circumstances.

See also Bruce L. Miller, "Michigan Medical Treatment Decision Act," in Cynthia B. Wong and Judith P. Swazey, *Dilemmas of Dying: Policies and Procedures for Decisions Not to Treat*, G.K. Hall Med. Pub., Boston (1981) at 161.
63. Cal. Health & Safety Code §§ 7187(e), 7191(b) (Deering Supp. 1982). . . .
64. Note, "The California Natural Death Act: An Empirical Study of Physicians' Practices," 31 *Stan. L. Rev.* 913, 928 (1979). Only two of the statutes passed since California's have followed that state's lead on these provisions. Although they differ in details, both Oregon and Texas treat only those directives executed after the patient has been informed that he or she has a terminal illness as "conclusively presumptive" of the patient's desires regarding the withholding or withdrawal of life-sustaining procedures. . . .
65. A.M. Capron, "The Development of Law on Human Death," 315 *Annals N.Y. Acad. Sci.* 45, 55 (1978).
66. See state statutes for Alabama, California, Delaware, the District of Columbia, Idaho, Kansas, New Mexico, Oregon, Texas, Vermont, and Washington in Appendix D [not reprinted in this volume]. . . .
67. See Table D1 [in Appendix D of this Report]. . . .

68. Del. Code Ann. tit. 16, § 2501(e) (1982). . . .
69. The California statute . . . refers to a patient advocate or ombudsman "as may be designated by the State Department of Aging for this purpose pursuant to any other applicable provision of law." A companion statute providing for such a service was not approved by the legislature, however, precluding residents of California nursing homes effectively from making valid directives. See Capron, supra note 65, at 56.
70. Note, "The California Natural Death Act," supra note 64, at 938–39.
71. McCormick and Hellegers, supra note 47. McCormick has since withdrawn his opposition to "living will" legislation, despite continuing concern with overtreatment of those who have not signed. See John J. Paris and Richard A. McCormick, "Living-Will Legislation, Reconsidered," 145 *America* 86, (1981):

    > Our experience of recent rulings by the . . . Courts on the need for legislative direction on these questions, and the fact that an overwhelming number of physicians, attorneys and legislation continue to believe an individual's statement has no legitimacy without a statutory enactment, force us to revise our previous opposition to this legislation (86–87).

72. Leon R. Kass, "Ethical Dilemmas in the Care of the Ill: II. What Is the Patient's Good?", 244 *J.A.M.A.* 1946, 1948 (1980).
73. A California Medical Association study of the effects of the California Natural Death Act, conducted one year after it went into effect, emphasized that "the Act has been a positive force in encouraging patients and their families to discuss the subject of terminal illness." Murray Klutch, "Survey Result After One Year's Experience with the National Death Act," 128 *West. J. Med.* 329, 330 (1978).
74. Del. Code Ann. tit. 16, § 2502(b) (1982). In the 1981 legislative session in Michigan, House Bill No. 4492 contained provisions designed to authorize the appointment of an agent for medical decisionmaking. . . .
75. See Appendix E [not reprinted in this volume].
76. See *Restatement (Second) of Agency*, American Law Institute Publishers, St. Paul, Minn. (1957) § 122.
77. Virtually all the durable power of attorney statutes enacted in approximately 40 states have been modeled on three acts: (1) Virginia Code Sections 11-9.1 to .2 (1950), (2) Model Special Power of Attorney for Small Property Interests Act (Uniform Law Commissioners, 1964), and (3) Uniform Probate Code Section 5-501 to 502 (1969). In 1979, the National Conference of Commissioners on Uniform State Law promulgated a Uniform Durable Power of Attorney Act, which has been enacted in four states as of February 1983. . . .

    The provisions of the Uniform Durable Power of Attorney Act are typical. Its basic provisions provide for the appointment of an attorney whose authority continues notwithstanding the principal's subsequent disability or incapacity (Sections 1 and 2). Other provisions protect those who engage in transactions with an attorney in fact (a proxy) by ensuring that, in the absence of the proxy knowing of the principal's death and provided the proxy acts in good faith, the authority to act is not revoked by the principal's death (Sections 4 and 5).
78. Four states—California, Kansas, Massachusetts, and Wisconsin—have adopted the Uniform Durable Power of Attorney Act, which creates a strong presumption for conservator of person but does not establish that power. . . .
79. National Conference of Commissioners on Uniform State Laws, *Handbook and Proceedings of the Annual Conference Meeting* 1964 (1964) at 273–74.
80. Yale Law School Legislative Services Project, *Medical Treatment Decision Act*, Society for the Right to Die, New York (1981) [and reprinted in Appendix D of this Report].
81. *Model Health Care Consent Act* (draft), National Conference of Commissioners on Uniform State Laws, Chicago (1982) [and reprinted in Appendix E of this Report].
82. *Uniform Right to Refuse Treatment Act* (draft), Concern for Dying, New York (May 1982) [and reprinted in Appendix E of this Report].
83. Michigan House Bill 4492 (March 26, 1981), [and reprinted in Appendix E]; see also Arnold S. Relman, "Michigan's Sensible 'Living Will'," 300 *New Eng. J. Med.* 1270 (1979).
84. These considerations were developed at greater length in *Making Health Care Decisions*, supra note 2, at 155–66.
85. [For example] (s)tatutes of Alabama, Delaware, Kansas . . . the Medical Treatment Decision Act . . . and the Uniform Right to Refuse Treatment Act . . . [Appendixes D and E of this Report, not reprinted in this volume.]
86. See state statutes for California, the District of Columbia, Kansas, Oregon, and Texas, Appendix D [not reprinted in this volume.]
87. There are no cases known to the Commission of penalties being imposed under any of the natural death acts that provide for them.
88. See . . . supra [the discussion "Determination of Incapacity," (Chapter 4, at the beginning)].
89. See, e.g., the California statute . . . .
90. For example, the *Model Health Care Consent Act*, . . . provides for a limited delegation of power by some individuals, authorized to consent to health care for another. The only proxies who may delegate their decisional authority are family members. Nonfamily health care representatives, who may be appointed according to the terms of the Act, are not authorized to delegate their decisional authority. All delegations must be in writing, and unless the writing so specifies, no further delegation of decisional authority is permitted. Any delegated authority terminates six months after the effective date of the writing.
91. See . . . supra [the subsection] *Substituted Judgment*, in "Surrogate Decisionmaking," [in chapter 4].
92. See Table D1 [in Appendix D of this Report].
93. Ibid.
94. Appendix D [of this Report].
95. An exception might be the patient who knows that foregoing a treatment is likely to bring about a period of incompetence prior to death, during which the patient might ask for the treatment. If such a patient wants to bind all parties concerned—health care professionals, family, and patient—in a promise to act in accord with the preferences expressed by the patient while competent, such a request might be honored. See Gail Povar, "Case #11," in James F.

Childress, *Who Should Decide? Paternalism and Health Care*, Oxford Univ. Press, New York (1982) at 224–25.

96. See . . . infra [subsequent discussions in Chapter 4; not reprinted in this volume].

5. Patients with Permanent Loss of Consciousness

1. Sometime after she ceased breathing for unknown reasons, Karen Quinlan was brought, unconscious, to a hospital emergency room. After her condition stabilized, feeding required a nasogastric tube and breathing required a respirator. She never experienced irreversible cessation of all brain functions (that is, death) but rather retained function of the brain stem and was diagnosed as being in a "persistent vegetative state," a condition that has not changed. Joseph Quinlan and Julia Quinlan, with Phyllis Battelle, *Karen Ann: The Quinlans Tell Their Story*, Doubleday & Co., Garden City, N.Y. (1977).
2. Karen Quinlan's father sought court appointment as guardian of her person for the express purpose of authorizing the removal of her respirator, whether or not she died as a consequence. He was opposed not only by Karen's physicians but by the local prosecutor and the state attorney general. The New Jersey Supreme Court, however, granted his request. Her physicians gradually discontinued the respirator during May of 1976 and she was able to breathe on her own; at this writing she is alive, cared for in a New Jersey nursing home. *In re* Quinlan, 70 N.J. 10, 355 A. 2d 647, *cert. denied* 429 U.S. 922, (1976); *In the Matter of Karen Quinlan* (2 vol.), Univ. Publications of America, Frederick, Md. (1977).
3. See, e.g., Lawrence K. Altman, "Princess Death: U.S. Physicians Raise Questions," *N.Y. Times*, Sept. 21, 1982, at C-1; Glenn Collins, "When Life Is a Matter for Debate," *N.Y. Times*, Aug. 16, 1982, at B-12.

   In addition to the well-known *Quinlan* case, there have been several other court reviews of the case of comatose patients. *Dockery v. Dockery*, 559 S.W. 2d 952 (Tenn. App. 1977) (appeal of chancery court order, which appointed husband as guardian for purposes of authorizing removal of respirator from comatose wife, mooted by wife's death); *In re* Piotrowicz, No. 1948 (Essex Cty., Mass. Probate Ct., Dec. 23, 1977) (husband appointed guardian of 56-year-old comatose wife for purposes of authorizing withdrawal of respirator); *In re* Nichols, No. A99511, Orange Cty. Calif. Super. Ct. (March 21, 1979) discussed in Note, "Comatose Conservatee—Restrictions of Legal Capacity—Substance or Procedure?" 7 *Wash St. U. L. Rev.* 205 (1980); *Leach v. Akron General Medical Center*, 426 N.E.2d 809 (Ohio Com. Pl. 1980) (family sought directive to disconnect life support); *In re* Storar 52 N.Y.2d 363, 420 N.E.2d 64 (1981), *modifying* Eichner v. Dillon, 426 N.Y.S.2d 527 (App. Div. 1980) (in which a comatose Catholic priest, Brother Joseph Fox, was allowed to have treatment stopped because he had given strong advance directives); *Severns v. Wilmington Medical Center, Inc.*, 421 A.2d 1334 (Del. 1980) (comatose woman with substantial advance deliberation allowed to stop all treatment); *In re* Lydia Hall Hospital, No. 23730182 (Special Term, Part II, Sup. Ct., Nassau County, N.Y., Oct. 22, 1982) (Peter Cinque, while competent, asked to cease dialysis and then became comatose after a resuscitation effort and court ordered discontinuation of treatment on family request); *In re* Cruse, No. J914419 and *In re* Guardianship of Cruse No. P645318 (Sup. Ct., Los Angeles, Cal., Feb. 15, 1979) (3-year-old child in coma, life-support discontinuance authorized); *In re* Young, No. A100863 (Sup. Ct., Orange County, Cal., Sept. 11, 1979) (removal of respirator allowed for comatose automobile accident victim).
4. President's Commission for the Study of Ethical Problems in Medicine and Biomedical and Behavioral Research, *Defining Death*, U.S. Government Printing Office, Washington (1981).
5. About 12%, typically those whose coma was due to drug intoxication, made a good to moderate recovery, and about an equal number were left with severe disability, though they regained consciousness. Ibid. at 94.
6. Ad Hoc Committee of the Harvard Medical School to Examine the Definition of Brain Death, "A Definition of Irreversible Coma," 205 *J.A.M.A.* 377 (1968).
7. See Julius Korein, "Terminology, Definitions and Usage," 315 *Annals N. Y. Acad. Sci.* 6 (1978); testimonies of Dr. Lawrence Pitts, Dr. Robert Kaiser, and Mr. Leslie Rothenberg, transcript of 12th meeting of the President's Commission (Sept. 12, 1981) at 348–65; testimony of Dr. David Levy, transcript of 15th meeting of the President's Commission (Dec. 12, 1981) at 275–82.
8. A determination of unconsciousness will therefore generally be based upon evidence that the person lacks any responsiveness to the internal or external environment (excepting unmodulated reflex responses), does not engage in purposive action, and manifests no other signs of mental activity.
9. Two other terms could have been used: "coma" and "vegetative state." But "coma" has often been used imprecisely and both terms might connote only a subset of the relevant group. Sometimes coma is graded to reflect all possible degrees of impaired consciousness. See, e.g., Graham Teasdale and Bryan Jennett, "Assessment of Coma and Impaired Consciousness—A Practical Scale," 1 *Lancet* 81 (1974); Bruce D. Snyder et al., "Neurologic Prognosis after Cardiopulmonary Arrest: II. Level of Consciousness," 30 *Neurology* 52 (1980). Others have insisted upon a more restrictive definition that includes absence of eye opening. "Coma is complete unresponsiveness with eyes closed." Fred Plum, "Consciousness and Its Disturbances: Introduction," in Paul B. Beeson, Walsh McDermott, and James B. Wyngaarden, eds., *Cecil Textbook of Medicine*, W.B. Saunders Co., Philadelphia (15th ed. 1979) at 640. The first usage is overly inclusive for the present discussion, as it includes responsive and sentient individuals; the second definition is overly restrictive as it excludes unconscious patients whose eyes open, like those in a "vegetative state," a large subgroup of patients with permanent unconsciousness.

   The term "vegetative state" (or, more anatomically, "apallic syndrome") denotes unconsciousness with persistent brain-stem functions that maintain subsistence functions and often wakefulness. It includes patients with the appearance of wakefulness but conversely excludes those who are more deeply comatose with closed eyes. See David H. Ingvar et al., "Survival after Severe Cerebral Anoxia with Destruction of the Cerebral Cortex: The Apallic Syndrome," 35 *Annals N.Y. Acad. Sci.* 184 (1978). The term needed for the discussion in this Report was selected to include deep coma and vegetative state but to exclude patients with partial impairments of consciousness. "Permanent loss of consciousness" accomplishes this.

10. Some hold that such a patient ought not to be considered a "person." See Joseph Fletcher, "Indicators of Humanhood," 2 *Hastings Ctr. Rep.* 1, 3 (Nov. 1972); Lawrence C. Becker, "Human Being: The Boundaries of the Concept," 4 *Phil. & Pub. Affairs* 334 (Summer 1975); John Lachs, "Humane Treatment and the Treatment of Humans," 294 *New Eng. J. Med.* 838 (1976). Rather than attempt to define "person," the Commission has concentrated on delineating the obligations to provide care to patients who have permanently lost consciousness, since it had earlier concluded that such patients are living human beings. *Defining Death*, supra note 4, at 7, 38–41.
11. Fred Plum and Jerome B. Posner, *The Diagnosis of Stupor and Coma*, F.A. Davis Co., Philadelphia (3rd ed. 1980) at 6.
12. Medical science has been unable to detect or postulate neurologic damage to the brain that would result in a functioning cerebrum capable of consciousness but able to perform absolutely no purposeful actions. At the least, to have consciousness a person must have some functioning cerebrum connected to adequate activating structures in the midbrain. Neurological findings indicate that having that much of a functioning central nervous system entails having at least the ability to blink voluntarily or move the eyes deliberately, and usually much more. Patients with the rare neurologic syndrome termed "locked-in state" retain only the ability to control movements of the eyes or eyelids. See, e.g., Martin H. Feldman, "Physiological Observations in a Chronic Case of 'Locked-in Syndrome'," 21 *Neurology* 459 (1971); Plum and Posner, supra note 11, at 6, 24.
13. The term "permanent" could have been replaced by "persistent," "irreversible," or "judged to be permanent." "Persistent" was rejected because it can apply to situations that are not permanent. Ordinarily a situation is persistent when it lasts a long time, but not necessarily forever. However, repeated evaluations over a period of persistence is often essential to a reliable prognostication of permanence.

    "Irreversible" not only conveys permanence but also focuses upon the prognostication of therapeutic possibilities, which might be a beneficial additional nuance. However, using "irreversible" to refer to this class of patients is virtually precluded by its inappropriate use in the phrase "irreversible coma" to describe neurologically dead bodies maintained on artificial circulatory and respiratory support. See notes 6 and 7, supra.

    The phrase "judged to be permanent" would highlight the irreducible element of probabilistic judgment that is part of the diagnosis of permanent unconsciousness. However, since such judgment is an essential part of every scientific prognostication, it is redundant and unnecessarily awkward. See, e.g., Alvan R. Feinstein, *Clinical Judgment*, Robert Kreiger Pub. Co., Huntington, N. Y. (1967); Mark Siegler, "Pascal's Wager and the Hanging of Crepe," 292 *New Eng. J. Med.* 853 (1975).
14. *Compact Edition of the Oxford English Dictionary*, Oxford University Press, New York (1971) at 710.
15. The only prevalence survey available estimates that Japan has about 2000 permanently unconscious patients in long-term care, which, if the prevalence were the same (and if differing definitions of terms did not cause substantial error), would imply less than 5000 at any one time in the United States. S. Sato et al., "Epidemiological Survey of Vegetative State Patients in Tokuhu District in Japan," 8 *Neurologia Medico-Chirurgia* (Tokyo) 141 (1978). See also, Peter Perl, "Silent Epidemic: Modern Medicine Saves Victims of Crash but Creates Dilemma: Coma," *Wash. Post*, March 18, 1982, at A-1; William D. Kalsbeek et al, "National Head Injury and Spinal Cord Injury Survey: Major Findings," 53 *J. Neurosurg.* 19 (Supp. 1980); *Defining Death*, supra note 4, at 92–95. Dr. Ake Grenvik reports between 500 and 1000 patients at Presbyterian-University Hospital in Pittsburgh have had life-sustaining treatment withdrawn because of permanent loss of the important cortical layers of the brain. Letter to Joanne Lynn, Dec. 14, 1981.
16. The longest case of coma on record is that of Elaine Esposito, who never recovered consciousness after receiving general anesthesia for surgery on August 6, 1941. She died 37 years and 111 days later. Norris McWhirter, ed., *The Guinness Book of World Records*, Bantam Books, New York (1981) at 42. See also the description of a woman injured at age 27 who neither regained consciousness nor left the hospital during the remaining 18 years of her life. Robert E. Field and Raymond J. Romanus, "A Decerebrate Patient: Eighteen Years of Care," 151 *Ill. Med. J.* 121 (1977).
17. Letter from Dr. Fred Plum, Neurologist-in-Chief, New York Hospital-Cornell Medical Center, New York, Dec. 22, 1981, reprinted in Appendix G [of this Report]. See also, "Predicting Outcome After Severe Brain Damage" (Editorial), 1 *Lancet* 523 (1973); *Eichner v. Dillon*, 426 N.Y.S.2d 517, 527–529, *modified in, In re* Storar, 420 N.E.2d 64 (1981).
18. Bryan Jennett and Fred Plum, "The Persistent Vegetative State: A Syndrome in Search of a Name," 1 *Lancet* 734 (1972); K. Higashi et al., "Epidemiological Studies on Patients with a Persistent Vegetative State," 40 *J. Neurol., Neurosurg. & Psychiatry* 876 (1977); Plum and Posner, supra note 11, at 338–40.
19. Testimony of Dr. Lawrence Pitts, transcript of 12th meeting of the President's Commission (Sept. 12, 1981) at 348–64; Bryan Jennett et al., "Severe Head Injuries in Three Countries," 40 *J. Neurol., Neurosurg., & Psychiatry* 291 (1977).
20. Bryan Jennett et al., "Prognosis of Patients with Severe Head Injury," 4 *Neurosurgery* 283 (1979); Thomas W. Langfitt, "Measuring the Outcome from Head Injuries," 48 *J. Neurosurg.* 673 (1978); *Defining Death*, supra note 4, at 89–107.
21. See David Bates et al., "A Prospective Study of Nontraumatic Coma: Methods and Results in 310 Patients," 2 *Annals Neurol.* 211 (1977); David E. Levy et al., "Prognosis in Nontraumatic Coma," 94 *Annals Int. Med.* 293 (1981); Higashi, supra note 18; *Defining Death*, supra note 4, at 92–95.

22. In one case, cognitive abilities became normal, although the patient suffered from emotional instability and paralysis of three limbs and remained completely dependent upon others for the rest of his life. Gary A. Rosenberg, Stephen F. Johnson, and Richard P. Brenner, "Recovery of Cognition after Prolonged Vegetative State," 2 *Ann. Neurol.* 167 (August 1977). The other case has recovered only to a locked-in status, with all communication by eyeblink. Lewis Cope, "Doctors Think Mack 'in vegetative state'," *Minneapolis Tribune*, March 20, 1980, at A-1; David Peterson, "Shooting Case Turns into Vigil," *Minneapolis Tribune*, March 7, 1980, at A-1; telephone interviews with Ronald Cranford, M.D., consultant neurologist on this case, Hennepin County Hospital, Minneapolis, Minn., March 8, 1982, and Dec. 2, 1982.
23. "Outcome of Non-Traumatic Coma" (Editorial), 2 *Lancet* 507 (1981); J.A. Bell and H.J.F. Hodgson, "Coma after Cardiac Arrest", 97 *Brain* 361 (1974); Fred Plum and John J. Caronna, "Can One Predict Outcome of Medical Coma?, Outcome of Severe Damage to the Central Nervous System," *CIBA Foundation Symposium* #34, Elsevier-North Holland, Amsterdam, (1975) at 121; Bruce D. Snyder, Manuel Ramirez-Lassepas, and D.M. Lippert, "Neurologic Status and Prognosis after Cardiopulmonary Arrest: I. A Retrospective Study," 27 *Neurology* 807 (1977); Bruce D. Snyder, et al., "Neurologic Prognosis after Cardiopulmonary Arrest: II. Level of Consciousness," 30 *Neurology* 52 (1980). Jorgensen and Malchow-Moller contend that recovery of consciousness before death can be reliably predicted from careful attention to the time course of EEG and brain stem reflex activity in the first 10 to 36 hours. E.O. Jorgensen and A. Malchow-Moller, "Natural History of Global and Critical Brain Ischaemia: Part III: Cerebral Prognostic Signs After Cardiopulmonary Resuscitation. Cerebral Recovery Course and Rate during the First Year after Global and Critical Ischaemia Monitored and Predicted by EEG and Neurological Signs," 9 *Resuscitation* 175 (1981). Snyder et al. state that "Reliable predictions of survival and outcome can often be based up on LOC [level of consciousness] within 2 days after CPA [cardiopulmonary arrest]." Bruce D. Snyder et al., "Neurologic Prognosis after Cardiopulmonary Arrest: II. Level of Consciousness," 30 *Neurology* 52 (1980). Evoked potentials may add to the reliability of these early prognostications. Richard Paul Greenberg and Donald Paul Becker, "Clinical Applications and Results of Evoked Potential Data in Patients with Severe Head Injury," 26 *Surg. Forum* 484 (1975).
24. This caution might be especially appropriate in children. See, e.g., "The brains of infants and young children have increased resistance to damage and may recover substantial functions even after exhibiting unresponsiveness on neurological examination for longer periods compared with adults." Medical Consultants on the Diagnosis of Death to the President's Commission for the Study of Ethical Problems in Medicine and Biomedical and Behavioral Research, "Guidelines for the Determination of Death," 246 *J.A.M.A.* 2184, 2186 (1981).
25. See, e.g., Snyder, Ramirez-Lassepas, and Lippert, supra note 22; Bell and Hodgson, supra note 22; *Defining Death*, supra note 4, at 92–95.
26. See Gayle C. Windham and Larry D. Edmonds, "Current Trends in the Incidence of Neural Tube Defects," 70 *Pediatrics* 333 (1982); Lewis B. Holmes, "The Health Problem: Neural Tube Defects," in National Center for Health Care Technology, *Maternal Serum Alphafetoprotein: Issues in Prenatal Screening and Diagnosis of Neural Tube Defects*, U.S. Government Printing Office, Washington (1980). The annual number of live births used to calculate incidence is from U.S. Department of Health and Human Services, *Health United States 1981*, U.S. Government Printing Office, Washington (1981).
27. One recent court case points out the conceptual and practical conundrums that arise in defining the interests of a person devoid of all mental life or conscious experience. The suit was brought on behalf of such a plaintiff, seeking damages for loss of enjoyment of life as a result of loss of customary activities. One of the questions for the court was whether it must be shown that the plaintiff is conscious of the fact that he has lost any enjoyment of life. The court answered that, under the disability law, conscious awareness of injuries need not be shown. *Flannery v. U.S.*, 51 U.S.L.W 2293, 2293 (W. Va. Sup. Ct., 1982).

    However, other legal questions are even more vexing: [Thus] Laurence H. Tribe, *American Constitutional Law*, Foundation Press, Mineola, N.Y. (1978):

    > Someone who has died cannot be said to have "rights" in the usual sense; although a person may have a right to determine how her body is dealt with after death, even that is a troublesome concept. . . . To be sure, Karen Quinlan was not "dead" in most of the increasingly multiple senses of that term, but the task of giving content to the notion that she had rights, in the face of the recognition that she could make no decisions about how to exercise any such rights, remains a difficult one (at 936, n 11).

28. John A. Robertson, "The Courts and Non-treatment Criteria," in Cynthia B. Wong and Judith P. Swazey, eds., *Dilemmas of Dying: Policies and Procedures for Decisions Not to Treat*, G.K. Hall Med. Pub., Boston (1981):

    > There is a small, finite chance that she [Karen Quinlan] could recover, so keeping her alive for that reason might be a benefit to her, for it at least leaves open the possibility of recovery. This is not to say that Karen Quinlan has a very great chance of recovery, but even a small possibility suggests that it may be in her interests to continue to be alive (at 105).

29. See note 22 supra. See also Martin Lasden, "Coming Out of Coma," *N.Y. Times*, June 27, 1982 (Magazine) at 29.
30. Testimony of Earl Appleby, transcript of 25th meeting of the President's Commission (Oct. 9, 1982) at 383–85.
31. When, some six weeks after the New Jersey Supreme Court opinion authorizing the discontinuance of the respirator for Karen Quinlan, the family asked her attending physician, Dr. Robert J. Morse, why the respirator care was still being continued, Dr. Morse explained, "I have tried to explain to you, I am following medical protocol." When asked how long he would keep her on the respirator if she could not successfully be weaned, Dr. Morse replied,

"For as long as it takes. Forever" (Quinlan and Quinlan, supra note 1, at 287).

Dr. Marshall Brumer, Abe Perlmutter's physician when Perlmutter requested the Florida courts to authorize removal of his life-supporting ventilator, told the Commission: "[The Court-ordered removal of the respirator] was an execution, as the day, location, time, and mode of death were all chosen by the court." When asked how he would have treated a respirator-dependent Karen Quinlan, Dr. Brumer replied, "My opinion of the Karen Ann Quinlan case is that I would support her with whatever technologies are available" (Testimony of Dr. Marshall Brumer, transcript of 8th meeting of the President's Commission [April 19, 1981] at 16).

32. The New Jersey Supreme Court recognized this interest, in a case involving a blood transfusion for a 23-year-old Jehovah's Witness who had been rendered incompetent and in need of blood as a result of an accident: "The medical and nursing professions are consecrated to preserving life. That is their professional creed. To them, a failure to use a simple established procedure in the circumstances of this case would be malpractice." *John F. Kennedy Memorial Hospital v. Heston*, 279 A.2d 670, 673 (1971).

More recently, however the Massachusetts Supreme Judicial Court denied that an independent interest of health professionals exists that would go against what patients want or will find beneficial. [See] *Superintendent of Belchertown School v. Saikewicz*, 370 N.E.2d 417 426 (1977):

> Recognition of the right to refuse necessary treatment in appropriate circumstances is consistent with existing medical mores; such a doctrine does not threaten either the integrity of the medical profession, the proper role of hospitals in caring for such patients or the State's interests in protecting the same. It is not necessary to deny a right of self-determination to a patient in order to recognize the interests of doctors, hospitals, and medical personnel in attendance on the patient. Also, if the doctrines of informed consent and right of privacy have as their foundations the right to bodily integrity and control of one's own fate, then those rights are superior to the institutional considerations.

33. Two unusual circumstances present additional considerations for the interests of others. First, occasionally a permanently unconscious woman is pregnant. If the pregnancy can be continued to the stage of viability for the infant, the interests of the child and the family would usually provide adequate justification for vigorous life-support and therapy until delivery. See *Wash. Post*, March 2, 1982, at A-2, noting the case of a 23-year-old Oregon woman who gave birth to a 7 lb. 13 oz. child after being comatose and on life-support systems for four months. But see *Pettit v. Chester County Hospital*, No. 322, August Term 1982 (Court of Common Pleas, Chester County, Pa.); Mark Butler, "Judge Rules Comatose Woman Can Have Abortion," *Phil. Inquirer*, Aug. 26, 1982, at A-1. See generally William P. Dillon et al., "Life Support and Maternal Brain Death During Pregnancy," 248 *J.A.M.A.* 1089 (1982).

Second, permanently unconscious patients may be desirable subjects for research. When the research offers prospect of even distant benefit to the subject, it might be approved in the usual way. When the research is not intended to benefit the subject, it would probably be very difficult to secure legally effective consent from a surrogate. See President's Commission, *Protecting Human Subjects*, U.S. Government Printing Office, Washington (1981) at 74–76; Task Force on Research on Senile Dementia, Vijaya Melnick, ed., *Guidelines for Research on Senile Dementia of the Alzheimer's Type*, submitted to National Institutes on Aging (Nov. 1982). Since it would be so easy to overuse these patients in research, great caution is probably appropriate before considering any weakening of the protection involved in the requirement for valid consent.

34. At least one court has specifically denied a state interest in preserving such a patient's life: "Such a patient has no health and, in the true sense, no life for the state to protect." *Eichner v. Dillon*, 426 N.Y.S.2d 517, 543 (1980) *modified in, In re* Storar, 420 N.E.2d 64 (1981).

35. In 1968 Henry Beecher estimated it would cost $25,000 to $30,000 per year for hospital care for each permanently unconscious patient. Henry K. Beecher, "Ethical Problems Created by the Hopelessly Unconscious Patient," 278 *New Eng. J. Med.* 1425 (1968). While these costs are mitigated by providing care in a skilled nursing facility, inflation must also be taken into account. Even skilled nursing facilities can now cost over $25,000 per year. Telephone survey of Washington, D.C., area nursing homes (Dec. 1982).

Reported cases provide striking cost estimates. A comatose Tennessee woman who was maintained on a respirator because her death without it might lead to a murder prosecution was costing $1000 per day. David Meyers, "The California Natural Death Act: A Critical Appraisal," 52 *Cal. St. Bar J.* 326 (1977). Four months of care for a comatose child cost about $40,000. *In re* Benjamin Cruse. Nos. J9 14419 and P6 45318 (Los Angeles Superior Ct., Feb. 15, 1979). The first two years of care for an adolescent with persistent vegetative state cost $280,000. Ronald E. Cranford and Harmon L. Smith, "Some Critical Distinctions between Brain Death and Persistent Vegetative State," 6 *Ethics in Sci. & Med.* 199, 203 (1979). See also note 115, in Chapter Four.

36. The disruption of family life, together with the emotional drain on families which elect to care for these patients at home, can be very significant. Moreover, sensational but unverified reports from the lay literature regarding miraculous recovery in patients with irreversible brain damage are often unsettling to the families and a source of false hope and further emotional turmoil.

6. Seriously Ill Newborns

1. *See* pp. 179–81 *supra*, and the President's Commission for the Study of Ethical Problems in Medicine and Biomedical and Behavioral Research, *Making Health Care Decisions*, U.S. Government Printing Office, Washington (1982) at 181–88, for a general discussion of the designation and role of surrogates.

2. There are any number of explanations for this societal allocation of authority: respect for the family and a desire to foster the diversity which it brings; the fitness of giving the power to decide to the same people who created the child

> and have the duty to support and protect him; the belief that a child cannot be much harmed by parental choices which fall within the range permitted by society and a willingness to bear the risks of harm this allocation entails or a belief that in most cases "harm" would be hard for society to distill and measure anyway; or simply the conclusion that the administrative costs of giving authority to anyone but the parents outweigh the risks for children and for society unless the parents are shown to be unable to exercise their authority adequately.

A. M. Capron, "Legal Considerations Affecting Clinical Pharmacological Studies in Children," 21 *Clinical Research* 141, 146 (1972).

3. Margaret O'Brien Steinfels, "Children's Rights, Parental Rights, Family Privacy, and Family Autonomy," in Willard Gaylin and Ruth Macklin, eds., *Who Speaks for the Child*, Plenum Press, New York (1982) at 223.
4. Although some of the earlier cases were rooted in religious claims, others—including a companion case to *Pierce*—were rooted in liberty interests. *See Pierce v. Hill Military Academy*, 268 U.S. 510 (1925). Since the enunciation of a constitutional right of privacy in Griswold v. Connecticut, 381 U.S. 479 (1965), and its subsequent growth, claims of parental autonomy now seem more appropriate to be couched in those terms.
5. *Prince v. Massachusetts*, 321 U.S. 158, 166 (1944).
6. *See, e.g.*, Herman A. Hein, Christina Christopher, and Norma Ferguson, "Rural Perinatology," 55 *Pediatrics* 769 (1975); Herman A. Hein, "Evaluation of a Rural Perinatal Care System," 66 *Pediatrics* 540 (1980).
7. John C. Fletcher, *Coping with Genetic Disorders: A Guide for Clergy and Parents*, Harper & Row, New York (1982).
8. John A. Robertson, "Dilemma in Danville," 11 *Hastings Ctr. Rep.* 5, 6 (Oct. 1981).
9. There are no reported appellate cases of this type, but a few trial court decisions have overridden parental refusals of treatment of their defective newborn children. *See, e.g.*, Maine Medical Center v. Houle, No. 74–145 (Cumberland County Super. Ct., Maine, Feb. 14, 1974) (court order to repair meningomyelocele mooted by baby's death); *In re* Cicero, 101 Misc.2d 699, 421 N.Y.S.2d 965 (Sup. Ct. Bronx County, 1979) (parental refusal to treat meningomyelocele overridden). *In re* Elin Daniel, Case No. 81–15577 FJO1 (Miami, Fla., June 23, 1981); "Court-Ordered Surgery on Baby Held Success," *N.Y. Times*, Sept. 18, 1981, at A-9.
10. With some exceptions . . . the staff's assessment of parents and parents' dispositions toward their babies and the degree to which parents are understanding what is being told to them is often inaccurate. Most assessments of parents are based on limited knowledge, derived mainly from short observations, limited conversations, or secondhand reporting of incidents and information. What is known is episodic, not informed by the context of the perinatal experience in the lives of the parents.

Robert Bogdan, Mary Alice Brown, and Susan Bannerman Foster, "Be Honest but Not Cruel: Staff/Parent Communication on a Neonatal Unit," 41 *Human Organization* 11 (1982).

11. The importance of adopting the viewpoint of the incompetent patient, see pp. 181–82 *supra*, is especially well illustrated regarding newborns. For many adults, life with severe physical or mental handicap would seem so burdensome as to offer no benefits. However, this assessment arises largely from the adults' existing hopes and aspirations that would be forever unfulfilled. From the perspective of an infant who can be helped to develop realistic goals and satisfactions, such frustrations need not occur. In fact, many severely handicapped persons are quite successful in finding and creating meaningful lives despite various limitations. Adopting the infant's point of view requires valuing these successes equally with a more conventional ideal. *See, e.g.*, Karen M. Metzler, "Human and Handicapped," in Samuel Gorovitz *et al.*, eds., *Moral Problems in Medicine*, Prentice-Hall, Inc., Englewood Cliffs, N.J. (1976) at 358.
12. For a discussion of discrimination against handicapped, see Institute of Medicine, *Health Care in the Context of Civil Rights*, National Academy of Sciences, Washington (1981). *Cf.* Helge H. Mansson, "Justifying the Final Solution," 3 *Omega* 79 (May 1972).
13. People differ in their assessment of when a potential prolongation of life is to be taken as meaningful. The analysis in this section applies to babies whose lives will end in infancy and are likely be measured in hours or days, not years.

> Medicine may *never* have all the solutions to all the problems that occur at birth. I personally foresee no medical solution to a cephalodymus or an anencephalic child. The first is a one-headed twin; the second, a child with virtually no functioning brain at all. In these cases the prognosis is an early and merciful death by natural causes. There are no so-called "heroic measures" possible and intervention would merely prolong the patient's process of dying. Some of nature's errors are extraordinary and frightening . . . but nature also has the kindness to take them away. For such infants, neither medicine nor law can be of any help. And neither medicine nor law should prolong these infants' process of dying.

Dr. C. Everett Koop, Statement before Hearing on Handicapped Newborns, Subcomm. on Select Education Comm. on Education and Labor, U.S. House of Representatives (Sept. 16, 1982).

14. *See* pp. 91–94 of original report (not reprinted in this volume).
15. Uncertainty about the course is partly the consequence of the rapidly expanding ability to save newborns who until recently could not have survived. Neonatal intensive care is a rapidly developing field and long-term follow-up on much of the most modern treatment is not yet available. Limited experience also compromises the ability to assess the effects—especially long-term physical and psychological effects—of medicine's effort to create a womb-like environment for the premature infant. *See* Albert R. Jonsen, "Justice and the Defective Newborn," in Earl E. Shelp, ed., *Justice and Health Care*, D. Reidel Pub. Co., Boston (1981) at 95.
16. John Lorber, "Early Results of Selective Treatment of Spina Bifida Cystica," 4 *Brit. Med. J.* 201 (1973); John Lorber, "Results of Treatment of Myelomeningocele," 13 *Dev. Med. & Child Neurol.* 279 (1971). *See also* Terrence

F. Ackerman, "Meningomyelocele and Parental Commitment: A Policy Proposal Regarding Selection for Treatment," 5 *Man & Med.* 291 (1980).

17. John M. Freeman, "The Shortsighted Treatment of Myelomeningocele: A Long-Term Case Report," 53 *Pediatrics* 311 (1974); Robert Reid, "Spina Bifida: The Fate of the Untreated," 7 *Hastings Ctr. Rep.* 16 (Aug. 1977).
18. Robert M. Veatch, "The Technical Criteria Fallacy," 7 *Hastings Ctr. Rep* 4. 15, 16 (Aug. 1977).
19. Courts, for example, sometimes automatically assume the priority of the value of a longer life. In the case of Kerri Ann McNulty, a Massachusetts probate judge ruled that corrective surgery had to be done on a month-old infant diagnosed as having congenital rubella, cataracts on both eyes, deafness, congenital heart failure, respiratory problems, and probable severe retardation. After reviewing the medical testimony, the court explicitly eschewed "quality of life" considerations, stating: "I am persuaded that the proposed cardiac surgery is not merely a life prolonging measure, but indeed is for the purpose of saving the life of this child, *regardless of the quality of that life.*" In the Matter of Kerri Ann McNulty, No. 1960 (Probate Ct., Essex Co., Mass., Feb. 15, 1978).
20. Veatch, *supra* note 18, at 15. *But see* Stuart F. Spicker and John R. Raye, "The Bearing of Prognosis on the Ethics of Medicine: Congenital Anomalies, the Social Context and the Law," in Stuart F. Spicker, Joseph M. Healy, Jr., and H. Tristam Engelhardt, Jr., eds., *The Law-Medicine Relation: A Philosophical Exploration*, D. Reidel Pub. Co., Boston (1981) at 189, 202–05, 212.
21. Many have noted that diffusion of responsibility often acts to make no one feel responsible. *See. e.g.*, R. B. Zachary. "Commentary: On the Death of a Baby," 7 *J. Med. Ethics* 5, 11 (1981).

7. Resuscitation Decisions

1. *See*, "Doctor Sees Trend Not to Resuscitate," *Wash. Post*, June 13, 1982, at A-4.
2. *See* pp. 26–27 of original report.
3. Although the attending physician bears the responsibility, often others among the care giving professionals, religious advisors, or family members are in a good or better position to discuss the issues and convey the information. This is to be encouraged, but the physician is still obliged to see that it is done well.
4. Contrary to the Commission's conclusions, some have contended that involving the patient is unnecessary:

> Consent of the patient is irrelevant because we are dealing with a situation in which there is no course of treatment for which to secure consent. This is different from the case in which there is a medically accepted course of treatment, but the patient does not wish to be subjected to this care.

William G. Ketterer, Senior Attorney, NIH, in a letter to James H. Erickson, Assistant Surgeon General and Joel M. Mangel, Deputy Assistant General Counsel for Public Health (April 8, 1977) at 6. The Commission finds it necessary for the patient or surrogate to have given valid consent to any plan of treatment, whether involving omissions or actions, and rejects this claim. *See* pp. 66–73 and 126–31 *supra*.

5. *See, e.g.*, "Such explanations to the patient, on the other hand, are thoughtless to the point of being cruel, unless the patient inquires, which he is extremely unlikely to do." Steven S. Spencer, "'Code' or 'No Code': A Non Legal Opinion," 300 *New Eng. J. Med.* 138, 139 (1979). *But see* "The physician and family often underestimate the patient's ability to handle this issue and participate in the decision." Steven H. Miles, Ronald E. Cranford, and Alvin L. Schultz, "The Do-Not-Resuscitate Order in a Teaching Hospital," 96 *Annals Int. Med.* 660, 661 (1982).
6.

> Sometimes it seems cruel and unnecessary. Other times it is just difficult, in the midst of what is usually a very emotional and difficult time, to get around to the question of whether you want us pumping on your chest when you die. . . . Having taken care of someone for some period of time has usually generated prior tacit, if not overt, understanding between the patient and me on these issues.

Michael Van Scoy-Mosher, "An Oncologist's Case for No-Code Orders," in A. Edward Doudera and J. Douglas Peters, eds., *Legal and Ethical Aspects of Treating Critically and Terminally Ill Patients*, AUPHA Press, Ann Arbor, Mich. (1982) at 16; *see also* Ronald A. Carson and Mark Siegler, "Does 'Doing Everything' Include CPR?" 12 *Hastings Ctr. Rep.* 27 (Oct. 1982); John J. Paris, "Comfort Measures Only for 'DNR' Orders," 46 *Conn. Med.* 195 (April 1982).

7. President's Commission for the Study of Ethical Problems in Medicine and Biomedical and Behavioral Research, *Securing Access to Health Care*, U.S. Government Printing Office, Washington (1983) at 4.
8. "[W]hether one month's additional cost of acute hospital care should or should not be incurred . . . is an important and relevant ingredient in the decisionmaking process . . [W]e as a society must face the issue not of whether to preserve life but rather for how long." Letter from Joel May, Health Research and Educational Trust of New Jersey, to Joanne Lynn (May 11, 1982). "[T]he prolongation of life in hopeless situations must truly be viewed in the context of family resources and societal resources." Letter from Leo F. Greenawalt, President, Washington State Hospital Association, to Austin Ross, Vice-President, Virginia Mason Hospital, Seattle, WA (June 10, 1982). "Obviously, we must be very careful not to waste precious resources and money when it is to no avail." Letter from Dr. Ake Grenvik, Professor of Anesthesiology and Surgery, Univ. of Pittsburgh, to Joanne Lynn (March 30, 1982).

Proposals have been made that patients with advanced and irreversible diseases and organ system failures, including dementia, should not be offered resuscitation, principally because the expense and the necessary shifting of resources from other important uses are considered so disproportionate to the benefits. *E.g.*, in 1967 BBC-TV reported the following notice in a London hospital: "The following patients are not to be resuscitated: very elderly, over 65, malignant disease. Chronic chest disease. Chronic renal disease." In the controversy that ensued the physician who posted the notice received public support from a number of his colleagues. Louis Lasagna, "Physicians' Behavior Toward the Dying Patient," in Orville Brim, Jr., *et al.*, eds., *The Dying Patient*, Russell Sage Foundation, New York (1970) at 87.

9. Resuscitation efforts themselves commonly cost over $1000 and usually entail substantial derivative costs in caring for the surviving patients who suffer side effects.
10. *See* pp. 97–98 of original report.
11. *See* pp. 98–100 of original report. See also, *Securing Access to Health Care*, *supra* note 7, at 185–90.
12. For a discussion of the rationale and procedures for prior directives *see* pp. 182–88 *supra*. The weight assigned to such written or oral instructions—in other words, the extent to which a presently *incompetent* patient is treating as expressing a *competent* preference through an advance directive—depends on the facts of each case.

    If a patient while competent anticipated a later incompetence and medical condition, understood what should be entailed in a decision for or against resuscitation, and made firm and explicit statements regarding the decision, then those directives should be honored provided there is no reason to think that the patient's choice had changed or would have changed. Advance directives can be in the form of written instructions or of statements made to health care professionals, members of a patient's family, or others.

    The physician will have to assess whether the patient adequately understood the ramifications of the choice and clearly stated his or her decision.
13. *See* Comment, "Medico-Legal Implications of 'Orders Not to Resuscitate,'" 31 *Cath. U. L. Rev.* 515, 535 (1982).
14. *See* pp. 160–70 of original report.
15. *See* pp. 30–32, 39 of original report. To stop recourse to the courts from becoming routine, the courts could decline DNR cases involving competent patients unless the circumstances were unusual. Particularly to be discouraged are cases in which physicians or hospitals desire court review of decisions that are actually uncontroversial, simply to shield themselves from liability.
16. See pp. 235–36 of original report.
17. *See generally* Theodore R. LeBlang, "Does Your Hospital Have a Policy for No-Code Orders?" Part 2, 9 *Leg. Aspects Med. Practice* 5, 6–7 (April 1981); No Code Subcommittee of the Medical-Legal Interprofessional Committee, sponsored by the San Francisco Medical Society and the Bar Association of San Francisco, *Final Report*, July 20, 1982 . . . . *infra*. Miles, Cranford, and Schultz, *supra* note 5; "No-Code Orders," 7 *L. Rep.* 1 (March 1982); Aileen McPheil et al., "One Hospital's Experience With a 'Do No Resuscitate' Policy," 125 *Canadian Med. Assoc. J.* 830 (1980).
18. Concerns about resuscitation practices are not, however, limited to the hospital settings. "All information available on CPR deals with hospital settings. I am concerned about long term care facilities because the population is different and I feel their age and condition preclude mandatory blanket CPR. . . . The usual policy is to let the nurse on the scene make a decision." A nurse quoted in Jane Greenlaw, "Orders Not to Resuscitate: Dilemma for Acute Care as Well as Long-Term Care Facilities," 10 *L. Med. & Health Care* 29 (Feb. 1982).
19. Since the principles governing decisionmaking about resuscitation are the same as for decisionmaking generally, such a policy might well include other decisions. Indeed, at Northwestern Memorial Hospital near Chicago, the policy covers all orders that preclude "the use of extraordinary or 'heroic' measures to maintain life." Reprinted in Appendix I pp. 511–13 of original report. The policy at the University of Wisconsin's hospital covers decisionmaking generally. . . .
20. Mila Aroskar, Josephine M. Flaherty, and James M. Smith, "The Nurse and Orders Not to Resuscitate," 7 *Hastings Ctr. Rep.* 27 (Aug. 1977); Leah Curtin, "CPR: Optimal Care vs. Maximal Treatment," 10 *Supervisor Nurse* 16 (Aug. 1979).
21. "The physician must discuss his/her opinion and decision concerning both competence and DNR orders with the nursing staff from the outset and frequently thereafter." *Guidelines: Orders Not to Resuscitate*, Somerville Hospital, Mass., Memorandum #80-7, (Feb. 27, 1980), *reprinted in* Appendix I, pp. 507–10 of original report.
22. > [The use of partial codes] represents a tempting act of rationalization that is neither medically nor ethically sound. At best it is a waste of time and a failure to face reality and hard decisionmaking; at worst, it is an ethical fraud. I doubt that "partial codes" can be justified, but I see them frequently . . .

    John Goldenring, Letter, 300 *New Eng. J. Med.* 1057, 1058 (1979).
23. > There are many forms of "codes": slow code, chemical code, partial code. In my opinion, there is a time and a place for a limited code. Recently, I took care of an Hassidic rabbi. Because Hassidic Jews are very uncomfortable with DNR orders or anything that might hasten death, such a course of action was not acceptable to him. We decided that it was reasonable to make some effort to resuscitate, but not necessarily all efforts. Setting such a limit on resuscitative efforts was acceptable to the family. In this case we decided that it would not be acceptable to intubate him nor to leave him on a respirator. So, there is a way of giving what I will call a partial code—some attempt at resuscitation, but not applying everything known to man.

    Michael Van Scoy-Mosher, *supra* note 6, at 15 (citation omitted). *See also* Marc D. Basson, "Introduction: The Decision to Resuscitate-Slowly," in Marc D. Basson, Rachel Lipson, and Doreen Ganos, eds., *Troubling Problems in Medical Ethics*, Alan R. Liss, Inc., New York (1981) at 117; Paris, *supra* note 6.
24. The no-resuscitation status is compatible with maximal and aggressive medical care, and does not imply that current treatment will be withdrawn or that additional therapy will not be initiated. Decisions as to the choice and level of treatment should be based on continued evaluation of clinical information and the patient's condition regardless of a do-not-resuscitate order.

    Miles, Cranford, and Schultz, *supra* note 5, at 661. *But see* David Baror, "The Do Not Resuscitate Order" (Letter),

97 *Annals Int. Med.* 280 (1982); George Spelvin (pseudonym), "Should a 'No-Code' Be a Death Sentence?," *Med. World News* 64 (April 27, 1981).

25. *See* pp. 94–95 of original report.
26. In one series of 48 cases, two patients whose cardiac arrests resulted directly from biomedical procedures survived resuscitation to go home. Francis P. Arena, Martin Perkin and Alan Turnbull, "Initial Experience with a 'code-no code' Resuscitation System in Cancer Patients," 8 *Critical Care Medicine* 734 (1980). In particular, policies should encourage consideration of this potential dilemma when especially risky procedures are being discussed with a patient who otherwise would have a DNR order.
27. Comment, "Medico-Legal Implications of 'Orders Not to Resuscitate,'" supra note 13, at 518 n.9; Testimony of Dr. Mitchell Rabkin, transcript of 10th meeting of the President's Commission (June 4, 1981) at 65–69.

IN THE MATTER OF CLAIRE CONROY: THE SUPREME COURT, STATE OF NEW JERSEY (1985)

INTRODUCTION. *Almost a decade after Quinlan and Saikewicz, people were more willing to entertain the possibility of forgoing ventilators, major cancer treatment, and other high tech, complex efforts to prolong the dying process. Reasoning about the potential benefits and harms of life support was now applied to more everyday, routine procedures: medications, CPR, and medical means to supply nutrition and hydration. Key court cases and legislation in the mid-1980s dealt with decisions to forgo nasogastric tubes, gastrostomies, and intravenous fluids.*

Claire Conroy had a reputation of disliking physicians. Suffering from organic brain syndrome, she developed gangrene that led her physician to recommend an amputation of her leg. Her nephew, her nearest relative, refused on the grounds that his aunt would not want the surgery. It was a sign of the social change in the past decade that the nephew's decision was accepted. But then Ms. Conroy's nutritional status deteriorated leading to the placing of a nasogastric tube. When her nephew attempted to refuse consent to the tube, his decision was challenged. Ms. Conroy died before the New Jersey Supreme Court was able to rule, but the court, recognizing that similar problems were likely to arise, identified three conditions under which nutrition and hydration could be foregone: (1) if it is clear that the particular patient would have refused the treatment under the circumstances involved, (2) if there is evidence that the patient would have refused the treatment and the burdens markedly outweigh the benefits, or (3) if the net burdens markedly outweigh the benefits and continuing treatment would be inhumane.

In 1979 Claire Conroy, who was suffering from an organic brain syndrome that manifested itself in her exhibiting periodic confusion, was adjudicated an incompetent, and plaintiff, her nephew, was appointed her guardian. The guardian had Ms. Conroy placed in the Parkview Nursing Home, a small nursing facility with thirty beds. There she came under the care of Dr. Kazemi, a family practitioner, and Catherine Rittel, a registered nurse, who was the nursing home administrator. Upon her admission, Ms. Conroy, although confused, could converse and follow directions, was ambulatory, and was in relatively good physical condition. Thereafter, she became increasingly confused, disoriented, and physically dependent.

Ms. Conroy was hospitalized on two occasions at Clara Maas Hospital, once between July 23, 1979 and August 8, 1979, for dehydration and a urinary tract infection, and later between July 21, 1982 and November 17, 1982, for an elevated temperature and dehydration. During the latter hospitalization the diagnostic evaluation showed that Ms. Conroy had necrotic gangrenous ulcers on her left foot. Two orthopedic surgeons recommended that to save her life, her leg should be amputated. However, her nephew refused to consent to the surgery because he was confident that she would not have wanted it. Contrary to the doctors' prognosis, Ms. Conroy did not die from the gangrene.

During this second hospitalization, Dr. Kazemi observed that Ms. Conroy was not eating adequately, and therefore, on July 23, he inserted a nasogastric tube that extended from her nose through her esophagus to her stomach. Medicines and food were then given to her through this tube. On October 18, the tube was removed, and Ms. Conroy was fed by hand through her mouth for two weeks. However, she was unable to eat a sufficient amount in this manner, and the tube was reinserted on November 3.

Excerpts from *In re Conroy*, 98 N.J. 321, 486 A.2D 1209 (1985).

When Ms. Conroy was discharged from the hospital to the nursing home on November 17, 1982, the tube was left in place. It continued to be used for the same purposes thereafter. A second attempt to feed Ms. Conroy through her mouth about January, 1983 failed because Ms. Conroy was incapable of swallowing sufficient amounts of nutrients and water. According to the testimony of Dr. Kazemi, Ms. Conroy had such difficulty swallowing that even a person with great time and patience could probably not have coaxed her into absorbing enough fluids and solid food by mouth to sustain herself.

At the time of trial, Ms. Conroy was no longer ambulatory and was confined to bed, unable to move from a semi-fetal position. She suffered from arteriosclerotic heart disease, hypertension, and diabetes mellitus; her left leg was gangrenous to her knee; she had several necrotic decubitus ulcers (bed sores) on her left foot, leg, and hip; an eye problem required irrigation; she had a urinary catheter in place and could not control her bowels; she could not speak; and her ability to swallow was very limited. On the other hand, she interacted with her environment in some limited ways: she could move her head, neck, hands, and arms to a minor extent; she was able to scratch herself, and had pulled at her bandages, tube, and catheter; she moaned occasionally when moved or fed through the tube, or when her bandages were changed; her eyes sometimes followed individuals in the room; her facial expressions were different when she was awake from when she was asleep; and she smiled on occasion when her hair was combed, or when she received a comforting rub.

Dr. Kazemi and Dr. Davidoff, a specialist in internal medicine who observed Ms. Conroy before testifying as an expert on behalf of the guardian, testified that Ms. Conroy was not brain dead, comatose, or in a chronic vegetative state. They stated, however, that her intellectual capacity was very limited, and that her mental condition probably would never improve. Dr. Davidoff characterized her as awake, but said that she was severely demented, was unable to respond to verbal stimuli, and, as far as he could tell, had no higher functioning or consciousness. Dr. Kazemi, in contrast, said that although she was confused and unaware, "she responds somehow."

The medical testimony was inconclusive as to whether, or to what extent, Ms. Conroy was capable of experiencing pain. Dr. Kazemi thought that Ms. Conroy might have experienced some degree of pain from her severely contracted limbs, or that the contractures were a reaction to pain, but that she did not necessarily suffer pain from the sores on her legs. According to Dr. Davidoff, it was unclear whether Ms. Conroy's feeding tube caused her pain, and it was "an open question whether she [felt] pain" at all; however, it was possible that she was experiencing a great deal of pain. Dr. Davidoff further testified that she responded to noxious or painful stimuli by moaning. The trial court determined that the testimony of a neurologist who had examined Ms. Conroy would not be necessary, since it believed that it had sufficient evidence about her medical condition on which to base a decision.

Both doctors testified that if the nasogastric tube were removed, Ms. Conroy would die of dehydration in about a week. Dr. Davidoff believed that the resulting thirst could be painful but that Ms. Conroy would become unconscious long before she died. Dr. Kazemi concurred that such a death would be painful.

Dr. Kazemi stated that he did not think it would be acceptable medical practice to remove the tube and that he was in favor of keeping it in place. As he put it, "she's a human being and I guess she has a right to live if it's possible." Ms. Rittel, the nurse, also thought the tube should not be removed since in her view it was not an extraordinary treatment. The nursing home had taken no position on the subject.

Dr. Davidoff said that if he had been the treating physician and the case had not come to court, he would have removed the tube with the family's consent. In his opinion, although Ms. Conroy seemed to be receiving excellent care, she did not have long to live, perhaps a few months. In those circumstances, he considered nasogastric feeding an extraordinary, or optional, medical treatment, because it went "beyond the necessities of life." He analogized the nasogastric tube to a respirator that supplies oxygen and said that since Ms. Conroy was "hopelessly ill with no possibility of returning to any sort of cognitive function, in the face of possibly [*sic*] suffering taking place at the moment," he could recommend that the feeding tube be removed.

Ms. Conroy had lived a rather cloistered life. She had been employed by a cosmetics company from her teens until her retirement at age 62 or 63. She had lived in the same home from her childhood until she was placed in the nursing home, had never married, and had very few friends. She had been very close to her three sisters, all of whom had died.

Ms. Conroy's only surviving blood relative was her nephew, the guardian, Thomas Whittemore. He had known her for over fifty years, had visited her approximately once a week for four or five years prior to her commitment to the nursing home, and had continued to visit her regularly at the nursing home for some time. The record contained additional evidence about the nephew's and aunt's financial situations and the history of their relationship. Based on the details of that record, there was no question that the nephew had good intentions and had no real conflict of interest due to possible inheritance when he sought permission to remove the tube.

Mr. Whittemore testified that Ms. Conroy feared and avoided doctors and that, to the best of his knowledge, she had never visited a doctor until she became incompetent in 1979. He said that on the couple of occasions that Ms. Conroy had pneumonia, "[y]ou couldn't bring a doctor in," and his wife, a registered nurse, would "try to get her through whatever she had." He added that once, when his wife took Ms. Conroy to the hospital emergency room, "as foggy as she was she snapped out of it, she would not sign herself in and she would have signed herself out immediately." According to the nephew, "[a]ll [Ms. Conroy and her sisters] wanted was to . . . have their bills paid and die in their own house." He also stated that he had refused to consent to the amputation of her gangrenous leg in 1982 and that he now sought removal of the nasogastric tube because, in his opinion, she would have refused the amputation and "would not have allowed [the nasogastric tube] to be inserted in the first place."

Ms. Conroy was a Roman Catholic. The Rev. Joseph Kukura, a Roman Catholic priest and an associate professor of Christian Ethics at the Immaculate Conception Seminary in Mahwah, New Jersey, testified that acceptable church teaching could be found in a document entitled "Declaration of Euthanasia" published by the Vatican Congregation for the Doctrine of the Faith, dated June 26, 1980. The test that this document espoused required a weighing of the burdens and the benefits to the patient of remaining alive with the aid of extraordinary life-sustaining medical treatment. Father Kukura said that life-sustaining procedures could be withdrawn if they were extraordinary, which he defined to embrace "all procedures, operations or other interventions which are excessively expensive, burdensome or inconvenient or which offer no hope of benefit to a patient." Here, he said, the hope of recovery and of returning to cognitive life, even with the nasogastric feeding, was not a reasonable possibility. The means of care were not adding to the value of her life, which was outweighed by the burdens of that life. He therefore considered the use of the nasogastric tube extraordinary. It was his judgment that removal of the tube would be ethical and moral, even though the ensuing period until her death would be painful.

The trial court decided to permit removal of the tube. 188 *N.J.Super.* 523, (Ch.Div.1983). It reasoned that the focus of inquiry should be whether life has become impossibly and permanently burdensome to the patient. If so, the court held, prolonging life becomes pointless and perhaps cruel. It determined that removal of the tube would lead to death by starvation and dehydration within a few days, and that the death might be painful. Nevertheless, it found that Ms. Conroy's intellectual functioning had been permanently reduced to a very primitive level, that her life had become impossibly and permanently burdensome, and that removal of the feeding tube should therefore be permitted.

The guardian *ad litem* appealed. While the appeal was pending, Ms. Conroy died with the nasogastric tube intact. Nevertheless, the Appellate Division decided to resolve the meritorious issues, finding that they were of significant public importance and that this type of case was capable of repetition but would evade review because the patients involved frequently die during litigation. 190 *N.J.Super.* 453, 459–60 (1983).

The Appellate Division viewed the ultimate question to be whether Claire Conroy's right of privacy outweighed the State's interest in preserving life. *Id.*, 190 *N.J.Super.* at 460. It held that the right to terminate life-sustaining treatment based on a guardian's judgment was limited to incurable and terminally ill patients who are brain dead, irreversibly comatose, or vegetative, and who would gain no medical benefit from continued treatment. *Id.*, 190 *N.J.Super.* at 466. As an alternative ground for its decision, it held that a guardian's decision may never be used to withhold nourishment, as opposed to the treatment or attempted curing of a disease, from an incompetent patient who is not comatose, brain dead, or vegetative, and whose death is not irreversibly imminent. *Id.*, 190 *N.J.Super.* at 469–70. Depriving a patient of a basic necessity of life, such as food, under those circumstances, the court stated, would hasten death rather than simply allow the illness to take its natural course. *Id.*, 190 *N.J.Super.* at 473. The court concluded that withdrawal of Ms. Conroy's nasogastric tube would be tantamount to killing her—not simply letting her die—and that such active euthanasia was ethically impermissible. *Id.*, 190 *N.J.Super.* at 475. The Appellate Division therefore reversed the trial court's judgment.

* * *

In view of the case law, we have no doubt that Ms. Conroy, if competent to make the decision and if resolute in her determination, could have chosen to have her nasogastric tube withdrawn. Her interest in freedom from nonconsensual invasion of her bodily integrity would outweigh any state interest in preserving life or in safeguarding the integrity of the medical profession. In addition, rejecting her artificial means of feeding would not constitute attempted suicide, as the decision would probably be based on a wish to be free of medical intervention, rather than a specific intent to die, and her death would result, if at all, from her underlying medical condition, which included her inability to swallow. Finally, removal of her feeding tube would not create a public health or safety hazard, nor would her death leave any minor dependents without care or support.

It should be noted that if she were competent, Ms. Conroy's right to self-determination would not be affected by her medical condition or prognosis. Our Legislature has recognized that an institutionalized, elderly person, whatever his physical and mental limitations and life expectancy, has the same right to receive medical treatment as a competent young person whose physical functioning is basically intact. *See N.J.S.A.* 52:27G-1 (declaring "that it is the public policy of this State to secure for elderly patients, residents and clients of health care facilities serving their specialized needs and problems, *the same civil and human rights guaranteed to all citizens*") (emphasis added). Moreover, a young, generally healthy person, if competent, has the same right to decline life-saving medical treatment as a competent elderly person who is terminally ill. Of course, a patient's decision to accept or reject medical treatment may be influenced by his medical condition, treatment, and prognosis; nevertheless, a competent person's common-law and constitutional rights do not depend on the quality or value of his life.

More difficult questions arise in the context of patients who, like Claire Conroy, are incompetent to make particular treatment decisions for themselves. Such patients are unable to exercise directly their own right to accept or refuse medical treatment. In attempting to exercise that right on their behalf, substitute decision-makers must seek to respect simultaneously both aspects of the patient's right to self-determination—the right to live, and the right, in some cases, to die of natural causes without medical intervention. . . .

In light of these rights and concerns, we hold that life-sustaining treatment may be withheld or withdrawn from an incompetent patient when it is clear that the particular patient would have refused the treatment under the circumstances involved. The standard we are enunciating is a subjective one, consistent with the notion that the right that we are seeking to effectuate is a very personal right to control one's own life. The question is not what a reasonable or average person would have chosen to do under the circumstances but what the particular patient would have done if able to choose for himself.

The patient may have expressed, in one or more ways, an intent not to have life-sustaining medical intervention. Such an intent might be embodied in a written document, or "living will," stating the person's desire not to have certain types of life-sustaining treatment administered under certain circumstances.[1] It might also be evidenced in an oral directive that the patient gave to a family member, friend, or health care provider. It might consist of a durable power of attorney or appointment of a proxy authorizing a particular person to make the decisions on the patient's behalf if he is no longer capable of making them for himself. *See N.J.S.A.* 46:2B-8 (providing that principal may confer authority on agent that is to be exercisable "notwithstanding later disability or incapacity of the principal at law or later uncertainty as to whether the principal is dead or alive"). It might take the form of reactions that the patient voiced regarding medical treatment administered to others. *See, e.g., Storar, supra,* 52 *N.Y.*2d 363, 420 *N.E.*2d 64, 438 *N.Y.S.*2d 266 (withdrawal of respirator was justified as an effectuation of patient's stated wishes when patient, as member of Catholic religious order, had stated more than once in formal discussions concerning the moral implications of the *Quinlan* case, most recently two months before he suffered cardiac arrest that left him in an irreversible coma, that he would not want extraordinary means used to keep him alive under similar circumstances).[2] It might also be deduced from a person's religious beliefs and the tenets of that religion, *id.* at 378, 420 *N.E.*2d at 72, 438 *N.Y.S.*2d at 274, or from the patient's consistent pattern of conduct with respect to prior decisions about his own medical care. Of course, dealing with the matter in advance in some sort of thoughtful and explicit way is best for all concerned.

Any of the above types of evidence, and any other information bearing on the person's intent, may be appropriate aids in determining what course of treatment the patient would have wished to pursue. In this respect, we now believe that we were in error in *Quinlan, supra,* 70 *N.J.* at 21, 41, to disregard evidence of statements that Ms. Quinlan made to friends concerning artificial prolongation of the lives of others who were terminally ill. See criticism of this portion of *Quinlan* opinion in Collester, *supra,* 30 *Rutgers L.Rev.* at 318; Smith, *supra,* 12 *Tulsa L.J.* at 163; and *D. Meyers, supra,* at 282 n. 65. Such evidence is certainly relevant to shed light on whether the patient would have consented to the treatment if competent to make the decision.

Although all evidence tending to demonstrate a person's intent with respect to medical treatment should properly be considered by surrogate decision-makers, or by a court in the event of any judicial proceedings, the probative value of such evidence may vary depending on the remoteness, consistency, and thoughtfulness of the prior statements or actions and the maturity of the person at the time of the statements or acts. *Colyer, supra,* 99 *Wash.*2d at 131, 660 *P.*2d at 748. Thus, for example, an offhand remark about not wanting to live under certain circumstances made by a person when young and in the peak of health would not in itself constitute clear proof twenty years later that he would want life-sustaining treatment withheld under those circumstances. In contrast, a carefully considered position, especially if written, that a person had maintained over a number of years or that he had acted upon in comparable circumstances might be clear evidence of his intent.

Another factor that would affect the probative value of a person's prior statements of intent would be their specificity. Of course, no one can predict with accuracy the precise circumstances with which he ultimately might be faced. Nevertheless, any details about the level of impaired functioning and the forms of medical treatment that one would find tolerable should be incorporated into advance directives to enhance their later usefulness as evidence.

Medical evidence bearing on the patient's condition, treatment, and prognosis, like evidence of the patient's wishes, is an essential prerequisite to decision-making under the subjective test. The medical evidence must establish that the patient fits within the Claire Conroy pattern: an elderly, incompetent nursing-home resident with severe and permanent mental and physical impairments and a life expectancy of approximately one year or less. In addition, since the goal is to effectuate the patient's right of informed consent, the surrogate decision-maker must have at least as much medical information upon which to base his decision about what the patient would have chosen as one would expect a competent patient to have before consenting to or rejecting treatment. Such information might include evidence about the patient's present level of physical, sensory, emotional, and cognitive functioning; the degree of physical pain resulting from the medical condition, treatment, and termination of treatment, respectively; the degree of humiliation, dependence, and loss of dignity probably resulting from the condition and treatment; the life expectancy and prognosis for recovery with and without treatment; the various treatment options; and the risks, side effects, and benefits of each of those options. Particular care should be taken not to base a decision on a premature diagnosis or prognosis. *See Colyer, supra*, 99 *Wash.*2d at 143–45, 660 *P.*2d at 754–55 (Dore, J., dissenting).

We recognize that for some incompetent patients it might be impossible to be clearly satisfied as to the patient's intent either to accept or reject the life-sustaining treatment. Many people may have spoken of their desires in general or casual terms,[3] or, indeed, never considered or resolved the issue at all. In such cases, a surrogate decision-maker cannot presume that treatment decisions made by a third party on the patient's behalf will further the patient's right to self-determination, since effectuating another person's right to self-determination presupposes that the substitute decision-maker knows what the person would have wanted. Thus, in the absence of adequate proof of the patient's wishes, it is naive to pretend that the right to self-determination serves as the basis for substituted decision-making. *See Storar, supra*, 52 *N.Y.*2d at 378-380, 420 *N.E.*2d at 72–73, 438 *N.Y.S.*2d at 274–75; Veatch, "An Ethical Framework for Terminal Care Decisions: A New Classification of Patients," 32(9) *J.Am. Geriatrics Soc'y* 665, 666 (1984).

We hesitate, however, to foreclose the possibility of humane actions, which may involve termination of life-sustaining treatment, for persons who never clearly expressed their desires about life-sustaining treatment but who are now suffering a prolonged and painful death. An incompetent, like a minor child, is a ward of the state, and the state's *parens patriae* power supports the authority of its courts to allow decisions to be made for an incompetent that serve the incompetent's best interests, even if the person's wishes cannot be clearly established. This authority permits the state to authorize guardians to withhold or withdraw life-sustaining treatment from an incompetent patient if it is manifest that such action would further the patient's best interests in a narrow sense of the phrase, even though the subjective test that we articulated above may not be satisfied. We therefore hold that life-sustaining, treatment may also be withheld or withdrawn from a patient in Claire Conroy's situation if either of two "best interests" tests—a limited-objective or a pure-objective test—is satisfied.

Under the limited-objective test, life-sustaining treatment may be withheld or withdrawn from a patient in Claire Conroy's situation when there is some trustworthy evidence that the patient would have refused the treatment, and the decision-maker is satisfied that it is clear that the burdens of the patient's continued life with the treatment outweigh the benefits of that life for him. By this we mean that the patient is suffering, and will continue to suffer throughout the expected duration of his life, unavoidable pain, and that the net burdens of his prolonged life (the pain and suffering of his life with the treatment less the amount and duration of pain that the patient would likely experience if the treatment were withdrawn) markedly outweigh any physical pleasure, emotional enjoyment, or intellectual satisfaction that the patient may still be able to derive from life. This limited-objective standard permits the termination of treatment for a patient who had not unequivocally expressed his desires before becoming incompetent, when it is clear that the treatment in question would merely prolong the patient's suffering.

Medical evidence will be essential to establish that the burdens of the treatment to the patient in terms of pain and suffering outweigh the benefits that the patient is experiencing. The medical evidence should make it clear that the treatment would merely prolong the patient's suffering and not provide him with any net benefit. Information is particularly important with respect to the degree, expected duration, and constancy of pain with and without treatment, and the possibility that the pain could be reduced by drugs or other means short of terminating the life-sustaining treatment. The same types of medical evidence that are relevant to the subjective analysis, such as the patient's life expectancy, prognosis, level of functioning, degree of humiliation and dependency, and treatment options, should also be considered.

This limited-objective test also requires some trustworthy evidence that the patient would have wanted the treatment terminated. This evidence could take any one or more of the various forms appropriate to prove the patient's intent under the subjective test. Evidence that, taken as a whole, would be too vague, casual, or remote to constitute the clear proof of the patient's subjective intent that is necessary to satisfy the subjective test—for example, informally expressed reactions to other people's medical conditions and treatment—might be sufficient to satisfy this prong of the limited-objective test.

In the absence of trustworthy evidence, or indeed any evidence at all, that the patient would have declined the treatment, life-sustaining treatment may still be withheld or withdrawn from a formerly competent person like Claire Conroy if a third, pure-objective test is satisfied. Under that test, as under the limited-objective test, the net burdens of the patient's life with the treatment should clearly and markedly outweigh the benefits that the patient derives from life. Further, the recurring, unavoidable and severe pain of the patient's life with the treatment should be such that the effect of administering life-sustaining treatment would be inhumane. Subjective evidence that the patient would not have wanted the treatment is not necessary under this pure-objective standard. Nevertheless, even in the context of severe pain, life-sustaining treatment should not be withdrawn from an incompetent patient who had previously expressed a wish to be kept alive in spite of any pain that he might experience.

Although we are condoning a restricted evaluation of the nature of a patient's life in terms of pain, suffering, and possible enjoyment under the limited-objective and pure-objective tests, we expressly decline to authorize decision-making based on assessments of the personal worth or social utility of another's life, or the value of that life to others. We do not believe that it would be appropriate for a court to designate a person with the authority to determine that someone else's life is not worth living simply because, to that person, the patient's "quality of life" or value to society seems negligible. The mere fact that a patient's functioning is limited or his prognosis dim does not mean that he is not enjoying what remains of his life or that it is in his best interests to die. *But cf. In re Dinnerstein*, 6 *Mass.App.Ct.* 466, 473, 380 *N.E.*2d 134, 138 (1978) (indicating, in reference to possible resuscitation of half-paralyzed, elderly victim of Alzheimer's disease, that prolongation of life is not required if there is no hope of return to a "normal, integrated, functioning, cognitive existence"); *see also President's Commission Report, supra*, at 135 (endorsing termination of treatment whenever surrogate decision-maker in his discretion believes it is in the patient's best interests, defined broadly to "take into account such factors as the relief of suffering, the preservation or restoration of functioning, and the quality as well as the extent of life sustained"). More wide-ranging powers to make decisions about other people's lives, in our view, would create an intolerable risk for socially isolated and defenseless people suffering from physical or mental handicaps.

* * *

We emphasize that in making decisions whether to administer life-sustaining treatment to patients such as Claire Conroy, the primary focus should be the patient's desires and experience of pain and enjoyment—not the type of treatment involved. Thus, we reject the distinction that some have made between actively hastening death by terminating treatment and passively allowing a person to die of a disease as one of limited use in a legal analysis of such a decision-making situation.

Characterizing conduct as active or passive is often an elusive notion, even outside the context of medical decision-making.

> Saint Anselm of Canterbury was fond of citing the trickiness of the distinction between "to do" (*facere*) and "not to do" (*non facere*). In answer to the question "What's he doing?" we say "He's just sitting there" (positive), really meaning something negative: "He's not doing anything at all." [*D. Walton, supra*, at 234 (footnote omitted).]

The distinction is particularly nebulous, however, in the context of decisions whether to withhold or withdraw life-sustaining treatment. In a case like that of Claire Conroy, for example, would a physician who discontinued nasogastric feeding be actively causing her death by removing her primary source of nutrients; or would he merely be omitting to continue the artificial form of treatment, thus passively allowing her medical condition, which includes her inability to swallow, to take its natural course? *See President's Commission Report, supra*, at 65–66. The ambiguity inherent in this distinction is further heightened when one performs an act within an over-all plan of non-intervention, such as when a doctor writes an order not to resuscitate a patient. *Id.* at 67.

> Consequently, merely determining whether what was done involved a fatal act or omission does not establish whether it was morally acceptable. . . . [In fact, a]ctive steps to terminate life-sustaining interventions may be permitted, indeed required, by the patient's authority to forego therapy even when such steps lead to death. [*President's Commission Report, supra*, at 67, 72.]

For a similar reason, we also reject any distinction between withholding and withdrawing life-sustaining treatment. Some commentators have suggested that discontinuing life-sustaining treatment once it has been commenced is morally more problematic than merely failing to begin the treatment. *See* Clouser, "Allowing or Causing: Another Look," 87 *Annals Internal Med.* 622, 624 (1977) ("To stop [therapy] . . . seems different in principle from refusing to initiate a therapy in response to a new crisis."). Discontinuing life-sustaining treatment, to some, is an "active" taking of life, as opposed to the more "passive" act of omitting the treatment in the first instance. In the words of one writer, "[T]he difference between taking away that which one has come to count on as normal support for life and not instituting therapy when a new crisis begins . . . fits nicely a basic moral distinction throughout life—we are not morally obligated to help another person, but we are morally obligated not to interfere with his life-sustaining routines." *Id.*

This distinction is more psychologically compelling than logically sound. As mentioned above, the line between active and passive conduct in the context of medical decisions is far too nebulous to constitute a principled basis for decision-making. Whether necessary treatment is withheld at the outset or withdrawn later on, the consequence—the patient's death—is the same. Moreover, from a policy standpoint, it might well be unwise to forbid persons from discontinuing a treatment under circumstances in which the treatment could permissibly be withheld. Such a rule could discourage families and doctors from even attempting certain types of care and could thereby force them into hasty and premature decisions to allow a patient to die. *See* Lynn & Childress, "Must Patients Always Be Given Food and Water?," 13 *Hastings Center Rep.* 17, 19–20 (1983).

* * *

Because of the special vulnerability of mentally and physically impaired, elderly persons in nursing homes and the potential for abuse with unsupervised institutional decision-making in such homes, life-sustaining treatment should not be withdrawn or withheld from a nursing-home resident like Claire Conroy in the absence of a guardian's decision, made in accordance with the procedure outlined below, that the elements of the subjective, limited-objective, or pure-objective test have been satisfied. A necessary prerequisite to surrogate decision-making is a judicial determination that the patient is incompetent to make the decision for himself and designation of a guardian for the incompetent patient if he does not already have one.

Substitute decision-making by a guardian is not permissible unless the patient has been proven incompetent to make the particular medical treatment decision at issue. *See* Veatch, "An Ethical Framework for Terminal Care Decisions: A New Classification of Patients," 32(9) *J. Am. Geriatrics Soc'y* 665, 668 (1984) ("[O]ne cannot simply presume that a patient is incompetent. There must be some sort of due process, and if the patient has not been adjudicated to be incompetent, he must be treated as . . . competent . . . ."). A patient may be incompetent because he lacks the ability to understand the information conveyed, to evaluate the options, or to communicate a decision. Medical evidence bearing on these capabilities should be furnished to a court by at least two doctors with expertise in relevant fields who have personally examined the patient. *See R.* 4:83-2(b). The proof must be clear and convincing that the patient does not have and will not regain the capability of making the decision for himself. *Cf. Grady, supra,* 85 *N.J.* at 265 (requiring clear and convincing proof of incompetence of mentally retarded adult before allowing guardian to consent to sterilization of such incompetent person).

Determining whether the patient is competent to make the medical decision at issue is necessary even if the patient previously had been adjudicated an incompetent and had a general guardian appointed pursuant to *N.J.S.A.* 3B:12-25. Here, for example, the plaintiff, Mr. Whittemore, had been appointed Ms. Conroy's guardian in 1979, when she entered the nursing home, at which time she was still lucid sporadically and could speak. That designation was made pursuant to Rule 4:83, which requires medical proof that "the alleged incompetent is unfit and unable to govern himself and to manage his affairs." *R.* 4:83-2(b); *see also N.J.S.A.* 3B:12-25 (providing that the Superior Court may determine "mental incompetency" and "appoint a guardian" for the incompetent's person and estate). Such a general appointment does not necessarily mean that the incompetent cannot make an informed judgment regarding a particular medical treatment. *See Grady, supra,* 85 *N.J.* at 265 ("The fact that a person is legally incompetent for some purposes, *cf. R.* 4:83 (action for guardianship of incompetent), does not mean that he lacks the capacity to make a decision about sterilization."); *In re Schiller,* 148 *N.J.Super.* 168, 180-81 (Ch. 1977) (stating that test for mental capacity to consent to medical treatment is whether the patient has "sufficient mind to reasonably understand the condition, the nature and effect of the proposed treatment, [and the] attendant risks in pursuing . . . and not pursuing the treatment"). The inability to "govern" one's self and manage one's other affairs does not necessarily preclude the ability to make a decision to forego further medical treatment.

If the patient already has a general guardian, the court should determine whether that guardian is a suitable person to represent the patient with respect to the medical decision in question. Such a determination necessitates an inquiry into the guardian's knowledge of the patient and motivations or possible conflicts of interest. If the patient, although incompetent to make the treatment decision for himself, does not yet have a guardian, a suitable person should be appointed as guardian for him.

We hold that to determine whether withholding or withdrawing life-sustaining treatment from an elderly nursing-home resident who is incompetent to make the decision for himself is justified under any of the three tests articulated above, the following procedure is required. A person who believes that withholding or withdrawing life-sustaining treatment would effectuate an incompetent patient's wishes or would be in his "best interests" should notify the Office of the Ombudsman of the contemplated action. Such notification may be undertaken by the patient's guardian, or by another interested party, such as a close family member, an attending physician, or the nursing home in which the patient resides. Any person who believes the contrary, that is, who has reasonable cause to suspect that withholding or withdrawing the life-sustaining treatment would be an abuse of that patient, should also report such information to the ombudsman.

We believe the ombudsman should be involved in the process at this stage. The ombudsman should treat every notification that life-sustaining treatment will be withheld or withdrawn from an institutionalized, elderly patient as a possible "abuse." Under *N.J.S.A.* 52:27G-7.2a, the ombudsman would then be required to investigate the situation and to report it within twenty-four hours to the Commissioner of Human Services and to any other government agency that regulates or operates the facility.

Evidence concerning the patient's condition should be furnished by the attending physician and nurses. Two other physicians, unaffiliated with the nursing home and with the attending physician, should then be appointed to confirm the patient's medical condition and prognosis. We recommend that the ombudsman exercise his discretionary authority under *N.J.S.A.* 52:27G-5b to appoint the physicians. In the event that the ombudsman chooses not to exercise his authority in this regard, application may be made to the assignment judge of the appropriate vicinage for designation of the two physicians. Depending upon the circumstances of a particular case, the physicians may be compensated by the patient's estate, the guardian, the family, or the nursing home. If the funds from these sources are insufficient, the guardian may seek reimbursement from the ombudsman or possibly from Medicare.

Provided that the two physicians supply the necessary medical foundation, the guardian, with the concurrence of the attending physician,[4] may withhold or withdraw life-sustaining medical treatment if he believes in good faith, based on the medical evidence and any evidence of the patient's wishes, that it is clear that the subjective, limited-objective, or pure-objective test is satisfied. In addition, the ombudsman must concur in that decision. This role would be consonant with his legislative responsibilities. Finally, if the limited-objective or pure-objective test is being used, the family—that is, the patient's spouse, parents, and children, or, in their absence, the patient's next of kin, if any—must also concur in the decision to withhold or withdraw life-sustaining treatment.

In the absence of bad faith, no participant in the decision-making process shall be civilly or criminally liable for actions taken in accordance with the procedures set forth in this opinion. *Cf. Quinlan, supra,* 70 *N.J.* at 54 (providing for complete civil and criminal immunity for guardians, physicians, hospitals, and others, who, after complying with the procedures articulated in *Quinlan,* participate in a decision to withhold life support treatment). However, the decision-making procedure that we have outlined does not necessarily immunize its participants entirely from judicial oversight. As previously noted, the ombudsman can refer cases of questionable criminal abuse to the county prosecutor. *N.J.S.A.* 52:27G-7.2d.

As noted above, *supra* at 381, the guardian will resolve the issues in these matters and make the ultimate decision with such concurrences as we have required. Ordinarily, court involvement will be limited to the determination of incompetency, and the appointment of a guardian unless a personal guardian has been previously appointed, who will determine whether the standards we have prescribed have been satisfied. The record in this case did not satisfy those standards. The evidence that Claire Conroy would have refused the treatment, although sufficient to meet the lower showing of intent required under the limited-objective test, was certainly not the "clear" showing of intent contemplated under the subjective test. More information should, if possible, have been obtained by the guardian with respect to Ms. Conroy's intent. What were her ethical, moral, and religious beliefs? She did try to refuse initial hospitalization, and indeed had "scorned medicine." 188 *N.J.Super.* at 525. However, she allowed her nephew's wife, a registered nurse, to care for her during several illnesses. It was not clear whether Ms. Conroy permitted the niece to administer any drugs or other forms of medical treatment to her during these illnesses. Although it may often prove difficult, and at times impossible, to ascertain a person's wishes, the Conroy case illustrates the sources to which the guardian might turn. For example, in more than eight decades of life in the same house, it is possible that she revealed to persons other than her nephew her feelings regarding medical treatments, other values, and her goals in life. Some promising avenues for such an inquiry about her personal values included her response to the illnesses and deaths of her sisters and others, and her statements with respect to not wanting to be in a nursing home.

Moreover, there was insufficient information concerning the benefits and burdens of Ms. Conroy's life to satisfy either the limited-objective or pure-objective test. Although the treating doctor and the guardian's expert testified as to Claire Conroy's condition, neither testified conclusively as to whether she was in pain or was capable of experiencing pain or thirst. There was medical agreement that removal of the tube would have caused pain during the period of approximately one week that would have elapsed before her death, or at least until she were to lapse into a coma. On the other hand, there was little, if any, evidence of the discomfort, suffering, and pain she would endure if she continued to be fed and medicated through the tube during her remaining life—contemplated to be up to one year. Apparently her feedings sometimes occasioned moaning, but it remains unclear whether these were reflex responses or expressions of discomfort. Moreover, although she tried to remove the tube, it is not clear that this was intentional, and there was little evidence that she was in distress. Her treating physician also offered contradictory views as to whether the contractures of her legs caused pain or whether, indeed, they might be the result of pain, without offering any evidence on that issue. The trial court rejected as superfluous the offer to present as an expert witness a neurologist, who might have been able to explain what Ms. Conroy's reactions to the environment indicated about her perception of pain.

The evidence was also unclear with respect to Ms. Conroy's capacity to feel pleasure, another issue as to which the information supplied by a neurologist might have been helpful. What was known of her awareness of the world? Although Ms. Conroy had some ability to smile and scratch, the relationship of these activities to external stimuli apparently was quite variable.

The trial transcript reveals no exploration of the discomfort and risks that attend nasogastric feedings. A casual mention by the nurse/administrator of the need to restrain the patient to prevent the removal of the tube was not followed by an assessment of the detrimental impact, if any, of those restraints. Alternative modalities, including gastrostomies, intravenous feeding, subcutaneous or intramuscular hydration, or some combination, were not investigated. Neither of the expert witnesses presented empirical evidence regarding the treatment options for such a patient.

It can be seen that the evidence at trial was inadequate to satisfy the subjective, the limited-objective, or the pure-objective standard that we have set forth. Were Claire Conroy still alive, the guardian would have been required to explore these issues prior to reaching any decision. Guardians—and courts, if they are involved—should act cautiously and deliberately in deciding these cases. The consequences are most serious—life or death.

We have not attempted to set forth guidelines for decision-making with respect to life-sustaining treatment in a variety of other situations that are not currently before us. Innumerable variations are possible. However, each case—such as that of the severely deformed newborn, of the never-competent adult suffering from a painful and debilitating illness, and of the mentally alert quadriplegic who has given up on life—poses its own unique difficulties. We do not deem it advisable to attempt to resolve all such human dilemmas in the context of this case. It is preferable, in our view, to move slowly and to gain experience in this highly sensitive field. As we noted previously, the Legislature is better equipped than we to develop and frame a comprehensive plan for resolving these problems.

The judgment of the Appellate Division is reversed. In light of Ms. Conroy's death, we do not remand the matter for further proceedings.

NOTES

1. The Legislature has not enacted a statute recognizing the validity of living wills or prescribing the means to execute such wills . . . [though there is] pending legislation. Whether or not they are legally binding, however, such advance directives are relevant evidence of the patient's intent. *John F. Kennedy Memorial Hosp., Inc. v. Bludworth*, 452 So.2d 921, 926 (Fla.1984).
2. None of these forms of evidence need be excluded as hearsay from a court proceeding, if there be one, since oral and written expressions of a person's reactions or desires fit within the "existing state of mind" exception to the hearsay rule. *Evid.R.* 63(12); *see State v. Ready*, 78 *N.J.L.* 599. 609 (E. & A. 1910) (testator's oral statements admissible to show his testamentary design); *Woll v. Dugas*, 104 *N.J.Super.* 586, 592–93 (Ch.Div.1969) (decedent's statements to lawyer about testamentary intent may fall within "state of mind" exception to hearsay rule), aff'd, 112 *N.J.Super.* 366 (App.Div.1970); *D. Meyers, supra*, at 282 n. 65; *Smith, supra*, 12 *Tulsa L.J.* at 163.
3. For example, someone may have said orally or in writing merely that he would not want to be "artificially sustained" by "heroic measures" if his condition was "hopeless," or that he would not want to have doctors apply life-sustaining procedures "that would serve only to artificially prolong the dying process" if he were "terminally ill." Such a general statement might not in itself provide clear guidance to a surrogate decision-maker in all situations. *See* Cantor, *supra*, 30 *Rutgers L.Rev.* at 262; Hilfiker, *supra*, 308 *New Eng.J. Med.* at 718.
4. *See Quinlan, supra*, 70 *N.J.* at 54 (authorizing the guardian to replace the attending physician with one whose views may be different).

CRUZAN V. DIRECTOR, MISSOURI DEPARTMENT OF HEALTH: 110 S.CT. 2841 (1990)

INTRODUCTION. *A second major case involving refusal of nutrition and hydration involved Nancy Beth Cruzan, a young woman and accident victim who was left permanently vegetative, and who was being fed with a gastrostomy. The State of Missouri claimed a state interest in preserving her life. Her parents claimed that she would not want to be maintained in this condition. The controversy, which at times appeared to be intertwined with the state's abortion tensions, sometimes appeared to be cast in a way that would apply to all life-prolonging whether involving nutrition or any other means of life support. At times the argument was even cast in a form that would have applied to conscious, competent patient's refusing life-support. At other times the state was claiming the right to insist on "clear and convincing evidence" of the patient's wishes, the highest legal evidentiary standard for such cases. After several hearings at the state level, the case reached the U.S. Supreme Court where the court supported the right of the state to insist on clear and convincing evidence, but implied that if the patient's wishes are established at the state's chosen standard, then a constitutional right of refusal does extend to a surrogate's interpretation of the patient's wishes. After the U.S. Supreme Court decision, the state withdrew its opposition to Nancy's parents and a state court eventually determined at a "clear and convincing" level, based on testimony from friends, that Nancy would not want the medical feeding. She died within days of its withdrawal.*

ON THE NIGHT of January 11, 1983, Nancy Cruzan lost control of her car as she traveled down Elm Road in Jasper County, Missouri. The vehicle overturned, and Cruzan was discovered lying face down in a ditch without detectable respiratory or cardiac function. Paramedics were able to restore her breathing and heartbeat at the accident site, and she was transported to a hospital in an unconscious state. An attending neurosurgeon diagnosed her as having sustained probable cerebral contusions compounded by significant anoxia (lack of oxygen). The Missouri trial court in this case found that permanent brain damage generally results after 6 minutes in an anoxic state; it was estimated that Cruzan was deprived of oxygen from 12 to 14 minutes. She remained in a coma for approximately three weeks and then progressed to an unconscious state in which she was able to orally ingest some nutrition. In order to ease feeding and further the recovery, surgeons implanted a gastrostomy feeding and hydration tube in Cruzan with the consent of her then husband. Subsequent rehabilitative efforts proved unavailing. She now lies in a Missouri state hospital in what is commonly referred to as a persistent vegetative state: generally, a condition in which a person exhibits motor reflexes but evinces no indications of significant cognitive function.[1] The State of Missouri is bearing the cost of her care.

After it had become apparent that Nancy Cruzan had virtually no chance of regaining her mental faculties her parents asked hospital employees to terminate the artificial nutrition and hydration procedures. All agree that such a removal would cause her death. The employees refused to honor the request without court approval. The parents then sought and received authorization from the state trial court for termination. The court found that a

---

Cite as *Cruzan v. Director, Missouri Dept. of Health*, 110 S.Ct. 2841 (1990). The text reprinted here is the U.S. Supreme Court's affirmation "on writ of certiorari to the Supreme Court of Missouri." Chief Justice Rehnquist delivered the opinion of the court.

person in Nancy's condition had a fundamental right under the State and Federal Constitutions to refuse or direct the withdrawal of "death prolonging procedures." App. to Pet. for Cert. A99. The court also found that Nancy's "expressed thoughts at age twenty-five in somewhat serious conversation with a housemate friend that if sick or injured she would not wish to continue her life unless she could live at least halfway normally suggests that given her present condition she would not wish to continue on with her nutrition and hydration." *Id.*, at A97–A98.

The Supreme Court of Missouri reversed by a divided vote. The court recognized a right to refuse treatment embodied in the common-law doctrine of informed consent, but expressed skepticism about the application of that doctrine in the circumstances of this case. *Cruzan v. Harmon*, 760 S. W. 2d 408, 416–417 (Mo. 1988) (en banc). The court also declined to read a broad right of privacy into the State Constitution which would "support the right of a person to refuse medical treatment in every circumstance," and expressed doubt as to whether such a right existed under the United States Constitution. *Id.*, at 417–418. It then decided that the Missouri Living Will statute, Mo. Rev. Stat. § 459.010 *et seq.* (1986), embodied a state policy strongly favoring the preservation of life. 760 S. W. 2d, at 419–420. The court found that Cruzan's statements to her roommate regarding her desire to live or die under certain conditions were "unreliable for the purpose of determining her intent," *id.*, at 424, "and thus insufficient to support the co-guardians claim to exercise substituted judgment on Nancy's behalf." *Id.*, at 426. It rejected the argument that Cruzan's parents were entitled to order the termination of her medical treatment, concluding that "no person can assume that choice for an incompetent in the absence of the formalities required under Missouri's Living Will statutes or the clear and convincing, inherently reliable evidence absent here." *Id.*, at 425. The court also expressed its view that "[b]road policy questions bearing on life and death are more properly addressed by representative assemblies" than judicial bodies. *Id.*, at 426.

We granted certiorari to consider the question of whether Cruzan has a right under the United States Constitution which would require the hospital to withdraw life-sustaining treatment from her under these circumstances.

At common law, even the touching of one person by another without consent and without legal justification was a battery. See W. Keeton, D. Dobbs, R. Keeton, & D. Owen, Prosser and Keeton on Law of Torts §9, pp. 39–42 (5th ed. 1984). Before the turn of the century, this Court observed that "[n]o right is held more sacred, or is more carefully guarded, by the common law, than the right of every individual to the possession and control of his own person, free from all restraint or interference of others, unless by clear and unquestionable authority of law." *Union Pacific R. Co.* v. *Botsford*, 141 U.S. 250, 251 (1891). This notion of bodily integrity has been embodied in the requirement that informed consent is generally required for medical treatment. Justice Cardozo, while on the Court of Appeals of New York, aptly described this doctrine: "Every human being of adult years and sound mind has a right to determine what shall be done with his own body; and a surgeon who performs an operation without his patient's consent commits an assault, for which he is liable in damages." *Schloendorff* v. *Society of New York Hospital*, 211 N.Y. 125, 129–30, 105 N. E. 92, 93 (1914). The informed consent doctrine has become firmly entrenched in American tort law. See Dobbs, Keeton, & Owen, *supra*, § 32, pp. 189–192; F. Rozovsky, Consent to Treatment, A Practical Guide 1-98 (2d ed. 1990).

The logical corollary of the doctrine of informed consent is that the patient generally possesses the right not to consent, that is, to refuse treatment. Until about 15 years ago and the seminal decision in *In re Quinlan*, 70 N.J. 10, 355 A.2d 647, cert. denied *sub nom.*, *Garger* v. *New Jersey*, 429 U.S. 922 (1976), the number of right-to-refuse-treatment decisions were relatively few.[2] Most of the earlier cases involved patients who refused medical treatment forbidden by their religious beliefs, thus implicating First Amendment rights as well as common law rights of self-determination.[3] More recently, however, with the advance of medical technology capable of sustaining life well past the point where natural forces would have brought certain death in earlier times, cases involving the right to refuse life-sustaining treatment have burgeoned. See 760 S.W.2d, at 412, n. 4 (collecting 54 reported decisions from 1976–1988).

In the *Quinlan* case, young Karen Quinlan suffered severe brain damage as the result of anoxia, and entered a persistent vegetative state. Karen's father sought judicial approval to disconnect his daughter's respirator. The New Jersey Supreme Court granted the relief, holding that Karen had a right of privacy grounded in the Federal Constitution to terminate treatment. *In re Quinlan*, 70 N.J., at 38–42, 355 A.2d at 662–664. Recognizing that this right was not absolute, however, the court balanced it against asserted state interests. Noting that the State's interest "weakens and the individual's right to privacy grows as the degree of bodily invasion increases and the prognosis dims," the court concluded that the state interests had to give way in that case. *Id.*, at 41, 355 A.2d, at 664. The court also concluded that the "only practical way" to prevent the loss of Karen's privacy right due to her incompetence was to allow her guardian and family to decide "whether she would exercise it in these circumstances." *Ibid.*

After *Quinlan*, however, most courts have based a right to refuse treatment either solely on the common law right to informed consent or on both the common law right and a constitutional privacy right. See L. Tribe, American Constitutional Law § 15-11, p. 1365 (2d ed. 1988). In *Superintendent of Belchertown State School* v. *Saikewicz*, 373 Mass. 728, 370 N.E.2d 417 (1977), the Supreme Judicial

Court of Massachusetts relied on both the right of privacy and the right of informed consent to permit the withholding of chemotherapy from a profoundly-retarded 67-year-old man suffering from leukemia. *Id.*, at 737–738, 370 N.E.2d, at 424. Reasoning that an incompetent person retains the same rights as a competent individual "because the value of human dignity extends to both," the court adopted a "substituted judgment" standard whereby courts were to determine what an incompetent individual's decision would have been under the circumstances. *Id.*, at 745, 752–753, 757–758, 370 N.E.2d, at 427, 431, 434. Distilling certain state interests from prior case law—the preservation of life, the protection of the interests of innocent third parties, the prevention of suicide, and the maintenance of the ethical integrity of the medical profession—the court recognized the first interest as paramount and noted it was greatest when an affliction was curable, "as opposed to the State interest where, as here, the issue is not whether, but when, for how long, and at what cost to the individual [a] life may be briefly extended." *Id.*, at 742, 370 N.E.2d, at 426.

In *In re Storar* 52 N.Y.2d 363, 420 N.E.2d 64, cert. denied, 454 U.S. 858 (1981), the New York Court of Appeals declined to base a right to refuse treatment on a constitutional privacy right. Instead, it found such a right "adequately supported" by the informed consent doctrine. *Id.*, at 376–377, 420 N.E.2d, at 70. In *In re Eichner* (decided with *In re Storar, supra*) an 83-year-old man who had suffered brain damage from anoxia entered a vegetative state and was thus incompetent to consent to the removal of his respirator. The court, however, found it unnecessary to reach the question of whether his rights could be exercised by others since it found the evidence clear and convincing from statements made by the patient when competent that he "did not want to be maintained in a vegetative coma by use of a respirator." *Id.*, at 380, 420 N.E 2d, at 72. In the companion *Storar* case, a 52-year-old man suffering from bladder cancer had been profoundly retarded during most of his life. Implicitly rejecting the approach taken in *Saikewicz, supra*, the court reasoned that due to such life-long incompetency, "it is unrealistic to attempt to determine whether he would want to continue potentially life prolonging treatment if he were competent." 52 N.Y.2d, at 380, 420 N.E.2d, at 72. As the evidence showed that the patient's required blood transfusions did not involve excessive pain and without them his mental and physical abilities would deteriorate, the court concluded that it should not "allow an incompetent patient to bleed to death because someone, even someone as close as a parent or sibling, feels that this is best for one with an incurable disease." *Id.*, at 382, 420 N.E.2d, at 73.

Many of the later cases build on the principles established in *Quinlan, Saikewicz* and *Storar/Eichner*. For instance, in *In re Conroy*, 98 N.J. 321, 486 A.2d 1209 (1985), the same court that decided *Quinlan* considered whether a nasogastric feeding tube could be removed from an 84-year-old incompetent nursing-home resident suffering irreversible mental and physical ailments. While recognizing that a federal right of privacy might apply in the case, the court, contrary to its approach in *Quinlan*, decided to base its decision on the common-law right to self-determination and informed consent. 98 N.J., at 348, 486 A.2d, at 1223. "On balance, the right to self-determination ordinarily outweighs any countervailing state interests, and competent persons generally are permitted to refuse medical treatment, even at the risk of death. Most of the cases that have held otherwise, unless they involved the interest in protecting innocent third parties, have concerned the patient's competency to make a rational and considered choice." *Id.*, at 353–354, 486 A.2d, at 1225.

Reasoning that the right of self-determination should not be lost merely because an individual is unable to sense a violation of it, the court held that incompetent individuals retain a right to refuse treatment. It also held that such a right could be exercised by a surrogate decisionmaker using a "subjective" standard when there was clear evidence that the incompetent person would have exercised it. Where such evidence was lacking, the court held that an individual's right could still be invoked in certain circumstances under objective "best interest" standards. *Id.*, at 361–368, 486 A.2d, at 1229–1233. Thus, if some trustworthy evidence existed that the individual would have wanted to terminate treatment, but not enough to clearly establish a person's wishes for purposes of the subjective standard, and the burden of a prolonged life from the experience of pain and suffering markedly outweighed its satisfactions, treatment could be terminated under a "limited-objective" standard. Where no trustworthy evidence existed, and a person's suffering would make the administration of life-sustaining treatment inhumane, a "pure-objective" standard could be used to terminate treatment. If none of these conditions obtained, the court held it was best to err in favor of preserving life. *Id.*, at 364–368, 486 A.2d, at 1231–1233.

The court also rejected certain categorical distinctions that had been drawn in prior refusal-of-treatment cases as lacking substance for decision purposes: the distinction between actively hastening death by terminating treatment and passively allowing a person to die of a disease; between treating individuals as an initial matter versus withdrawing treatment afterwards; between ordinary versus extraordinary treatment; and between treatment by artificial feeding versus other forms of life-sustaining medical procedures. *Id.*, at 369–374, 486 N.E.2d, at 1233–1237. As to the last item, the court acknowledged the "emotional significance" of food, but noted that feeding by implanted tubes is a "medical procedur[e] with inherent risks and possible side effects, instituted by skilled health-care providers to compensate for impaired physical functioning" which analytically was equivalent to artificial breathing using a respirator. *Id.*, at 373, 486 A.2d, at 1236.[4]

In contrast to *Conroy*, the Court of Appeals of New York recently refused to accept less than the clearly expressed wishes of a patient before permitting the exercise of her right to refuse treatment by a surrogate decisionmaker. *In re Westchester County Medical Center on behalf of O'Connor*, 531 N.E.2d 607 (1988) *(O'Connor)*. There, the court, over the objection of the patient's family members, granted an order to insert a feeding tube into a 77-year-old woman rendered incompetent as a result of several strokes. While continuing to recognize a common-law right to refuse treatment, the court rejected the substituted judgment approach for asserting it "because it is inconsistent with our fundamental commitment to the notion that no person or court should substitute its judgment as to what would be an acceptable quality of life for another. Consequently, we adhere to the view that, despite its pitfalls and inevitable uncertainties, the inquiry must always be narrowed to the patient's expressed intent, with every effort made to minimize the opportunity for error." *Id.*, at 530, 531 N.E.2d, at 613 (citation omitted). The court held that the record lacked the requisite clear and convincing evidence of the patient's expressed intent to withhold life-sustaining treatment. *Id.*, at 531–534, 531 N.E.2d, at 613–615.

Other courts have found state statutory law relevant to the resolution of these issues. In *Conservatorship of Drabick*, 200 Cal. App. 3d 185, 245 Cal. Rptr. 840, cert. denied, ____ U.S. ____ (1988), the California Court of Appeal authorized the removal of a nasogastric feeding tube from a 44-year-old man who was in a persistent vegetative state as a result of an auto accident. Noting that the right to refuse treatment was grounded in both the common law and a constitutional right of privacy, the court held that a state probate statute authorized the patient's conservator to order the withdrawal of life-sustaining treatment when such a decision was made in good faith based on medical advice and the conservatee's best interests. While acknowledging that "to claim that [a patient's] 'right to choose' survives incompetence is a legal fiction at best," the court reasoned that the respect society accords to persons as individuals is not lost upon incompetence and is best preserved by allowing others "to make a decision that reflects [a patient's] interests more closely than would a purely technological decision to do whatever is possible."[5] *Id.*, at 208, 245 Cal.Rptr., at 854–855. See also *In re Conservatorship of Torres*, 357 N.W.2d 332 (Minn. 1984) (Minnesota court had constitutional and statutory authority to authorize a conservator to order the removal of an incompetent individual's respirator since in patient's best interests).

In *In re Estate of Longeway*, 123 Ill.2d 33, 549 N.E.2d 292 (1989), the Supreme Court of Illinois considered whether a 76-year-old woman rendered incompetent from a series of strokes had a right to the discontinuance of artificial nutrition and hydration. Noting that the boundaries of a federal right of privacy were uncertain, the court found a right to refuse treatment in the doctrine of informed consent. *Id.*, at 43–45, 549 N.E.2d, at 296–297. The court further held that the State Probate Act impliedly authorized a guardian to exercise a ward's right to refuse artificial sustenance in the event that the ward was terminally ill and irreversibly comatose. *Id.*, at 45–47, 549 N.E.2d, at 298. Declining to adopt a best interests standard for deciding when it would be appropriate to exercise a ward's right because it "lets another make a determination of a patient's quality of life," the court opted instead for a substituted judgment standard. *Id.*, at 49, 549 N.E.2d, at 299. Finding the "expressed intent" standard utilized in *O'Connor, supra*, too rigid, the court noted that other clear and convincing evidence of the patient's intent could be considered. 133 Ill.2d, at 50–51, 549 N.E.2d, at 300. The court also adopted the "consensus opinion [that] treats artificial nutrition and hydration as medical treatment." *Id.*, at 42, 549 N.E.2d, at 296. Cf. *McConnell* v. *Beverly Enterprises-Connecticut, Inc.*, 209 Conn. 692, 705, 553 A.2d 596, 603 (1989) (right to withdraw artificial nutrition and hydration found in the Connecticut Removal of Life Support Systems Act, which "provid[es] functional guidelines for the exercise of the common law and constitutional rights of self-determination"; attending physician authorized to remove treatment after finding that patient is in a terminal condition, obtaining consent of family, and considering expressed wishes of patient).[6]

As these cases demonstrate, the common-law doctrine of informed consent is viewed as generally encompassing the right of a competent individual to refuse medical treatment. Beyond that, these decisions demonstrate both similarity and diversity in their approach to decision of what all agree is a perplexing question with unusually strong moral and ethical overtones. State courts have available to them for decision a number of sources—state constitutions, statutes, and common law—which are not available to us. In this Court, the question is simply and starkly whether the United States Constitution prohibits Missouri from choosing the rule of decision which it did. This is the first case in which we have been squarely presented with the issue of whether the United States Constitution grants what is in common parlance referred to as a "right to die." We follow the judicious counsel of our decision in *Twin City Bank* v. *Nebeker*, 167 U.S. 196, 202 (1897), where we said that in deciding "a question of such magnitude and importance . . . it is the [better] part of wisdom not to attempt, by any general statement, to cover every possible phase of the subject."

The Fourteenth Amendment provides that no State shall "deprive any person of life, liberty, or property, without due process of law." The principle that a competent person has a constitutionally protected liberty interest in refusing unwanted medical treatment may be inferred from our prior decisions. In *Jacobson* v. *Massachusetts*, 197 U.S. 11, 24–30 (1905), for instance, the Court balanced an individual's liberty interest in declining an unwanted smallpox vaccine against the State's interest in preventing disease. Decisions prior to the incorporation of the Fourth Amendment into the Fourteenth Amendment analyzed searches and seizures involving the body under the Due Process Clause and were thought to implicate substantial liberty interests. See, e.g., *Breithaupt* v. *Abrams*, 352 U.S. 432, 439 (1957) ("As against the right of an individual that his person be held inviolable . . . must be set the interests of society . . .").

Just this Term, in the course of holding that a State's procedures for administering antipsychotic medication to prisoners were sufficient to satisfy due process concerns, we recognized that prisoners possess "a significant liberty interest in avoiding the unwanted administration of antipsychotic drugs under the Due Process Clause of the Fourteenth Amendment." *Washington* v. *Harper*, ___ U.S. ___, ___ (1990) (slip op., at 9); see also *id.*, at ___ (slip op., at 17) ("The forcible injection of medication into a nonconsenting person's body represents a substantial interference with that person's liberty"). Still other cases support the recognition of a general liberty interest in refusing medical treatment. *Vitek* v. *Jones*, 445 U.S. 480, 494 (1980) (transfer to mental hospital coupled with mandatory behavior modification treatment implicated liberty interests); *Parham* v. *J.R.*, 442 U.S. 584, 600 (1979) ("a child, in common with adults, has a substantial liberty interest in not being confined unnecessarily for medical treatment").

But determining that a person has a "liberty interest" under the Due Process Clause does not end the inquiry;[7] "whether respondent's constitutional rights have been violated must be determined by balancing his liberty interests against the relevant state interests." *Youngberg* v. *Romeo*, 457 U.S. 307, 321 (1982). See also *Mills* v. *Rogers*, 457 U.S. 291, 299 (1982).

Petitioners insist that under the general holdings of our cases, the forced administration of life-sustaining medical treatment, and even of artificially-delivered food and water essential to life, would implicate a competent person's liberty interest. Although we think the logic of the cases discussed above would embrace such a liberty interest, the dramatic consequences involved in refusal of such treatment would inform the inquiry as to whether the deprivation of that interest is constitutionally permissible. But for purposes of this case, we assume that the United States Constitution would grant a competent person a constitutionally protected right to refuse lifesaving hydration and nutrition.

Petitioners go on to assert that an incompetent person should possess the same right in this respect as is possessed by a competent person. They rely primarily on our decisions in *Parham* v. *J.R.*, *supra*, and *Youngberg* v. *Romeo*, 457 U.S. 307 (1982). In *Parham*, we held that a mentally disturbed minor child had a liberty interest in "not being confined unnecessarily for medical treatment," 442 U.S., at 600, but we certainly did not intimate that such a minor child, after commitment, would have a liberty interest in refusing treatment. In *Youngberg*, we held that a seriously retarded adult had a liberty interest in safety and freedom from bodily restraint, 457 U.S., at 320. *Youngberg*, however, did not deal with decisions to administer or withhold medical treatment.

The difficulty with petitioners' claim is that in a sense it begs the question: an incompetent person is not able to make an informed and voluntary choice to exercise a hypothetical right to refuse treatment or any other right. Such a "right" must be exercised for her, if at all, by some sort of surrogate. Here, Missouri has in effect recognized that under certain circumstances a surrogate may act for the patient in electing to have hydration and nutrition withdrawn in such a way as to cause death, but it has established a procedural safeguard to assure that the action of the surrogate conforms as best it may to the wishes expressed by the patient while competent. Missouri requires that evidence of the incompetent's wishes as to the withdrawal of treatment be proved by clear and convincing evidence. The question, then, is whether the United States Constitution forbids the establishment of this procedural requirement by the State. We hold that it does not.

Whether or not Missouri's clear and convincing evidence requirement comports with the United States Constitution depends in part on what interests the State may properly seek to protect in this situation. Missouri relies on its interest in the protection and preservation of human life, and there can be no gainsaying this interest. As a general matter, the States—indeed, all civilized nations—demonstrate their commitment to life by treating homicide as serious crime. Moreover, the majority of States in this country have laws imposing criminal penalties on one who assists another to commit suicide.[8] We do not think a State is required to remain neutral in the face of an informed and voluntary decision by a physically-able adult to starve to death.

But in the context presented here, a State has more particular interests at stake. The choice between life and death is a deeply personal decision of obvious and overwhelming finality. We believe Missouri may legitimately seek to safeguard the personal element of this choice through the imposition of heightened evidentiary requirements. It cannot be disputed that the Due Process Clause protects an interest in life as well as an interest in refusing life-sustaining medical treatment. Not all incompetent patients will have loved ones available to serve as surrogate decisionmakers. And even where family members are present, "[t]here will, of course, be some unfortunate situations in which family members will not act to protect a patient." *In re Jobes*, 108 N.J. 394, 419, 529 A.2d 434, 477 (1987). A State is entitled to guard against potential abuses in such situations. Similarly, a State is entitled to consider that a judicial proceeding to make a determination regarding an incompetent's wishes may very well not be an adversarial one, with the added guarantee of accurate factfinding that the adversary process brings with it.[9] See *Ohio* v. *Akron Center for Reproductive Health*, ___ U.S. ___, ___ (1990) (slip op., at 10–11). Finally, we think a State may properly decline to make judgments about the "quality" of life that a particular individual may enjoy, and simply assert an unqualified interest in the preservation of human life to be weighed against the constitutionally protected interests of the individual.

In our view, Missouri has permissibly sought to advance these interests through the adoption of a "clear and convincing" standard of proof to govern such proceedings. "The function of a standard of proof, as that concept is embodied in the Due Process Clause and in the realm of factfinding, is to 'instruct the factfinder concerning the degree of confidence our society thinks he should have in the correctness of factual conclusions for a particular type of adjudication.'" *Addington* v. *Texas*, 441 U.S. 418, 423 (1979) (quoting *In re Winship*, 397 U.S. 358, 370 (1970) (Harlan, J., concurring)). "This Court has mandated an intermediate standard of proof—'clear and convincing evidence'—when the individual interests at stake in a state proceeding are both 'particularly important' and 'more substantial than mere loss of money.'" *Santosky* v. *Kramer*, 455 U.S. 745, 756 (1982) (quoting *Addington, supra*, at 424). Thus, such a standard has been required in deportation proceedings, *Woodby* v. *INS*, 385 U.S. 276 (1966), in denaturalization proceedings, *Schneiderman* v. *United States*, 320 U.S. 118 (1943), in civil commitment proceedings, *Addington, supra*, and in proceedings for the termination of parental rights. *Santosky, supra.*[10] Further, this level of proof, "or an even higher one, has traditionally been imposed in cases involving allegations of civil fraud, and in a variety of other kinds of civil cases involving such issues as . . . lost wills, oral contracts to make bequests, and the like." *Woodby, supra*, at 285, n. 18.

We think it self-evident that the interests at stake in the instant proceedings are more substantial, both on an individual and societal level, than those involved in a run-of-the-mine civil dispute. But not only does the standard of proof reflect the importance of a particular adjudication, it also serves as "a societal judgment about how the risk of error should be distributed between the litigants." *Santosky, supra*, 455 U.S. at 755; *Addington, supra*, at 423. The more stringent the burden of proof a party must bear, the more that party bears the risk of an erroneous decision. We believe that Missouri may permissibly place an increased risk of an erroneous decision on those seeking to terminate an incompetent individual's life-sustaining treatment. An erroneous decision not to terminate results in a maintenance of the status quo; the possibility of subsequent developments such as advancements in medical science, the discovery of new evidence regarding the patient's intent, changes in the law, or simply the unexpected death of the patient despite the administration of life-sustaining treatment, at least create the potential that a wrong decision will eventually be corrected or its impact mitigated. An erroneous decision to withdraw life-sustaining treatment, however, is not susceptible of correction. In *Santosky*, one of the factors which led the Court to require proof by clear and convincing evidence in a proceeding to terminate parental rights was that a decision in such a case was final and irrevocable. *Santosky, supra*, at 759. The same must surely be said of the decision to discontinue hydration and nutrition of a patient such as Nancy Cruzan, which all agree will result in her death.

It is also worth noting that most, if not all, States simply forbid oral testimony entirely in determining the wishes of parties in transactions which, while important, simply do not have the consequences that a decision to terminate a person's life does. At common law and by statute in most States, the parole evidence rule prevents the variations of the terms of a written contract by oral testimony. The statute of frauds makes unenforceable oral contracts to leave property by will, and statutes regulating the making of wills universally require that those instruments be in writing. See 2 A. Corbin, Contracts § 398, pp. 360–361 (1950); 2 W. Page, Law of Wills §§ 19.3-19.5, pp. 61–71 (1960). There is no doubt that statutes requiring wills to be in writing, and statutes of frauds which require that a contract to make a will be in writing, on occasion frustrate the effectuation of the intent of a particular decedent, just as Missouri's requirement of proof in this case may have frustrated the effectuation of the not-fully-expressed desires of Nancy Cruzan. But the Constitution does not require general rules to work faultlessly; no general rule can.

In sum, we conclude that a State may apply a clear and convincing evidence standard in proceedings where a guardian seeks to discontinue nutrition and hydration of a person diagnosed to be in a persistent vegetative state. We note that many courts which have adopted some sort of substituted judgment procedure in situations like this, whether they limit consideration of evidence to the prior expressed wishes of the incompetent individual, or whether they allow more general proof of what the individual's decision would have been, require a clear and convincing standard of proof for such evidence. See, *e.g.*, *Longeway*, 133 Ill.2d, at 5051, 549 N.E.2d at 300; *McConnell*, 209 Conn., at 707–710, 553 A.2d at 604–605; *O'Connor*, 72 N.Y.2d, at 529–530, 531 N.E.2d, at 613; *In re Gardner*, 534 A. 2d 947, 952–953 (Me. 1987); *In re Jobes*, 108 N.J., at 412–413, 529 A.2d, at 443; *Leach* v. *Akron General Medical Center*, 68 Ohio Misc. 1, 11, 426 N.E.2d 809, 815 (1980).

The Supreme Court of Missouri held that in this case the testimony adduced at trial did not amount to clear and convincing proof of the patient's desire to have hydration and nutrition withdrawn. In so doing, it reversed a decision of the Missouri trial court which had found that the evidence "suggest[ed]" Nancy Cruzan would not have desired to continue such measures, App. to Pet. for Cert. A98, but which had not adopted the standard of "clear and convincing evidence" enunciated by the Supreme Court. The testimony adduced at trial consisted primarily of Nancy Cruzan's statements made to a housemate about a year before her accident that she would not want to live should she face life as a "vegetable," and other observations to the same effect. The observations did not deal in terms with withdrawal of medical treatment or of hydration and nutrition. We cannot say that the Supreme Court of Missouri committed constitutional error in reaching the conclusion that it did.[11]

Petitioners alternatively contend that Missouri must accept the "substituted judgment" of close family members even in the absence of substantial proof that their views reflect the views of the patient. They rely primarily upon our decisions in *Michael H.* v. *Gerald D.*, 491 U.S. ____ (1989), and *Parham* v. *J.R.*, 442 U.S. 584 (1979). But we do not think these cases support their claim. In *Michael H.*, we *upheld* the constitutionality of California's favored treatment of traditional family relationships; such a holding may not be turned around into a constitutional requirement that a State *must* recognize the primacy of those relationships in a situation like this. And in *Parham*, where the patient was a minor, we also *upheld* the constitutionality of a state scheme in which parents made certain decisions for mentally ill minors. Here again petitioners would seek to turn a decision which allowed a State to rely on family decisionmaking into a constitutional requirement that the State recognize such decisionmaking. But constitutional law does not work that way.

No doubt is engendered by anything in this record but that Nancy Cruzan's mother and father are loving and caring parents. If the State were required by the United States Constitution to repose a right of "substituted judgment" with anyone, the Cruzans would surely qualify. But we do not think the Due Process Clause requires the State to repose judgment on these matters with anyone but the patient herself. Close family members may have a strong feeling—a feeling not at all ignoble or unworthy, but not entirely disinterested, either—that they do not wish to witness the continuation of the life of a loved one which they regard as hopeless, meaningless, and even degrading. But there is no automatic assurance that the view of close family members will necessarily be the same as the patient's would have been had she been confronted with the prospect of her situation while competent. All of the reasons previously discussed for allowing Missouri to require clear and convincing evidence of the patient's wishes lead us to conclude that the State may choose to defer only to those wishes, rather than confide the decision to close family members.[12]

The judgment of the Supreme Court of Missouri is *Affirmed*.

NOTES

1. The State Supreme Court, adopting much of the trial court's findings, described Nancy Cruzan's medical condition as follows:

> ". . . (1) [H]er respiration and circulation are not artificially maintained and are within the normal limits of a thirty-year-old female; (2) she is oblivious to her environment except for reflexive responses to sound and perhaps painful stimuli; (3) she suffered anoxia of the brain resulting in a massive enlargement of the ventricles filling with cerebrospinal fluid in the area where the brain has degenerated and [her] cerebral cortical atrophy is irreversible, permanent, progressive and ongoing; (4) her highest cognitive brain function is exhibited by her grimacing perhaps in recognition of ordinarily painful stimuli, indicating the experience of pain and apparent response to sound; (5) she is a spastic quadriplegic; (6) her four extremities are contracted with irreversible muscular and tendon damage to all extremities; (7) she has no cognitive or reflexive ability to swallow food or water to maintain her daily essential needs and . . . she will never recover her ability to swallow sufficient [sic] to satisfy her needs. In sum, Nancy is diagnosed as in a persistent vegetative state. She is not dead. She is not terminally ill. Medical experts testified that she could live another thirty years." *Cruzan* v. *Harmon*, 760 S.W.2d 408, 411 (Mo. 1989) (en banc) (quotations omitted; footnote omitted).

In observing that Cruzan was not dead, the court referred to the following Missouri statute:

> "For all legal purposes, the occurrence of human death shall be determined in accordance with the usual and customary standards of medical practice, provided that death shall not be determined to have occurred unless the following minimal conditions have been met:
>
> "(1) When respiration and circulation are not artificially maintained, there is an irreversible cessation of spontaneous respiration and circulation; or
>
> "(2) When respiration and circulation are artificially maintained, and there is total and irreversible cessation of all brain function, including the brain stem and that such determination is made by a licensed physician." Mo. Rev. Stat. § 194.005 (1986).

Since Cruzan's respiration and circulation were not being artificially maintained, she obviously fit within the first proviso of the statute.

Dr. Fred Plum, the creator of the term "persistent vegetative state" and a renowned expert on the subject, has described the "vegetative state" in the following terms:

> "'Vegetative state describes a body which is functioning entirely in terms of its internal controls. It maintains temperature. It maintains heart beat and pulmonary ventilation. It maintains digestive activity. It maintains reflex activity of muscles and nerves for low level conditioned responses. But there is no behavioral evidence of either self-awareness or awareness of the surroundings in a learned manner.'" *In re Jobes*, 108 N.J. 394, 403, 529 A.2d 434, 438 (1987).

See also Brief for American Medical Association et al., as *Amici Curiae*, 6 ("The persistent vegetative state can best be understood as one of the conditions in which patients have suffered a loss of consciousness").

2. See generally Karnezis, Patient's Right to Refuse Treatment Allegedly Necessary to Sustain Life, 93 A.L.R.3d 67 (1979) (collecting cases); Cantor, A Patient's Decision to Decline Life-Saving Medical Treatment: Bodily Integrity

Versus the Preservation of Life, 26 Rutgers L. Rev. 228, 229, and n. 5 (1973) (noting paucity of cases).

3. See Chapman, The Uniform Rights of the Terminally Ill Act: Too Little, Too Late?, 42 Ark. L. Rev. 319, 324, n. 15 (1989); see also F. Rozovsky, Consent to Treatment, A Practical Guide 415–423 (2d ed. 1984).
4. In a later trilogy of cases, the New Jersey Supreme Court stressed that the analytic framework adopted in *Conroy* was limited to elderly, incompetent patients with shortened life expectancies, and established alternative approaches to deal with a different set of situations. See *In re Farrell*, 108 N.J. 335, 529 A.2d 404 (1987) (37-year-old competent mother with terminal illness had right to removal of respirator based on common law and constitutional principles which overrode competing state interests); *In re Peter*, 108 N.J. 365, 529 A.2d 419 (1987) (65-year-old woman in persistent vegetative state had right to removal of nasogastric feeding tube—under *Conroy* subjective test, power of attorney and hearsay testimony constituted clear and convincing proof of patient's intent to have treatment withdrawn); *In re Jobes*, 108 N.J. 394, 529 A.2d 434 (1987) (31-year-old woman in persistent vegetative state entitled to removal of jejunostomy feeding tube—even though hearsay testimony regarding patient's intent insufficient to meet clear and convincing standard of proof, under *Quinlan*, family or close friends entitled to make a substituted judgment for patient).
5. The *Drabick* court drew support for its analysis from earlier, influential decisions rendered by California courts of appeal. See *Bouvia* v. *Superior Court*, 179 Cal. App.3d 1127, 225 Cal. Rptr. 297 (1986) (competent 28-year-old quadriplegic had right to removal of nasogastric feeding tube inserted against her will); *Bartling* v. *Superior Court*, 163 Cal. App.3d 186, 209 Cal. Rptr. 220 (1984) (competent 70-year-old, seriously-ill man had right to the removal of respirator); *Barber* v. *Superior Court*, 147 Cal. App.3d 1006, 195 Cal. Rptr. 484 (1983) (physicians could not be prosecuted for homicide on account of removing respirator and intravenous feeding tubes of patient in persistent vegetative state).
6. Besides the Missouri Supreme Court in *Cruzan* and the courts in *McConnell, Longeway, Drabick, Bouvia, Barber, O'Connor, Conroy, Jobes*, and *Peter, supra*, appellate courts of at least four other States and one Federal District Court have specifically considered and discussed the issue of withholding or withdrawing artificial nutrition and hydration from incompetent individuals. See *Gray* v. *Romeo*, 697 F.Supp. 580 (RI 1988); *In re Gardner*, 534 A.2d 947 (Me. 1987); *In re Grant*, 109 Wash. 2d 545, 747 P.2d 445 (Wash. 1987); *Brophy* v. *New England Sinai Hospital, Inc.*, 398 Mass. 417, 497 N.E.2d 626 (1986); *Corbett* v. *D'Alessandro*, 487 So.2d 368 (Fla. App. 1986). All of these courts permitted or would permit the termination of such measures based on rights grounded in the common law, or in the State or Federal Constitution.
7. Although many state courts have held that a right to refuse treatment is encompassed by a generalized constitutional right of privacy, we have never so held. We believe this issue is more properly analyzed in terms of a Fourteenth Amendment liberty interest. See *Bowers* v. *Hardwick*, 478 U.S. 186, 194–195 (1986).
8. See Smith, All's Well That Ends Well: Toward a Policy of Assisted Rational Suicide or Merely Enlightened Self-Determination?, 22 U.C. Davis L. Rev. 275, 290–291, n. 106 (1989) (compiling statutes).
9. Since Cruzan was a patient at a state hospital when this litigation commenced, the State has been involved as an adversary from the beginning. However, it can be expected that many of these types of disputes will arise in private institutions, where a guardian *ad litem* or similar party will have been appointed as the sole representative of the incompetent individual in the litigation. In such cases, a guardian may act in entire good faith, and yet not maintain a position truly adversarial to that of the family. Indeed, as noted by the court below, "[t]he guardian *ad litem* [in this case] finds himself in the predicament of believing that it is in Nancy's 'best interest to have the tube feeding discontinued,' but 'feeling that an appeal should be made because our responsibility to her as attorneys and guardians *ad litem* was to pursue this matter to the highest court in the state in view of the fact that this is a case of first impression in the State of Missouri.'" 760 S.W. 2d, at 410, n. 1. Cruzan's guardian *ad litem* has also filed a brief in this Court urging reversal of the Missouri Supreme Court's decision. None of this is intended to suggest that the guardian acted the least bit improperly in this proceeding. It is only meant to illustrate the limits which may obtain on the adversarial nature of this type of litigation.
10. We recognize that these cases involved instances where the government sought to take action against an individual. See *Price Waterhouse* v. *Hopkins*, 490 U.S. ____, ____ (1989) (plurality opinion). Here, by contrast, the government seeks to protect the interests of an individual, as well as its own institutional interests, in life. We do not see any reason why important individual interests should be afforded less protection simply because the government finds itself in the position of defending them. "[W]e find it significant that . . . the defendant rather than the plaintiff" seeks the clear and convincing standard of proof—"suggesting that this standard ordinarily serves as a shield rather than . . . a sword." *Id.*, at____. That it is the government that has picked up the shield should be of no moment.
11. The clear and convincing standard of proof has been variously defined in this context as "proof sufficient to persuade the trier of fact that the patient held a firm and settled commitment to the termination of life supports under the circumstances like those presented," *In re Westchester County Medical Center on behalf of O'Connor*, 72 N.Y.2d 517, 531, N.E.2d 607, 613 (1988) *(O'Connor)*, and as evidence which "produces in the mind of the trier of fact a firm belief or conviction as to the truth of the allegations sought to be established, evidence so clear, direct and weighty and convincing as to enable [the factfinder] to come to a clear conviction, without hesitancy, of the truth of the precise facts in issue." *In re Jobes*, 108 N.J., at 407–408, 529 A.2d, at 441 (quotation omitted). In both of these cases the evidence of the patient's intent to refuse medical treatment was arguably stronger than that presented here. The New York Court of Appeals and the Supreme Court of New Jersey, respectively, held that the proof failed to meet a clear and convincing threshold.

See *O'Connor, supra*, at 526–534, 531 N.E.2d, at 610–615; *Jobes, supra*, at 442–443.

12. We are not faced in this case with the question of whether a State might be required to defer to the decision of a surrogate if competent and probative evidence established that the patient herself had expressed a desire that the decision to terminate life-sustaining treatment be made for her by that individual.

Petitioners also adumbrate in their brief a claim based on the Equal Protection Clause of the Fourteenth Amendment to the effect that Missouri has impermissibly treated incompetent patients differently from competent ones, citing the statement in *Cleburne* v. *Cleburne Living Center, Inc.*, 473 U.S. 432, 439 (1985), that the clause is "essentially a direction that all persons similarly situated should be treated alike." The differences between the choice made *by* a competent person to refuse medical treatment, and the choice made *for* an incompetent person by someone else to refuse medical treatment, are so obviously different that the State is warranted in establishing rigorous procedures for the latter class of cases which do not apply to the former class.

CHILD ABUSE AND NEGLECT PREVENTION AND TREATMENT: FINAL RULE

INTRODUCTION. *The early controversies over foregoing life-sustaining treatments often involved newborns with serious, life-threatening conditions, some involving Down Syndrome, hydrocephaly, or other conditions that lead to some degree of mental retardation. The controversy centered on parental refusals of life-support. Two major attempts were made at the federal level to write regulations, often referred to as the Baby Doe Regulations, to prohibit refusals of treatment in such cases. The first effort was based on Section 504 of the Disabilities Act of 1973, which prohibited discrimination on the basis of handicap. Its proponents argued that refusals of treatment were actually based on the mental handicap and that babies with similar physical problems unaccompanied by mental disorder would not be refused life support. This approach was later rejected by the courts on a technicality and dropped in favor of a second effort grounded in the claim that refusal of treatment constituted child neglect or abuse. Federal regulations promulgated in 1985 required any state receiving federal child abuse funds to have protections of infants against parental refusal of life-support in place. Three exceptions in which life support may be refused were recognized: inevitable terminal condition, coma, and conditions in which it was virtually futile in terms of preserving life and inhumane to make the attempt. Even when these three conditions were met, "appropriate" nutrition, hydration, and medication had to be provided. This leads to an anomaly: the courts recognize refusal of nutrition and hydration in adults, even in some cases based solely on surrogate decisions, while comparable refusal in infants violates federal regulations. Unless no medical feeding is deemed "appropriate" in such babies, families must presently feed infants while older family members who are equally incapable of expressing their own wishes are able to have treatment foregone.*

§ 1340.15—Services and Treatment for Disabled Infants

(a) Purpose. The regulations in this section implement certain provisions of the Child Abuse Amendments of 1984, including section 4(b)(2)(K) of the Child Abuse Prevention and Treatment Act governing the protection and care of disabled infants with life-threatening conditions.

(b) Definitions. (1) The term "medical neglect" means the failure to provide adequate medical care in the context of the definitions of "child abuse and neglect" in section 3 of the Act and § 1340.2(d) of this part. The term "medical neglect" includes, but is not limited to, the withholding of medically indicated treatment from a disabled infant with a life-threatening condition.

(2) The term "withholding of medically indicated treatment" means the failure to respond to the infant's life-threatening conditions by providing treatment (including appropriate nutrition hydration, and medication) which, in the treating physician's (or physicians') reasonable medical judgment, will be most likely to be effective in ameliorating or correcting all such conditions, except that the term does not include the failure to provide treatment (other than appropriate nutrition, hydration, or medication) to an infant when, in the treating physician's (or physicians') reasonable medical judgment any of the following circumstances apply:

(i) The infant is chronically and irreversibly comatose;
(ii) The provision of such treatment would merely prolong dying, not be effective in ameliorating or correcting all

Reprinted from the Final Rule: 45 CFR 1340. U.S. Department of Health and Human Services (1985). Published in 50 *Federal Register* 72, 14887-92. The table of contents, citation of authority, and revision of § 1340.14 (to require 1340.15) have been omitted.

of the infant's life-threatening conditions, or otherwise be futile in terms of the survival of the infant; or

(iii) The provision of such treatment would be virtually futile in terms of the survival of the infant and the treatment itself under such circumstances would be inhumane.

(3) Following are definitions of terms used in paragraph (b)(2) of this section:

(i) The term "infant" means an infant less than one year of age. The reference to less than one year of age shall not be construed to imply that treatment should be changed or discontinued when an infant reaches one year of age, or to affect or limit any existing protections available under State laws regarding medical neglect of children over one year of age. In addition to their applicability to infants less than one year of age, the standards set forth in paragraph (b)(2) of this section should be consulted thoroughly in the evaluation of any issue of medical neglect involving an infant older than one year of age who has been continuously hospitalized since birth, who was born extremely prematurely, or who has a long-term disability.

(ii) The term "reasonable medical judgment" means a medical judgment that would be made by a reasonably prudent physician, knowledgeable about the case and the treatment possibilities with respect to the medical conditions involved.

(c) Eligibility requirements. (1) In addition to the other eligibility requirements set forth in this Part, to qualify for a grant under this section, a State must have programs, procedures, or both, in place within the State's child protective service system for the purpose of responding to the reporting of medical neglect, including instances of withholding of medically indicated treatment from disabled infants with life-threatening conditions.

(2) These programs and/or procedures must provide for:

(i) Coordination and consultation with individuals designated by and within appropriate health care facilities;

(ii) Prompt notification by individuals designated by and within appropriate health care facilities of cases of suspected medical neglect (including instances of the withholding of medically indicated treatment from disabled infants with life-threatening conditions); and

(iii) The authority, under State law, for the State child protective service system to pursue any legal remedies, including the authority to initiate legal proceedings in a court of competent jurisdiction, as may be necessary to prevent the withholding of medically indicated treatment from disabled infants with life-threatening conditions.

(3) The programs and/or procedures must specify that the child protective services system will promptly contact each health care facility to obtain the name, title, and telephone number of the individual(s) designated by such facility for the purpose of the coordination, consultation, and notification activities identified in paragraph (c)(2) of this section, and will at least annually recontact each health care facility to obtain any changes in the designations.

(4) These programs and/or procedures must be in writing and must conform with the requirements of section 4(b)(2) of the Act and § 1340.14 of this part.

In connection with the requirement of conformity with the requirements of section 4(b)(2) of the Act and § 1340.14 of this part, the programs and/or procedures must specify the procedures the child protective services system will follow to obtain, in a manner consistent with State law:

(i) Access to medical records and/or other pertinent information when such access is necessary to assure an appropriate investigation of a report of medical neglect (including instances of withholding of medically indicated treatment from disabled infants with life threatening conditions); and

(ii) A court order for an independent medical examination of the infant, or otherwise effect such an examination in accordance with processes established under State law, when necessary to assure an appropriate resolution of a report of medical neglect (including instances of withholding of medically indicated treatment from disabled infants with life threatening conditions).

(5) The eligibility requirements contained in this section shall be effective October 9, 1985.

(d) Documenting eligibility. (1) In addition to the information and documentation required by and pursuant to § 1340.12(b) and (c), each State must submit with its application for a grant sufficient information and documentation to permit the Commissioner to find that the State is in compliance with the eligibility requirements set forth in paragraph (c) of this section.

(2) This information and documentation shall include:

(i) A copy of the written programs and/or procedures established by, and followed within, the State for the purpose of responding to the reporting of medical neglect, including instances of withholding of medically indicated treatment from disabled infants with life-threatening conditions:

(ii) Documentation that the State has authority, under State law, for the State child protective service system to pursue any legal remedies, including the authority to initiate legal proceedings in a court of competent jurisdiction, as may be necessary to prevent the withholding of medically indicated treatment from disabled infants with life-threatening conditions. This documentation shall consist of:

(A) A copy of the applicable provisions of State statute(s); or

(B) A copy of the applicable provisions of State rules or regulations, along with a copy of the State statutory provisions that provide the authority for such rules or regulations; or

(C) A copy of an official, numbered opinion of the Attorney General of the State that so provides, along with a copy of the applicable provisions of the State statute that provides a basis for the opinion, and a certification that the official opinion has been distributed to interested parties within the State, at least including all hospitals; and

(iii) Such other information and documentation as the Commissioner may require.

(e) Regulatory construction. (1) No provision of this section or part shall be construed to affect any right, protection, procedures, or requirement under 45 CFR Part 84, Nondiscrimination in the Basis of Handicap in Programs and Activities Receiving or Benefiting from Federal Financial Assistance.

(2) No provision of this section or part may be so construed as to authorize the Secretary or any other governmental entity to establish standards prescribing specific medical treatments for specific conditions, except to the extent that such standards are authorized by other laws or regulations.

* * *

5. 45 CFR Part 1340 is further amended by adding at the end thereof the following . . .

Appendix to Part 1340—Interpretative Guidelines Regarding 45 CFR 1340.15—Services and Treatment for Disabled Infants

This appendix sets forth the Department's interpretative guidelines regarding several terms that appear in the definition of the term "withholding of medically indicated treatment" in section 3(3) of the Child Abuse Prevention and Treatment Act, as amended by section 121(3) of the Child Abuse Amendments of 1984. This statutory definition is repeated in § 1340.15(b)(2) of the final rule.

The Department's proposed rule to implement those provisions of the Child Abuse Amendments of 1984 relating to services and treatment for disabled infants included a number of proposed clarifying definitions of several terms used in the statutory definition. The preamble to the proposed rule explained these proposed clarifying definitions, and in some cases used examples of specific diagnoses to elaborate on meaning.

During the comment period on the proposed rule, many commenters urged deletion of these clarifying definitions and avoidance of examples of specific diagnoses. Many commenters also objected to the specific wording of some of the proposed clarifying definitions, particularly in connection with the proposed use of the word "imminent" to describe the proximity in time at which death is anticipated regardless of treatment in relation to circumstances under which treatment (other than appropriate nutrition, hydration and medication) need not be provided. A letter from the six principal sponsors of the "compromise amendment" which became the pertinent provisions of the Child Abuse Amendments of 1984 urged deletion of "imminent" and careful consideration of the other concerns expressed.

After consideration of these recommendations, the Department decided not to adopt these several proposed clarifying definitions as part of the final rule. It was also decided that effective implementation of the program established by the Child Abuse Amendments would be advanced by the Department stating its interpretations of several key terms in the statutory definition. This is the purpose of this appendix.

The interpretative guidelines that follow have carefully considered comments submitted during the comment period on the proposed rule. These guidelines are set forth and explained without the use of specific diagnostic examples to elaborate on meaning.

Finally, by way of introduction, the Department does not seek to establish these interpretative guidelines as binding rules of law, nor to prejudge the exercise of reasonable medical judgment in responding to specific circumstances. Rather, this guidance is intended to assist in interpreting the statutory definition so that it may be rationally and thoughtfully applied in specific contexts in a manner fully consistent with the legislative intent.

1. In general: the statutory definition of "withholding of medically indicated treatment." Section 1340.15(b)(2) of the final rule defines the term "withholding of medically indicated treatment" with a definition identical to that which appears in section 3(3) of the Act (as amended by section 121(3) of the Child Abuse Amendments of 1984).

This definition has several main features. First, it establishes the basic principle that all disabled infants with life-threatening conditions must be given medically indicated treatment, defined in terms of action to respond to the infant's life-threatening conditions by providing treatment (including appropriate nutrition, hydration or medication) which, in the treating physician's (or physicians') reasonable medical judgment will be most likely to be effective in ameliorating or correcting all such conditions.

Second, the statutory definition spells out three circumstances under which treatment is not considered "medically indicated." These are when, in the treating physician's (or physicians') reasonable medical judgment:

- The infant is chronically and irreversibly comatose;
- The provision of such treatment would merely prolong dying, not be effective in ameliorating or correcting all of

the infant's life-threatening conditions, or otherwise be futile in terms of survival of the infant; or

- The provision of such treatment would be virtually futile in terms of survival of the infant and the treatment itself under such circumstances would be inhumane.

The third key feature of the statutory definition is that even when one of these three circumstances is present, and thus the failure to provide treatment is not a "withholding of medically indicated treatment," the infant must nonetheless be provided with appropriate nutrition, hydration, and medication.

Fourth, the definition's focus on the potential effectiveness of treatment in ameliorating or correcting life-threatening conditions makes clear that it does not sanction decisions based on subjective opinions about the future "quality of life" of a retarded or disabled person.

The fifth main feature of the statutory definition is that its operation turns substantially on the "reasonable medical judgment" of the treating physician or physicians. The term "reasonable medical judgment" is defined in § 1340.15(b)(3)(ii) of the final rule, as it was in the Conference Committee Report on the Act, as a medical judgment that would be made by a reasonably prudent physician, knowledgeable about the case and the treatment possibilities with respect to the medical conditions involved.

The Department's interpretations of key terms in the statutory definition are fully consistent with these basic principles reflected in the definition. The discussion that follows is organized under headings that generally correspond to the proposed clarifying definitions that appeared in the proposed rule but were not adopted in the final rule. The discussion also attempts to analyze and respond to significant comments received by the Department.

2. The term "life-threatening condition." Clause (b)(3)(ii) of the proposed rule proposed a definition of the term "life-threatening condition." This term is used in the statutory definition in the following context:

> [T]he term "withholding of medically indicated treatment" means the failure to respond to the infant's *life-threatening conditions* by providing treatment (including appropriate nutrition, hydration, and medication) which, in the treating physician's or physicians' reasonable medical judgment, will be most likely to be effective in ameliorating or correcting all such conditions [, except that] . . . . [Emphasis supplied].

It appears to the Department that the applicability of the statutory definition might be uncertain to some people in cases where a condition may not, strictly speaking, by itself be life-threatening, but where the condition significantly increases the risk of the onset of complications that may threaten the life of the infant. If medically indicated treatment is available for such a condition, the failure to provide it may result in the onset of complications that, by the time the condition becomes life-threatening in the strictest sense, will eliminate or reduce the potential effectiveness of any treatment. Such a result cannot, in the Department's view, be squared with the Congressional intent.

Thus, the Department interprets the term "life-threatening condition" to include a condition that, in the treating physician's or physicians' reasonable medical judgment, significantly increases the risk of the onset of complications that may threaten the life of the infant.

In response to comments that the proposed rule's definition was potentially overinclusive by covering any condition that one could argue "may" become life-threatening, the Department notes that the statutory standard of "the treating physician's or physicians' reasonable medical judgment" is incorporated in the Department's interpretation, and is fully applicable.

Other commenters suggested that this interpretation would bring under the scope of the definition many irreversible conditions for which no corrective treatment is available. This is certainly not the intent. The Department's interpretation implies nothing about whether, or what, treatment should be provided. It simply makes clear that the criteria set forth in the statutory definition for evaluating whether, or what, treatment should be provided are applicable. That is just the start, not the end, of the analysis. The analysis then takes fully into account the reasonable medical judgment regarding potential effectiveness of possible treatments, and the like.

Other comments were that it is unnecessary to state any interpretation because reasonable medical judgment commonly deems the conditions described as life-threatening and responds accordingly. HHS [Health and Human Services] agrees that this is common practice followed under reasonable medical judgment, just as all the standards incorporated in the statutory definition reflect common practice followed under reasonable medical judgment. For the reasons stated above, however, the Department believes it is useful to say so in these interpretative guidelines.

3. The term "treatment" in the context of adequate evaluation. Clause (b)(3)(ii) of the proposed rule proposed a definition of the term "treatment." Two separate concepts were dealt with in clause (A) and (B, respectively, of the proposed rule. Both of these clauses were designed to ensure that the Congressional intent regarding the issues to be considered under the analysis set forth in the statutory definition is fully effectuated. Like the guidance regarding "life-threatening condition," discussed above, the Department's interpretations go to the applicability of the statutory analysis, not its result.

The Department believes that Congress intended that the standard of following reasonable medical judgment regarding the potential effectiveness of possible courses of action should apply to issues regarding adequate medical evaluation, just as it does to issues regarding adequate medical intervention. This is apparent Congressional intent because Congress adopted, in the Conference Report's definition of "reasonable medical judgment," the standard of adequate knowledge about the case and the treatment possibilities with respect to the medical condition involved.

Having adequate knowledge about the case and the treatment possibilities involved is, in effect, step one of the process, because that is the basis on which "reasonable medical judgment" will operate to make recommendations regarding medical intervention. Thus, part of the process to determine what treatment, if any, "will be most likely to be effective in ameliorating or correcting" all life-threatening conditions is for the treating physician or physicians to make sure they have adequate information about the condition and adequate knowledge about treatment possibilities with respect to the condition involved. The standard for determining the adequacy of the information and knowledge is the same as the basic standard of the statutory definition: reasonable medical judgment. A reasonably prudent physician faced with a particular condition about which he or she needs additional information and knowledge of treatment possibilities would take steps to gain more information and knowledge by, quite simply, seeking further evaluation by, or consultation with, a physician or physicians whose expertise is appropriate to the condition(s) involved or further evaluation at a facility with specialized capabilities regarding the conditions(s) involved.

Thus, the Department interprets the term "treatment" to include (but not be limited to) any further evaluation by, or consultation with, a physician or physicians whose expertise is appropriate to the condition(s) involved or further evaluation at a facility with specialized capabilities regarding the condition(s) involved that, in the treating physician's or physicians' reasonable medical judgment, is needed to assure that decisions regarding medical intervention are based on adequate knowledge about the case and the treatment possibilities with respect to the medical conditions involved.

This reflects the Department's interpretation that failure to respond to an infant's life-threatening conditions by obtaining any further evaluations or consultations that in the treating physician's reasonable medical judgment, are necessary to assure that decisions regarding medical intervention are based on adequate knowledge about the case and the treatment possibilities involved constitutes a "withholding of medically indicated treatment." Thus, if parents refuse to consent to such a recommendation that is based on the treating physician's reasonable medical judgment that, for example, further evaluation by a specialist is necessary to permit reasonable medical judgments to be made regarding medical intervention, this would be a matter for appropriate action by the child protective services system.

In response to comments regarding the related provision in the proposed rule, this interpretative guideline makes quite clear that this interpretation does not deviate from the basic principle of reliance on reasonable medical judgment to determine, the extent of the evaluations necessary in the particular case. Commenters expressed concerns that the provision in the proposed rule would intimidate physicians to seek transfer of seriously ill infants to tertiary level facilities much more often than necessary, potentially resulting in diversion of the limited capacities of these facilities away from those with real needs for the specialized care, unnecessary separation of infants from their parents when equally beneficial treatment could have been provided at the community or regional hospital, inappropriate deferral of therapy while time-consuming arrangements can be affected, and other counterproductive ramifications. The Department intended no intimidation, prescription or similar influence on reasonable medical judgment, but rather, intended only to affirm that it is the Department's interpretation that the reasonable medical judgment standard applies to issues of medical evaluation, as well as issues of medical intervention.

4. The term "treatment" in the context of multiple treatments. Clause (b)(3)(iii)(B) of the proposed rule was designed to clarify that, in evaluating the potential effectiveness of a particular medical treatment or surgical procedure that can only be reasonably evaluated in the context of a complete potential treatment plan, the "treatment" to be evaluated under the standards of the statutory definition includes the multiple medical treatments and/or surgical procedures over a period of time that are designed to ameliorate or correct a life- threatening condition or conditions. Some commenters stated that it could be construed to require the carrying out of a long process of medical treatments or surgical procedures regardless of the lack of success of those done first. No such meaning is intended.

The intent is simply to characterize that which must be evaluated under the standards of the statutory definition, not to imply anything about the results of the evaluation. If parents refuse consent for a particular medical treatment or surgical procedure that by itself may not correct or ameliorate all life-threatening conditions, but is recommended as part of a total plan that involves multiple medical treatments and/or surgical procedures over a period of time that, in the treating physician's reasonable medical judgment, will be most likely to be effective in ameliorating or correcting all such conditions, that would be a matter for appropriate action by the child protective services system.

On the other hand, if, in the treating physician's reasonable medical judgment, the total plan will, for example, be virtually futile and inhumane, within the meaning of the statutory term, then there is no "withholding of medically indicated treatment." Similarly,if a treatment plan is commenced on the basis of a reasonable medical judgment that there is a good chance that it will be effective, but due to a lack of success, unfavorable complications, or other factors, it becomes the treating physician's reasonable medical judgment that further treatment in accord with the prospective treatment plan, or alternative treatment, would be futile, then the failure to provide that treatment would not constitute a "withholding of medically indicated treatment." This analysis does not divert from the reasonable medical judgment standard of the statutory definition: it simply makes clear the Department's interpretation that the failure to evaluate the potential effectiveness of a treatment plan as a whole would be inconsistent with the legislative intent.

Thus, the Department interprets the term "treatment" to include (but not be limited to) multiple medical treatments and/or surgical procedures over a period of time that are designed to ameliorate or correct a life-threatening condition or conditions.

5. The term "merely prolong dying." Clause (b)(3)(v) of the proposed rule proposed a definition of the term "merely prolong dying," which appears in the statutory definition. The proposed rule's provision stated that this term "refers to situations where death is imminent and treatment will do no more than postpone the act of dying."

Many commenters argued that the incorporation of the word "imminent," and its connotation of immediacy, appeared to deviate from the Congressional intent, as developed in the course of the lengthy legislative negotiations, that reasonable medical judgments can and do result in nontreatment decisions regarding some conditions for which treatment will do no more than temporarily postpone a death that will occur in the near future, but not necessarily within days. The six principal sponsors of the compromise amendment also strongly urged deletion of the word "imminent."

The Department's use of the term "imminent" in the proposed rule was not intended to convey a meaning not fully consonant with the statute. Rather, the Department intended that the word "imminent" would be applied in the context of the condition involved, and in such a context, it would not be understood to specify a particular number of days. As noted in the preamble to the proposed rule, this clarification was proposed to make clear that the "merely prolong dying" clause of the statutory definition would not be applicable to situations where treatment will not totally correct a medical condition but will give a patient many years of life. The Department continues to hold to this view.

To eliminate the type of misunderstanding evidenced in the comments, and to assure consistency with the statutory definition, the word "imminent" is not being adopted for purposes of these interpretative guidelines.

The Department interprets the term "merely prolong dying" as referring to situations where the prognosis is for death and, in the treating physician's (or physicians') reasonable medical judgment, further or alternative treatment would not alter the prognosis in an extension of time that would not render the treatment futile.

Thus, the Department continues to interpret Congressional intent as not permitting the "merely prolong dying" provision to apply where many years of life will result from the provision of treatment, or where the prognosis is not for death in the near future, but rather the more distant future. The Department also wants to make clear it does not intend the connotations many commenters associated with the word "imminent." In addition, contrary to the impression some commenters appeared to have regarding the proposed rule, the Department's interpretation is that reasonable medical judgments will be formed on the basis of knowledge about the condition(s) involved, the degree of inevitability of death, the probable effect of any potential treatments, the projected time period within which death will probably occur, and other pertinent factors.

6. The term "not be effective in ameliorating or correcting all of the infant's life threatening conditions" in the context of a future life-threatening condition. Clause (b)(3)(vi) of the proposed rule proposed a definition of the term "not be effective in ameliorating or correcting all the infant's life-threatening conditions" used in the statutory definition of "withholding of medically indicated treatment."

The basic point made by the use of this term in the statutory definition was explained in the Conference Committee Report:

> Under the definition, if a disabled infant suffers from more than one life-threatening condition and, in the treating physician's or physicians' reasonable medical judgment, there is no effective treatment for one of those conditions, then the infant is not covered by the terms of the amendment (except with respect to appropriate nutrition, hydration, and medication) concerning the withholding of medically indicated treatment. H. Conf. Rep. No. 1038, 98th Cong., 2d Sess. 41 (1980).

This clause of the proposed rule dealt with the application of this concept in two contexts: first, when the nontreatable condition will not become life-threatening in the near future, and second, when humaneness makes palliative treatment medically indicated.

With respect to the context of a future life-threatening condition, it is the Department's interpretation that the term "not be effective in ameliorating or correcting all of the infant's life-threatening conditions" does not permit the withholding of treatment on the grounds that one or more of the infant's life-threatening conditions, although not life-threatening in the near future, will become life-threatening in the more distant future.

This clarification can be restated in the terms of the Conference Committee Report excerpt, quoted just above, with the italicized words indicating the clarification, as follows: Under the definition, if a disabled infant suffers from more than one life-threatening condition and, in the treating physician's or physicians' reasonable medical judgment, there is no effective treatment for one of these conditions *that threatens the life of the infant in the near future*, then the infant is not covered by the terms of the amendment (except with respect to appropriate nutrition, hydration, and medication) concerning the withholding of medically indicated treatment: *but if the nontreatable condition will not become life-threatening until the more distant future, the infant is covered by the terms of the amendment.*

Thus, this interpretative guideline is simply a corollary to the Department's interpretation of "merely prolong dying," stated above, and is based on the same understanding of Congressional intent, indicated above, that if a condition will not become life-threatening until the more distant future, it should not be the basis for withholding treatment.

Also for the same reasons explained above, the word "imminent" that appeared in the proposed definition is not adopted for purposes of this interpretative guideline. The Department makes no effort to draw an exact line to separate "near future" from "more distant future." As noted above in connection with the term "merely prolong dying," the statutory definition provides that it is for reasonable medical judgment, applied to the specific condition and circumstances involved, to determine whether the prognosis of death, because of its nearness in time, is such that treatment would not be medically indicated.

7. The term "not be effective in ameliorating or correcting all life-threatening conditions" in the context of palliative treatment. Clause (b)(3)(iv)(B) of the proposed rule proposed to define the term "not be effective in ameliorating or correcting all life-threatening conditions" in the context where the issue is not life-saving treatment, but rather palliative treatment to make a condition more tolerable. An example of this situation is where an infant has more than one life-threatening condition, at least one of which is not treatable and will cause death in the near future. Palliative treatment is available, however, that will, in the treating physician's reasonable medical judgment, relieve severe pain associated with one of the conditions. If it is the treating physician's reasonable medical judgment that this palliative treatment will ameliorate the infant's *overall* condition, taking all individual conditions into account, even though it would not ameliorate or correct *each* condition, then this palliative treatment is medically indicated. Simply put, in the context of ameliorative treatment that will make a condition more tolerable, the term "not be effective in ameliorating or correcting *all* life-threatening conditions" should not be construed as meaning *each and every* condition, but rather as referring to the infant's *overall* condition.

HHS believes Congress did not intend to exclude humane treatment of this kind from the scope of "medically indicated treatment." The Conference Committee Report specifically recognized that "it is appropriate for a physician, in the exercise of reasonable medical judgment, to consider that factor [humaneness] in selecting among effective treatments." H. Conf. Rep. No. 1038, 98th Cong., 2d Sess. 41 (1984). In addition, the articulation in the statutory definition of circumstances in which treatment need not be provided specifically states that "appropriate nutrition, hydration, and medication" must nonetheless be provided. The inclusion in this proviso of medication, one (but not the only) potential palliative treatment to relieve severe pain, corroborates the Department's interpretation that such palliative treatment that will ameliorate the infant's overall condition, and that in the exercise of reasonable medical judgment is humane and medically indicated, was not intended by Congress to be outside the scope of the statutory definition.

Thus, it is the Department's interpretation that the term "not be effective in ameliorating or correcting all of the infant's life-threatening conditions" does not permit the withholding of ameliorative treatment that, in the treating physician's or physicians' reasonable medical judgment, will make a condition more tolerable, such as providing palliative treatment to relieve severe pain, even if the overall prognosis, taking all conditions into account, is that the infant will not survive.

A number of commenters expressed concerns about some of the examples contained in the preamble of the proposed rule that discussed the proposed definition relating to this point, and stated that, depending on medical complications, exact prognosis, relationships to other conditions, and other factors, the treatment suggested in the examples might not necessarily be the treatment that reasonable medical judgment would decide would be most likely to be effective. In response to these comments, specific diagnostic examples have not been included in this discussion, and this interpretative guideline makes clear that the "reasonable medical judgment" standard applies on this point as well.

Other commenters argued that an interpretative guideline on this point is unnecessary because reasonable medical judgment would commonly provide ameliorative or palliative treatment in the circumstances described. The Department agrees that such treatment is common in the exercise of reasonable medical judgment, but believes it useful, for the reasons stated, to provide this interpretative guidance.

8. The term "virtually futile." Clause (b)(3)(vii) of the proposed rule proposed a definition of the term "virtually futile" contained in the statutory definition. The context of this term in the statutory definition is:

> [T]he term "withholding of medically indicated treatment" . . . does not include the failure to provide treatment (other than appropriate nutrition, hydration, or medication) to an infant when in the treating physician's or physicians' reasonable medical judgment. . . . the provision of such treatment would be *virtually futile* in terms of the survival of the infant and the treatment itself under such circumstances would be inhumane. Section 3(3)(C) of the Act [emphasis supplied].

The Department interprets the term "virtually futile" to mean that the treatment is highly unlikely to prevent death in the near future.

This interpretation is similar to those offered in connection with "merely prolong dying" and "not be effective in ameliorating or correcting all life-threatening conditions" in the context of a future life-threatening condition, with the addition of a characterization of likelihood that corresponds to the statutory word "virtually." For the reasons explained in the discussion of "merely prolong dying," the word "imminent" that was used in the proposed rule has not been adopted for purposes of this interpretative guideline.

Some commenters expressed concern regarding the words "highly unlikely," on the grounds that such certitude is often medically impossible. Other commenters urged that a distinction should be made between generally utilized treatments and experimental treatments. The Department does not believe any special clarifications are needed to respond to these comments. The basic standard of reasonable medical judgment applies to the term "virtually futile." The Department's interpretation does not suggest an impossible or unrealistic standard of certitude for any medical judgment. Rather, the standard adopted in the law is that there be a "reasonable medical judgment." Similarly, reasonable medical judgment is the standard for evaluating potential treatment possibilities on the basis of the actual circumstances of the case. HHS does not believe it would be helpful to try to establish distinctions based on characterizations of the degree of general usage, extent of validated efficacy data, or other similar factors. The factors considered in the exercise of reasonable medical judgment, including any factors relating to human subjects experimentation standards, are not disturbed.

9. The term "the treatment itself under such circumstances would be inhumane." Clause (b)(3)(viii) of the proposed rule proposed a definition of the term "the treatment itself under such circumstances would be inhumane," that appears in the statutory definition. The context of this term in the statutory definition is that it is not a "withholding of medically indicated treatment" to withhold treatment (other than appropriate nutrition, hydration, or medication) when, in the treating physician's reasonable medical judgment, "the provision of such treatment would be virtually futile in terms of the survival of the infant and the treatment itself under such circumstances would be inhumane." § 3(3)(C) of the Act.

The Department interprets the term "the treatment itself under such circumstances would be inhumane" to mean the treatment itself involves significant medical contraindications and/or significant pain and suffering for the infant that clearly outweigh the very slight potential benefit of the treatment for an infant highly unlikely to survive. (The Department further notes that the use of the term "inhumane" in this context is not intended to suggest that consideration of the humaneness of a particular treatment is not legitimate in any other context; rather, it is recognized that it is appropriate for a physician, in the exercise of reasonable medical judgment, to consider that factor in selecting among effective treatments.)

Other clauses of the statutory definition focus on the expected *result* of the possible treatment. This provision of the statutory definition adds a consideration relating to the *process* of possible treatment. It recognized that in the exercise of reasonable medical judgment, there are situations where, although there is some slight chance that the treatment will be beneficial to the patient (the potential treatment is considered *virtually* futile, rather than futile), the potential benefit is so outweighed by negative factors relating to the process of the treatment itself that, under the circumstances, it would be inhumane to subject the patient to the treatment.

The Department's interpretation is designed to suggest the factors that should be taken into account in this difficult balance. A number of commenters argued that the interpretation should permit, as part of the evaluation of whether treatment would be inhumane, consideration of the infant's future "quality of life."

The Department strongly believes such an interpretation would be inconsistent with the statute. The statute specifies that the provision applies only where the treatment would be "virtually futile in terms of the survival of the infant," and the "treatment *itself* under such circumstances would be inhumane." (Emphasis supplied.) The balance is clearly to be between the very slight chance that treatment will allow the infant to survive and the negative factors relating to the process of the treatment. These are the circumstances under which reasonable medical judgment could decide that the treatment itself would be inhumane.

Some commenters expressed concern about the use of terms such as "clearly outweigh" in the description of this balance on the grounds that such precision is impractical. Other commenters argued that this interpretation could be construed to mandate useless and painful treatment. The Department believes there is no basis for these worries because "reasonable medical judgment" is the governing standard. The interpretative guideline suggests nothing other than application of this standard. What the guideline does is set forth the Department's interpretation that the statute directs the reasonable medical judgment to considerations relating to the slight chance of survival and the negative factors regarding the process of treatment and to the balance between them that would support a conclusion that the treatment itself would be inhumane.

Other commenters suggested adoption of a statement contained in the Conference Committee Report that makes clear that the use of the term "inhumane" in the statute was not intended to suggest that consideration of the humaneness of a particular treatment is not legitimate in any other context. The Department has adopted this statement as part of its interpretative guideline.

10. Other terms. Some comments suggested that the Department clarify other terms used in the statutory definition of "withholding of medically-indicated treatment," such as the term "appropriate nutrition hydration or medication" in the context of treatment that may not be withheld, notwithstanding the existence of one of the circumstances under which the failure to provide treatment is not a "withholding of medically indicated treatment." Some commenters stated, for example, that very potent pharmacologic agents, like other methods of medical intervention, can produce results accurately described as accomplishing no more than to merely prolong dying, or be futile in terms of the survival of the infant, or the like, and that, therefore, the Department should clarify that the proviso regarding "appropriate nutrition, hydration or medication" should not be construed entirely independently of the circumstances under which other treatment need not be provided.

The Department has not adopted an interpretative guideline on this point because it appears none is necessary. As noted above in the discussion of palliative treatment the Department recognizes that there is no absolutely clear line between medication and treatment other than medication that would justify excluding the latter from the scope of palliative treatment that reasonable medical judgment would find medically indicated, notwithstanding a very poor prognosis.

Similarly, the Department recognizes that in some circumstances, certain pharmacologic agents, not medically indicated for palliative purposes, might, in the exercise of reasonable medical judgment also not be indicated for the purpose of correcting or ameliorating any particular condition because they will for example, merely prolong dying. However, the Department believes the word "appropriate" in this proviso of the statutory definition is adequate to permit the exercise of reasonable medical judgment in the scenario referred to by these commenters.

At the same time, it should be clearly recognized that the statute is completely unequivocal in requiring that all infants receive "appropriate nutrition hydration and medication," regardless of their condition or prognosis.

IN THE MATTER OF BABY K, 1993

INTRODUCTION. *While the Baby Doe Regulations established three exceptions to the general policy of treating refusal of life-sustaining treatment as child abuse, they raise an as yet unresolved question. The regulations establish the right of parents to refuse treatment when it merely prolongs a terminal illness, is keeping a comatose baby alive, or when it is virtually futile and inhumane. But does the right of the parent to refuse such treatment imply that this refusal is also the parent's duty? Put in other words, do health professionals or health care institutions have the right unilaterally to refuse to treat such patients?*

Arguments are emerging that claim that such treatments are "medically futile." The literature has challenged the meaning of the term. Some people argue that if a treatment sustains life even temporarily, it is having a physiological effect on the patient, and thus is not futile, at least in a physiological sense. If such treatment is futile, it is futile normatively: it involves a moral value judgment about which lives are worth preserving. But about this judgment physicians have no special expertise.

Others have argued that physicians have the right to refuse to preserve such lives either because of scarcity of resources or because it violates the integrity of the provider to be forced to deliver such care. Baby K was born with anencephaly. She had a brain stem, but no capacity for conscious life, and survival for more than a few months was unprecedented. Yet her mother insisted on maximal ventilatory support, believing all human life is precious and to be preserved. The federal district court in Alexandria, Virginia, supported the mother's claim, at least in the case when an insurer is willing to pay the bill and when the baby was unconscious and therefore beyond pain and suffering. The opinion presented here reviews the legal arguments, which have been upheld by a Court of Appeals. An appeal to the U.S. Supreme Court is contemplated.

Findings of Fact

1. Plaintiff Hospital is a general acute care hospital located in Virginia that is licensed to provide diagnosis, treatment, and medical and nursing services to the public as provided by Virginia law. Among other facilities, the Hospital has a Pediatric Intensive Care Department and an Emergency Department.

2. The Hospital is a recipient of federal and state funds including those from Medicare and Medicaid and is a "participating hospital" pursuant to 42 U.S.C. § 1395cc.

3. The Hospital and its staff (including emergency doctors, pediatricians, neonatologists and pediatric intensivists) treat sick children on a daily basis.

4. Defendant Ms. H, a citizen of the Commonwealth of Virginia, is the biological mother of Baby K, an infant girl born by Caesarean section at the Hospital on October 13, 1992. Baby K was born with anencephaly.

5. Anencephaly is a congenital defect in which the brain stem is present but the cerebral cortex is rudimentary or absent. There is no treatment that will cure, correct, or ameliorate anencephaly. Baby K is permanently unconscious and cannot hear or see. Lacking a cerebral function, Baby K does not feel pain. Baby K has brain stem functions primarily limited to reflexive actions such as feeding reflexes (rooting, sucking, swallowing), respiratory reflexes (breathing, coughing), and reflexive responses to sound or touch. Baby K has a normal heart rate, blood pressure, liver function, digestion, kidney function, and bladder function and has gained weight since her birth. Most anencephalic infants die within days of birth.

6. Baby K was diagnosed prenatally as being anencephalic. Despite the counselling of her obstetrician and neonatologist that she terminate her pregnancy, Ms. H refused to have her unborn child aborted.

7. A Virginia court of competent jurisdiction has found defendant Mr. K, a citizen of the Commonwealth of Virginia, to be Baby K's biological father.

8. Ms. H and Mr. K have never been married.

Reprinted from *In the Matter of Baby K.* 832 F.Supp. 1022 (E.D. Va. 1993).

9. Since Baby K's birth, Mr. K has, at most, been only distantly involved in matters relating to the infant. Neither the Hospital nor Ms. H ever sought Mr. K's opinion or consent in providing medical treatment to Baby K.

10. Because Baby K had difficulty breathing immediately upon birth, Hospital physicians provided her with mechanical ventilator treatment to allow her to breathe.

11. Within days of Baby K's birth, Hospital medical personnel urged Ms. H to permit a "Do Not Resuscitate Order" for Baby K that would discontinue ventilator treatment. Her physicians told her that no treatment existed for Baby K's anencephalic condition, no therapeutic or palliative purpose was served by the treatment, and that ventilator care was medically unnecessary and inappropriate. Despite this pressure, Ms. H continued to request ventilator treatment for her child.

12. Because of Ms. H's continued insistence that Baby K receive ventilator treatment, her treating physicians requested the assistance of the Hospital's "Ethics Committee" in overriding the mother's wishes.

13. A three person Ethics Committee subcommittee, composed of a family practitioner, a psychiatrist, and a minister, met with physicians providing care to Baby K. On October 22, 1992, the group concluded that Baby K's ventilator treatment should end because "such care is futile" and decided to "wait a reasonable time for the family to help the caregiver terminate aggressive therapy." If the family refused to follow this advice, the committee recommended that the Hospital should "attempt to resolve this through our legal system."

14. Ms. H subsequently rejected the committee's recommendation. Before pursuing legal action to override Ms. H's position, the Hospital decided to transfer the infant to another health care facility.

15. Baby K was transferred to a nursing home ("Nursing Home") in Virginia on November 30, 1992 during a period when she was not experiencing respiratory distress and thus did not need ventilator treatment. A condition of the transfer was that the Hospital agreed to take the infant back if Baby K again developed respiratory distress to receive ventilator treatment which was unavailable at the Nursing Home. Ms. H agreed to this transfer.

16. Baby K returned to the Hospital on January 15, 1993 after experiencing respiratory distress to receive ventilator treatment. Hospital officials again attempted to persuade Ms. H to discontinue ventilator treatment for her child. Ms. H again refused. After Baby K could breathe on her own, she was transferred back to the Nursing Home on February 12, 1993.

17. Baby K again experienced breathing difficulties on March 3, 1993 and returned to the Hospital to receive ventilator treatment.

18. On March 15, 1993, Baby K received a tracheotomy, a procedure in which a breathing tube is surgically implanted in her windpipe, to facilitate ventilator treatment. Ms. H agreed to this operation.

19. After no longer requiring ventilator treatment, Baby K was transferred back to the Nursing Home on April 13, 1993 where she continues to live.

20. Baby K will almost certainly continue to have episodes of respiratory distress in the future. In the absence of ventilator treatment during these episodes, she would suffer serious impairment of her bodily functions and soon die.

21. Ms. H visits Baby K daily. The mother opposes the discontinuation of ventilator treatment when Baby K experiences respiratory distress because she believes that all human life has value, including her anencephalic daughter's life. Ms. H has a firm Christian faith that all life should be protected. She believes that God will work a miracle if that is his will. Otherwise, Ms. H believes, God, and not other humans, should decide the moment of her daughter's death. As Baby K's mother and as the only parent who has participated in the infant's care, Ms. H believes that she has the right to decide what is in her child's best interests.

22. On the Hospital's motion, a guardian *ad litem* to represent Baby K was appointed pursuant to Virginia Code § 8.01-9.

23. Both the guardian *ad litem* and Mr. K share the Hospital's position that ventilator treatment should be withheld from Baby K when she experiences respiratory distress.

24. The Hospital has stipulated that it is not proposing to deny ventilator treatment to Baby K because of any lack of adequate resources or any inability of Ms. H to pay for the treatment.

Conclusions of Law

Pursuant to the Declaratory Judgment Act, 28 U.S.C. § 2201, the Hospital has sought declaratory and injunctive relief under four federal statutes and one Virginia statute: the Emergency Medical Treatment and Active Labor Act, 42 U.S.C. § 1395dd; the Rehabilitation Act of 1973, 29 U.S.C. § 794; the Americans with Disabilities Act of 1990, 42 U.S.C. § 12101 *et seq.*; the Child Abuse Amendments of 1984, 42 U.S.C. § 5102 *et seq.*; and the Virginia Medical Malpractice Act, Va.Code § 8.01-581.1 *et seq*. This court has federal question jurisdiction under the four federal statutes and supplemental jurisdiction regarding the Virginia statute. 28 U.S.C. §§ 1331, 1367.

EMERGENCY MEDICAL TREATMENT AND ACTIVE LABOR ACT

Plaintiff seeks a declaration that its refusal to provide Baby K with life-supporting medical care would not transgress the Emergency Medical Treatment and Active Labor Act, 42 U.S.C. § 1395dd ("EMTALA"). EMTALA requires that participating hospitals provide stabilizing medical treatment to any person who comes to an emergency department in an "emergency medical condition" when treatment is requested on that person's behalf. An "emergency medical condition" is defined in the statute as "acute symptoms of sufficient severity . . . such that the absence of immediate medical attention could reasonably be expected to result in . . . serious impairment to bodily functions, or serious dysfunction of any bodily organ or part." 42 U.S.C. § 1395dd(e)(1)(A). "Stabilizing" medical treatment is defined as "such medical treatment of the condition as may be necessary to assure, within reasonable medical probability, that no material deterioration of the condition" will result. *Id.* § 1395dd(e)(3)(A). The statute's legislative history includes a position paper by the American College of Emergency Physicians stating that "stabilization" should include "[e]stablishing and assuring an adequate airway and adequate ventilation." H.R.Rep. No. 241 (Pt. 3), 99th Cong., 1st Sess. 26 (1985).

The Hospital admits that Baby K would meet these criteria if she is brought to the Hospital while experiencing breathing difficulty. As stated in the Hospital's complaint, when Baby K is in respiratory distress, that condition is "such that the absence of immediate medical attention could reasonably be expected to cause serious impairment to her bodily functions"—*i.e.*, her breathing difficulties constitute an "emergency medical condition." The Hospital also concedes in its complaint that ventilator treatment is required in such circumstances to assure "that no material deterioration of Baby K's condition is likely to occur"—*i.e.*, a ventilator is necessary to "stabilize" the baby's condition. These admissions establish that the Hospital would be liable under EMTALA if Baby K arrived there in respiratory distress (or some other emergency medical condition) and the Hospital failed to provide mechanical ventilation (or some other medical treatment) necessary to stabilize her acute condition.

The Hospital would also have an obligation to continue to provide stabilizing medical treatment to Baby K even if she were admitted to the pediatric intensive care unit or other unit of the Hospital and to provide the treatment until she could be transferred back to the Nursing Home or to another facility willing to accept her. *See Thornton v. Southwest Detroit Hosp.*, 895 F.2d 1131, 1135 (6th Cir.1990) ("emergency care does not always stop when a patient is wheeled from the emergency room into the main hospital"); *McIntyre v. Schick*, 795 F.Supp. 777, 781 (E.D.Va.1992) (rationale behind "anti-dumping statute is not based upon the door of the hospital through which a patient enters, but rather upon the notion of proper medical care for those persons suffering medical emergencies, whenever such emergencies occur at a participating hospital. Indeed, it is a ridiculous distinction, one which places form over substance, to state that the care a patient receives depends on the door through which the patient walks").

Despite EMTALA's clear requirements and in the face of the Hospital's admissions, the Hospital seeks an exemption from the statute for instances in which the treatment at issue is deemed "futile" or "inhumane" by the hospital physicians. The plain language of the statute requires stabilization of an emergency medical condition. The statute does not admit of any "futility" or "inhumanity" exceptions. Any argument to the contrary should be directed to the U.S. Congress, not to the Federal Judiciary. *Cf. Baber v. Hospital Corporation of America*, 977 F.2d 872, 878 (4th Cir.1992) (rejecting argument that EMTALA provides private cause of action against physicians on grounds that "it is not our role to rewrite legislation passed by Congress. When a statute is clear and unambiguous, we must apply its terms as written instead of varying its terms to accommodate a perceived legislative intent").

Even if EMTALA contained the exceptions advanced by the Hospital, these exceptions would not apply here. The use of a mechanical ventilator to assist breathing is not "futile" or "inhumane" in relieving the *acute* symptoms of respiratory difficulty which is the emergency medical condition that must be treated under EMTALA. To hold otherwise would allow hospitals to deny emergency treatment to numerous classes of patients, such as accident victims who have terminal cancer or AIDS, on the grounds that they eventually will die anyway from those diseases and that emergency care for them would therefore be "futile."

REHABILITATION ACT

Section 504 of the Rehabilitation Act prohibits discrimination against an "otherwise qualified" handicapped individual, solely by reason of his or her handicap, under any program or activity receiving federal financial assistance. Hospitals such as plaintiff that accept Medicare and Medicaid funding are subject to the Act. *United States v. Baylor Univ. Medical Center*, 736 F.2d 1039, 1049 (5th Cir.1984), *cert. denied*, 469 U.S. 1189, 105 S.Ct. 958, 83 L.Ed.2d 964 (1985). Baby K is a "handicapped" and "disabled" person within the meaning of the Rehabilitation Act of 1973. A "handicapped individual" under the Rehabilitation Act "includes an infant who is born with a congenital defect." *Bowen v. American Hospital Ass'n*, 476 U.S. 610, 624, 106 S.Ct. 2101, 2110, 90 L.Ed.2d 584 (1986).

Section 504's plain text spells out the necessary scope of inquiry: Is Baby K otherwise qualified to receive ventilator treatment and is ventilator treatment being threatened with being denied because of an unjustified consideration of her anencephalic handicap? The Hospital has admitted that the sole reason it wishes to withhold ventilator treatment for Baby K over her mother's objections, is because of Baby K's anencephaly—her handicap and disability.

To evade this textual mandate, the Hospital relies on two cases which held that a hospital's decision not to override the desire of the parents of babies with congenital defects to withhold treatment did not violate section 504. *Johnson v. Thompson*, 971 F.2d 1487, 1493 (10th Cir.1992), *cert. denied*, ____ U.S. ____, 113 S.Ct. 1255, 122 L.Ed.2d 654 (1993); *United States v. University Hospital, State U. of New York*, 729 F.2d 144, 156–57 (2d Cir.1984). Because the parents in *Johnson* and *University Hospital* consented to the withholding of treatment, the two cases are factually distinguishable from this case.[1]

When the Rehabilitation Act was passed in 1973, Congress intended that discrimination on the basis of a handicap be treated in the same manner that Title VI of the Civil Rights Act treats racial discrimination. *University Hospital*, 729 F.2d at 161–163 (Winter, J., dissenting). This analogy to race dispels any ambiguity about the extent to which Baby K has statutory rights not to be discriminated against on the basis of her handicap. It also shatters the Hospital's contention that ventilator treatment should be withheld because Baby K's recurring breathing troubles are intrinsically related to her handicap. No such distinction would be permissible within the context of racial discrimination. In addition, the Hospital was able to perform a tracheotomy on Baby K. This surgery was far more complicated than linking her to a ventilator to allow her to breathe. *Cf. Bowen*, 476 U.S. at 655, 106 S.Ct. at 2127 ("if an otherwise normal child would be given the identical treatment, so should the handicapped child") (White, J., dictum in dissent). Just as an AIDS patient seeking ear surgery is "otherwise qualified" to receive treatment despite poor long-term prospects of living, Baby K is "otherwise qualified" to receive ventilator treatment despite similarly dismal health prospects. *Cf. Glanz v. Vernick*, 750 F.Supp. 39, 45–46 (D.Mass.1990). Thus, the Hospital's desire to withhold ventilator treatment from Baby K over her mother's objections would violate the Rehabilitation Act.

AMERICANS WITH DISABILITIES ACT

Section 302 of the Americans with Disabilities Act ("ADA") prohibits discrimination against disabled individuals by "public accommodations." 42 U.S.C. § 12182. A "disability" is "a physical or mental impairment that substantially limits one or more of the major life activities" of an individual. 42 U.S.C. § 12102(2). This includes any physiological disorder or condition affecting the neurological system, musculoskeletal system, or sense organs, among others. 28 C.F.R. § 36.104 (definition of "physical or mental impairment"). Anencephaly is a disability, because it affects the baby's neurological functioning, ability to walk, and ability to see or talk. "Public accommodation" is defined to include a "professional office of a health care provider, hospital, or other service establishment." 42 U.S.C. § 12181(7). The Hospital is a public accommodation under the ADA. 28 C.F.R. § 36.104.

Section 302(a) of the ADA states a general rule of nondiscrimination against the disabled:

> General rule. No individual shall be discriminated against on the basis of disability in the full and equal enjoyment of the goods, services, facilities, privileges, advantages, or accommodation of any place of public accommodations by any person who owns, leases (or leases to), or operates a place of public accommodation.

42 U.S.C. § 12182(a). In contrast to the Rehabilitation Act, the ADA does not require that a handicapped individual be "otherwise qualified" to receive the benefits of participation. Further, section 302(b)(1)(A) of the ADA states that "[i]t shall be discriminatory to subject an individual or class of individuals on the basis of a disability . . . to a denial of the opportunity of the individual or class to participate in or benefit from the goods, services, facilities, privileges, advantages, or accommodations of an entity." 42 U.S.C. § 12182(b)(1)(A)(i).

The Hospital asks this court for authorization to deny the benefits of ventilator services to Baby K by reason of her anencephaly. The Hospital's claim is that it is "futile" to keep alive an anencephalic baby, even though the mother has requested such treatment. But the plain language of the ADA does not permit the denial of ventilator services that would keep alive an anencephalic baby when those life-saving services would otherwise be provided to a baby without disabilities at the parent's request. The Hospital's reasoning would lead to the denial of medical services to anencephalic babies as a class of disabled individuals. Such discrimination against a vulnerable population class is exactly what the American with Disabilities Act was enacted to prohibit. The Hospital would therefore violate the ADA if it were to withhold ventilator treatment from Baby K.

CHILD ABUSE ACT

Plaintiff seeks a declaration that it may refuse to provide life-supporting medical care to Baby K without incurring liability under the Child Abuse Amendments of 1984, 42 U.S.C. § 5101 *et seq.* ("Child Abuse Act"). This request for relief must be denied because the Hospital has failed to join a necessary party—the Virginia Child Protective Services.

There is no private right of action against a health care provider under the Child Abuse Act. *Jensen v. Conrad*, 570 F.Supp. 91, 113 (D.S.C.1983) (citing *Perry v. Housing Authority of Charleston*, 664 F.2d 1210, 1213 (4th Cir.1981)), *aff'd*, 747 F.2d 185 (4th Cir.1984), *cert. denied*, 470 U.S. 1052, 105 S.Ct. 1754, 84 L.Ed.2d 818 (1985). The Act only authorizes states which receive federal grants for child abuse and neglect programs to bring legal action through their child protective services agencies to prevent the medical neglect of disabled infants. 42 U.S.C. § 5106a(b)(10)(C); 45 C.F.R. § 1340.15(c)(2)(iii).

Because the Virginia Child Protective Services has an interest in a declaratory judgment regarding the Child Abuse Act and is the only party that can enforce the Act, it is a necessary party. This court must have the sole enforcing authority party before it before considering the declaratory judgment issue. *ARW Exploration Corp. v. Aguirre*, 947 F.2d 450, 454 (10th Cir.1991). Without the Virginia Child Protective Services as a party, no actual controversy exists as to this issue as required by the Declaratory Judgment Act. 28 U.S.C. § 2201. Thus, the Hospital's request for declaratory and injunctive relief under the Child Abuse Amendments must be denied. *See White v. National Union Fire Ins. Co.*, 913 F.2d 165, 167168 (4th Cir.1990).

VIRGINIA MEDICAL MALPRACTICE ACT

The Hospital seeks a declaration that its refusal to provide Baby K with ventilator treatment does not constitute malpractice under the Virginia Medical Malpractice Act, Va.Code § 8.01-581.1 *et seq*. Under the Declaratory Judgment Act, 28 U.S.C. § 2201, a federal court has discretion to assert jurisdiction to render a declaration. *Mitcheson v. Harris*, 955 F.2d 235 (4th Cir.1992); Wright & Miller, *Federal Practice and Procedure* § 2759 (1983). This discretion is related to the interest in having states decide questions of state law, an interest having jurisprudential roots in *Erie R.R. Co. v. Tompkins*, 304 U.S. 64, 58 S.Ct. 817, 82 L.Ed. 1188 (1938). *Mitcheson*, 955 F.2d at 237. In the Declaratory Judgment Act, Congress has afforded federal courts a freedom to consider the state interest in having state courts determine questions of state law. *Id.* at 238. Virginia courts have not addressed the question of the appropriate standard of care for anencephalic infants and whether an exception to the general standard of care applies to them. Besides the Malpractice Act's general rule, Virginia's legislature has also been silent on the issue. Moreover, the determination of the standard of care under Virginia's Medical Malpractice Act involves a review panel appointed by the Chief Justice of the Virginia Supreme Court. This review panel mechanism is "so intimately bound up with the rights and obligations being asserted as to require their application in federal courts under the doctrine of *Erie Railroad Co. v. Tompkins.*" *DiAntonio v. Northampton-Accomack Memorial Hospital*, 628 F.2d 287, 290 (4th Cir.1980). Because of the significant state interests manifested by this review process as well as the Commonwealth's interest in resolving this contentious and unsettled social issue for itself, this court declines to "elbow its way" into Virginia medical malpractice standards. *Cf. Mitcheson*, 955 F.2d at 238 (quoting *Pennhurst State School & Hosp. v. Halderman*, 465 U.S. 89, 122 n. 32, 104 S.Ct. 900, 920 n. 32, 79 L.Ed.2d 67 (1984)).

Constitutional and Common Law Issues

Baby K's parents disagree over whether or not to continue medical treatment for her. Mr. K and Baby K's guardian *ad litem* join the Hospital in seeking the right to override the wishes of Ms. H, Baby K's mother. Regardless of the questions of statutory interpretation presented in this case, Ms. H retains significant legal rights regarding her insistence that her daughter be kept alive with ventilator treatment. A parent has a constitutionally protected right to "bring up children" grounded in the Fourteenth Amendment's due process clause. *Meyer v. Nebraska*, 262 U.S. 390, 399, 43 S.Ct. 625, 626, 67 L.Ed. 1042 (1923); *Pierce v. Society of Sisters*, 268 U.S. 510, 534–535, 45 S.Ct. 571, 573, 69 L.Ed. 1070 (1925). Parents have the "primary role" in the "nurture and upbringing of their children." *Wisconsin v. Yoder*, 406 U.S. 205, 232, 92 S.Ct. 1526, 1541, 32 L.Ed.2d 15 (1972); *Prince v. Massachusetts*, 321 U.S. 158, 166, 64 S.Ct. 438, 442, 88 L.Ed. 645 (1944). Decisions for children can be based in the parent's free exercise of religion, protected by the First Amendment. *Pierce*, 268 U.S. at 534–535, 45 S.Ct. at 573; *Yoder*, 406 U.S. at 234, 92 S.Ct. at 1542.

These constitutional principles extend to the right of parents to make medical treatment decisions for their minor children. Absent a finding of neglect or abuse, parents retain plenary authority to seek medical care for their children, even when the decision might impinge on a liberty interest of the child. *Parham v. J.R.*, 442 U.S. 584, 603–604, 99 S.Ct. 2493, 2504, 61 L.Ed.2d 101 (1979) (commitment of child to mental health hospital). Indeed, there is a "presumption that the parents act in the best interests of their child" because the "natural bonds of affection lead parents to act in the best interests of their children." *Id.* at 602, 99 S.Ct. at 2504.

State law rights to make medical and surgical treatment decisions for a minor child are grounded in the common law and can also be inferred from state statutes. *See* Va.Code § 54.1-2969(B) (procedure governing consent to treatment of minors when parents are unavailable); Va.Code § 16.1334(1) (right of emancipated minor to make her own medical care decisions without parental consent).

Based on Ms. H's "natural bonds of affection," *Parham*, 442 U.S. at 602, 99 S.Ct. at 2504, and the relative noninvolvement of Baby K's biological father, the constitutional and common law presumption must be that Ms. H is the appropriate decision maker. "[W]hen parents do not agree on the issue of termination of life support . . . this Court must yield to the presumption in favor of life." *In re Jane Doe, A Minor*, Civ. No. D93064, mem. op. at 18 (Super.Ct. Fulton Co., Ga., October 17, 1991), *aff'd*, 262 Ga. 389, 418 S.E.2d 3 (1992). This presumption arises from the explicit guarantees of a right to life in the United States Constitution, Amendments V and XIV, and the Virginia Constitution, Article 1, Sections 1 and 11.

The presumption in favor of life in this case is also based on Ms. H's religious conviction that all life is sacred and must be protected, thus implicating her First Amendment rights. When an individual asserts "the Free Exercise Clause in conjunction with other constitutional protections, such as . . . the right of parents," only a clear and compelling governmental interest can justify a statute that interferes with the person's religious convictions. *Employment Div., Department of Human Resources of Oregon v. Smith*, 494 U.S. 872, 881 n. 1, 110 S.Ct. 1595, 1601 n. 1, 108 L.Ed.2d 876 (1990); *Yoder*, 406 U.S. at 233, 92 S.Ct. at 1542.

The Hospital cannot establish any "clear and compelling" interest in this case. The Supreme Court has not decided whether the right to liberty encompasses a right to refuse medical treatment, often called a "right to die." *Cruzan v. Director, Missouri Dept. of Health*, 497 U.S. 261, 277279, 110 S.Ct. 2841, 2850–51, 111 L.Ed.2d 224 (refusing to decide this question). Parents have standing to assert the constitutional rights of their minor children. *Eisenstadt v. Baird*, 405 U.S. 438, 446 n. 6, 92 S.Ct. 1029, n. 6, 31 L.Ed.2d 349 (1972). When one parent asserts the child's explicit constitutional right to life as the basis for continuing medical treatment and the other is asserting the nebulous liberty interest in refusing life-saving treatment on behalf of a minor child, the explicit right to life must prevail. *See In re Jane Doe, supra*.

Reflecting the constitutional principles of family autonomy and the presumption in favor of life, courts have generally scrutinized a family's decision only where the family has sought to terminate or withhold medical treatment for an incompetent minor or incompetent adult. *See, e.g., Cruzan*, 497 U.S. at 270–75, 110 S.Ct. at 2847-49 (and cases cited therein). In a recent case in which a hospital sought to terminate life-supporting ventilation over the objections of the patient's husband, a Minnesota state court refused to remove decisionmaking authority from the husband. *In re Wanglie*, No. PX-91-283 (Prob.Ct., Hennepin Co., Minn., June 28, 1991). Likewise, where parents disagreed over whether to continue life-supporting mechanical ventilation, nutrition, and hydration for a minor child in an irreversible stupor or coma, a Georgia state court gave effect to the decision of the parent opting in favor of life support. *In re Jane Doe, supra*.[2]

At the very least, the Hospital must establish by clear and convincing evidence that Ms. H's treatment decision should not be respected because it would constitute abuse or neglect of Baby K. This clear and convincing evidence standard has been adopted by numerous courts and was upheld by the Supreme Court in *Cruzan* in authorizing the withdrawal of life-supporting treatment from an incompetent patient. *See Cruzan*, 497 U.S. at 284–85, 110 S.Ct. at 2854–55. In this case, where the choice essentially devolves to a subjective determination as to the quality of Baby's K's life, it cannot be said that the continuation of Baby K's life is so unreasonably harmful as to constitute child abuse or neglect.

For the foregoing reasons, the Hospital's request for a declaratory judgment that the withholding of ventilator treatment from Baby K would not violate the Emergency Medical Treatment and Active Labor Act, the Rehabilitation Act of 1973, the Americans with Disabilities Act, the Child Abuse Amendments of 1984, and the Virginia Medical Malpractice Act should be DENIED. Under the Emergency Medical Treatment and Active Labor Act, the Rehabilitation Act of 1973, and the Americans with Disabilities Act, the Hospital is legally obligated to provide ventilator treatment to Baby K. The court makes no ruling as to any rights or obligations under the Child Abuse Amendments of 1984 and under the Virginia Medical Malpractice Act.

An appropriate order shall issue.

NOTES

1. Department of Health and Human Services guidelines addressing hospital reporting obligations under the Act if parents seek to withhold treatment from anencephalic infants are similarly inapplicable because of their silence regarding whether hospitals are allowed to terminate care in spite of a parent's wishes to the contrary. See 45 C.F.R. Part 84, App. C., paragraph (a)(5)(iii) (1992).
2. Although the court in *Jane Doe* had appointed a guardian *ad litem* because of the parents' disagreement, the guardian's view (if any) was not discussed in the court's ruling. This is consistent with the limited role of a guardian *ad litem* as an independent fact finder and not a surrogate decisionmaker where family members are involved. Under Virginia law, the role of a guardian *ad litem* appointed under Va.Code § 8.01–9(A) is to "investigate thoroughly the facts" and "carefully examine[] the facts surrounding the case." *Ruffin v. Commonwealth*, 10 Va.App. 488, 393 S.E.2d 425 (Va.App.1990). The recommendation of Baby K's court-appointed guardian *ad litem* is thus irrelevant to the disposition of this case.

Part III

ETHICAL ISSUES IN HUMAN GENETICS

ISSUES IN GENETICS

LeRoy Walters

THE SECOND HALF of the twentieth century has been the golden age of human genetics. This era was presaged in 1949 by the establishment of a new journal, the *American Journal of Human Genetics*, edited by classical geneticist Hermann J. Muller. Four years later, in 1953, James Watson and Francis Crick launched the field of molecular biology by describing the double-helical structure of DNA. In 1972, the discovery by Paul Berg and his coworkers that DNA from bacteria could be spliced into a simian virus—to form "recombinant DNA"—gave further impetus to research in molecular biology around the world (Jackson et al. 1972).

This chapter begins by examining the ethical and public-policy response to two applications of new knowledge in genetics and molecular biology: genetic testing and screening and gene therapy. The chapter concludes with excerpts from two reports on a global research effort that began in the late 1980s—the attempt to map and sequence the human genome.

Genetic Testing and Screening

Genetic testing and the use of genetic testing in mass screening programs can occur at any of four stages of life: (1) prenatally; (2) in the neonatal period; (3) when a couple is considering marriage or reproduction; or (4) when a person, on the basis of family history, recognizes that he or she has a higher-than-average risk of developing a genetic disease later in life. These four types of genetic testing are frequently called, respectively: (1) prenatal diagnosis; (2) newborn screening; (3) carrier screening; and (4) predictive or presymptomatic testing.

Historically, the capacity to test newborns for phenylketonuria (PKU) was the first to be used in a mass genetic screening program. PKU is characterized by abnormally-high levels of an amino acid, phenylalanine, in an infant's blood. The result of this "inborn error of metabolism," unless it is compensated for by a low phenylalanine diet is severe mental retardation. In 1961, Dr. Robert Guthrie published a letter describing a simple blood test in newborns that could determine their phenylalanine levels. One year later an early version of the Guthrie test was used in a voluntary screening program in Massachusetts. Three "positives" were discovered among the first 8,000 tests. The following year, 1963, at the urging of advocacy groups for the mentally retarded, Massachusetts passed the nation's first mandatory newborn PKU-screening law. With strong support from the National Association for Retarded Children, similar mandatory programs were adopted in 42 other states by the early 1970s (U.S., President's Commission 1983, 12–14).

Unfortunately, several questions had been inadequately answered before the Guthrie test began to be used in mass screening programs. The cutoff point for high phenylalanine levels was originally set too low, with the result that newborns not at risk for developing mental retardation were erroneously classified as affected. Further, by the late 1960s it was clear that some children with PKU were being overtreated, that is, that their diets were now providing insufficient levels of phenylalanine. This insufficiency led in some cases to retarded growth. In addition, it was known from the beginning of PKU screening that, especially in the first few days of life, newborns with PKU might not be diagnosed by the Guthrie test; that is, there would be a small percentage of false negatives (National Research Council 1975, 26–30).

Prenatal diagnosis also began to be employed in the 1960s. In 1966 researchers reported that they had succeeding in studying the chromosomes withdrawn from the amniotic fluid by amniocentesis. In the following two years prenatal diagnosis of a chromosomal disorder and an inborn error of metabolism was reported in the scientific literature (U.S., President's Commission 1983, 23). Generally speaking, only women of advanced maternal age or women in whom there was a family history of chromosomal abnormalities underwent prenatal diagnosis. Because the diagnosis occurred late in the mid-trimester of pregnancy and because a positive finding often led to a decision to abort, prenatal diagnosis became the focus of searching ethical analysis (Fletcher 1972). A further technological development occurred in the early 1970s. British researchers reported that neural-tube defects like spina bifida and anencephaly were correlated with elevated levels of alpha fetoprotein in the sera of pregnant women. This finding raised at least the possibility that large numbers of pregnant women might be offered prenatal testing on the basis of a simple blood test (National Research Council 1975, 133–138; U.S., President's Commission 1983, 23–31).

A third type of genetic screening, carrier screening, raised more profound public-policy problems than prenatal diagnosis. Here one can tell "a tale of two screening programs." In the Baltimore-Washington area, physician Michael Kaback launched a voluntary education and testing program for Tay-Sachs carriers in 1971. The program was focused on members of the Ashkenazi-Jewish community, who were at higher-than-average risk of carrying the gene that causes Tay-Sachs disease. This program was regarded as highly beneficial by the members of the community. In contrast, carrier-testing programs for sickle-cell anemia were introduced in the early 1970s, sometimes on a mandatory basis, without adequate planning and to the detriment of many persons who were tested. Well-meaning policymakers supported and even mandated the test but failed in many cases to draw the important distinction between carrying a recessive genetic trait and being afflicted with a recessive genetic disease. In addition, those who rushed into mass sickle-cell screening programs did not adequately consider the kind of stigmatization that could occur through carrier testing of children or adolescents (U.S., President's Commission 1983, 17–23).

The ethical response to genetic testing and screening began with a research group on "Ethical, Social, and Legal Issues in Genetic Counseling and Genetic Engineering" at the Hastings Center. In 1972 this group published an influential position statement in the *New England Journal of Medicine* entitled "Ethical and Social Issues in Screening for Genetic Disease" (Lappé et al. 1972). In the same year a new committee of the National Research Council (NRC) met for the first time and began work on a report that would address, in particular, the problems encountered in the early years of newborn PKU screening and in recent programs of carrier screening for sickle-cell trait (National Research Council 1975). Several members of the Hastings Center research group were also members of the NRC committee or participated in the committee's work. The NRC committee's report was published in 1975.

Almost a decade later the President's Commission on Bioethics reviewed again many of the issues considered by the NRC Committee. In the meantime some testing technologies had advanced, in particular, the assay for maternal-serum alpha fetoprotein (MSAFP). Equally important, federal legislation and the impact of the 1975 NRC committee report had moved most genetic testing and screening, except for newborn screening, toward a voluntary approach. The 1983 report of the President's Commission reiterated many of the findings of the 1975 report and provided a more comprehensive ethical and legal framework for the discussion of genetic testing and screening.

By the early 1990s, and in the absence of any federal Ethics Advisory Board, the Institute of Medicine (IOM) found it necessary to reconsider the topic of genetic testing and screening. In the intervening decade MSAFP testing had come into widespread use in the United Kingdom and in several regions of the United States. Among the states of the United States, California pioneered in offering MSAFP testing to every pregnant woman at a reasonable cost (California 1994). The 1994 report of the IOM committee reflected the preceding decade of rapid progress in genetic research and the increasing number of genetic disorders, or even predispositions, that could be diagnosed. The new report also devoted substantial attention to the possible implications of genetic testing and screening for employment and insurance (Institute of Medicine 1994).

Substantial excerpts from the 1975 NRC report, the 1983 President's Commission report, and the 1994 IOM report are reprinted in the first section of this chapter.

Gene Therapy

During the 1960s a few scientists, theologians, and philosophers engaged in a debate about the genetic engineering of human beings (Wolstenholme 1963; Ramsey 1966; Rahner 1967; Golding 1968; Manier 1968). However, it was only in the 1970s that the gene-therapy discussion began to take on the shape that is still with us in the 1990s (Davis 1970; Hamilton 1972). On a parallel track, the recombinant DNA debate began in 1973 and evolved with a dynamic all its own (Singer and Soll 1973; Berg et al. 1974; Berg et al. 1975; *Research* 1977; Jackson and Stich 1979). While there were important points of contact between these two debates in the 1970s (see, for example, Lappé and Morison 1976), for the most part the recombinant-DNA discussion and the gene-therapy discussion were carried on independently. In the early 1980s, as public concern about the potential biohazards of laboratory research with recombinant DNA abated, public and political attention shifted to the prospects for gene therapy in human beings. Two documents from the year 1982 helped to signal this shift: the recommendation on genetic engineering by the Parliamentary Assembly of the Council of Europe and the *Splicing Life* report of the U.S. President's Commission on Bioethics. In addition, beginning in 1983, the principal U.S. advisory body established to deal with recombinant DNA research gradually turned its primary focus toward the emerging technology of gene therapy (Juengst and Walters 1995).

Europeans produced the first position statement on gene therapy and genetic engineering in January of 1982. Perhaps because of their tragic experience with Nazi programs of racial hygiene during the Hitler era, the members of the Parliamentary Assembly of the Council of Europe accented the right of every human being to a genetic inheritance that has not been artificially manipulated (Council of Europe 1982). In contrast, the *Splicing Life* report published by the President's Commission in November of the same year focused on the continuities between everyday medical practice and gene therapy in non-reproductive cells and sought to de-dramatize the objections that some critics had seemed to raise against all types of human genetic intervention (U.S., President's Commission 1982). Recommendation 934 (1982) on Genetic Engineering and substantial excerpts of *Splicing Life* are reprinted below.

In the United States, the *Splicing Life* report profoundly affected an existing public advisory body. Established by the National Institutes of Health in 1974 during the early stages of the recombinant DNA debate, the NIH Recombinant DNA Advisory Committee (RAC) had published cautious guidelines for laboratory research with recombinant DNA in 1976. By the early 1980s concern about the accidental escape of novel pathogens had subsided. The NIH RAC therefore had sufficient time to review the *Splicing Life* report of the President's Commission on Bioethics and to consider what role, if any, it might play in the evolution of the gene therapy field. In stepwise fashion, the Committee first declared its willingness, in principle, to review human gene therapy protocols on a case-by-case basis. It then accepted the notion of establishing an interdisciplinary working group to provide initial review of gene therapy protocols. The Working Group on Human Gene Therapy was in fact established in the fall of 1984 and immediately set to work preparing guidelines for what was then thought to be the imminent submission of the first clinical gene therapy protocol (Walters 1991). The introduction to an early version of those guidelines, called the "Points to Consider," is reprinted below, together with a summary of the major questions in the "Points to Consider" translated into the language of laypeople (U.S., National Institutes of Health 1985; U.S., National Institutes of Health 1990).

In 1988 the NIH RAC and its working group (now called the Human Gene Therapy Subcommittee) reviewed their first clinical protocol, which was technically a gene-marking study rather than a gene-therapy study in the strict sense. During the same year the medical research councils of eleven European countries continued the discussion that had been initiated by the Parliamentary Assembly of the Council of Europe in 1980 and carried forward in reports from national advisory committees in Denmark, Sweden, and the Federal Republic of Germany. The statement of the European medical research councils reflects the moderate international consensus of the late 1980s—namely, that gene therapy in somatic (non-reproductive) cells was scientifically and ethically acceptable with appropriate safeguards but that "Germline gene therapy should not be contemplated" (European 1988). The 1988 statement by the European medical research councils is reprinted in the volume.

In the 1980s, but especially in the early 1990s, some commentators had begun to question whether germ-line genetic intervention for the cure or prevention could be morally justified (Fletcher 1983; Anderson 1989; Fowler et al. 1989; Cook-Deegan 1990; Walters 1991; Juengst 1991). This academic questioning found its first expression in a policy statement in the Declaration of Inuyama, formulated in July of 1990 by an international group of participants in a conference sponsored by the Council for International Organizations of Medical Sciences (XXIVth Round Table 1990). The full text of the declaration is reprinted in this chapter.

The first clinical gene therapy protocol in the United States was approved by the NIH RAC a few days after the conclusion of the CIOMS conference, on July 31, 1990. The target disease in this initial protocol was severe combined immune deficiency caused by the malfunctioning of the gene that produces adenosine deaminase (ADA). In September 1990 the first patient was treated by means of gene therapy under this protocol (ADA 1990; Culver 1993; Thompson 1993; Thompson 1994). During the next several years many additional somatic-cell gene therapy protocols were submitted to the RAC. By late 1994 more than 70 gene therapy protocols had been approved by the Committee.

Genome Mapping and Sequencing

The quest to map and sequence several complex genomes in a coordinated research program emerged as a concept in 1985 and 1986 (Cook-Deegan 1994, 79–116). The principal goal of the effort was to understand more fully which parts of the human genome, in particular, are most closely correlated with normal physiological functioning and, conversely, with abnormal functioning and disease. Given the fact that the human genome is comprised of approximately 50,000–100,000 genes and approximately three billion base pairs, the task of mapping and sequencing this huge terrain appears daunting, to say the least.

In September 1986 two independent groups were charged with the task of studying the concept of a human genome project (or multiple genome projects). The first group was a committee appointed by the National Research Council. The NRC Committee on Mapping and Sequencing the Human Genome was comprised primarily of eminent scientists from the United Kingdom and the United States (Cook-Deegan 1994, 125–134). Almost simultaneously, the United States Congress asked its research arm, the Office of Technology Assessment (OTA), to conduct a study of the genome project idea and to outline options for legislative action (Cook-Deegan 1994, 147–160). The task of coordinating the OTA study fell to a physician with strong public-policy interests, Robert M. Cook-Deegan.

Early in 1988 both the NRC report (February) and the OTA report (April) were published. The NRC report urged that a carefully-planned program for mapping and sequencing the human genome be undertaken as a matter of national policy (National Research Council 1988). Although OTA reports generally outline policy options rather than making recommendations, the report on *Mapping Our Genes* also seemed to favor proceeding with multiple coordinated genome projects (Office of Technology Assessment 1988). Each report included an ethics chapter in which committee members and consultants (for the NRC committee) and OTA staff members sought to provide a survey of ethical, legal, and social issues that might arise if the project or projects were in fact undertaken. These ethics chapters, in turn, laid the groundwork for research programs in ethics and human genetics that were later established at the National Institutes of Health and the Department of Energy. The two ethics chapters are reprinted below.

REFERENCES

"ADA Human Gene Therapy Clinical Protocol." *Human Gene Therapy* 1(3): 327–329, 331–362; Fall 1990.

Anderson, W. French. "Human Gene Therapy: Why Draw a Line?" *Journal of Medicine and Philosophy* 14 (6): 681–693; December 1989.

Berg, Paul, et al. "Potential Biohazards of Recombinant DNA Molecules" [Letter]. *Science* 185(4148): 303; 26 July 1974.

Berg, Paul, et al. "Asilomar Conference on Recombinant DNA Molecules." *Science* 188(4192): 991–994; 6 June 1975.

California, State Department of Health Services, Genetic Disease Branch. *The California Alpha Fetoprotein Screening Program*. Berkeley: Genetic Disease Branch, 1994.

Cook-Deegan, Robert M. "Human Gene Therapy and Congress." *Human Gene Therapy* 1(2): 163–170; Summer 1990.

Cook-Deegan, Robert. *The Gene Wars: Science, Politics, and the Human Genome*. New York: W.W. Norton, 1994.

Council of Europe, Parliamentary Assembly. "Recommendation 934 (1982) on Genetic Engineering." *Texts Adopted by the Assembly*, 33rd Ordinary Session, Third Part, 22nd Sitting, January 26, 1982 (Strasbourg: the Council, 1982).

Culver, Kenneth W. "Splice of Life: Genetic Therapy Comes of Age." *The Sciences* 33(1): 18–24; January/February 1993.

Davis, Bernard D. "Prospects for Genetic Intervention in Man." *Science* 170(3964): 1279–1283; 18 December 1970.

European Medical Research Councils. "Gene Therapy in Man: Recommendations of European Medical Research Councils." *Lancet* 2(8597): 1271–1272; 4 June 1988.

Fletcher, John C. "The Brink: The Parent-Child Bond in the Genetic Revolution." *Theological Studies* 33(3): 457–485; September 1972.

Fletcher, John C. "Moral Problems and Ethical Issues in Prospective Human Gene Therapy." *Virginia Law Review* 69(3): 515–546; April 1983.

Fowler, Gregory, et al. "Germ-Line Gene Therapy and the Clinical Ethos of Medical Genetics." *Theoretical Medicine* 10(2): 151–165; June 1989.

Golding, Martin P. "Ethical Issues in Biological Engineering." *UCLA Law Review* 15(2): 443–479; February 1968.

Hamilton, Michael P., ed. *The New Genetics and the Future of Man*. Grand Rapids, MI: Eerdmans, 1972.

Institute of Medicine, Committee on Assessing Genetic Risks. *Assessing Genetic Risks: Implications for Health and Social Policy*, edited by Lori B. Andrews, et al. Washington, DC: National Academy Press, 1994.

Jackson, David A., et al. "Biochemical Method for Inserting New Genetic Information into DNA of Simian Virus 40." *Proceedings of the National Academy of Sciences, USA* 69(10): 2904–2909; October 1972.

Jackson, David A., and Stich, Stephen P., eds. *The Recombinant DNA Debate*. Englewood Cliffs, NJ: Prentice-Hall, 1979.

Juengst, Eric T., ed. "Human Germ-Line Engineering." *Journal of Medicine and Philosophy* 16(6): 587–694; December 1991.

Juengst Eric T., and Walters, LeRoy. "Gene Therapy: II. Ethical and Social Issues." In *Encyclopedia of Bioethics*, 2nd ed., edited by Warren T. Reich. New York: Macmillan, 1995: 914–922.

Lappé, Marc, et al. "Ethical and Social Issues in Screening for Genetic Disease." *New England Journal of Medicine* 286(21): 1129–1132; 25 May 1972.

Lappé, Marc, and Morison, Robert S. "Ethical and Scientific Issues Posed by Human Uses of Molecular Genetics." *Annals of the New York Academy of Sciences* 265: 1–208; 23 January 1976.

Manier, Edward. "Genetics and the Future of Man: Scientific and Ethical Possibilities." *Proceedings of the American Catholic Philosophical Association* 42: 183–192; 1968.

National Research Council, Committee for the Study of Inborn Errors of Metabolism. *Genetic Screening: Programs, Principles, and Research*. Washington, DC: National Academy Press, 1975.

National Research Council, Committee on Mapping and Sequencing the Human Genome, *Mapping and Sequencing the Human Genome*. Washington, DC: National Academy Press, 1988.

Rahner, Karl. "Zum Problem der genetischen Manipulation." In his *Schriften zur Theologie*, Bd. VIII. Einsiedeln, Federal Republic of Germany: Benziger Verlag, 1967: 286–321.

Ramsey, Paul. "Moral and Religious Implications of Genetic Control." In *Genetics and the Future of Man*, edited by John D. Roslansky. Amsterdam: North-Holland Publishing Company, 1966: 109–169.

Research with Recombinant DNA: An Academy Forum, March 7–9, 1977. Washington, DC: National Academy of Sciences, 1977.

Singer, Maxine, and Soll, Dieter. "Guidelines for DNA Hybrid Molecules." [Letter]. *Science* 181(4105): 1114; 21 September 1973.

Thompson, Larry. "The First Kids with New Genes." *Time,* 7 June 1993, 50–53.

Thompson, Larry. *Correcting the Code: Inventing the Genetic Cure for the Human Body.* New York: Simon & Schuster, 1994.

United States, National Institutes of Health, Recombinant DNA Advisory Committee, Working Group on Human Gene Therapy. "Points to Consider in the Design and Submission of Human Somatic-Cell Gene Therapy Protocols." *Federal Register* 50(160): 33463–33467; 19 August 1985.

United States, National Institutes of Health, Recombinant DNA Advisory Committee and Human Gene Therapy Subcommittee. *Gene Therapy for Human Patients: Information for the General Public.* Bethesda, Maryland: NIH, April 1990.

United States, Congress, Office of Technology Assessment. *Mapping Our Genes: The Genome Projects—How Big, How Fast?* Washington, DC: OTA, April 1988.

United States, President's Commission for the Study of Ethical Problems in Medicine and Biomedical and Behavioral Research. *Screening and Counseling for Genetic Conditions: A Report on the Ethical, Social, and Legal Implications of Genetic Screening, Counseling, and Education Programs.* Washington, DC: U.S. Government Printing Office, February 1983.

United States, President's Commission for the Study of Ethical Problems in Medicine and Biomedical and Behavioral Research. *Splicing Life: The Social and Ethical Issues of Genetic Engineering with Human Beings.* Washington, DC: U.S. Government Printing Office, November 1982.

Walters, LeRoy. "Human Gene Therapy: Ethics and Public Policy." *Human Gene Therapy* 2(2): 115–122; Summer 1991.

Wolstenholme, Gordon, ed. *Man and His Future.* London: J. & A. Churchill, 1963.

XXIVth Round Table Conference, Council for International Organizations of Medical Sciences (CIOMS). "The Declaration of Inuyama." In *Genetics, Ethics and Human Values: Proceedings of the XXIVth CIOMS Conference,* edited by Z. Bankowski and A. M. Capron. Geneva: CIOMS, 1991: 1–3.

GENETIC SCREENING: PROGRAMS, PRINCIPLES, AND RESEARCH

INTRODUCTION. *The Committee for the Study of Inborn Errors of Metabolism was established in response to a letter from the Chairman of the Social Issues Committee of the American Society of Human Genetics to the President of the National Academy of Sciences. In his letter, the chairman requested "an investigation into the origins, history, and current standing of screening for phenylketonuria (PKU) and into the effectiveness of its use" (p. iv). In response, the National Research Council appointed the Committee for the Study of Inborn Errors of Metabolism and broadened its mandate to include screening for other genetic diseases and traits. In particular, the committee focused considerable attention on carrier screening for the gene that causes Tay-Sachs disease and on screening for sickle-cell anemia and sickle-cell trait. The committee met for the first time in August 1972; its final meeting was held September 9, 1974. One of the central recommendations of the committee's report was that genetic screening programs be voluntary rather than mandatory. This report was the first of three major U.S. documents on ethical and public-policy issues in genetic testing and screening.*

Recommendations

GENERAL

1. Genetic screening, when carried out under controlled conditions, is an appropriate form of medical care when the following *criteria* are met:

a. There is evidence of substantial public benefit and acceptance, including acceptance by medical practitioners.
b. Its feasibility has been investigated and it has been found that benefits outweigh costs; appropriate public education can be carried out; test methods are satisfactory; laboratory facilities are available; and resources exist to deal with counseling, follow-up, and other consequences of testing.
c. An investigative pretest of the program has shown that costs are acceptable; education is effective; informed consent is feasible; aims of the program with regard to the size of the sample to be screened, the age of the screenees, and the setting in which the testing is to be done have been defined; laboratory facilities have been shown to fulfill requirements for quality control; techniques for communicating results are workable; qualified and effective counselors are available in sufficient number; and adequate provision for effective services has been made.
d. The means are available to evaluate the effectiveness and success of each step in the process.

2. Screening for phenylketonuria should be continued, and additional studies directed to its improvement should be supported. Although hindsight reveals that screening programs for phenylketonuria were instituted before the validity and effectiveness of all aspects of treatment, including appropriate dietary treatment, were thoroughly tested, current assessment reveals that case finding methods are reasonably efficient, the means for moving from test to definitive management are adequate, and the appropriate dietary treatment is harmless and effective. Experiences in screening for phenylketonuria, both favorable and adverse, constitute a valuable resource for guidance in the design and operation of future programs. It is important that these experiences be kept in mind and used where appropriate.

From the National Research Council, Committee for the Study of Inborn Errors of Metabolism, *Genetic Screening: Programs, Principles, and Research* (Washington, D.C.: National Academy Press, 1975). Note that the Committee's use of italics to introduce its recommendations (in the numbered paragraphs) has not been retained in this excerpt.

ORGANIZATIONAL

3. Responsibility for the organization and control of genetic screening programs should be lodged in some agency representative of both the public and the health professions. This is necessary because of the public nature of genetic screening and its use of public facilities. It is also essential because such screening carries some potential for invasion of privacy, "labeling," breach of confidentiality, and psychological abuse. The agency might take its authority from local or state government or from regional representation of a federal program.

4. Public representation is necessary both in determining that a new screening program is clearly in the public interest and also in the design and operation of any such program. This is because genetic screening is likely to affect, for one test or another and perhaps for many, every member of the population.

5. Screening agencies should consult regularly with local medical societies, stimulating their cooperation and participation. This is important in order to give genetic screening the maximum public and professional acceptance.

6. The aims of genetic screening should be clearly formulated and spelled out by the initiators of any screening program and should be publicly articulated with precision and candor. Thus there will be no possibility of a mistaken impression that the program is intended to be an instrument of discrimination or is devoted to any "eugenic" cause.

7. Some degree of standardization of screening projects is desirable. Demographic diversity, inequality of financial and educational resources of the various states, and the individuality of initiators of screening projects all lead to variation in the design, quality, and cost of screening programs. Standardization might be achieved by some national agency that could act as a clearinghouse for ideas and techniques, set standards, and exert quality control.

8. Regional programs with laboratories and other facilities based on population numbers rather than political subdivisions should be developed to make screening services of high quality available equally to all. Such programs would avoid the low priority currently given to genetic screening in states of low population density and low budget and would prevent the hardship otherwise suffered by the relatively few persons in such states to whom screening would be beneficial.

9. In the future, genetic screening should be regarded as one among several preventive health measures and its development should take place in the context of the evolution of health care in general. New projects should be dictated by general principles governing genetic screening rather than by pressures originating in the special qualities of particular diseases.

EDUCATIONAL

10. It is essential to begin the study of human biology, including genetics and probability, in primary school, continuing with a more health-related curriculum in secondary school because

a. In the absence of sufficient public knowledge of human biology and genetics, the difficulties of arousing concern over genetic diseases cannot be overcome, since even longstanding attempts to educate the public regarding traditional preventive health measures have had variable success.
b. In the short run, the educational aspects of genetic screening must consist of special campaigns devoted to each program. Sufficient knowledge of genetics, probability, and medicine leading to appropriate perceptions of susceptibility to and seriousness of genetic disease and of carrier status cannot be acquired as a consequence of incidental, accidental, or haphazard learning.

11. Screening authorities could improve the effectiveness of public education by studying and employing methods devised and tested by professional students of health behavior and health education. The use of the mass communication media and other techniques to change attitudes and behavior has not been particularly successful, partly because of failure to follow the appropriate precepts.

12. Continuing education courses for physicians should place emphasis on human genetics and particularly on the practical application of population genetics. In medical schools the study of genetics should be included in courses of epidemiology and preventive medicine, as well as in courses of medicine, pediatrics, and obstetrics. Such emphasis would raise the level of genetic knowledge of physicians and would increase their orientation toward preventive medicine so that they would be able to take an active role in genetic screening.

13. Schools of medicine, public health and hygiene, and allied health sciences, as well as universities, should receive support for programs to set standards and train persons to inform and counsel participants in screening programs. Such counselors are already in short supply.

LEGAL

14. Participation in a genetic screening program should not be made mandatory by law, but should be left to the discretion of the person tested or, if a minor, of the parents or legal guardian.

15. Identifying information obtained through genetic screening should not be made available to anyone other than the screenee except with the permission of the

screenee or, in the case of a minor, with the permission of the parents or legal guardian.

16. Screening authorities should consult regularly with lawyers and other persons knowledgeable in ethics to avoid social consequences of screening that may be damaging. These take the form of invasion of privacy, breach of confidentiality, and other transgressions of civil rights, as well as psychological damage resulting from being "labeled" or from misunderstandings about the significance of diseases and carrier states. The usefulness of or need for legislation to protect the participants in screening programs from such dangers should be reviewed from time to time.

17. For states considering legislation mandating genetic screening, the Committee recommends examination of a law creating a Board on Hereditary Disorders such as that proposed by the Council of State Governments' Committee on Suggested State Legislation.

RESEARCH

18. Research in genetic screening should be governed by the rigorous standards employed in laboratory investigation. Special efforts should be made to evaluate all aspects, even of routine procedures, and the social and ethical ramifications of screening in the lives of the persons tested should be investigated. So far, experience in genetic screening is insufficient to foresee and to forestall all possible untoward side effects. Accordingly, it should be approached in an experimental mood. At present, it is impressions that prevail, rather than data collected and analyzed according to scientific rules.

19. It is important that screening be used to study the natural history of genetic disorders for which there is no treatment at this time. Such research, in which the object of screening is to discover the full range of expression of the disease, will further the development of new methods of treatment and can provide the control data needed to evaluate proposed treatments. Particular effort must be exerted to protect individuals identified by such screening against the psychological and social hazards that attend all screening programs, but whose impact may be enhanced by the lack of an effective treatment.

20. Research should be supported in adapting discoveries of new genetic characteristics for screening purposes. This research includes increasing the number and quality of tests, reducing their cost, building regional networks of laboratories and other facilities to broaden and improve service, and designing simple, inexpensive, and effective treatments for newly discovered diseases. The acquisition of genetic knowledge is proceeding exponentially, and much of it is germane to the aims of genetic screening.

21. Research to discover polymorphic alleles occurring in high frequency should receive more substantial support. Certain common alleles have been shown to be associated with disease, and it is predictable that many more will also be implicated.

SCREENING AND COUNSELING FOR GENETIC CONDITIONS

INTRODUCTION. *The President's Commission for the Study of Ethical Problems in Medicine and Biomedical and Behavioral Research was established in 1979 and began work in January 1980. This report was a response to a congressional request to study the ethical and legal implications of "voluntary testing, counseling, and information and education programs with respect to genetic diseases and conditions" (Title III, Public Law 95-622, enacted November 9, 1978). The Commission's study began with a public hearing on May 8, 1981, at which several participants in the 1975 National Research Council study testified. An important achievement of this report was its update on changes in testing and screening technology since 1975. Its major recommendation was that individuals and families at risk should be educated about the potential benefits and harms of genetic testing. The individuals and families should then freely decide whether and how to participate in genetic testing. This report was the second of three key reports on genetic testing and screening that have been published at roughly ten-year intervals in the United States.*

INTRODUCTION

The rapid advances now occurring in genetic screening techniques and the increased resources devoted to genetic counseling give Americans new opportunities to understand their biological heritage and to make their health care and reproductive plans accordingly. In this Report, the President's Commission responds to its legislative mandate to study the ethical and legal implications of these programs for genetic screening, counseling, and education.[1] On the whole, the Commission finds that advances in genetics have greatly enhanced health and well-being. Nevertheless, due regard for the subtle interplay of social norms and individual choices is required as genetic screening and counseling become increasingly important.

The new prominence of the human genetics field has already heightened public awareness of the significant issues that genetic procedures may soon raise for individual patients and their families, for health care providers, and for the public and its representatives.[2] In responding to the Congressional request, the Commission in this Report makes specific recommendations to guide those charged with designing and providing genetics programs, and reaches several general conclusions about the ethical issues at stake.

The Report

Scope of Screening Covered In genetic screening, an asymptomatic population is tested to identify people who may possess a particular genotype.[3] The term "screening" is often used to connote the initial step toward a definitive diagnosis, which then requires repeated or more precise testing of anyone identified as possibly having the condition. Sometimes, however, the term is used for more specific tests in individuals at risk for a condition when further analysis is not needed to yield a diagnosis or prognosis.[4]

Genetic testing often requires only a simple blood test and laboratory analysis. Some forms of screening, however, are performed on cells that have been grown in a laboratory. This is true of most diagnoses done during pregnancy, which usually involve analysis of cells found in a sample of amniotic fluid surrounding a fetus, although some prenatal

President's Commission for the Study of Ethical Problems in Medicine and Biomedical and Behavioral Research, *Screening and Counseling for Genetic Conditions: A Report on the Ethical, Social, and Legal Implications of Genetic Screening, Counseling, and Education Programs* (Washington, D.C.: U.S. Government Printing Office, 1993). Note that bold emphases (on the Commission's recommendations) have generally been omitted.

diagnoses rely on examinations of the fetus by sonography, fetoscopy, or other techniques.

A number of the reasons screening is done are research-related. These include the testing of new genetic screening methods; attempts to establish a relationship between a particular genotype and a medical disorder or propensity; surveillance to detect the impact of environmental factors on genes (particularly on egg or sperm cells); and epidemiological studies of the frequency with which a gene or a chromosome abnormality occurs in a population. This Report does not explore the issues raised especially by screening for research purposes.

The possibility of screening to determine workers' susceptibility to disease from certain chemical factors in the workplace has received considerable attention from public and private groups. The U.S. Congress's Office of Technology Assessment is studying its potential uses and misuses, the Hastings Center is exploring its ethical implications, and some industries are examining its possible applications.[5] Because this issue is receiving extensive study already, the Commission decided not to address it at this time. Nevertheless, it is important not to separate these types of screening conceptually. The various reasons for screening and counseling or the settings in which they take place do not in themselves provide any basis for the adoption of different policies toward participants. Some of the Commission's conclusions will be equally relevant to the workplace.

The Commission has focused instead on genetic screening undertaken either to permit medical intervention (for example, through newborn screening) or to provide information about risks of genetic disease in natural-born children (through carrier screening or prenatal diagnosis). Both types sometimes occur as part of an individual provider-patient relationship, although screening is more frequently offered at a central genetics center (usually in a university medical center) under the auspicies of a public health department or in conjunction with a community outreach effort such as a health fair or a special school, church, or synagogue program.

Genetic screening to uncover a person's need for medical care is similar to nongenetic screening (such as routine blood pressure or tuberculin tests) in that the goal is to determine whether remedial or preventive health care is needed. Whether a condition arises from a genetic or a nongenetic source is usually of less immediate consequence than the need for medical attention. Indeed, it may be difficult to draw a medical distinction between genetic and nongenetic conditions.[6] Genetic screening differs from other routine tests, however, in that the information produced is often relevant to medical decisions by individuals other than the person screened, even when this is not the primary reason for obtaining the information. For example, the discovery of a rare genetic defect in one person will usually lead physicians to suggest that the person's relatives also be screened.

Screening for reproductive reasons, on the other hand, is inherently genetic; information is sought primarily because of its impact on future generations. The difference between these two types of screening has important ethical and social consequences in certain cases. By revealing information about a person's genotype, screening undertaken to identify people in need of preventive or remedial treatment may, of course, raise questions of personal responsibility for ill health, along with feelings of guilt, because genes, unlike infectious or environmental causes of illness, are part of each individual's body. But these concerns are likely to be magnified when screening is done for reproductive reasons because the information provided—and the decisions based on it—have significance not only for people's own health, but also for the health of their children.

Scope of Counseling Covered Genetic counseling helps people with a potential or manifest genetic problem understand and, if possible, adjust to genetic information; when necessary, it aids them in making decisions about what course to follow.[7] It is an individualized process in which a specialist in medical genetics confers with an individual, a couple, or sometimes a group seeking additional information or assistance. Before genetic screening tests enabled individuals to be tested prospectively, assessments of risks were based only on known genetic disease in the family. For example, following the birth of an affected child, the parents (and sometimes the extended family) might have sought genetic counseling. Since screening tests exist for only a very few genetic conditions, this retrospective counseling remains an important aspect of genetic counseling today.

For the most part, this Report considers counseling in conjunction with screening tests and programs. The demand for such counseling has grown dramatically in the past decades and promises to become increasingly important as new screening tests are developed. Nevertheless, the conclusions and recommendations in this Report are equally applicable to genetic counseling in other circumstances.

Organization of the Study The Report is fairly brief for two reasons. First, it draws on other reports by the Commission that treat in more detail the subjects of informed consent and access to health care.[8] In those studies the Commission discusses the principles of well-being, self-determination, and equity and it therefore does not reiterate that analysis here. Second, the Report examines only those types of genetic screening and counseling that involve personal health risks and risks to any natural-born children. It leaves for the attention of others (and perhaps for future attention by the Commission) several forms of screening, such as tests for susceptibility or resistance to disease, that are beginning to attract researchers' attention.

The Report does look to the future, however, as it applies its findings about the ethical and legal implications of genetics programs to a frequently heralded genetic test for cystic fibrosis. Research now under way is likely to lead to such a test in the near future. This condition is the most prevalent inherited lethal disorder in the United States. Among Caucasians, one person in 20 carries the gene for cystic fibrosis and one in every 1500–2000 infants is born with the disease.[9] If a test becomes available to identify these carriers, the demand for genetic screening and counseling could quickly become overwhelming.

To accommodate such an increase in an acceptable fashion, more than technical resources would be needed. Public understanding of the possible pitfalls of genetic testing as well as its potential benefits—of its human as well as its scientific implications—is essential if new screening capabilities are to yield safe, effective, equitable, and ultimately beneficial results.

The Commission hopes in this Report to further such public understanding. After sketching in Chapter One the basic facts about past genetic screening and counseling efforts, the Commission reaches a number of conclusions and recommendations in Chapter Two about how education, screening, and counseling programs should take account of important ethical and legal concerns. In Chapter Three, these points are applied to cystic fibrosis screening as a hypothetical test case; the issues that would be of concern there could also be expected to arise regarding tests developed for other genetic conditions.

The Commission held a hearing on this topic in May 1981 and discussed it at several other Commission meetings.[10] A partial draft of this Report was reviewed by the Commission with a panel of experts in March 1982; two months later, a revised draft was discussed, at which time the principal conclusions were approved by the Commissioners. On October 8, 1982, the Commission discussed and approved a revised draft, subject to editorial revisions.

Summary of Conclusions and Recommendations

The Commission's basic conclusion is that programs to provide genetic education, screening, and counseling provide valuable services when they are established with concrete goals and specific procedural guidelines founded on sound ethical and legal principles. The major conclusions fall into five categories.

CONFIDENTIALITY

(1) Genetic information should not be given to unrelated third parties, such as insurers or employers, without the explicit and informed consent of the person screened or a surrogate for that person.

(2) Private and governmental agencies that use data banks for genetics-related information should require that stored information be coded whenever that is compatible with the purpose of the data bank.

(3) The requirements of confidentiality can be overridden and genetic information released to relatives (or their physicians) if and only if the following four conditions are met: (a) reasonable efforts to elicit voluntary consent to disclosure have failed; (b) there is a high probability both that harm will occur if the information is withheld and that the disclosed information will actually be used to avert harm; (c) the harm that identifiable individuals would suffer if the information is not disclosed would be serious; and (d) appropriate precautions are taken to ensure that only the genetic information needed for diagnosis and/or treatment of the disease in question is disclosed.

- When it is known in advance that the results of a proposed screening program could be uniquely helpful in preventing serious harm to the biological relatives of individuals screened, it may be justifiable to make access to that program conditional upon prior agreement to disclose the results of the screening.

(4) Law reform bodies, working closely with professionals in medical genetics and organizations interested in adoption policies, should urge changes in adoption laws so that information about serious genetic risks can be conveyed to adoptees or their biological families. Genetic counselors should mediate the process by which adoptive records are unsealed and newly discovered health risks are communicated to affected parties.

AUTONOMY

(5) Mandatory genetic screening programs are only justified when voluntary testing proves inadequate to prevent serious harm to the defenseless, such as children, that could be avoided were screening performed. The goals of "a healthy gene pool" or a reduction in health costs cannot justify compulsory genetic screening.

(6) Genetic screening and counseling are medical procedures that may be chosen by an individual who desires information as an aid in making personal medical and reproductive choices.

- Professionals should generally promote and protect patient choices to undergo genetic screening and counseling, although the use of amniocentesis for sex selection should be discouraged.
- The value of the information provided by genetic screening and counseling would be diminished if available reproductive choices were to be restricted. (This is a factual conclusion that is not intended to involve the Commission in the national debate over abortion).

KNOWLEDGE

(7) Decisions regarding the release of incidental findings (such as nonpaternity) or sensitive findings (such as diagnosis of an XY-female) should begin with a presumption in favor of disclosure, while still protecting a client's other interests, as determined on an individual basis. In the case of nonpaternity, accurate information about the risk of the mother and putative father bearing an affected child should be provided even when full disclosure is not made.

(8) Efforts to develop genetics curricula for elementary, secondary, and college settings and to work with educators to incorporate appropriate materials into the classroom are commendable and should be furthered. The knowledge imparted is not only important in itself but also promotes values of personal autonomy and informed public participation.

(9) Organizations such as the Association of American Medical Colleges, the American Medical Association, and the American Nursing Association should encourage the upgrading of genetics curricula for professional students. Professional educators, working with specialty societies and program planners, should identify effective methods to educate professionals about new screening tests. Programs to train health professionals, pastoral counselors, and others in the technical, social, and ethical aspects of genetic screening deserve support.

WELL-BEING

(10) A genetic history and, when appropriate, genetic screening should be required of men donating sperm for artificial insemination; professional medical associations should take the lead in identifying what genetic information should be obtained and in establishing criteria for excluding a potential donor.

- Records of sperm donors are necessary, but should be maintained in a way that preserves confidentiality to the greatest extent possible.
- Women undergoing artificial insemination should be given genetic information about the donor as part of the informed consent process.

(11) Screening programs should not be undertaken unless the results that are produced routinely can be relied upon.

- Screening programs should not be implemented until the test has first demonstrated its value in well-conducted, large-scale pilot studies.
- Government agencies involved in introducing new screening projects should require appropriate pilot studies as a prerequisite to approval of the product or to the funding of services.
- Government regulators, funding organizations, private industry, and medical researchers should meet to discuss their respective roles in ensuring that a prospective test is studied adequately before genetic screening programs are introduced.

(12) A full range of prescreening and follow-up services for the population to be screened should be available before a program is introduced.

- Community leaders and local organizations should play an integral part in planning community-based screening programs.
- State governments should consider establishing a review group with professional and public members to oversee genetic services.
- New screening programs should include an evaluation component.

EQUITY

(13) Access to screening may take account of the incidence of genetic disease in various racial or ethnic groups within the population without violating principles of equity, justice, and fairness.

(14) When a genetic screening test has moved from a research to a service delivery setting, a process should exist for reviewing implicit or explicit policies that limit access to the genetic service; the review should be responsive to the full range of relevant considerations, to changes in relevant facts over time, and to the needs of any groups excluded.

- The time has come for such a review of the common medical practice of limiting amniocentesis for "advanced maternal age" to women 35 years or older.

(15) Determination of such issues as which groups are at high enough risk for screening or at what point the predictive value of a test is sufficiently high require ethical as well as technical analyses.

(16) Cost-benefit analysis can make a useful contribution to allocational decisionmaking, provided that the significant limitations of the method are clearly understood; it does not provide a means of avoiding difficult ethical judgments.

* * *

ETHICAL AND LEGAL IMPLICATIONS

The prevention and treatment of genetic disease has become an increasingly important component of health care.

A growing number of genetic diseases can be accurately diagnosed, and more genetic information of potential value to individuals and families is now available. By providing this important information, well-designed and carefully implemented genetic screening and counseling programs give individuals greater opportunities to make informed, autonomous decisions about their own health and about reproduction. Screening and counseling programs can also make major contributions to public health and personal well-being by reducing the incidence of genetic disease and by facilitating more-effective management and treatment.

Successful programs require concrete goals and specific procedural guidelines that are founded on sound ethical and public policy principles. In this chapter, the Commission articulates these principles and uses them to clarify some of the more important ethical and legal issues presented by the ever-increasing role of genetic screening and counseling in medical care and public programs. The main ethical principles are autonomy, beneficence (including the prevention of harm), justice (including equity and fairness), and privacy (including confidentiality). The chief public policy principles are efficiency (or economy) and public participation (through democratic political institutions). These principles are neither controversial nor peculiar to genetic screening and counseling. Disagreement arises only when there is a conflict among some of them, and their content and relative weight must be specified more precisely.

Because the ethical, social, and legal issues raised by genetic screening and counseling are so diverse and are at various stages of development as matters of public policy, the Commission's conclusions about them take different forms. On some points, the Commission has reached general conclusions that may be of interest to all concerned citizens and not just to patients, health care providers, or public officials. On other points, the Commission recommends that guidelines be adopted for genetic screening and counseling programs or that other steps be taken by legislative bodies. In each case, the Commission attempts to address its conclusions to particular groups among the wide range of players—from Federal officials to community organizers, from professional medical societies to primary school teachers. Some recommendations will best be carried out by professional medical organizations, such as medical specialty groups or medical school curriculum committees. Others are within the purview of state or Federal officials who have authority to allocate funds for screening and counseling programs. Still others apply to nonprofit organizations concerned with education, treatment, and research for genetic diseases.

Confidentiality

There are three main areas of concern over confidentiality in genetic screening and counseling: (1) disclosure of information to unrelated third parties, such as employers or insurers; (2) access to material stored in data banks; and (3) disclosure of information to relatives of the screenee, either to advise them that they or their offspring are at risk for genetic disease or to gain information about them for a more accurate diagnosis of the person originally screened.

Questions about disclosure of genetic information to third parties sound familiar notes in the debates over medical confidentiality. Because of the potential for misuse as well as unintended social or economic injury, information from genetic testing should be given to people such as insurers or employers only with the explicit consent of the person screened.[1] Further, the agencies in question should develop forms for specific rather than blanket consent, to prevent unnecessary disclosures and to ensure the screenee selective control over access. The screenee should be told which information has been disclosed, to whom, and for what purpose.

The confidentiality of material stored in data banks is also not peculiar to genetics. Concerns about privacy are particularly acute regarding genetics, however, both because the potential information involves particularly sensitive matters (such as personal identity and reproductive "fitness") and because, in the case of "banks" of actual cell samples, it may be impossible at the time the material is placed in the system to know all the information that new tests might someday reveal. Private and government agencies that use data banks for genetics-related information should require that stored information be coded, whenever coding is compatible with the reasons the information is stored, both to preserve anonymity and to minimize the risk of unauthorized computer access.

The Commission focuses its attention in this Report on the release of information to relatives of the screenee, which in some cases raises issues of special significance in the context of medical genetics.

Involuntary Disclosure to Relatives The issue of disclosing the results of genetic screening to relatives is raised when serious harm could be prevented by providing the relatives with information they would not otherwise be likely to obtain in a timely fashion. One example of this situation is the clinical diagnosis of multiple polyposis of the colon, a condition that is a precursor to cancer. Early detection and treatment—before the onset of symptoms—greatly improves the prognosis. Once the condition is detected clinically in one family member, therefore, the question is whether the physician, guided by the knowledge that the disease is genetic, should try to advise others in the family to be screened.

The issues raised by a patient's refusal to allow test results to be used as a basis for contacting relatives depend on the circumstances. The narrowest claim for involuntary disclosure to relatives at increased risk would apply when it is known in advance that a test's results could be uniquely helpful in preventing serious physical harm to relatives of the person tested. In such circumstances prospective screenees should be advised prior to testing of the value of informing at-risk relatives and efforts should be made to elicit their voluntary consent to disclosure. Making access to the test conditional upon prior agreement to disclose information may be justifiable. Conditional access would be easiest to justify in programs funded by private organizations. Since such groups are under no obligation to provide the service in the first place, it seems reasonable that they should be able to require a disclosure agreement as a condition of participation. In the case of publicly funded programs, the same policy might be justified on the grounds that even if citizens have a right to participate in the testing program, the right is not absolute and is limited by the state's interest in protecting others from harm. Such a policy, however, might deter some people from participating. Consequently, a decision to require consent to disclosure must take into account the harm that might be done or the benefits that might be foregone if some individuals chose not to participate.

A more difficult case arises when such an advance agreement has not been reached, as when genetic testing produces unexpected information that could benefit a person's relatives. People may oppose disclosure of results of their tests because they fear that the positive findings—or even their participation in the screening—could lead to stigmatization by relatives. In some cases, people may choose to withhold information because they believe their relatives would not want it. And some people are estranged from their families and do not want to do anything that might help their relatives or bring them back into contact with each another.

It might seem that a genetic counselor ought never to disclose information against the wishes of a client, because the counselor's professional obligation is to the client, not to others. Both the law and morality recognize, however, that a professional's primary obligation is in some circumstances subsumed by the need to prevent harm to others. Perhaps the clearest medical application of this principle is that of health providers' obligation to report communicable diseases. Genetic disease is not strictly analogous to communicable diseases, although it might be argued that the major difference is that transmission is "horizontal" in the one case and "vertical" in the other. Yet the relevant similarity is that in both cases the duty to prevent harm to others may in some instances place limits on the professional's duty of confidentiality.[2]

A professional's ethical duty of confidentiality to an immediate patient or client can be overridden only if several conditions are satisfied: (1) reasonable efforts to elicit voluntary consent to disclosure have failed; (2) there is a high probability both that harm will occur if the information is withheld and that the disclosed information will actually be used to avert harm; (3) the harm that identifiable individuals would suffer would be serious; and (4) appropriate precautions are taken to ensure that only the genetic information needed for diagnosis and/or treatment of the disease in question is disclosed.[3] The individual's family history (pedigree) should be carefully analyzed to identify accurately any relatives at increased risk so that information is presented only to the appropriate individuals, and anonymity should be preserved wherever possible. Since the decision to breach professional confidentiality is such a weighty one, it may also be advisable to seek review by an appropriate third party.

With improved public education about genetics, however, and appropriate genetic counseling in individual cases, it is hoped that involuntary disclosure will be infrequent. When a person understands that there is nothing shameful about a genetic disease or trait and that the information may be invaluable to relatives, either for their own health care or for their decisions about childbearing, willingness (or even eagerness) to share the information with relatives should increase.

Medical history is replete with examples of conditions once considered shameful or private and now openly discussed. The increased public awareness and education that led patients and physicians to say the word "tuberculosis" rather than refer vaguely to "a spot on the lung" and that has made the discussion of cancer more open could also reduce the stigma associated with genetic diseases.

Release of Information in Case of Adoption

Disclosure of information to relatives is more complicated when a sealed adoption record must be opened to locate the individual(s) at risk for a genetic condition. This may arise when a genetic condition identified in an adoptee bears on the health of members of the biological family or, the reverse, when a condition diagnosed in the biological family has implications for the health of the adoptee.

The laws governing adoption in all 50 states, the District of Columbia, Puerto Rico, and the Virgin Islands require adoption records to be sealed following adoption decrees as a way of protecting the confidentiality of both the biological and adoptive families. A family medical history typically is part of the required record, although specific reference to genetic information is generally not made. Moreover, sometimes a genetic condition does not become apparent until after the adoptive process is complete. For example, Huntington's disease, myotonic dystrophy, and other serious conditions may be diagnosed after the adoption proceeding; genetic counselors would then be concerned about the 50% risk that any child the person had given up for adoption has of developing such a disease. Such information can be conveyed to the relative at risk only if the adoptive record is unsealed.

Some adoption agencies or county courts that maintain adoption records may conclude that new genetic information renders the existing medical record incomplete and, therefore, that the record should be unsealed and the information communicated to the adoptive family.[4] But most adoption laws were not written with such contingencies in mind; existing provisions may be inadequate to address the circumstances or to provide procedures under which the record can be unsealed so that genetic information can be communicated to either the biological or adoptive family. The U.S. Department of Health and Human Services' recent model state statute for "children with special needs" (that is, children with characteristics that constitute a barrier to adoption of the child) would require inclusion of a genetic history and provides for supplementing this material for at least 60 years after the child reaches the age of majority.[5] Provisions like these are needed for all adoptions. The Commission recommends that law reform bodies, working closely with genetic professionals and organizations interested in adoption policies, seek changes in the adoption laws to ensure that information about serious genetic risks can be conveyed to adoptees or their biological families.

The Commission further finds that the goals of preserving confidentiality and preventing harm can best be advanced if genetic counselors act as mediators in the process of identifying relatives at risk and communicating relevant information. The counselor already is part of a confidential relationship in which sensitive information about the risks of genetic disease are discussed. That "circle of secrecy" need only be extended slightly to the confidentiality that surrounds an adoption record if important genetic information is provided to the relatives by the counselor.[6] In most cases, the biological and adoptive families would not need to communicate personally or be identified. When such safeguards are in place, it seems likely that screenees would be willing to have genetic information released to relatives at risk on either side of an adoption.

Autonomy

The Commission believes that the principle of autonomy, which holds a high place in Western ethical and legal traditions, is important not only in the relationships of individual patients and health care professionals (through the requirement of informed consent) but also in the choices that people make about the use of genetic services. Ethical and legal implications would therefore arise immediately were participation made compulsory by law, but they can also arise as a result of more subtle forms of pressure.

Voluntary Programs One of the central ethical issues in screening and counseling is that of voluntariness. There are two main questions: Should participation in screening and counseling programs always be voluntary? Should treatment of genetic disease detected through screening always be voluntary? If the general legal and ethical requirement of informed consent for medical procedures is applied here, the answer to both questions would seem to be yes. Although four major arguments have been offered to justify compulsion, the Commission finds that only one—the protection of those unable to protect themselves—has any merit, and then only under special circumstances.

To save society money. Some might argue that compulsion is warranted if it is necessary for the control of health care costs. That is, individuals may rightly be compelled to participate in genetic screening and counseling and to undergo prenatal therapy or even abortion in order to minimize society's burden in caring for individuals with serious genetic defects. The chief objection to this argument is that it rests upon a general principle that few, if any, would wish to see consistently implemented—namely, that a person's freedom to make the most intimate choices, and even a person's very existence, depends upon the degree to which social utility is maximized. Even were it morally permissible to employ utilitarian calculations in the extreme circumstances of so-called lifeboat or triage situations, it would not follow that it is permissible to do so in a society as affluent as the United States, especially when other means of husbanding resources are available that do not pose such a direct and profound threat to the commitment to equal respect for individuals. The Commission finds no basis in the maximization of social utility that justifies compulsory participation in genetics programs. Rather than finding utilitarianism particularly appropriate in determining social policy on genetics programs, the contrary appears to be the case, in light of the especially strong reasons to preserve individual liberty on matters of medical treatment and reproduction.

To allocate resources fairly. Alternatively, an attempt might be made to rest compulsory screening and treatment on an appeal to fairness rather than to social utility. Specifically, some may argue that it is unfair for an individual to exercise his or her freedom of choice so as to impose upon others the burden of caring for someone whose condition was avoidable. Those who fail to prevent genetic disease might be said to take unfair advantage of the contributions that others make to minimizing human suffering.

Though this argument avoids assuming that utilitarianism is the appropriate moral theory, it is unpersuasive for other reasons, particularly because it assumes that an individual who fails to undergo screening or treatment thereby *imposes* a burden on others. Two cases must be distinguished: those in which an adult will not voluntarily undergo screening to detect a genetic condition that, if undetected, may result in a deterioration of his or her own health, and those in which a genetic condition will adversely affect the health of an individual's children.

At present there may be few instances of the first sort of case, in which early detection through screening of an adult would allow preventive intervention or less-costly management of a late-onset disease, though future research may make this increasingly possible. An individual who refuses to be screened could argue that the refusal does not impose a burden on other people because it is up to them to decide whether or not to provide the additional care needed due to the disease not being detected at an earlier stage. Others may assume the burden if they wish, but if they do assume it then the individual cannot be said to impose it on them.

Similarly, since society may choose whether or not to allocate resources for the care of those with unhealthy lifestyles, it is wrong to say that those individuals impose a burden on society. Society can either assume the responsibility of treating the heavy smoker's lung cancer or refrain from doing so and allow the burden to fall upon the smoker. If a person knowingly acts in a way that incurs avoidable medical expenses for his or her own care, and would not have done so had he or she not been counting on society to pay the bill, the person is taking unfair advantage of the generosity of others. However, if a person waives any right to social support and is willing to bear the consequences of the behavior, then it cannot be said that the person is taking unfair advantage of society's generosity or that society has a right to prevent that behavior, so long as others are not directly harmed by it.

Nonetheless, even if the very great practical problems could be overcome of establishing a system in which individuals could waive their rights to public support for health care in order to avoid having to undergo procedures they object to, the public might find it difficult if not impossible to turn a cold shoulder once the consequences are manifest. Although it may be true that a society can choose whether to assume the burden of an individual's illness, or that an individual can relieve society of that burden, it does not necessarily follow that the society will have either the will to follow through on the implications of such a decision or the ability to do so in a manner that seems fair. Society has been notably unwilling to deny care (or even to place conditions on it) for cigarette-smoking patients who develop lung cancer. Nor, to cite another example, have any head injuries of motorcyclists who failed to wear helmets been left unattended.

In the second type of case—a genetic risk that manifests itself only in offspring—the "fairness" argument for compulsory screening and treatment is totally unconvincing because a parent cannot waive a child's rights. Although it may be irresponsible and unfair for an individual to create an *avoidable* drain on resources that could be used to relieve other instances of suffering, it would be even more unfair to punish children because of their parents' choices.

Again, it is important to distinguish two morally distinct cases of parental choice: those in which the costs to society of caring for a child with a genetic disease are reduced or avoided entirely through carrier testing and a decision not to conceive, and those in which the social costs in question are to be avoided by abortion following a positive prenatal test. For people with firm convictions against abortion, the latter course of action is never a morally permissible way to avoid social costs. Moreover, most people who do not oppose abortion when chosen by a pregnant woman herself would still reject a policy that might require other people to act contrary to their fundamental moral convictions for the sake of achieving a fairer distribution of social costs.

The "fairness" argument in the case of carrier testing is not so easy to dismiss, however, because foregoing conception would not require a woman to terminate a pregnancy. In fact, if artificial insemination or adoption are available and acceptable to the individual, the experience of parenting need not even be forfeited. Some couples, however, may place great value on the opportunity to bear and raise children that are biologically their own, even at the risk of genetic disease. In such cases, it is not at all clear that considerations of fairness in the distribution of social burdens would justify overriding this deep personal preference.

Even in other, less controversial areas, society has generally not restricted individual liberty on the grounds that certain behavior would result in avoidable social costs, unless the behavior is directly dangerous to others. Though personal responsibility for health is increasingly advocated, no serious attempt has been made to implement policies that would place the costs of smoking, alcohol use, or other dangers to health on the individuals who expose themselves to such risks or that would prohibit people from running these risks. Moreover, while experts disagree about whether smoking and alcohol consumption are voluntary enough to say that they represent free choices about behavior, being at risk for genetic disease is clearly not voluntary. Consequently, the case for compulsory screening and treatment of genetic diseases seems even more dubious than for restrictions on other risks.

Finally, there is a strong American tradition to give the benefit of doubt to the value of individual liberty, especially in matters of reproductive choice. For this reason, compulsory genetic screening and treatment seems the least likely place to begin a policy of coercion in the name of a fair distribution of the costs of health care. Although the "fairness" argument raises issues that deserve consideration in defining the scope of individual choice, it does not provide adequate grounds for mandatory genetic screening and treatment.

To protect the helpless from harm. The most plausible case for compulsory participation in genetic screening and further interventions as necessary rests on the premise that society has an obligation to minimize serious and unambiguous harm to identifiable individuals who are unable to protect themselves.[7] Most states mandate screening for PKU and, in some cases, for other diseases as well.[8] But these tests only involve the taking of a small blood sample and are performed on the infants themselves, with the aim of preventing harm to them. The justification here is the same as for compulsory education, the assumption being that the state may act so as to protect the basic interests of minors; as in the case of education, the law in most states also explicitly recognizes valid grounds (such as religious objections) on which parents may resist such tests. Although a strong presumption prevails in favor of voluntary screening programs, the Commission concludes that programs requiring the performance of low-risk, minimally intrusive procedures may be justified if voluntary testing would fail to prevent an avoidable, serious injury to people —such as children—who are unable to protect themselves.

When screening involves only the child's body (for example, newborn screening), it is not ethically acceptable to fail to prevent or relieve serious, irreversible harm to a child merely because parents refuse to allow the screening. A legislature following this principle could mandate newborn screening for genetic conditions if some proportion of parents consistently withheld their consent, even though they have been given appropriate information about the purpose, benefits, and extremely small risks of a test that yields information of great importance to the well-being of children. Determining the number of refusals that ought to trigger imposition of mandatory screening is a delicate public policy issue that turns on an ethical evaluation of facts and assumptions. A study of the effects of a voluntary program for PKU screening, instituted in Maryland in 1976, found that the rate of parental refusal was only .05%; the chance of missing a case because of parental refusal is 100 times less than missing one from false negatives that occur because of problems with the time of testing and so forth.[9]

An ethically more difficult case is raised when the contemplated intervention is prenatal or preconceptual and thus would involve the body of one or both prospective parents. On a personal level it would, of course, be appropriate to give prospective parents moral counsel and as much practical assistance as possible in order to prevent or ameliorate any avoidable harm to their children. But the justification of protecting defenseless third parties would have to be very weighty before parents' bodily integrity could be invaded over their objections. As the degree of bodily invasion increases (ranging from a premarital blood test that could alert a person to the need for voluntary steps to correct a reversible condition, for example, to amniocentesis in order to diagnose an untreatable condition), the severity of the predicted harm and the certainty that the intervention will prevent it must likewise increase for an unconsented intervention to be ethically acceptable. As a legal matter, the constitutional right of privacy may erect an even more formidable barrier to forced testing.

The Commission has not found that any government programs of involuntary genetic screening and counseling of adults are presently being undertaken. Were such programs to be proposed as a means of protecting children, the first response should be to try to achieve the desired results through improvements in education and information for the public and health professionals and in the services available in voluntary genetics programs. Public efforts would be better directed at reducing infant morbidity associated with inadequate maternal nutrition or prenatal health care than at requiring genetic interventions simply because they are technologically available.

Similarly, even in the testing of children themselves for "protective" reasons, good results may depend more on the adequacy of support for planning and execution of the program than they do on its mandatory nature. In PKU testing and other screening that depends on subsequent tests to eliminate initial false positives, adequate follow-up is essential to meet screening goals. Deciding whether screening should be voluntary or mandatory should reflect, therefore, the expected ability not only to reach the target population for the initial test but also to provide needed follow-up services.

To improve society's "genetic health." Some people might contend that individuals may be compelled to participate in screening programs not only for the sake of preventing unambiguous, serious harms to particular individuals, but also in order to achieve a societal standard of "genetic health" or "genetic normality." The weaknesses of this line of argument are manifold. Perhaps most importantly, the very notions of "genetic health" and "genetic normality" are extremely vague and elastic slogans that disguise controversial ideals of human excellence as value-free medical categories. Recent history illustrates how these notions, in the hands of repressive and exploitative political movements, can be used to justify extreme eugenic measures. Sound public policy—especially when it involves the curtailment of individual liberties—cannot be based on such loose and abusable notions. The Commission concludes that mandatory screening cannot be justified on grounds of achieving a "genetically healthy society" or other similarly vague and politically abusable social ideals.

Subtle Societal Pressures. Direct compulsion (through the imposition of economic burdens or through laws) is not the only way in which people may find their freedom restricted regarding genetics programs. Indeed, the attitudes and policies of health professionals and widely held social expectations may be more significant factors in determining the choices people are able—or feel themselves able—to make. Reciprocally, the choices made by many independent individuals form new societal norms that are not the conscious creation of any one person. These in turn may not only impose significant limitations on people's choices in the future but may also alter basic societal attitudes and presumptions.

The ethical problems presented by this interplay of individual choices and social norms may be as unanticipated as the emergence of new social norms is unintended. In addressing this subject, the Commission does not believe it would be either wise or feasible to attempt to freeze social norms and individual options just as they are today. But an awareness of the manifestations of this synergistic relationship that it finds undesirable can help society take appropriate corrective steps, especially to preserve the voluntariness of genetics programs.

Tensions between autonomy and collective goals. Human genetics has passed through a period when the most personal reproductive choices were manipulated for social and political ends.[10] Genetic screening came of age when those memories were very fresh and that early history affects programs even now. Nondirective counseling is widely extolled and, except in isolated instances where a child could suffer severe injury or death, it is generally recognized that choosing whether to participate in screening and how to use the results should be fully voluntary.

Thus in principle genetic screening and counseling closely resemble other medical interventions that individuals choose to use to a greater or lesser extent, depending on the relevance of the information to their personal decisionmaking. As already discussed, there is also a decided public health aspect to genetic disease, however. Society has been much more willing to limit individual freedom in the service of protecting people from certain communicable diseases (through mandatory vaccinations, for example) than from equally serious genetic diseases. This difference occurs in part because the likelihood of transmission is often less certain in the case of genetic disease and because genetic transmission occurs within the family, rather than the public at large. But more fundamentally, it reflects the facts that the prevention of genetic disease can impinge on reproductive freedom and that modern means of genetic screening developed just as this freedom was receiving increasingly explicit and extensive protection as a facet of a constitutional "right of privacy."[11]

For genetic screening and counseling to contribute to the public health goals of reducing the incidence and impact of inherited disorders, however, a subtle tension must arise between those goals and the special place accorded to the right of individuals to obtain and use screening information as their personal values dictate, whether or not their decisions result in a reduction in genetic disease.[12] While acknowledging the need for some balancing with public health goals, the Commission strongly endorses the emphasis on genetic screening and counseling as medical interventions to be elected by an individual who desires information to aid in making personal medical and reproductive choices.

Contradictory pressures on the use of genetic services. Decisions about whether and how to use genetic services are not made in a vacuum. If voluntariness is to be maintained, therefore, attention must be paid to the pressures exerted by social attitudes as well as by official limitations regarding policies that bear on decisions about genetic diseases. At the moment, reproductive decisions involving genetic information are subject to pressures from opposite poles.

On the one hand, efforts have been made to limit genetic services because certain uses of genetic information are deemed unacceptable.[13] For example, some couples may find themselves faced with the difficult decision of whether to forego natural conception or to terminate a pregnancy. Yet screening results may also prompt a couple to prepare specialized medical or surgical treatment for an expected child; and screening information is more likely in the future to facilitate the intrauterine treatment of disorders.[14] Moreover, for most couples genetic screening (particularly prenatal diagnosis) and counseling relieve fears of transmitting certain serious diseases to their offspring. Indeed, the vast majority of women undergoing amniocentesis receive that reassurance; prenatal screening has facilitated the birth of at least hundreds of children who, but for the test, might never have been born.[15] In sum, the fundamental value of genetic screening and counseling is their ability to enhance the opportunities for individuals to obtain information about their personal health and childbearing risks and to make autonomous and noncoerced choices based on that information. Abridgement of that autonomy —explicitly or implicitly—would diminish the value of genetic screening and counseling and undermine the achievement of their goals. Efforts to inform the public about genetic screening and counseling, and to ensure services for those who wish to participate, promote such autonomous decisionmaking.

On the other hand, parents who fail to take advantage of prenatal diagnosis and who bear a child with an "avoidable" disease may consider themselves—or may be considered by others—to be "responsible" for the disease in a way that contradicts the older notion that genetic diseases are solely a matter of fate for which individuals are not responsible.[16] Fear has been expressed about societal disapproval translating into a negative attitude toward such children, including an unwillingness to allocate adequate resources for their care or for research into the causes and prevention of their diseases.[17] Such a response would be indefensible; the claims of a handicapped child on societal resources should not be dependent on the decision of the child's parents to undergo screening. Such a response would also be out of keeping with current efforts to assure rights and opportunities for the handicapped.

The silence of the law on many areas of individual choice reflects the value this country places on pluralism. Nowhere is the need for freedom to pursue divergent conceptions of the good more deeply felt than in decisions concerning reproduction. It would be a cruel irony, therefore, if technological advances undertaken in the name of providing information to expand the range of individual choice resulted in unanticipated social pressures to pursue a particular course of action. Someone who feels compelled to undergo screening or to make particular reproductive choices at the urging of health care professionals or others or as a result of implicit social pressure is deprived of the choice-enhancing benefits of the new advances. The Commission recommends that those who counsel patients and those who educate the public about genetics should not only emphasize the importance of preserving choice but also do their utmost to safeguard the choices of those they serve.

The special case of sex selection. Despite the strong reasons for not precluding individuals from having access to genetic services on the basis of what they may do with the information, society may sometimes be warranted in discouraging certain uses. A striking example would be the use of prenatal diagnosis solely to determine the sex of the fetus and to abort a fetus of the unwanted sex.

Denying a woman access to the service for this purpose is sometimes defended on the ground of resource scarcity, since being the "wrong sex" is not a disease or even a condition that merits the limited time and facilities of genetic programs, as would conditions generally classified as genetic diseases. Nevertheless, parents bent on learning the sex of the fetus can probably do so, either by having another, acceptable reason for prenatal screening or by inventing one (such as claiming that the woman is over 35 years old).[18] The ethical concern about using knowledge of fetal sex as the reason for terminating a pregnancy thus goes beyond the resource issue, since even if resources were not scarce, the question of whether this is an acceptable ground for medical intervention would remain.

In a society in which women terminate pregnancies for a wide variety of reasons, it might seem indefensible to exclude sex selection, as a matter of public policy, or even to make it an object of informal social disapproval. As already noted, the Commission generally believes that medical options ought to be enhanced, not diminished. In the Commission's view, however, the question of sex selection raises special moral problems apart from the general issue of the morality of abortion. The willingness to undergo in the second trimester of pregnancy an invasive procedure that entails a risk of maternal morbidity as well as fetal morbidity and mortality, and perhaps to terminate a pregnancy intentionally, merely in order to satisfy a preference for choosing the sex of a child, calls into question the values underlying such a decision.

There are several reasons that using amniocentesis and abortion for this purpose is morally suspect. In some cases, the prospective parents' desire to undertake the procedures is an expression of sex prejudice. Such attitudes are an affront to the notion of human equality and are especially inappropriate in a society struggling to rid itself of a heritage of such prejudices. There is no evidence that amniocentesis is being sought widely to determine fetal sex.[19] Surveys of parents and prospective parents do indicate, however, a preference for sons (especially as the first-born child).[20] If it became an accepted practice, the selection of sons in preference to daughters would be yet another means of assigning greater social value to one sex over the other and of perpetuating the historical discrimination against women. Of course, in some instances the judgment may be relative rather than absolute (for example, a couple with several girls who want a boy to complete their family) and in some instances the preference may be for a daughter rather than a son.

Another issue in sex selection is that parental concern with the sex of the fetus (to the point of aborting one of the undesired sex) seems incompatible with the attitude of virtually unconditional acceptance that developmental psychologists have found to be essential to successful parenting. For the good of all children, society's efforts should go into promoting the acceptance of each individual—with his or her particular strengths and weaknesses—rather than reinforcing the negative attitudes that lead to rejection.

The idea that it is morally permissible to terminate pregnancy simply on the ground that a fetus of that sex is unwanted may also rest on the very dubious notion that virtually any characteristic of an expected child is an appropriate object of appraisal and selection. Taken to an extreme, this attitude treats a child as an artifact and the reproductive process as a chance to design and produce human beings according to parental standards of excellence, which over time are transformed into collective standards.

Although every reproductive decision based on information gained from genetic screening involves the conscious acceptance of certain characteristics and the rejection of others, a distinction can be made between seeking genetic information in order to correct or avoid unambiguous disabilities or to improve the well-being of a fetus, and seeking such information merely to satisfy parental preferences that are not only idiosyncratic but also unrelated to the good of the fetus.

Although in some cases it will be difficult to draw a clear line between these two types of interventions, sex selection appears to fall in the latter class. This is not to say that every decision to undergo amniocentesis solely for purposes of sex selection is subject to moral criticism. Nonetheless, widespread use of amniocentesis for sex selection would be a matter of serious moral concern. Therefore, the Commission concludes that although individual physicians are free to follow the dictates of conscience, public policy should discourage the use of amniocentesis for sex selection. The Commission recognizes, however, that a legal prohibition would probably be ineffective[21] and, worse, offensive to important social values (because vigorous enforcement of any such statute might depend on coercive state inquiries into private motivations).

Once new genetic technologies are in wide use, the emergence of new social norms about their proper use, and any corresponding limitations on individual choice, may be difficult or impossible to control. This is all the more reason to ensure that decisions to make available new uses of genetic services—such as sex selection—are guided by a serious effort to anticipate the moral implications of the subtle interplay of individual choices and the social norms they create and by which they are shaped.

Knowledge

Genetic screening and counseling have the same central purpose: to make people into informed decisionmakers about their genetic constitution, to the extent it is relevant to choices about their own well-being or that of their family. Thus providing information in a way the participant can understand would plainly seem to be a goal of any genetics program and would also seem more likely if there is appropriate education of the public and of health professionals about current genetic knowledge. A commitment to disseminate information does not require policymakers or practitioners to ignore other values, such as well-being, confidentiality, or equity.

Disclosure of Incidental Findings A genetic screening test undertaken to detect a particular genetic condition sometimes uncovers other information that could be very traumatic to the screenee. Genetic counselors and providers must decide whether such incidental information should be revealed to the individuals screened and, if so, how to reveal it.

Findings of nonpaternity. The finding that the putative father of a child is unlikely to be the biological father may arise during several types of medical screening. Screening family members to locate a suitable organ or bone marrow donor, for example, can incidentally yield strong evidence of nonpaternity. In these cases, however, the finding of nonpaternity has no bearing on personal medical decisionmaking (although it indirectly affects medical management, in that half-siblings and putative fathers may be excluded as donors because of an inadequate tissue match). Consequently, controversy has not arisen about the customary practice of not mentioning the possibility of nonpaternity to the potential organ donors. Findings of nonpaternity in the context of reproductive screening and counseling, however, present problems that are not so easily dismissed. The decisions based upon such screening and counseling rest on knowledge of the genetic makeup of the biological father. When doubts about paternity arise, therefore, they have direct ramifications for the counseling and decisionmaking process.

Following the birth of an affected child, parents often seek genetic counseling to know the likelihood that a subsequent child will also have the disease. If a carrier test for the disorder is available and has not already been done, this would be one way for the parents to obtain the information. If the condition in question is autosomal recessive, such as sickle-cell trait or Tay-Sachs disease, and the father is shown not to be a carrier, there is strong evidence of nonpaternity. Although explanations such as a spontaneous mutation, laboratory error, or even a mixup of newborns at the hospital could conceivably account for the unanticipated outcome, such occurrences are very rare. Genetic counselors have several choices for dealing with suspicions of nonpaternity.

First, they might choose not to inform the couple of the actual recurrence risk (the "bottom line") in order to shield them from information that the father was not a carrier. The actual risk of bearing a child with the disease with only one carrier parent is typically near zero (that is, dependent only on the mutation rate); the risk if the father were a carrier would be 25%. The harm of this deception is that the couple may make inappropriate decisions about future childbearing based on inaccurate information. If the couple mistakenly believes they are both carriers and therefore have a 25% chance of bearing another affected child, they may try artificial insemination or decide to forego future pregnancies; if they conceived another child they might needlessly incur the risk and expense of prenatal diagnosis; or they might divorce and perhaps each seek noncarrier mates. (Of course, if the woman suspected that another man fathered the child, she might separately seek additional information about recurrence risks and not pursue any of these options.)

Second, counselors could convey the actual risk but withhold information about genetic transmission that would explain the reason for the risk and raise the suspicion of nonpaternity. There is no way for counselors to prevent a couple (or either partner) from obtaining such information from another source, however; the chance of this happening is increased if the attempt at deception leaves the couple feeling confused and anxious.

Third, spontaneous mutation could be presented as the explanation for the outcome, without suggesting any other reasons. Although less likely than the second deception to be a goad to independent inquiry, this strategy is also vulnerable to being overturned by outside sources of information that could indicate the infrequency of spontaneous mutations compared with nonpaternity. Fourth, nondisclosure might be a matter not of what is revealed, but to whom: the counselors could discuss the situation with the woman (who would probably suspect nonpaternity) without the putative father being present. Finally, the counselors might disclose their findings, including the conclusion that recurrence risk in any future pregnancy with the putative father is virtually nil because the child is almost certainly illegitimate.

None of the alternatives that rely on incomplete or inaccurate information are fully compatible with genetic counselors' basic role as information-givers. The fourth approach involves partial disclosure, but excluding the putative father might make counselors feel they have become a party to the woman's intentional deception. Yet they may feel this is justified when they have reason to fear that the family or some of its members will suffer greater physical or psychological harm from disclosure of the suspicion of nonpaternity. One cogent argument against this line of reasoning is that the deception will often not succeed for long and that any hope the counselors have of supporting the family unit over the long term (and, in particular, in maximizing the child's prospects for well-being) may be seriously jeopardized by their deception of one or both parents.

The ethical argument against nondisclosure goes beyond these practical considerations. Although the possibility of nonpaternity may not necessarily arise during genetic counseling, counselors would seem to have an obligation to both partners counseled. Certainly, if the man were to *ask* about the possibility of nonpaternity, it is difficult to maintain that the counselors ought to withhold the information they have unless disclosure would probably result in a serious and irreversible harm (for example, a life-threatening attack by a husband on his wife). Even then, the obligation would seem to be to provide adequate protection for the parties at risk and then to disclose the information to the man in a way that minimizes the harm to him and the risk to others.

A basically different approach would be to inform all couples, prior to a test, that nonpaternity may be discovered. Knowing this possibility, screenees could agree with the counselors in advance on the particular way the information will be handled; if a genetics center has a firm policy on disclosure that is not satisfactory to a couple, they could go elsewhere for their screening. Although this approach has the advantage of involving couples in the decision about disclosure, it may also unnecessarily provoke sensitive, sometimes harmful, discussions and could discourage some women who would like genetic information from participating in screening.

No strategy for addressing the sensitive issue of nonpaternity entirely avoids conflicts among professional goals and social norms and expectations. Full disclosure, combined with careful counseling that goes well beyond information-giving, would seem most likely to fulfill the principles of autonomy and beneficence. When circumstances preclude this, however, an approach that accurately provides information on the genetic risk, even when the individuals counseled are sometimes left with an incomplete understanding of the reasons, is generally preferable.

Sex chromosome abnormalities. Chromosomal studies sometimes uncover aberrations in the sex chromosomes. In a few rare cases, for example, instead of having the normal XX (female) or XY (male) pair of chromosomes, individuals have XO, XXY, or other abnormal combination. Some such disorders are associated with obvious physical or mental abnormalities; in other cases research is only beginning to provide data on the significance of the disorder in areas such as developmental effects and learning disabilities. When information about a sex chromosome aberration is disclosed to a patient or parent (particularly a prospective parent), it is important that any discussion of the limitations in present knowledge about the effects of the condition be made clear.

One incidental finding of genetic screening that raises especially sensitive issues concerning disclosure is the so-called XY-female, or testicular feminization syndrome. These individuals possess the chromosomal configuration of a male and undeveloped, undescended testes rather than female reproductive organs, yet they have all the secondary sexual characteristics of normal (XX) females.

Patients need to be informed of this finding for two important reasons. First, sterility is one feature of the XY-female condition, which could make a difference in an individual's life plan. Second, the accepted medical response to the condition is removal of the undeveloped gonads, since they pose a risk of cancer; this operation, like any other, requires the informed consent of the competent patient. Disclosure of the diagnosis here, as elsewhere, does not flow from any single-minded commitment to truth-telling for its own sake, without regard for its consequences, but rather serves the two values that underlie the requirement of informed consent generally: concern for patient well-being and respect for patient self-determination. Some practitioners, however, express grave doubts about the wisdom of full disclosure in such cases, stating that it would inflict unconscionable psychological harm to tell an unsuspecting patient that she is really a male.

Although the Commission appreciates the extreme sensitivity of this situation, it does not believe there are only two alternatives: deception through nondisclosure or a blunt, psychologically threatening revelation. Indeed, given that the concept of being a male (or a female) is in part biological and in part social and that even the purely biological concept is complex and multidimensional, it would be not only unnecessarily destructive but also misleading to tell an XY-female that she is mistaken about her sexual identity.[22] Instead, it might be more appropriate to convey to a patient the basic facts, which are relevant to decisions she must make, and elaborate further only in response to the patient's questions. How the information is presented depends, of course, on the patient's level of education and knowledge of human biology, but basically the person needs to be told that she did not develop a uterus and ovaries (and hence cannot bear children) and has nonfunctioning reproductive tissue that must be surgically removed in order to avoid a risk of cancer. The context in which the disclosure is made will be just as important as the choice of an accurate but sensitive way of expressing the needed information. As the Commission emphasized in its report *Making Health Care Decisions*, a sound relationship between patient and practitioner requires a continuing process of open communication, mutual trust, and a sensitivity to the particular values and needs of the patient.

Public and Professional Education People are not only patients whose informed consent is required for particular genetic services but also responsible citizens participating in the broader process by which policy decisions are made. To function effectively in either role they need to be well informed about the nature and value of genetic screening and counseling in the context of health care and public health programs.

The doctrine of informed consent has been examined by many scholars and practitioners from law, medicine, philosophy, and the social sciences. The Commission's own report on the subject, in line with the prevailing view, concluded that the goal of patient-provider interactions is a process of shared decisionmaking involving an informed patient and a conscientious health care provider. This reasoning applies with particular force to genetic screening and counseling in the context of health care and reproduction. In the setting of mass screening programs, the same ethical norms of information and consent apply. Prior education in some of the basic principles of genetics would enhance people's ability to interpret the information conveyed about particular genetic procedures, and thereby facilitate true informed consent.

Furthermore, the formulation of public policy about matters of health should not be the exclusive prerogative of a small group of medical or public health "experts." Active and informed political participation by people without specialized training in the fields of medicine and human genetics is needed if the public interest is to be effectively represented. Consequently, educational efforts should consist of more than just informing individual patients about specific medical genetic procedures.

Adequate professional education is also necessary for genetic screening and counseling to become accepted components of public health efforts and standard medical care. Physicians across a broad range of specialties must be knowledgeable about the detection and treatment of genetic disease if patients are to receive the most beneficial care. Studies show, for example, that about 30% of the children in pediatric hospitals have diseases with either a clearly genetic or multifactorial etiology.[23] Continuing professional education is essential if the potential of new advances in the diagnosis and treatment of genetic diseases is to be realized. Several recent judicial decisions have recognized the importance of genetics in medical care; the courts have held physicians liable for failing to inform patients of their risks for genetic disease and of the availability of screening tests.[24] To be alert to these genetic risks, physicians need to increase their knowledge in this field.

Public education on basic genetic concepts. Most people do not have an educational background in the modern concepts of human genetics, particularly concerning human genetic disorders,[25] and this has been shown to be a barrier to effective genetic counseling.[26] A committee of the National Academy of Sciences concluded that "it is essential to begin the study of human biology, including genetics and probability, in primary school, continuing with a more health-related curriculum in secondary school."[27] By teaching young children the concepts of human variability, genetics education can dispel unfounded fears and help people understand and respond appropriately to genetic differences among groups. The importance of early education in genetics was also underscored by the Biological Sciences Curriculum Study (BSCS):

> Because the study of human genetics is not exclusively a biological science, and because most of its content deals with values, feelings, and emotion, it is important to provide information on this subject to children at a time when their fundamental attitudes are being formed.[28]

The educational approaches should recognize that information on genetics sometimes raises troubling and sensitive issues for certain individuals and groups. People at increased risk for a disease or of being a carrier may fear or actually encounter stigmatization or may experience a loss of self-esteem. Material on genetic disease should be presented in a way that does not inappropriately and insensitively single out particular groups.

The BSCS represents an important effort to redress deficiencies in primary and secondary school genetics education. The Commission commends efforts to develop curricula and to work with educators to incorporate genetics material in the classroom. The knowledge imparted is not only important as a basic part of science education but also promotes values of autonomy and informed public participation.

The field of genetics is rapidly changing; even people who gain a sound knowledge of basic genetic principles while at school will need continuing sources of information. Groups like the March of Dimes and associations concerned with specific diseases, such as the Cystic Fibrosis Foundation and the National Committee to Combat Huntington's Disease, can play an important part in this public education effort. Their programs to prepare people to be autonomous decisionmakers and informed participants in the formation of policy on genetics deserve encouragement and support. The Commission also encourages individual genetics professionals to teach school and community groups and to write articles for general-circulation magazines and newspapers.

Professional education. Deficiencies in genetics education extend to the curriculum for many health professionals. Except for programs that specifically provide training for medical geneticists and nonphysician genetic counselors, human genetics is not uniformly taught in schools of medicine, nursing, and the other health professions. A report on medical school curricula found that 30% of the 104 medical schools studied offered no formal education in genetics.[29] The 70% that did provide training in genetics devoted varying degrees of emphasis to the subject. The paucity of medical school training was evident in National Board of Medical Examiners' scores: the ability to answer questions on medical genetics varied directly with the number of hours of training received in medical school. The Commission encourages the Association of American Medical Colleges and professional societies, such as the American Medical Association (AMA) and the American Nurses Association, to upgrade genetics education for professional students.

Postgraduate education is also important to make professionals aware of new developments in genetics and several organizations have promoted continuing education. The Council on Scientific Affairs of the AMA, for example, recently encouraged medical specialty societies to expand their efforts to train physicians in the newer techniques of prenatal diagnosis.[30] The Federal government and the March of Dimes sponsor fellowships to train medical geneticists. Blue Cross/Blue Shield of New York and the National Genetics Foundation operate a toll-free "hotline" for physicians seeking information on genetic disease;[31] the enthusiastic response to the service attests to professional interest in up-to-date genetic information. Continuing education is important not only for physicians, but also for health educators, genetic counselors, and others involved in the delivery of genetic information and services. Organizations like the March of Dimes and governmental bodies make important contributions to this goal of professional education and therefore deserve public support. It is important that these educational efforts go beyond technical matters in genetic screening and counseling and include instruction about the role of informed consent, the psychosocial implications of screening and counseling, and the central place that value preferences hold in personal decisionmaking.

Education for particular screening programs. Improved public and professional education in human genetics generally can help set the stage for education on programs targeted at specific potential screening populations. Information should be aimed at both professionals and the public, drawing on past experience with screening programs and current expertise in health education. Prominent lay and professional communications media are important vehicles for widespread exposure about screening programs. Again, it is essential that the programs be sensitive to possible public misconceptions and to the risk of personal stigma that might occur when a certain subgroup is identified as at high risk for a deleterious genetic condition. In light of the anxiety that can arise among candidates for screening, the way information about genetic diseases and tests is presented deserves careful attention.[32] Community leaders and organizations representing the population to be screened should play an integral part in program planning—without their involvement, a program is unlikely to be effective. Moreover, excluding such groups violates ideals of public participation and represents a paternalistic intervention that shows a lack of respect for individual and community autonomy.

Before launching a program, it is also important that all participating health care professionals are adequately educated about its purposes and procedures. As demonstrated by the study of physician education about AFP testing,[33] this can be a less straightforward task than might be assumed. Failure to educate professionals adequately could lead to poor-quality testing and counseling and result in serious harm to patients and their children. Professional education is thus a crucial link in the implementation of a screening program; it provides an essential ethical safeguard. Even professionals not directly involved in counseling or screening must be well informed if they are to be effective in referring individuals to the program and in responding to the concerns and questions of their patients. Therefore, the Commission believes that it is essential for professional educators, working with specialty societies and program planners, to identify effective methods to educate professionals about new screening tests.

Well-Being

The promotion of personal well-being is a major objective underlying all the facets of health care considered by the Commission. This goal—sometimes stated as the principle of beneficence—has definite application in the field of genetics both for the work of individual health care professionals and for the decisionmaking of officials of public and private bodies.

The Special Case of Artificial Insemination by Donor Almost 100 years after the first successful artificial insemination by donor (AID)[34] was performed in 1884, a host of legal, social, and ethical questions still surround the procedure. Although a comprehensive analysis of these issues is beyond the scope of this report, the Commission felt it was important to consider the role of genetic screening and counseling in AID.

Each year, an estimated 6000–10,000 infants are born in the United States as a result of AID. A recent study found that little, if any, information is obtained about the genetic history or genetic risks of the donor.[35] Moreover, recordkeeping on the source of semen samples is sparse.[36] This is largely due to a desire to provide donors with anonymity and protection against legal liability. However, this casual approach to obtaining donor samples poses several potentially serious problems.[37]

First, there is the risk of genetic disease in the offspring. Women who are Tay-Sachs or sickle-cell carriers, for example, might unknowingly receive sperm from another carrier and consequently bear a child with the condition. Similarly, serious problems could occur if a woman whose blood is Rh-negative is inseminated with sperm from a donor whose Rh factor has not been ascertained. Second, one effect of minimal recordkeeping is that when AID results in genetic disease, the source of the sample cannot be determined; semen from that donor may be used again and may result in another child with that disease. Indeed, the Commission heard testimony about just such a case, involving one woman who bore two children with the same serious genetic disorder.[38] Lack of recordkeeping also makes it impossible to alert the donor that any of his own offspring are at risk—information he might find useful for his plans about having children. Finally, there is the possibility that children conceived from the same donor (half-brothers and half-sisters) might marry. Children of such an unwittingly incestuous union would be at increased risk for rare genetic disorders. The likelihood of this occurring would probably be greatest if several individuals in a small town were inseminated with sperm from one donor.

As elaborated in the Commission's report *Making Health Care Decisions*, true informed consent in patient-provider relationships involves a discussion of the possible benefits and risks of a contemplated medical procedure and of the alternatives. Accordingly, a woman considering artificial insemination should be apprised of the risks being taken by conceiving a child with a donor's sample.[39] Clearly it is not feasible—or even possible—to enumerate the risk of the thousands of diseases of genetic origin. When a genetic history and genetic screening could provide useful data about the risks for particular diseases, however, this information is an important element of informed decisionmaking. For example, a black woman who is a sickle-cell carrier or a Jewish woman who carries a gene for Tay-Sachs disease should know the carrier status of the potential donor as part of her decisionmaking process; an Rh-negative woman should know the Rh status of the donor.[40] Women seeking AID are very eager to bear children. If no information is available on potential donors, they might nonetheless agree to the procedure. Providing them only with the options of inadequate information or no insemination is inconsistent with the values underlying informed consent.

The Commission concludes that a genetic history should be obtained on all potential sperm donors and, where appropriate, the results of genetic screening should be available to prospective recipients, with a view toward promulgating guidelines for those involved in obtaining samples and performing AID. Professional associations, such as the American Society of Human Genetics or the American College of Obstetrics and Gynecology, are probably best suited to develop and disseminate such criteria.[41]

Policies on recordkeeping involve balancing confidentiality interests with the prevention of harm. To prevent harm to future offspring and families from repeated use of samples in unfavorable circumstances, records of the source of the sample should be kept. Harm might also be prevented if donors were informed about any risks of genetic disease that were identified during the screening.

Recordkeeping does pose a potential risk that a paternity suit might be initiated, that a child might wish to locate his or her biological father, or that a donor might seek out his offspring. The Commission believes that safeguards could be put in place to minimize the risk that recordkeeping would violate confidentiality interests. Law reform groups, as part of a much-needed reformulation of law in this field, should include provisions that will allow the source of donor samples to be identified and the results of genetic tests to be recorded in a way that protects the confidentiality of the donor to the greatest extent possible.

The chance of unwittingly incestuous marriages can best be reduced if physicians take care to use samples from a variety of donors when inseminating women in one particular locale. This, of course, presumes that it is possible to determine that the source of the samples is different, a concern that should be addressed by the recordkeeping system recommended.

Ensuring Accuracy and Safety of All Programs The value of genetic screening lies in providing information that can assist people in making voluntary decisions about health care and reproduction that reflect their personal values. This information can have an enormous impact on the physical and emotional well-being of patients and of prospective parents and their children. Failure to provide accurate information not only thwarts the potential benefits of screening but can cause harm.

Pilot programs. Pilot studies are an essential means of determining the accuracy and reliability of a test before it is introduced to the general population. Public screening programs should not be implemented until they have first demonstrated their value in well-conducted pilot studies. The Food and Drug Administration (FDA) and other relevant government agencies should require such studies as a prerequisite to introducing new products for general use. These studies should yield information on the false positive and false negative rates associated with possible cutoff points and on the predictive power of the test in the populations to be screened. Ultimately, individual physicians and an informed public can act as the final check on the system by requiring that a test's value be established before they participate in a screening program.

Although pilot studies should precede the introduction of a screening test into the health care system, it is not clear who bears the responsibility for producing the data and funding the studies. If FDA classifies a test as a class III medical device, proof of its safety and efficacy is required before it is marketed.[42] In these cases, the companies seeking to market the product must provide FDA with data from human subjects research. Experience with AFP test kits, however, demonstrated a confusion about the extent and nature of the studies that commercial companies must provide and about the safety and efficacy standard that should be applied to genetic screening tests.[43] With these issues still unresolved and with other tests likely to raise similar questions, the parties involved—including regulators, funding agency administrators, industry representatives, researchers, and public health officials—should meet to discuss their respective roles in ensuring that a prospective test is studied adequately before genetic screening programs are introduced.

Monitoring long-term outcome. In addition to careful design and proper pilot studies, an evaluation of the long-term effects of genetic screening is important. Such monitoring may be necessary if the low-frequency adverse effects of screening are to be detected, since pilot studies involve only a limited population. A small but significant error rate, for example, may not become evident until a larger population undergoes the test. Some effects—both physical and psychosocial—may be so unanticipated that the initial evaluation procedures overlook them; other effects may not be manifested until after the pilot study.

Information about the medical and psychological consequences of screening gained from extended follow-up enhances the informed consent process and the overall determination of the risks and benefits of a program. Despite this value, follow-up research is too often neglected. This is in part due to the methodological difficulties and expense of following or locating screening participants, sometimes several years after they took part in the program. Federal funding for follow-up studies has been sparse. Research on stigmatization and other possible psychosocial effects of screening has for the most part been seriously inadequate. The Commission finds that if ethical and policy goals are to be promoted, every screening program should have an evaluation component. In some cases it may not be possible or even necessary to conduct extensive follow-up research, but needs of each particular program should be considered. Sometimes the scope of the studies, the significance for potential screenees throughout the country, and the involvement of programs in several states make this evaluation an appropriate function of the Federal government. However, officials administering more-limited programs should also be aware of the needs for long-term monitoring. In addition, follow-up of participants by a genetic counselor can provide a valuable service.

Professional and quality standards. Adapting a successful experimental procedure to wide-scale use often requires more than merely enlarging its scope. A broadly based pilot study provides important data on the effects of a genetic test, but it still benefits from the special preparation that health professionals, laboratory facilities, and others make for an experiment. Proper research, by definition, involves a carefully controlled situation. The real world is less ideal, and therein lie serious ethical and policy issues for those who initiate new screening efforts.

Questions both of quality and of quantity arise. The quality questions concern the ability of those in a genetic screening program to meet a necessary standard of performance. Laboratories are a prime focus of this concern. It is unrealistic to expect that laboratory errors can be avoided entirely. Samples can be labeled incorrectly, clerical mistakes can be made in reporting results, and other such "human errors" can occur. With well-trained, conscientious professionals, however, these should be very rare.

Another source of error relates to the diffusion of a new screening technology. Widespread use of a new screening technique can attract a large number of laboratories anticipating commercial advantages from the test and seeking to enlarge access to it in their locale. Yet some of them may serve a small population or a population with a low incidence of the disease; these laboratories will probably never gain extensive experience performing the test. Cases of PKU are less likely to be missed when tests are conducted by a more-skilled, centralized laboratory that processes a large number of samples than when they are done in a smaller facility that receives fewer samples.[44] But if screening samples are not stable over time and distances, the effect of laboratory centralization may be to restrict access to screening programs to the areas of high population density served by these larger laboratories.

These are not easy conflicts to resolve. Yet the underlying ethical and policy goals promoted by screening are undermined by inaccurate results. The Commission believes that screening should only be undertaken if results that are produced can be routinely relied upon. Thus, specific mechanisms must be in place to preclude involvement of laboratories, physicians, or other elements of a program that fail to meet these standards. Federal licensure of interstate laboratories and proficiency testing are important quality-control measures. State agencies and professional associations such as the Joint Commission on Accreditation of Hospitals, the College of American Pathologists, and the American Board of Medical Genetics can also play important roles in promoting sound laboratory performance.

Laboratory quality-control measures are targeted toward each specific genetic test. Performance standards for providers and counselors participating in particular screening programs are a far less familiar notion, however. As already noted, educational programs and evaluations of their effectiveness are important adjuncts to general professional standards and licensure. Existing norms of tort liability may provide a means of redress to individuals injured as a result of negligence, but the Commission finds this after-the-fact approach to quality control inadequate. Indeed, fear of liability may work in conflicting ways; it may cause those involved in testing to be more cautious, but it could also prompt an ill-prepared provider to perform a test. This problem is not restricted to lack of technical proficiency. Physicians may possess the skill to withdraw amniotic fluid, for example, but not understand the meaning of various outcomes, or they may lack the time or expertise to counsel patients in a way that would provide some balance of benefits and harms and help patients make decisions based on the information.

Much of the responsibility for establishing and enforcing performance standards for a particular test will fall to the professions themselves. Nevertheless, public officials, including those who fund programs or regulate screening products, share responsibility for seeing that the test is used in a way that will maximize benefits and minimize harm.

When a screening test is promoted by a laboratory or offered independently by physicians rather than as part of a coordinated program, overall responsibility for coordinating and assessing its availability and quality may be overlooked. As one leading physician-geneticist told the Commission:

> Most of the mistakes, most of the ethical transgressions, most of the failures to observe people's rights, most of the breaches of confidentiality and of informed consent and so on occurred early on when screening was being done by individual investigators or by interested lay groups, when it was being done in inappropriate places, and before the network of educators, counselors, physicians, health officers, and the like were set up.[45]

Some states have created bodies to oversee the execution and evaluation of genetic screening programs and to avert harm that can result when responsibility for coordinating programs is not clearly assigned. These organizations benefit from both public and professional input in policy-making.[46] Such bodies can provide an important focus for the successful provision of genetic services. Other states could benefit from such an arrangement. In its absence, medical specialty groups, state and local health officials, or others must assume these important responsibilities.

Requests for a new test can place demands not only on the performance quality of providers, but also on the quantity of adequate resources. Clearly these are related issues—demand that outstrips the capacity of qualified providers can prompt inadequately prepared groups to fill the gap. A genetic test performed or overseen by a physician is only one part of a network of prescreening and follow-up procedures and services. The unavailability of any part of this network can undermine the goals of a screening program. An inadequate laboratory capacity or roster of counselors to explain the test, interpret test results, and discuss options or follow-up studies can render the information from an initial screening test more harmful than beneficial to the screenee. Therefore, the Commission recommends that those who conduct or oversee screening programs ensure that the anticipated demand for the full range of services can be met before a test is offered. Yet if this principle is applied to the existing system—in which some groups lack access (for geographical or financial reasons) to certain of the necessary services or options for medical management—then access to genetic screening and counseling ought not to be provided to some people. From the viewpoint of well-being, this result seems sensible because of the network of prescreening and follow-up services that an effective genetic screening program requires. If all the services are not available, it may seem unwise to perform screening.

Yet in ethical terms, applying the net benefit principle to a group that lacks access to the full range of health services associated with genetic screening doubles the detriment those people experience in the area of health services. If policymakers accept that a low-income population at risk for a genetic disorder will be unable to avail themselves of a full range of services or treatment options because of a lack of private funds and because the medical procedures in question are not covered by Medicaid, then it would seem that these people should be denied that screening service. Thus, problems of access to genetic screening and counseling are inextricably connected with ethical issues in access to health care in general and with the still larger issue of distributive justice. When a screening program is needed but auxiliary services are unavailable, efforts to remedy resource limitations and improve access should be undertaken.

Equity

The concern that appropriate quality standards not leave already underserved populations without access to the genetics service that are made available to others has already pointed to the relevance to this field of a final ethical and legal concern—that of equity or fairness. In the context of highly sophisticated biomedical techniques, it is important to guard against the tendency to treat as matters of scientific expertise what are actually ethical decisions about the allocation of benefits and burdens.

Distributing Benefits The availability of services sometimes depends on factors other than economic resources, race, or place of residence. In the area of genetic screening, for example, it is now common practice for physicians to offer amniocentesis for "advanced maternal age" only to women age 35 years or over. In effect, this is a policy about the way in which this beneficial service should be distributed.

The medical literature today invariably lists maternal age of 35 or over as an indication for prenatal diagnosis through amniocentesis because such women have an increased risk of bearing a child with a chromosomal defect.[47] The courts have reinforced this policy by accepting this standard, articulated by medical professionals as the measure of "due care"; that is, physicians who have failed to inform 35-year-old pregnant women about the availability of amniocentesis may be found negligent and therefore be held liable if a patient of theirs bears a child with such a defect.[48] A pregnant patient who is 34, however, may well not be told about amniocentesis or may even be told, if she asks for it, that the procedure is unavailable or inappropriate.

The policy of counseling only women age 35 or over about the benefits and risks of amniocentesis has been adopted informally by many practitioners over the past ten years.[49] The practice has been institutionalized by some laboratories that do not accept amniotic fluid samples from women under age 35 (in the absence of other risk factors).[50] This disparity illustrates the questions of fairness and equity that arise in genetic screening and counseling: in what way, and for what reasons, is it ethically acceptable to limit access to genetic services? An answer to that question in the context of amniocentesis must begin with an examination of the origin (in about 1968) of the age-based distinction and a review of whether the factors relied on then remain relevant today as the basis for an ethically acceptable policy.

Although there was no formal process from which the 35-year-old cutoff arose, several factors apparently led to it in the early days of the procedure. First, data on the relationship between maternal age and Down Syndrome were then collated in five-year age intervals and a marked increase in risk occurred in the 35–40 year age-group (see Figure 1). Second, the risks of amniocentesis to the mother and the fetus—subsequently found to be less than 1% morbidity and mortality—were then regarded as potentially serious. The unknown risk argued for limiting the procedure to those most likely to have an affected pregnancy, meaning that the probability of harm from the procedure was less likely to be disproportionate to the risk of bearing an affected child. Third, from a public health perspective, the greatest impact in reducing the incidence of Down Syndrome with the least expenditure (that is, the most cost-effective method) was to concentrate resources in the 35-and-over age-group. Data cited in a 1969 meeting showed that women 35 and over accounted for 13.5% of all births but about 50% of Down Syndrome births.[51] Thus, theoretically, the incidence of the condition could be reduced significantly by screening this limited age-group. Finally, the specialized training, time, and expense required to analyze amniotic fluid samples assured that a significant start-up time would be required; the resource would be scarce, at least in the initial phases of the program, so some method for restricting access would be needed. The birth rate fell off markedly at age 34, making the group of women over that age a manageable one.

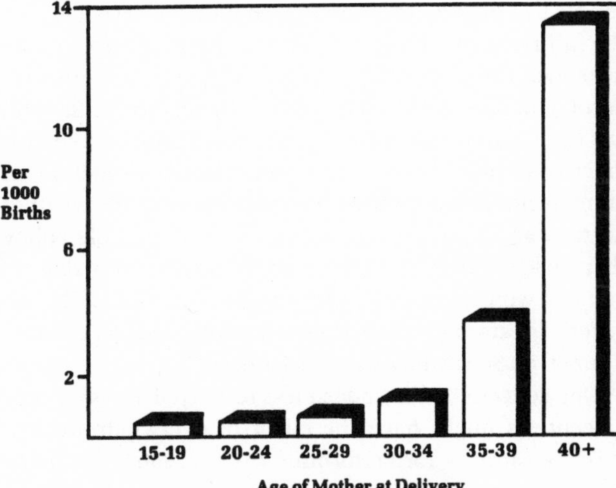

FIGURE 1. Prevalence of Down Syndrome by age of mother, in five-year maternal age intervals, 1954–1965

Source: Brian MacMahol and Thomas F. Pugh, *Epidemiology: Principles and Methods*, Little, Brown and Company, Boston (1970) at 328.

In light of these factors, concerns for fairness and equity argued in favor of concentrating resources on women who were at least 35. Moreover, since amniocentesis for prenatal diagnosis was initially a research procedure, it is not inappropriate that decisions about the selection of the population rested in the hands of the medical experts. However, each of these considerations is also subject to change over time. Sound decisionmaking calls for a process by which the policy can be reevaluated when changes occur in these or other factors that would alter the basis for the policy.

In fact, many of the factors have changed—or could be changed—in significant ways. Information is now available on the incidence of Down Syndrome by maternal age in single-year intervals. Whereas the five-year age-interval data showed a marked upward swing at age 35, the more detailed data show instead a steady increase in incidence with increasing age (see Figure 2). These data do not suggest the obvious cutoff point seen in the earlier chart.

In addition, the demographics of the childbearing population have shifted significantly in the last two decades; the economic justification for the policy in 1970, which was based on data from the 1950s and 1960s, weakens in light of recent data. The proportion of all births to women age 35 or over dropped from about 10% in the 1960s to about 4.5% by the mid-1970s. This decrease resulted in the percentage of Down Syndrome births that are to older mothers declining from about 44% in 1960 to 21% in 1978.[52] This decline in the proportion of these births that are to older women reflects demographic shifts (that is, the larger proportion of all births to younger women), not the impact of prenatal diagnosis. Amniocentesis was in very limited use at the time the data were collected. Therefore, although older mothers are at the highest risk of bearing infants with chromosomal abnormalities, and although the procedure offers beneficial information to them, it no longer seems possible to achieve marked reductions in the incidence of Down Syndrome by focusing resources solely on this limited population of pregnant women.

Recent research has also injected another consideration into the assessment of risks for Down Syndrome births relative to maternal age. Studies have shown that in about

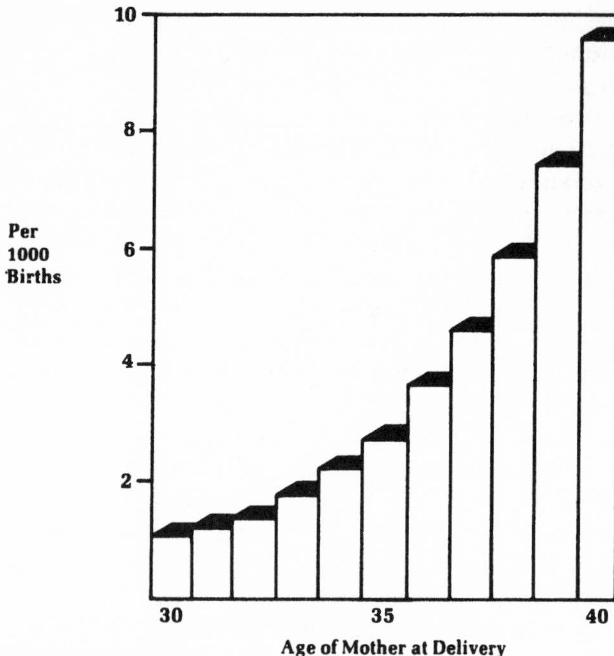

FIGURE 2. Prevalence of Down Syndrome for mothers aged 30–40, in single-year intervals (New York), 1974

Source: Derived from National Institute of Child Health and Human Development, *Antenatal Diagnosis: Report of a Consensus Development Conference*, Dept. of Health, Education, and Welfare, Washington (1979) at I-49.

24% of the cases the extra chromosome 21, which is frequently characteristic of the condition, is contributed by the father.[53] Although it is possible that the maternal environment plays a role in inducing that error, this discovery does raise the possibility that the effect of maternal age may be somewhat less than had been assumed.

Recent studies of the safety of amniocentesis also provide an opportunity to reconsider the benefits and risks of the procedure in relation to the risks of bearing an affected child. Reliance on strict benefit-risk analysis in genetic screening is problematic because many important benefits are intangible and subjective. Whether the benefits outweigh the risks, therefore, is largely a matter of personal values; not only must the mathematical probability of two events be compared but also a personal valuation of their relative severity must be made. A woman who desperately wants to continue her pregnancy (perhaps her first after many years of trying) may regard the risk of the procedure as higher than the risk of bearing a Down Syndrome child. In contrast, another woman (perhaps one who is already a mother) may strongly wish to avoid the risk of a Down Syndrome child, even when achieving that perceived benefit requires a diagnostic procedure with its own risks.

Subjective assessments of risk are particularly important when the mathematical probability of two events occurring is similar. For example, the probability of the most serious harm—fetal loss from amniocentesis—appears to be .5% or lower, while the probability of bearing an affected child ranges from about .13% at age 32 to .56% at age 38. The likelihood of losing a fetus is thus generally proportionate to the likelihood of bearing an affected child in this age range; in contrast, for very young mothers the likelihood of bearing an affected child is considerably less than that of harm through amniocentesis.

Finally, current policies regarding amniocentesis for "advanced age" mothers must be examined in relation to the availability and elasticity of resources. Amniocentesis is frequently termed a "scarce resource," and the need to ration its use justified on that basis. However, restricting demand for a service because the facilities and trained personnel to provide it are perceived to be limited can inhibit the possible expansion of the service, which would in turn accommodate a larger demand.[54] (This is particularly true with respect to the for-profit laboratories, but it also applies to state-operated facilities that have to compete for funds in legislative and bureaucratic arenas.) When amniocentesis first became available, the buildup of facilities was expected to be slow—perhaps slower than the buildup of demand. Although the number of amniocenteses performed has increased steadily in the past several years, only a small proportion of the potential candidates are using the service. This has been attributed to a lag in introducing the technology into clinical settings (including a failure of physicians to refer patients for the test), rather than refusal of the technique by informed women.[55] Moreover, women who obtain amniocentesis are disproportionately white and urban.[56]

This review of the "35-and-over" policy for amniocentesis leads to two conclusions, one general and the other specific. First, as limitations on access move from the research context to implicit (or explicit) policies on the availability of a genetic service they should be subjected to review by a broadly based process that will be responsive to the full range of relevant considerations, to changes in the facts over time, and to the needs of the excluded group(s). Second, in light of the facts concerning this particular policy the Commission believes that the common medical practice of only informing women age 35 or older about amniocentesis should be reevaluated to determine whether fairness and equity would support a more flexible policy that made amniocentesis more generally available to younger women. This need for a reconsideration of the age criteria for amniocentesis has been recognized by the AMA Council on Scientific Affairs and others.[57]

One concern is that sudden less restricted access to amniocentesis might have the effect of overwhelming the existing capacity for performing the procedure, with the result that some of the women who have the greatest need would fail to receive the test while those at lower risk do have it. Thus it is important that the elasticity of the capacity for amniocentesis is studied. A policy of increasing access for younger women should not interfere with the goal of making the test more available to women at highest risk who want to have access to it. Moreover, amniocentesis is a costly procedure; it may not be efficient or equitable in light of other demands on scarce resources to expend public funds for groups at low risk, although this should not preclude individuals from paying for the procedure with private funds.

Distributing Risks Inherent in the allocation of benefits is an allocation of their reciprocal risks (that is, the burdens that may befall people who do not receive the benefits). Sometimes, however, the distribution of risks is more apparent, as, for example, in decisions about the standards for genetic screening.

The appropriate requirement for a particular test depends on the objective of the screen. Screening tests that try to identify a high-risk population for subsequent preciser diagnostic testing need not achieve as high a degree of accuracy as must a test that is not followed by confirmatory studies. PKU screening is an example of the former type of test; some prenatal diagnostic procedures illustrate the latter category. Errors in any test could lead to unnecessary anxiety or unfounded reassurance, from either of which could follow consequences contrary to the intent and expectations of the families and physicians involved. But the danger is plainly much greater when no further diagnostic steps are usually employed.

Of special concern in evaluating a test's accuracy are its sensitivity and specificity. Sensitivity is a measure of the proportion of people with the disease who test positive, while a test's specificity is the proportion of those without the disease who test negative. The sensitivity and specificity of a test are inversely related. For example, increasing a test's sensitivity to pick up more cases decreases the specificity by labeling more unaffected people as affected. Striking a balance between sensitivity and specificity is not solely a technical matter. It requires value preferences to guide the distribution of the risks, as well as evaluation of the health care system's capacity to respond to the consequences of the policy chosen. The benefits and burdens of false positive and false negative findings for a particular test must be weighed and the sensitivity and specificity set so as to do the least harm and distribute the benefits and burdens most equitably. This amounts to an intersection of ethics and public policy since it requires an application of the principle of justice.

False positive results lead to needless anxiety and corrective steps, and—where the risk of such false results is recognized—also the cost, inconvenience, and possible danger of undergoing additional tests. Of greatest concern are the cases in which mistaken diagnoses are not identified in subsequent testing and individuals or couples may make difficult choices to forgo reproduction, terminate a pregnancy, or initiate arduous and sometimes harmful treatment regimens unnecessarily.

False negatives can also be harmful. The false reassurance they provide fails to prepare those involved medically, emotionally, or psychologically for a pregnancy outcome or manifestation of disease. False negative results are actually more harmful than having no test. In the latter case, a person who understands the probability of a genetic disease may take appropriate steps (for example, a couple at risk for an autosomal recessive disorder might decide not to conceive a child), while a false negative result effectively discourages recognition that the risk of the disease is a reality (as in newborn screening, when a false negative may mean that an infant who could have been spared the harmful effects of a genetic disease, if it had been identified and the child had started on an appropriate regimen early, is instead not treated and suffers premature death, mental retardation, or other severe consequences). Whereas false positive diagnoses can be corrected in subsequent tests, a false negative generally eliminates the individual from the screening protocol with the result that the error may not be recognized until it is too late for effective corrective action to be taken.

Frequently this weighing of benefits and harms leads public health officials to make a test "oversensitive." The intent is to have no false negatives even though a large number of false positives may result. PKU screening (which has a false positive rate of over 90%) illustrates the ethical and public policy considerations underlying the design of genetic screening programs. A positive result on an initial PKU test probably causes new parents anxiety and requires an additional test in the doctor's office. But PKU tests are simple, inexpensive, essentially painless, and without risk. Thus the anxiety, the need for a follow-up visit (which may add only a small financial and logistical burden if it coincides with a routine newborn checkup), and possibly a small fee are the major consequences of an initial false positive test. If the subsequent test establishes that the disease is not present, this is the extent of the harm. In contrast, a false negative result likely dooms the child to severe mental retardation that could have been averted had the disease been diagnosed and appropriate treatment initiated. As discussed in Chapter One, the development of an effective dietary treatment has drastically reduced the number of children suffering from mental retardation due to PKU.[58] False negative results prevent screenees from benefiting from this important therapeutic intervention.

Program planners should also consider the predictive power of a test for a prospective screening population. This is the proportion of all positive tests that are true cases. A test that yields many false positives to produce a true positive has a low predictive power and may be too costly or burdensome to initiate. For a given sensitivity and specificity, the rarer the disease, the lower the predictive power.

The nature of the test and the capacity of the system to obtain test results efficiently are important factors in determining acceptable sensitivity, specificity, and predictive power, however. In addition to a PKU test being simple, quick, essentially without pain or risk, and cheap, it can be automated, which facilitates the processing of large numbers of samples in a short time. These considerations have made it feasible to screen the entire population and to set the cutoff level such that a large number of false positives result. Furthermore, a second test is highly diagnostic, eliminating most false positives. These factors, together with the conclusion that the harms of false negatives on the initial test are more serious than those of false positives, provide the ethical grounds on which public officials initiated testing (even though the incidence of the disease and the predictive power of the test are low) and opted to make the PKU test "oversensitive" by setting the cutoff level very low.

Genetic diseases are rare. Thus in a screening program involving thousands of screenees, most of whom are normal, even a 1% false positive rate could result in a large number of misdiagnoses. Moreover, the stakes involved in genetic testing are high—decisions may be made about reproduction, and even in some cases about termination of a pregnancy, on the basis of test results. Screening ought, therefore, typically to be restricted to "high-risk" groups. This policy would also conform to goals of economy and efficiency, since the cost of a large-scale screening program can be substantial in proportion to the small number of cases detected when the population has a very low incidence of a disease.

Questions of equity and justice underlie a determination of which groups are at a high enough risk for screening and at what point the predictive value of a test is sufficiently high. Since the balance of benefits and harms from a test's false positives and false negatives will vary with the incidence of a disease within a group, the value of screening must be determined separately for different subpopulations. The principles of equity should be reflected in the design of all genetic screening programs. Equity is best served when a decision whether to promote screening for a particular population reflects a balancing of benefits and harms, given the incidence of the disease in the population, rather than an aim to give equal access to screening to all groups, regardless of the population-based incidence.

Uses and Limits of Cost-Benefit Analysis Cost-benefit analysis has become a recognized tool for making allocational decisions in a broad range of areas, including health care. It can help answer resource allocation and access questions concerning genetic screening and counseling, provided the significant limitations of the method are clearly understood.

Cost-benefit analysis is most useful when the costs and benefits of the action under consideration are tangible, can be measured by a common unit of measurement, and can be known with certainty. These conditions are rarely satisfied in public policy situations and they can be particularly elusive in genetic screening and counseling programs. For example, cost-benefit calculations can accurately evaluate the worth of a projected prenatal screening program if the only costs measured are the financial outlays (that is, administering a screening and counseling program and performing abortions when defects are detected) and the benefits measured are the dollars that would have been spent on care of affected children. But the calculations become both much more complex and much less accurate if an attempt is made to quantify the psychological "costs" and "benefits" to screenees, their families, and society.

A more fundamental limitation on cost-benefit analysis is that in its simplest form it assumes that the governing moral value is to maximize the general welfare (utilitarianism). Simply aggregating gains and losses across all the individuals affected omits considerations of equity or fairness. Indeed, cost-benefit methodology itself does not distinguish as to *whose* costs and benefits are to be considered. But in the case at hand, it is an ethical question as to whether the costs and benefits to the fetus are to be considered, and, if so, whether they are to be given the same weight as those of the mother and family.

It is possible, however, to incorporate considerations of equity or fairness and thereby depart from a strictly utilitarian form of cost-benefit analysis either by weighting some costs or benefits or by restricting the class of individuals who will be included in the calculation. In any case, cost-benefit analysis must be regarded as a technical instrument to be used within an ethical framework (whether utilitarian or otherwise), rather than as a method of avoiding difficult ethical judgments.

In general, the process of attempting to ascertain the costs and benefits of a given policy according to a common standard of measurement performs the useful function of forcing policymakers to envision as clearly as possible the consequences of a decision. For example, the health authorities in cities with few marriages between Ashkenazi Jews might decide not to mount a Tay-Sachs screening program, on the ground that the rarity of the expected occurrence would raise the cost-per-case-detected to a very high level in light of the expected savings. Yet their ethical analysis will need to recognize that the risk of a Tay-Sachs birth for an individual Ashkenazi couple is the same whether the benefits and burdens are distributed fairly or not.

More particularly, cost-benefit analysis can rule out some policy proposals, once ethical priorities have been fixed. It is now generally agreed, for example, that cost-benefit analysis of sickle-cell carrier screening of elementary school children would show that the benefits of the knowledge gained through screening do not outweigh the administration costs combined with the social stigma and psychological distress suffered by the screenees and their families.

The experience with sickle-cell testing and other genetic programs, together with the ethical principles discussed in this chapter, should provide policymakers with the basis for careful preparation for tests that could become available soon.

NOTES

Introduction

1. 42 U.S.C. § 300v-1(a)(1)(C)(1981).
2. *See, e.g.*, Don Kaercher, "Genetic Diseases and Birth Defects: What Every Family Needs to Know," *Better Homes and Gardens* 66 (March 1980); Graham Chedd, "Who Shall Be Born?", *Science 81*, 32 (Jan./Feb. 1981); Matt Clark, with Mariana Gosnell, "The New Gene Doctors," *Newsweek* 120 (May 18, 1981).
3. For definitions of technical terms throughout this Report, see "Glossary," Appendix A, pp. 105–08 *infra*; for further information on genetics and means of testing, see "Basic Concepts," Appendix B, pp. 109–15 *infra*.
4. *See* Committee for the Study of Inborn Errors of Metabolism, *Genetic Screening: Programs, Principles, and Research*, National Academy of Sciences, Washington (1975) at 9–13.
5. Office of Technology Assessment, *The Role of Genetic Testing in the Prevention of Occupational Illness*, U.S. Congress, Washington (forthcoming); Thomas H. Murray, Statement before the Committee on Science and Technology, Subcommittee on Investigations and Oversight, U.S. Congress, Oct. 6, 1982.
6. Genetic predispositions are being found behind many conditions long thought of as nongenetic, while some genetic conditions are only regarded as "diseases" because of particular environmental settings or stimuli.
7. Ad Hoc Committee on Genetic Counseling, "Genetic Counseling," 27 *Am. J. Human Genetics* 240–41 (1975).
8. President's Commission for the Study of Ethical Problems in Medicine and Biomedical and Behavioral Research, *Making Health Care Decisions*, U.S. Government Printing Office, Washington (1982); President's Commission for the Study of Ethical Problems in Medicine and Biomedical and Behavioral Research, *Securing Access to Health Care*, U.S. Government Printing Office, Washington (1983).
9. As explained in Appendix B, pp. 109–15 *infra*, it takes two genes to have the disease, one from each parent. The incidence of cystic fibrosis in other races is much lower.
10. The participants in the Commission's study are set forth in "The Commission Process," Appendix C, pp. 117–19 *infra*.

Ethical and Legal Implications

1. When screening (genetic or nongenetic) is undertaken in the industrial setting at company expense in order to monitor workplace safety or employee suitability, access to the resulting medical record—by third parties, and even by the person screened—raises special issues that are currently being studied by other groups, such as the Congressional Office of Technology Assessment.
2. *See, e.g.*, Almeta E. Cooper, "Duty to Warn Third Parties," 248 *J.A.M.A.* 431 (1982).
3. It is worth emphasizing that the harm-prevention argument for compelled disclosure merely shows that the commitment to confidentiality is not absolute in cases of the sort described. It does not establish that a general practice of breaching the confidentiality of genetic information would have acceptable consequences.
4. Gilbert S. Omenn, Judith G. Hall, and Kenneth D. Hansen, "Genetic Counseling for Adoptees at Risk for Specific Inherited Disorders," 5 *Am. J. Med. Genetics* 157, 158–59 (1980).
5. § 303(f)(5), Model Act for Adoption of Children with Special Needs; Final Legislation, 46 *Federal Register* 50022 (Oct. 8, 1981).
6. A.M. Capron, "Tort Liability in Genetic Counseling," 79 *Colum. L. Rev.* 619, 680 (1979).
7. *Compare* Ruth R. Faden, Neil A. Holtzman, and A. Judith Chwalow, "Parental Rights, Child Welfare, and Public Health: The Case of PKU Screening," 72 *Am. J. Pub. Health* 1396 (1982) (argues on moral grounds against parental consent for newborn screening), *with* George Annas, "Mandatory PKU Screening: The Other Side of the Looking Glass," 72 *Am. J. Pub. Health* 1401 (1982) (focuses on improving parental understanding, not on coercion).
8. National Clearinghouse for Human Genetic Diseases, *State Laws and Regulations on Genetic Disorders*, Dept. of Health and Human Services, Washington (1980). As of 1980, PKU screening was mandatory in 48 states; two states and the District of Columbia have voluntary programs. For a discussion of conditions for which newborns are sometimes screened, see pp. 12–17 *supra*.
9. Ruth R. Faden *et al.*, "A Survey to Evaluate Parental Consent as Public Policy for Neonatal Screening," 72 *Am. J. Pub. Health* 1347 (1982) (finds that shift to voluntary PKU screening, with parental consent, under Maryland statute did not make screening less persuasive or cost-effective; most mothers wanted to be informed of test in advance, although about half did not believe parental consent should be required).
10. *See, e.g.*, Kenneth M. Ludmerer, *Genetics and American Society*, Johns Hopkins Univ. Press, Baltimore (1972).
11. *See* Laurence H. Tribe, *American Constitutional Law*, Foundation Press, Mineola, N.Y. (1978) at 886–990. *See also*, Ludmerer, *supra* note 10.
12. This tension is also reflected in some aspects of the debate over directive and nondirective counseling. For a further discussion, see pp. 36–38 of original report.
13. The March of Dimes, for example, has been a target of some anti-abortionists because of the organization's support for genetic services. *See, e.g.*, Fr. John Dietzen, "Question Box," *Catholic Standard*, Jan. 22, 1981, at 36; "Dr. Wilkie Says March of Dimes Hasn't Totally Reformed," *National Right to Life News*, April 1978, at 3.
14. If the capacity to perform prenatal therapy expands, significant changes are likely to occur in social expectations about parental and societal obligations toward the unborn. The fetus becomes a patient, rather than the inaccessible and largely unknown predecessor of an infant. One aspect of this change would be more-demanding social expectations of parents in promoting the welfare of the fetus. So although developments in prenatal therapy increase the range of technically feasible options, social pressures may severely limit parents' freedom to refrain from choosing certain options.
15. *See, e.g.*, "Genetic Testing Imperfect but Is Still Valuable," *OB-GYN News*, Feb. 15–28, 1982, at 1; Aubrey Milunsky,

"Medico-Legal Issues in Prenatal Diagnosis," in Aubrey Milunsky and George J. Annas, eds., *Genetics and the Law*, Plenum Press, New York (1976) at 53.

16. The directors of a thalassemia screening program in Great Britain report that

> The existence of antenatal diagnosis has made things worse for couples of heterozygotes who are "missed". . . and so produce a thalassemic child. They now find the disease and its treatment much harder to accept than was formerly the case. Three out of five such couples known to us . . . express(ed) their conviction that once prevention methods are available, the continuing birth of affected children has become *someone's* responsibility.

B. Modell et al., "Population Screening for Carriers of Recessively Inherited Disorders" (Letter), 2 *Lancet* 806 (1980).

17. *See e.g.*, Arno G. Motulsky and Jeffrey Murray, "Will Prenatal Diagnosis with Selective Abortion Affect Society's Attitude toward the Handicapped?", in K. Berg, ed., *Research Ethics*, Alan R. Liss, Inc., New York (in press).
18. Even those prospective parents who do not start off with a particular desire to know the sex of their fetus may learn it as a routine part of the process, although not everyone chooses to learn this information when its disclosure is offered.
19. For example, one genetics center that has a publicized policy of performing amniocentesis for sex selection if, after counseling, the client requests it, reports only one request for this purpose in the six months since the policy was initiated. Haig H. Kazazian, "Prenatal Diagnosis for Sex Choice: A Medical View," 10 *Hastings Ctr. Rep.* 17 (Feb. 1980). The author notes, "Our overall experience during the past eight years leads us to believe that couples desiring sex selection who are willing to undergo midtrimester abortions are uncommon in American society." It is unclear how frequently unplanned pregnancies are terminated because parents do not want to take a chance that the infant is of the unwanted sex.
20. Amitai Etzioni, *Genetic Fix*, Macmillian Publishing Co., Inc., New York (1973) at 227–28.
21. Deception by patients would be easy, even if physicians fully endorsed such a statute. Even if a law prohibited reporting of fetal gender until very late in the pregnancy, enforcement would be difficult.
22. *Dorland's Medical Dictionary*, for example, includes psychological, social, and morphological as well as chromosomal definitions of "sex."
23. Judith G. Hall *et al.*, "The Frequency and Financial Burden of Genetic Disease in a Pediatric Hospital," 1 *Am. J. Med. Genetics* 417 (1978).
24. *Turpin v. Sortini*, 31 Cal.3d 220, 643 P.2d 954 (1982); *Becker v. Schwartz*, 46 N.Y.2d 401, 386 N.E.2d 807 (1978); *Howard v. Lecher*, 42 N.Y.2d 109, 366 N.E.2d 64 (1977). *See also*, Ellen Wright, "Father and Mother Know Best: Defining the Liability of Physicians for Inadequate Genetic Counseling," 87 *Yale L.J.* 1488 (1978); Capron, *supra* note 6.
25. Biological Sciences Curriculum Study, "Guidelines for Educational Priorities and Curricular Innovations in Human and Medical Genetics," 1 *BSCS Journal* 20, 28 (1978).
26. Clare O. Leonard, Gary A. Chase, and Barton Childs, "Genetic Counseling: A Consumer's View" (Special Article) 287 *New Eng. J. Med.* 433, 438 (1972).
27. Committee for the Study of Inborn Errors of Metabolism, *Genetic Screening: Programs, Principles, and Research*, National Academy of Sciences, Washington (1975) at 3.
28. "Guidelines for Education Priorities and Curricular Innovations in Human and Medical Genetics," *supra* note 25, at 21.
29. Barton Childs *et al.*, "Human Genetics Teaching in U.S. Medical Schools," 33 *Am. J. Human Genetics* 1 (1981).
30. Council on Scientific Affairs, "Council Report: Genetic Counseling and Prevention of Birth Defects," 248 *J.A.M.A.* 221 (1982).
31. "Genetics Hotline Established," *Fast Facts for Physicians* (Blue Cross/Blue Shield of Greater New York), April 1982, at 1.
32. For two views of psychosocial implications of public screening programs for Tay-Sachs disease, see Fred Massarik and Michael M. Kaback, *Genetic Disease Control: A Social Psychological Approach*, Sage Publications, Beverly Hills, Calif. (1981), and Madeleine J. Goodman and Lenn E. Goodman, "The Overselling of Genetic Anxiety," 12 *Hastings Ctr. Rep.* 20 (Dec. 1982).
33. *See* note 59, Chapter One of original report.
34. Artificial insemination is classified into three types, based on the source of the semen: by husband (AIH); by donor (AID), in which the semen comes from a third party; and by husband and donor (AIDH), in which semen from the two sources is combined. The Commission's discussion applies to the last two categories.
35. Martin Curie-Cohen, Lesleigh Luttrell, and Sander Shapiro, "Current Practice of Artificial Insemination by Donor in the United States," 300 *New Eng. J. Med.* 585 (1979).
36. F. Clarke Fraser and R. Allan Forse, "On Genetic Screening of Donors for Artificial Insemination," 10 *Am. J. Med. Genetics* 399 (1981).
37. The same concerns about a donor's genetic contribution also apply when a woman donates an egg for an *in vitro* fertilization procedure or when sperm from the husband of an infertile woman is used to impregnate a woman (a surrogate mother) who gestates an infant who will be returned at birth to the man and his wife. These procedures are far less common in the United States at this time.
38. Testimony of Dr. Kurt Hirschhorn, transcript of the 18th meeting of the President's Commission (March 12, 1982) at 227.
39. For example, recent data suggest that AID may be associated with an increased rate of birth defects. R. Allan Forse and F. Clarke Fraser, "Is AID Teratogenic?", 34 *Am. J. Hum. Genetics* 89A (1982). Further research in this area is needed to determine whether the process increases the likelihood of adverse germ-cell changes.
40. The obligation of the physician who performs the insemination to provide genetic information on the donor can be compared to an obstetrician's responsibility to identify possible genetic risks in the prospective parents of a traditional union. For example, a doctor is expected to inform a Jewish woman who is pregnant or who is considering hav-

ing a child about Tay-Sachs disease and the availability of screening tests for it. She and her husband would then have the option of obtaining carrier tests and, if appropriate, the prenatal test for Tay-Sachs. If the conception is going to occur with a third-party donor, the woman should likewise have the option of obtaining information about the chances of bearing a Tay-Sachs child; this is possible only if information on the carrier status of the donor is available.

41. Fraser and Forse, *supra* note 36, recently proposed a set of guidelines for donors that could serve as a starting point for general consideration.
42. The Medical Device Amendments of 1976 to the Federal Food, Drug, and Cosmetic Act establish three categories of medical devices for regulatory purposes—those requiring (1) general controls; (2) performance standards and (3) pre-market approval. 21 U.S.C. § 360c (a)(1)(1976).
43. David Dickson, "Alpha Fetoprotein: Too Hot to Handle?", 280 *Nature* 6 (1979). *See also* p. 29 of original report.
44. David L. Meryash, *et al.*, "Prospective Study of Early Neonatal Screening for Phenylketonuria," 304 *New Eng. J. Med.* 294 (1981); Neil A. Holtzman *et al.*, "Screening for Phenylketonuria" (Letter), 304 *New Eng. J. Med.* 1300 (1981).
45. Testimony of Dr. Barton Childs, transcript of 9th meeting of the President's Commission (May 8, 1981) at 9.
46. For a description of the Maryland Commission on Hereditary Disorders, see Neil A. Holtzman, "Public Participation in Genetic Policymaking," in Aubrey Milunsky, ed., *Genetics and the Law II*, Plenum Press, New York (1980).
47. A 1974 editorial in the *Journal of the American Medical Association*, for example, asserted that any pregnant patient more than 35 years old should have amniocentesis. Jack W. Pearson, "The Management of High-Risk Pregnancy" (Commentary), 229 *J.A.M.A.* 1439 (1974).
48. *Werth v. Paroly*, No. 74025162NM (Wayne Co., Mich. Ct., verdict, Jan. 12, 1979); *Call v. Kezirian*, 185 Cal. Rptr. 103 (1982).
49. The effect of this practice is to restrict access to the procedure to pregnant women older than 34. Younger women may be able to obtain the service if they pay for it. However, if they are not informed of its availability, if they must locate the service independently—sometimes with difficulty if restrictive state laboratories service the area—and if they must pay the full cost of several hundred dollars, then clearly they face significant barriers not encountered by older women.
50. For example, the Prenatal Diagnosis Laboratory of New York City has a policy against conducting cytogenetic studies on fluid from women younger than 35 unless other risk factors are present. Information provided by personal communication with Dr. Lillian Hsu, Director, Prenatal Diagnosis Laboratory of New York City (1982). *See also*, Diana Paul, "Access to Amniocentesis" (Letter), 303 *New Eng. J. Med.* 1005 (1980) describing her efforts to obtain amniocentesis at age 30 "even though the state of California has an implicit policy of denying that procedure to women under 35 unless there is a family history of chromosomal disorders."
51. John W. Littlefield, "Introductory Remarks" (at conference on Down's Syndrome (Mongolism), Nov. 24–26, 1969), 171 *Ann. N.Y. Acad. Sci.* 379 (1970).
52. Melissa M. Adams *et al.*, "Down's Syndrome: Recent Trends in the United States" (Special Communication), 246 *J.A.M.A.* 758 (1981); Lewis B. Holmes, "Genetic Counseling for the Older Pregnant Woman: New Data and Questions," 298 *New Eng. J. Med.* 419 (1978).
53. R.E. Magenis *et al.*, "Parental Origin of the Extra Chromosome in Down's Syndrome," 37 *Hum. Genetics* 7 (1977).
54. *See* National Institute of Child Health and Human Development, *Antenatal Diagnosis: Report of a Consensus Development Conference*, Dept. of Health, Education and Welfare, Washington (1979) at I-151–56.
55. David C. Sokal *et al.*, "Prenatal Chromosomal Diagnosis: Racial and Geographic Variation for Older Women in Georgia," 244 *J.A.M.A.* 1355 (1980); Abby Lippman-Hand and David I. Cohen, "Influence of Obstetricians' Attitudes on their Use of Prenatal Diagnosis for the Detection of Down's Syndrome," 122 *Canadian Med. J.* 1381 (1980).
56. Melissa M. Adams *et al.*, "Utilization of Prenatal Genetic Diagnosis in Women 35 Years of Age and Older in the United States," 139 *Am. J. Obstet. Gynecol.* 673 (1981).
57. Council on Scientific Affairs, "Council Report: Genetic Counseling and Prevention of Birth Defects," 248 *J.A.M.A.* 221 (1982); Lewis B. Holmes, "Genetic Counseling for the Older Pregnant Woman: New Data and Questions," 298 *New Eng. J. Med.* 1419 (1978).
58. M. L. Williamson *et al.*, "Correlates of Intelligence Test Results in Treated Phenylketonuric Children," 68 *Pediatrics* 2 (1981).

ASSESSING GENETIC RISKS: IMPLICATIONS FOR HEALTH AND SOCIAL POLICY

INTRODUCTION. *A close genetic relationship exists between this third important U.S. report on genetic testing and screening and the earlier two reports. Four members of the Committee for the Study of Inborn Errors of Metabolism (see the report on Screening: Programs, Principles, and Research) returned to serve on this more recent committee: Barton Childs, Neil A. Holtzman, Arno G. Motulsky, and Robert F. Murray. In addition, two members of the Institute of Medicine committee—Patricia A. King and Arno G. Motulsky—served on the President's Commission on Bioethics (see the report on Screening and Counseling for Genetic Conditions). The Institute of Medicine Committee did most of its work in 1992 and 1993; in 1992, it convened a series of workshops and held a public forum. Important new topics in the 1994 report concern preimplantation genetic testing, presymptomatic (or predictive) genetic testing and screening, and the potential role of genetic testing and screening in the employment and insurance arenas.*

EXECUTIVE SUMMARY

Approximately 3 percent of all children are born with a severe disorder that is presumed to be genetic in origin, and several thousand definite or suspected single-gene diseases have been described. Most of these diseases manifest themselves early in life, although some inherited diseases—and many others that have a genetic component—have their onset much later in life (e.g., diabetes mellitus or mental illness). Then there are many disorders in which both genetic and environmental factors play major roles (e.g., coronary heart disease, hypertension). These "complex" disorders are more common than single-gene diseases and thus, in the aggregate, constitute a greater public health burden. Many disease genes can be detected in individuals before symptoms occur, but for many common diseases with some genetic basis, such as heart disease and cancer, the detection of genetic alterations might only indicate susceptibility, not the certainty of disease.

Reprinted from Institute of Medicine, Committee on Assessing Genetic Risks, *Assessing Genetic Risks: Implications for Health and Social Policy*, edit. Lori B. Andrews, Jane E. Fullarton, Neil A. Holtzman, and Arno G. Motulsky. (Washington, D.C.: National Academy Press, 1994). Note that cross references in this excerpt are to the report itself and do not refer to material reprinted in this volume; and though the committee's recommendations (expressed as general principles) originally appeared in bold print, that convention has not been retained.

Promise and Problems in Genetic Testing

The ability to diagnose genetic disease has developed rapidly over the past 20 years, and the Human Genome Project, with its ambitious goal of mapping and sequencing the entire genome, will bring a further explosion in our knowledge of the structure and function of human genes. The ultimate goals of these scientific advances are the treatment, cure, and eventual prevention of genetic disorders, but effective interventions lag behind the ability to detect disease or increased susceptibility to disease. Thus, many genetic services today consist of diagnosis and counseling; effective treatment is rare. Nevertheless, as more genes are identified, there is growing pressure to broaden existing screening programs, and otherwise increase both the number of available genetic tests and the volume of genetic information they generate.

The rapidly changing science and practice of genetic testing raise a number of scientific, ethical, legal, and social issues. The national investment in the Human Genome Project will greatly increase the capacity to detect genes leading to disease susceptibility. It will also greatly increase the availability of genetic testing over the next 5 to 10 years, identifying the genetic basis for diseases—even some newly discovered to be genetic—and increasing the number of tests for detecting them. The emergence of the biotechnology industry increases the likelihood that these findings will be rapidly translated into widely available test kits and diagnostic products. Entrepreneurial pressure may also lead to the development of commercial and academic "genetic testing services" that would not be regulated under current Food and Drug Administration (FDA) procedures. Problems of laboratory quality control would be heightened by the introduction of "multiplex" tests that detect the presence of numerous genetic markers—for disease, carrier status, and susceptibility alike—at the same time. And the potential for generating all of this genetic information about individuals raises serious questions of informed consent, confidentiality, and discrimination. Over the next five to ten years, there will be an increasing number of personal and public policy decisions related to genetic testing; well-trained health professionals and an interested and informed public will both be key to that decision making.

As genetic screening becomes more widespread, these issues threaten to outrun current ethical and regulatory standards, as well as the training of health professionals. There will be a need for greater numbers of genetics specialists, but genetic testing is no longer just for specialists. Increasingly, primary care providers will be called upon to administer tests, counsel patients, and protect their privacy. Government officials and the broader public will also be called upon to participate in setting public policy for genetic testing and in making difficult decisions, public and private, based on the results of genetic tests. Consequently, there must be a significant increase in genetics education, both in the medical curriculum and for all Americans. Finally, there will be a need for centralized oversight to ensure that new genetic tests are accurate and effective, that they are performed and interpreted with close to "zero-error" tolerance, and that the results of genetic testing are not used to discriminate against individuals in employment or health insurance.

Committee on Assessing Genetic Risks

This study of the scientific, ethical, legal, and social issues implicit in the field of genetic diagnosis, testing, and screening was supported jointly by the National Center for Human Genome Research at the National Institutes of Health and the Department of Energy's Health Effects and Life Sciences Research Office. Supplemental funding was also provided by the Markey Charitable Trust and the Institute of Medicine. The Committee on Assessing Genetic Risks hopes that this report will be widely read, not only by various health professionals interested in genetics and preventive medicine, but by a wide-ranging audience who makes and influences public policy in the United States, including members of genetic support groups and the public.

The establishment of the Ethical, Legal, and Social Implications (ELSI) Program in the Human Genome Project (HGP) and the set-aside of the first 3 to 5 percent of the HGP research budget for the study of ethical, legal, and social issues are unique in the history of science. This support gives us the opportunity to "worry in advance" about the implications and impacts of the mapping and sequencing of the human genome, including several thousand human disease genes, *before* wide-scale genetic diagnosis, testing, and screening come into practice, rather than *after* the problems have presented themselves in full relief.

The committee took its starting point from the wise advice of the 1975 National Academy of Sciences study *Genetic Screening: Programs, Principles, and Research*:

> Screening programs for genetic diseases and characteristics . . . have multiplied rapidly in the past decade, and many have been begun without prior testing and evaluation and not always for reasons of health alone. Changes in disease patterns and a new emphasis on preventive medicine, as well as recent and rapid advances in genetics, indicate that screening for genetic characteristics will become more common in the future. These conditions, together with the mistakes already made, suggested the need for a review of current screening practices that would identify the problems and difficulties and give some procedural guidance, in order to minimize the shortcomings and maximize the effectiveness of future genetic screening programs.

These words, written almost 20 years ago, remain just as valid today for genetic testing and diagnosis. The committee reaffirms the sentiments expressed in the 1975 report and hopes to update and broaden their application for the 1990s and beyond.

As a result, the committee has posed its recommendations in terms of general principles that we hope will be useful today—and for some years into the future—for the evaluation of expanded genetic diagnosis, testing, and screening. Although these recommendations reflect what is known today, and what experts foresee for the next few years, the committee had no crystal ball and, therefore, tried to develop criteria and to suggest processes for assessing when new tests are ready for pilot introduction and for widespread application in the population.

The committee's fundamental ethical principles include *voluntariness, informed consent, and confidentiality,* which in turn derive from respect for autonomy, equity, and privacy. Other committee principles described in the report include the necessity of (1) *high-quality tests (of high specificity and sensitivity) performed with the highest level of proficiency and interpreted correctly*; and (2) *conveying information to clients—both before and after testing—in an easily understood manner through genetic education and counseling that is relevant to the needs and concerns of the client.* These principles are the absolute foundation of genetic testing.

It is the view of the committee that, *until benefits and risks have been defined, genetic testing and screening programs remain a form of human investigation.* Therefore, routine use of tests should be preceded by pilot studies that demonstrate their safety and effectiveness. Standard safeguards should be applied in conducting these pilot studies, and independent review of the pilot studies should be conducted to determine whether the test should be offered clinically. Publicly supported population-based screening programs are justified only for disorders of significant severity, impact, frequency, and distribution, and when there is consensus that the available interventions warrant the expenditure of funds. Informed consent should be an essential element of all screening. These principles and procedures described above should apply to genetic testing regardless of the setting, whether in primary medical practice, public programs, or any other settings.

Genetic Testing and Assessment

Genetic tests include the many different laboratory assays used to diagnose or predict a genetic condition or the susceptibility to genetic disease. *Genetic testing* denotes the use of specific assays to determine the genetic status of individuals already suspected to be at high risk for a particular inherited condition because of family history or clinical symptoms; *genetic screening* involves the use of various genetic tests to evaluate populations or groups of individuals independent of a family history of a disorder. However, these terms are commonly used interchangeably, and the committee has generally used the term *genetic testing* unless a specific aspect of genetic screening alone is being discussed. *Genetic counseling* refers to the communication process by which individuals and their family members are given information about the nature, recurrence risk, burden, risks and benefits of tests, and meaning of test results, including reproductive options of a genetic condition, as well as counseling and support concerning the implications of such genetic information.

TABLE 1. Genetic Disorders for Which Newborns Were Screened in the United States in 1990

Disorder	*No. of States That Provided Screening*[a]
Phenylketonuria	52
Congenital hypothyroidism[b]	52
Hemoglobinopathy	42[c]
Galactosemia	38
Maple syrup urine disorder	22
Homocysteinuria	21
Biotinidase deficiency	14
Adrenal hyperplasia	8
Tyrosinemia	5
Cystic fibrosis	3[d]

[a]Includes District of Columbia, Puerto Rico, and U.S. Virgin Islands.

[b]Only a proportion of cases have a genetic etiology.

[c]Utah's hemoglobinopathy pilot study (6-1-90 through 3-31-91) has been discontinued.

[d]Wisconsin's cystic fibrosis screening program is for research purposes only.

Source: Council of Regional Networks for Genetic Services, 1992.

Newborn Screening At the present time, there are 10 genetic conditions for which some states screen newborns, although the scope of such screening varies by state (see Table 1). It is also possible to extract DNA from the newborn blood "spots" that are used for these tests. There is increasing pressure to test old blood samples for a wide variety of disorders, as well as to do DNA testing on newborns for a wide variety of disorders in the future. As basic principles to govern newborn screening, the committee recommends that such screening take place only when (1) there is a clear indication of benefit to the newborn, (2) a system is in place to confirm the diagnosis, and (3) treatment and follow-up are available for affected newborns. In addition, the committee does not believe that newborns should be screened using multiplex testing for many disorders at one time unless all of the disorders meet the principles described by the committee in this report (see Chapters 2 and 8).

To determine clear benefit to the newborn, well-designed and peer-reviewed pilot studies are required to demonstrate the safety and effectiveness of the proposed screening program. In pilot studies for new population-based newborn screening programs, parents should be informed of the investigational nature of the test and have the opportunity to consent to the participation of their infant. Since some existing programs may not have been subject to careful evaluation, the committee recommends that ongoing programs be reviewed periodically, preferably by an independent body that is authorized to add, eliminate, or modify existing programs (see Chapters 1, 3, and 9). The need for ongoing review and revision also suggests that detailed statutory requirements for specific tests may be unduly inflexible; state statutes should provide guidance for standards—not prescriptions. The committee recommends that states with newborn screening programs for treatable disorders also have programs available to ensure that necessary treatment and follow-up services are provided to affected children identified through newborn screening without regard to ability to pay. Informed consent should also be an integral part of newborn screening, including disclosure of the benefits and risks of the tests and treatments. Finally, mandatory screening has not been shown to be essential to achieve maximum public health benefits; however, it is appropriate to mandate the *offering* of established tests (e.g., phenylketonuria, hypothyroidism) where early diagnosis leads to improved treatable outcomes. (See Chapter 8.)

Newborns should not be screened for the purpose of determining the carrier status of the newborn or its parents for autosomal recessive disorders. Instead, couples in high-risk populations who are considering reproduction should be offered carrier screening for themselves (see below). When carrier status may be incidentally determined in newborn screening (e.g., in sickle cell screening), parents should be informed in advance about the benefits and limitations of genetic information, and that this information is not relevant to the health of their child. If they ask for the results of the incidentally determined carrier status for their own reproductive planning, it should be communicated to them in the context of genetic counseling, and they should be informed that misattributed paternity could be revealed. Newborn screening programs should include provision for counseling of parents who are informed that the child is affected with a genetic disorder.

The committee recognizes the complexities of identifying information about misattributed paternity. On balance, the committee recommends that information on misattributed paternity be communicated to the mother, but not be volunteered to the woman's partner. There may be special circumstances that warrant such disclosure, but these situations present difficult counseling challenges (see Chapters 4 and 8).

Stored newborn blood spots should be made available for additional research only if identifiers have been removed. As with other research involving human subjects, research proposals for the subsequent use of newborn blood spots should be reviewed by an appropriate institutional review board. If identifiable information is to be disclosed, informed consent of the infant's parent or guardian should be obtained prior to use of the specimen (see Chapters 2 and 8 for further discussion). Although DNA typing will provide new tools for newborn screening, in general, the committee recommends that these tools be employed only (1) when genetic heterogeneity of conditions to be detected is small; (2) when the sensitivity of detecting disease-causing mutations is high; (3) when costs are reasonable; and (4) when the benefits to newborns of early detection are clear.

Carrier Identification Carrier testing is usually provided for purposes of reproductive planning. The committee recommends that couples in high-risk populations who are considering reproduction be offered carrier screening before pregnancy if possible. Standard safeguards such as institutional review and demonstrated safety and effectiveness should be applied in initiating any carrier detection program. First, the test should be accurate, sensitive, and specific. In the future, such screening will be done increasingly as part of routine medical care; the same principles should apply regardless of the setting. Carrier testing and screening should also be voluntary, with high standards of informed consent and attention to telling individuals or couples, in easily understood terms, the medical and social choices available to them should they be found at risk for disease in their offspring, including termination of the pregnancy. Research is needed to develop innovative methods for providing carrier testing in young adults before pregnancy and to evaluate these methods through pilot studies. The committee had reservations about carrier screening programs in the high school setting in the United States and about carrier screening of persons younger than age 18.

With improving technology, carrier status for many different rare autosomal and X-linked recessive disorders will be detectable by multiplex technology (see Chapters 1 and 8). Obtaining appropriate informed consent before testing for each of these disorders will be a challenge (see Chapter 4). Multiplexed tests should, therefore, be grouped into categories of tests (and disorders) that raise similar issues and implications for informed consent and for genetic education and counseling (see Chapters 1, 4, and 8). If carrier status is detected, individuals should be informed of their carrier status to allow testing and counseling to be offered to their partners. Usually, the partner will be found not to be a carrier; however, if both partners are carriers, they should be referred for genetic counseling to help them understand available reproductive options, including the possibility of abortion of an affected fetus identified through prenatal diagnosis.

Prenatal Diagnosis Anyone considering prenatal diagnosis must be fully informed about the risks and benefits of both the testing procedure and the possible outcomes, as well as alternative options that might be available. Disclosure should include full information concerning the spectrum of severity of the genetic disorders for which prenatal diagnosis is being offered (e.g., cystic fibrosis or fragile X). Furthermore, invasive prenatal diagnosis is only justified if the diagnostic procedures are accurate, sensitive, and specific for the disorder(s) for which prenatal diagnosis is being offered. Standards of care for prenatal screening and diagnosis should also include education and counseling before and after the test, either directly or by referral, and ongoing counseling should also be available following termination of pregnancies.

The committee believes that *offering* prenatal diagnosis is an appropriate standard of care in circumstances associated with increased risk of carrying a fetus with a diagnosable genetic disorder, including the increased risks associated with advanced maternal age. However, the committee was concerned about the use of prenatal diagnosis for identification of trivial characteristics or conditions. It was the consensus of this committee that prenatal diagnosis should only be offered for the diagnosis of genetic disorders and birth defects. A family history of a diagnosable genetic disorder warrants the offering of prenatal diagnosis, regardless of maternal age, as does determination of carrier status in both parents of an autosomal recessive disorder for which prenatal diagnosis is available. Prenatal diagnostic services for detection of genetic disease for which there is a family history should be reimbursed by insurers (see Chapters 2 and 7). Ability to pay should not restrict appropriate access to prenatal diagnosis or termination of pregnancy of an affected fetus.

The committee felt strongly that the use of fetal diagnosis for determination of fetal sex and the subsequent use of abortion for the purpose of preferential selection of the sex of the fetus represents a misuse of genetic services that is inappropriate and should be discouraged by health professionals. More broadly, reproductive genetic services should not be used to pursue eugenic goals, but should be aimed at increasing individual control over *reproductive options*. As a consequence, additional research is needed on the impact of prenatal diagnosis, particularly its immediate and long-term impact on women, and on the design and evaluation of genetic counseling techniques for prenatal diagnosis for the future.

Testing for Late-Onset Disorders Science is moving closer to defining the genetics of such adult disorders as Alzheimer disease, a variety of cancers, heart disease, and arthritis, to name a few (see Chapter 2). A combination of genetic and environmental factors plays a predominant role in most people afflicted with these disorders, but we do not yet understand why some people with a certain gene(s) develop a disease and others do not. Although further work may eventually elucidate the gene(s) involved, there may be long delays until the time when effective interventions are available for many disorders. Furthermore, not all affected individuals will have an identifiable genetic basis to their disorder. Thus, the complexities involved in determining and establishing susceptibility, sorting out potential environmental influences, and devising a strategy for counseling and treatment will pose tremendous challenges in the future.

Many of these diseases do not manifest clinically until adulthood and may become apparent only in middle age or later. *Predictive* or *presymptomatic* testing and screening can provide clues about genetic susceptibility or predisposition to genetic disorders. For monogenic disorders of late onset, such as Huntington disease, tests will usually be highly predictive. Many common diseases usually have multifactorial—or complex—causation, including both multiple genetic factors and environmental effects; for these disorders, prediction will be less certain. Many common diseases of adulthood, including coronary artery disease, some cancers, diabetes, high blood pressure, rheumatoid arthritis, and some psychiatric diseases, fall into this category. However, in rare forms of these common diseases, single genes may play the decisive role; screening for disease-causing alleles of these genes will be of much greater predictive value.

The committee therefore recommends caution in the use and interpretation of presymptomatic or predictive tests. The nature of these predictions will usually be probabilistic (i.e., with a certain degree of likelihood of occurrence) and not deterministic (i.e., not definite, settled, or without doubt). The dangers of stigmatization and discrimination are areas of concern, as is the potential for harm due to inappropriate preventive or therapeutic measures. Since environmental factors are often essential for the manifestation of complex diseases, the detection of those at high risk will identify certain individuals who will most benefit from certain interventions (e.g., dietary measures in coronary heart disease). Identification of some persons at high risk for certain cancers suggests that more frequent monitoring may identify the earliest manifestations of cancer when treatability is greatest (e.g., colon cancer); research is needed on the psychosocial implications of such testing in both adults and children.

Further research and the unfolding of the Human Genome Project are likely to reveal the underlying genes mediating predisposition to numerous common diseases, and genetic susceptibility testing will be increasingly possible. Certain environmental factors may interact with only one set of genes and not with another. There may also be interaction between the various genes involved, so that the effects of multiple gene action cannot be predicted by separate analyses of each of the single genes. In such cases, definitive prediction will rarely, if ever, be possible. When dealing with genetic testing for some non-Mendelian diseases, it will be impossible to group individuals into two distinct categories—those at no (or very low) risk and those at high risk. Extensive counseling and education will be essential in any testing for genetic susceptibility. The benefits of the various presymptomatic interventions must be weighed against the potential anxiety, stigmatization, and other possible harms to individuals who are informed that they are at increased risk of developing future disease.

Population screening for predisposition to late-onset monogenic diseases should only be considered for treatable or preventable conditions of relatively high frequency. Under such guidelines, population screening should only be offered after appropriate, reliable, sensitive, and specific tests become available. Such tests do not yet exist. The committee recommends that the predictive value of genetic tests be thoroughly validated in prospective studies of sufficient size and statistical power before their widespread application. Since there will be a considerable time lag before the appearance of confirmatory symptoms, these studies will require support for long periods of time (see Chapter 3).

In the case of predictive tests for mental disorders, results must be handled with stringent attention to confidentiality to protect an already vulnerable population. If no effective treatment is available, testing may not be appropriate since more harm than good could result from improper use of test results. On the other hand, future research might result in psychological or drug treatments that could prevent the onset of these diseases. Carefully designed pilot studies should be conducted to determine the effectiveness of such interventions and to measure the desirability and psychosocial impact of such testing. Interpretation and communication of predictive test results in psychiatry will be particularly difficult. To prepare for the issues associated with genetic testing for psychiatric diseases in the future, psychiatrists and other mental health professionals will need more training in genetics and genetic counseling; such training should include the ethical, legal, and social issues in genetic testing.

Because of their wide applicability, it is likely there will be strong commercial interests in the introduction of genetic tests for common, high-profile complex disorders. Strict guidelines for efficacy therefore will be necessary to prevent premature introduction of this technology.

Testing of Children or Minors Children should generally be tested only for genetic disorders for which there exists an effective curative or preventive treatment that must be instituted early in life to achieve maximum benefit. Childhood testing is not appropriate for carrier status, untreatable childhood diseases, and late-onset diseases that cannot be prevented or forestalled by early treatment. In general, the committee believes that testing of minors should be discouraged unless delaying such testing would reduce benefits of available treatment or monitoring. It is essential that the individual seeking testing understand the potential abuse of such information in society, including in employment or insurance practice, and that the provider should ensure that confidentiality is respected (see Chapter 8 for discussion of disclosure to relatives).

Because only certain types of genetic testing are appropriate for children, multiplex testing that includes tests specifically directed to obtaining information about carrier status, untreatable childhood diseases, or late-onset diseases should not be included in the multiplex tests offered to children. Research should be undertaken to determine the appropriate age for testing and screening for genetic disorders, both to maximize the benefits of therapeutic intervention and to avoid the possibility of generating genetic information about a child when there is no likely benefit and there is possibility of harm to the child.

* * *

Social, Legal, and Ethical Issues in Genetic Testing

The committee recommends that vigorous protection be given to *autonomy, privacy, confidentiality, and equity.* These principles should be breached only in rare instances and only when the following conditions are met: (1) the action must be aimed at an important goal—such as the protection of others from serious harm—that outweighs the value of autonomy, privacy, confidentiality, or equity in the particular instance; (2) it must have a high probability of realizing that goal; (3) there must be no acceptable alternatives that can also realize the goal without breaching those principles; and (4) the degree of infringement of the principle must be the minimum necessary to realize the goal.

Voluntariness Voluntariness should be the cornerstone of any genetic testing program. The committee found no justification for a state-sponsored *mandatory* public health program involving genetic testing of adults or for *unconsented-to* genetic testing of patients in the clinical setting. There is evidence that voluntary screening programs achieve a higher level of efficacy in screening, and there is no evidence that mandating newborn screening is necessary or sufficient to ensure that the vast majority of newborns are screened. Mandatory *offering* of newborn screening is appropriate for disorders with treatments of demonstrated efficacy where very early intervention is essential to improve health outcomes (e.g., phenylketonuria and congenital hypothyroidism). One benefit of voluntariness and informing parents about newborn screening is that of quality assurance: parents can check to see if the sample was actually drawn. In addition, since people will be facing the possibility of undergoing many more genetic tests in their lifetimes, the disclosure of information to parents about newborn screening prior to the event can be an important tool for education about genetics.

Informed Consent Obtaining informed consent should be the method of ensuring that genetic testing is voluntary. By *informed consent* the committee means a *process* of education and the opportunity to have questions answered—not merely the signing of a form. The patient or client should be given information about the risks, benefits, efficacy, and alternatives to the testing; information about the severity, potential variability, and treatability of the disorder being tested for; information about the subsequent decisions that will be likely if the test is positive (such as a decision about abortion); and information about any potential conflicts of interest of the person or institution offering the test (see Chapters 1, 3, and 8). Research should therefore also be undertaken to determine what patients *want* to know in order to make a decision about whether or not to undergo a genetic test. People often have less interest in the label for the disorder and its mechanisms of action than in how certainly the test predicts the disorder, what effects the disorder has on physical and mental functioning, and how intrusive, difficult, or effective any existing treatment protocol would be. Research is also necessary to determine the advantages and disadvantages of various means of conveying that information (e.g., through specialized genetic counselors, primary care providers, single disorder counselors, brochures, videos, audiotapes, computer programs).

Confidentiality All forms of genetic information should be considered confidential and should not be disclosed without the individual's consent (except as required by state law, or in rare instances discussed in Chapters 4 and 8). This includes genetic information that is obtained through specific genetic testing of a person, as well as genetic information about that person that is obtained in other ways (e.g., physical examination, past treatment, or a relative's genetic status). The confidentiality of genetic information should be protected no matter who obtains or maintains that information. This includes genetic information collected or maintained by health care professionals, health care institutions, researchers, employers, insurance companies, laboratory personnel, and law enforcement officials. To the extent that current statutes do not ensure such confidentiality, they should be amended.

Codes of ethics for professionals providing genetic services should contain specific provisions to protect autonomy, privacy, and confidentiality. The committee endorses the 1991 National Society of Genetic Counselors (NSGC) statement of guiding principles on confidentiality of test results:

> The NSGC supports individual confidentiality regarding results of genetic testing. It is the right and responsibility of the individual to determine who shall have access to medical information, particularly results of testing for genetic conditions.

Confidentiality should be breached and relatives informed about genetic risks *only* when (1) attempts to elicit voluntary disclosure fail, (2) there is a high probability of irreversible harm that the disclosure will prevent, and (3) there is no other reasonable way to avert the harm. When disclosure is to be attempted over the patient's refusal, the burden should be on the person who wishes to disclose to justify to the patient, to an ethics committee, and perhaps in court that the disclosure was necessary and met the committee's test. Thus, the committee has determined that the disadvantages of informing relatives over the patient's refusal generally outweigh the advantages, except in the rare instances described above (see Chapters 4 and 8). The committee recommends that health care providers not reveal genetic information about a patient's carrier status to the patient's spouse without the patient's permission, and that information on misattributed paternity should be given to the mother, but not be volunteered to her partner.

As a matter of general principle, the committee believes strongly that patients should disclose to relatives genetic information relevant to ensuring the health of those relatives. Patients should be encouraged and aided in sharing appropriate genetic information with spouses and relatives. To facilitate the disclosure of relevant genetic information to family members, accurate and balanced materials should be developed to assist individuals in informing their families, and in providing access to further information, as well as access to testing if relatives should choose to be tested. Under those rare circumstances where unauthorized disclosure of genetic information is deemed warranted, the genetic counselor should first try to obtain the permission of the person to release the information.

The committee also endorses the principles on the protection of DNA data and DNA data banking developed in 1990 by the ASHG Ad Hoc Committee on Identification by DNA Analysis. In short, patients' consent should be obtained before their names are provided to a genetic disease registry, and their consent should also be obtained before information is redisclosed. Each entity that receives or maintains genetic information or samples should have procedures in place to protect confidentiality. Information or samples should be kept free of identifiers and instead use encoding to link the information or sample to the individual's name. Finally, any entity that releases genetic information about an individual to someone other than that individual should ensure that the recipient of the genetic information has procedures in place to protect the confidentiality of the information.

Genetic Discrimination in Health Insurance Legislation should be adopted to prevent medical risks, including genetic risks, from being taken into account in decisions on whether to issue or how to price health care insurance. Because health insurance differs significantly from other types of insurance in that it regulates access to health care—an important social good—risk-based health insurance should be eliminated. Access to health care should be available to every American without regard to the individual's present health status or condition; in particular, the committee recommends that insurability decisions not be based on genetic status (see Chapters 7 and 8).

Some of the committee's concerns about genetic discrimination in health insurance would be obviated by current proposals for national health insurance reform that would eliminate most, if not all, aspects of medical underwriting. The committee recommends that insurance reform preclude the use of genetic information in establishing eligibility for health insurance. As health insurance reform proposals are developed, those concerned with genetic disorders will need to assess whether they adequately protect genetic information and persons with genetic disorders from health insurance discrimination and discrimination in the provision of medical services (see Chapters 7 and 8).

Genetic Discrimination in Employment

Legislation should be adopted that forbids employers to collect genetic information on prospective or current employees unless it is clearly job related. Sometimes employers will have employees submit to medical exams to see if they are capable of performing particular job tasks. If an individual consents to the release of genetic information to an employer or potential employer, the releasing entity should not release specific information, but instead answer only yes or no regarding whether the individual was fit to perform the job at issue.

The committee urges the Equal Employment Opportunity Commission to recognize that the language of the Americans with Disabilities Act (ADA) provides protection for presymptomatic people with genetic risks for late-onset disorders, unaffected carriers of disorders that might affect their children, and individuals with genetic profiles indicating the possibility of increased risk of a multifactorial disorder. State legislatures should adopt laws to protect people from genetic discrimination in employment. In addition, ADA should be amended (and similar state statutes adopted) to limit the type of medical testing employers can request and to ensure that the medical information they can collect is job related.

RECOMMENDATION 934: ON GENETIC ENGINEERING

INTRODUCTION. *This document stands at the head of the second section of Part 3, a consideration of the primary source materials on gene therapy. It represents the culmination of a two-year study by the Council of Europe's Parliamentary Assembly. In January 1980, Mr. B. Elmquist, a Danish member of the Legal Affairs Committee, requested that the Assembly pass a "recommendation on the protection of humanity against genetic engineering" (Document 4493). This request led, in turn, to a two-day parliamentary hearing in Copenhagen, Denmark, May 25–26, 1981. A report based on the hearing was published the following January (1982) under the title* Genetic Engineering: Risks and Chances for Human Rights. *In the same month, the Assembly's Legal Affairs Committee presented a report on genetic engineering and a draft recommendation to the full Assembly.*

Recommendation 934 argues that every human being has "the right to inherit a genetic pattern which has not been artificially changed." The Assembly adopted it on January 26, 1992. At the same time, however, the Assembly seemed to allow for the possibility of germ-line genetic intervention to prevent or cure disease. Thus, the right to a genetic inheritance that has not been artificially interfered with is recognized "except in accordance with certain principles which are recognised as being fully compatible with respect for human rights (as, for example, in the field of therapeutic applications)." This recommendation is the first statement on genetic intervention by a governmental or quasi-governmental body.

Text adopted by the Assembly on 26 January 1982

The Assembly,

1. Aware of public concern about the use of new scientific techniques for artificially recombining genetic material from living organisms, referred to as "genetic engineering";

2. Considering that these concerns fall into two distinct categories:

- those arising from uncertainty as to the health, safety and environmental implications of experimental research;
- those arising from the longer-term legal, social and ethical issues raised by the prospect of knowing and interfering with a person's inheritable genetic pattern;

3. Having regard, in respect of the health, safety and environmental implications of experimental research, to the following considerations:

i. the techniques of genetic engineering present an immense industrial and agricultural potential which in coming decades could help to solve world problems of food production, energy and raw materials;

ii. radical breakthroughs in scientific and medical understanding (university of the genetic code) are associated with the discovery and development of these techniques;

iii. freedom of scientific enquiry—a basic value of our societies and a condition of their adaptability to the changing world environment—carries with it duties and responsibilities, notably in regard to the health and safety of the general public and of fellow scientific workers and to the non-contamination of the environment;

iv. in the light of the then existing scientific knowledge and experience, uncertainties about the health, safety and environmental implications of experiments in

Council of Europe, Parliamentary Assembly. "Recommendation 934 (1982) on Genetic Engineering." *Texts Adopted by the Assembly*, 33rd Ordinary Session, Third Part, 22nd Sitting, January 26, 1982 (Strasbourg: the Council, 1982).

genetic engineering were a legitimate cause for concern in the early 1970s—to the point of giving rise to requests, at the time, from within the scientific community, for certain types of experiment not to be made;

v. in the light of new scientific knowledge and experience, uncertainties in regard to experimental research have in recent years been largely clarified and resolved—to the point of allowing substantial relaxation of the control and containment measures initially instituted or envisaged;

vi. strict and comparable levels of protection should be provided in all countries for the general public and for laboratory workers against risks involved in the handling of pathogenic micro-organisms in general, irrespective of whether techniques of genetic engineering are used;

4. Having regard, in respect of the legal, social and ethical issues, to the following considerations inspired by the Council of Europe's 7th Public Parliamentary Hearing (Copenhagen, 25 and 26 May 1981) on genetic engineering and human rights:

i. the rights to life and to human dignity protected by Articles 2 and 3 of the European Convention on Human Rights imply the right to inherit a genetic pattern which has not been artificially changed;

ii. this right should be made explicit in the context of the European Convention on Human Rights;

iii. the explicit recognition of this right must not impede development of the therapeutic applications of genetic engineering (gene therapy), which holds great promise for the treatment and eradication of certain diseases which are genetically transmitted;

iv. gene therapy must not be used or experimented with except with the free and informed consent of the person(s) concerned, or in cases of experiment with embryos, foetuses or minors with the free and informed consent of the parent(s) or legal guardian(s);

v. the boundaries of legitimate therapeutic application of genetic engineering techniques need to be clearly drawn, brought to the attention of research workers and experimentalists, and subjected to periodical reappraisal;

vi. outline regulations should be drawn up to protect individuals against non-therapeutic applications of these techniques;

5. Expressing the wish that the European Science Foundation should keep under review:

a. procedures and criteria for licensing the use of products of recombinant DNA techniques in medicine, in agriculture and industry;

b. the effects of the commercialisation of recombinant DNA techniques on the funding and orientations of fundamental research in molecular biology.

6. Invites member governments:

a. to take note of the reassessments which have taken place in recent years within the scientific community concerning levels of risk from research involving recombinant DNA techniques, and to adjust, in the light of these reassessments, their systems of supervision and control;

b. to provide for the periodical reassessment of levels of risk from research involving recombinant DNA techniques within the regulatory frameworks for assessing the risks from research involving the handling of micro-organisms in general;

7. Recommends that the Committee of Ministers:

a. draw up a European agreement on what constitutes legitimate application to human beings (including future generations) of the techniques of genetic engineering, align domestic regulations accordingly, and work towards similar agreements at a world level;

b. provide for explicit recognition in the European Convention on Human Rights of the right to a genetic inheritance which has not been artificially interfered with, except in accordance with certain principles which are recognised as being fully compatible with respect for human rights (as, for example, in the field of therapeutic applications);

c. provide for the drawing up of a list of serious diseases which may properly, with the consent of the person concerned, be treated by gene therapy (though certain uses without consent, in line with existing practice for other forms of medical treatment, may be recognised as compatible with respect for human rights in the probability of a very serious disease being transmitted to a person's offspring);

d. lay down principles governing the preparation, storage, safeguarding and use of genetic information on individuals, with particular reference to protecting the rights to privacy of the persons concerned in accordance with the Council of Europe conventions and resolutions on data protection;

e. examine whether levels of protection of the health and safety of the general public and of laboratory workers engaged in experiments or industrial applications involving microorganisms, including micro-organisms subject to recombinant DNA techniques, are adequate and comparable throughout Europe, and whether existing legislation and institutional machinery offer an adequate framework for their periodical verification and revision to this end;

f. ensure, by periodic reviews in liaison with the European Science Foundation, that national containment measures for recombinant DNA research and required laboratory safety practice continue to converge and to evolve (albeit by different routes) towards harmonisation in Europe, in the light of new research findings and risk evaluations;

g. examine the draft recommendation of the Council of the European Communities on the registration and notification to appropriate national and regional authorities of experiments involving recombinant DNA, with a view to the concerted implementation of its provisions in the countries of the Council of Europe;

h. examine the patentability of micro-organisms genetically altered by recombinant DNA techniques.

SPLICING LIFE: THE SOCIAL AND ETHICAL ISSUES OF GENETIC ENGINEERING WITH HUMAN BEINGS

INTRODUCTION. *Gene therapy, or genetic intervention, was not included in the original mandate that Congress gave to the President's Commission for the Study of Ethical Problems in Medicine and Biomedical and Behavioral Research. However, in June 1980, the general secretaries of three major religious organizations in the United States—organizations representing many Jews, Catholics, and Protestants—wrote a letter to then-President Jimmy Carter, expressing concern about the potential dangers of genetic engineering. In response, the Commission agreed at its September 1980 meeting to add a modest study of genetic engineering to its already-formidable list of reports. A preliminary analysis of the issues was prepared for the Commission and discussed in July 1981. During the ensuing months a draft report was prepared, which the committee considered at a hearing in July 1982. The final report,* Splicing Life, *was presented to the public at a congressional hearing on "Human Genetic Engineering," November 16–17, 1982. Then-Congressman Albert Gore, Jr., chaired the hearing before the Investigations and Oversight Subcommittee of the House Science and Technology Committee. The major conclusion of the report was that somatic-cell genetic intervention raises no qualitatively new ethical or public policy questions.*

Summary of Conclusions and Recommendations

This Report addresses some of the major ethical and social implications of biologists' newly gained ability to manipulate—indeed, literally to splice together—the material that is responsible for the different forms of life on earth. The Commission began this study because of an urgent concern expressed to the President that no governmental body was "exercising adequate oversight or control, nor addressing the fundamental ethical questions" of these techniques, known collectively as "genetic engineering," particularly as they might be applied directly to human beings [footnote deleted].

When it first examined the question of governmental activity in this area, in the summer of 1980, the Commission found that this concern was well founded. Not only was no single agency charged with exploring this field but a number of the agencies that would have been expected to be involved with aspects of the subject were unprepared to deal with it, and the Federal interagency body set up to coordinate the field was not offering any continuing leadership. Two years later, possibly because of the Commission's attention, it appears the Federal agencies are more aware of, and are beginning to deal with, questions arising from genetic engineering, although their efforts primarily address the agricultural, industrial, and pharmaceutical uses of gene splicing rather than its diagnostic and therapeutic uses in human beings [footnote deleted].

The Commission did not restrict its examination of the subject to the responses of Federal agencies, however, because it perceived more important issues of substance behind the expressed concern about the lack of Federal oversight. The Commission chose, therefore, to address these underlying issues, although certainly not to dispose of them. On many points, the Commission sees its contribution as stimulating thoughtful, long-term discussion

---

Excerpts from the President's Commission for the Study of Ethical Problems in Medicine and Biomedical and Behavioral Research, *Splicing Life: A Report on the Social and Ethical Issues of Genetic Engineering with Human Beings* (Washington, D.C.: U.S. Government Printing Office, 1982).

rather than truncating such thinking with premature conclusions.

This study, undertaken within the time limitations imposed by the Commission's authorizing statute, is seen by the Commission as a first step in what ought to be a continuing public examination of the emerging questions posed by developments and prospects in the human applications of molecular genetics. First, the report attempts to clarify concerns about genetic engineering and to provide technical background intended to increase public understanding of the capabilities and potential of the technique. Next, it evaluates the issues of concern in ways meaningful for public policy, and analyzes the need for an oversight mechanism.

To summarize, in this initial study the Commission finds that:

(1) Although public concern about gene splicing arose in the context of laboratory research with microorganisms, it seemed to reflect a deeper anxiety that work in this field might remake human beings, like Dr. Frankenstein's monster. These concerns seem to the Commission to be exaggerated. It is true that genetic engineering techniques are not only a powerful new tool for manipulating nature—including means of curing human illness—but also a challenge to some deeply held feelings about the meaning of being human and of family lineage. But as a product of human investigation and ingenuity, the new knowledge is a celebration of human creativity, and the new powers are a reminder of human obligations to act responsibly.

(2) Genetic engineering techniques are advancing very rapidly. Two breakthroughs in animal experiments during 1981 and 1982, for example, bring human applications of gene splicing closer: in one, genetic defects have been corrected in fruit flies; in another, artificially inserted genes have functioned in succeeding generations of mammals.

(3) Genetic engineering techniques are already demonstrating their great potential value for human well-being. The aid that these new developments may provide in the relief of human suffering is an ethical reason for encouraging them.

- Although the initial benefits to human health involve pharmaceutical applications of the techniques, direct diagnostic and therapeutic uses are being tested and some are already in use. Those called upon to review such research with human subjects, such as local Institutional Review Boards, should be assured of access to expert advice on any special risks or uncertainties presented by particular types of genetic engineering.
- Use of the new techniques in genetic screening will magnify the ethical considerations already seen in that field because they will allow a larger number of diseases to be detected before clinical symptoms are manifest and because the ability to identify a much wider range of genetic traits and conditions will greatly enlarge the demand for, and even the objectives of, prenatal diagnosis.

(4) Many human uses of genetic engineering resemble accepted forms of diagnosis and treatment employing other techniques. The novelty of gene splicing ought not to erect any automatic impediment to its use but rather should provoke thoughtful analysis.

- Especially close scrutiny is appropriate for any procedures that would create inheritable genetic changes; such interventions differ from prior medical interventions that have not altered the genes passed on to patients' offspring.
- Interventions aimed at enhancing "normal" people, as opposed to remedying recognized genetic defects, are also problematic, especially since distinguishing "medical treatment" from "nonmedical enhancement" is a very subjective matter; the difficulty of drawing a line suggests the danger of drifting toward attempts to "perfect" human beings once the door of "enhancement" is opened.

(5) Questions about the propriety of gene splicing are sometimes phrased as objections to people "playing God." The Commission is not persuaded that the scientific procedures in question are inherently inappropriate for human use. It does believe, nevertheless, that objections of this sort, which are strongly felt by many people, deserve serious attention and that they serve as a valuable reminder that great powers imply great responsibility. If beneficial rather than catastrophic consequences are to flow from the use of "God-like" powers, an unusual degree of care will be needed with novel applications.

(6) The generally very reassuring results of laboratory safety measures have led to a relaxation of the rules governing gene splicing research that were established when there was widespread concern about the potential risks of the research. The lack of definitive proof of danger or its absence has meant that the outcome—whether to restrict certain research—has turned on which side is assigned the burden of proving its case. Today those regulating gene splicing research operate from the assumption that most such research is safe, when conducted according to normal scientific standards; those opposing that position face the task of proving otherwise.

- The safety issue will arise in a wider context as gene splicing is employed in manufacturing, in agriculture and other activities in the general environment, and in medical treatment. As a matter of prudence, such initial steps should be accompanied by renewed attention to the issue of risk (and by continued research on that subject).
- Efforts to educate the newly exposed population to the appropriate precautions, whenever required, and serious efforts to monitor the new settings (since greater exposure increases the opportunity to detect low-frequency events) should be encouraged. In general, the questions

of safety concerning gene splicing should not be viewed any differently than comparable issues presented by other scientific and commercial activities.

(7) The Recombinant DNA Advisory Committee (RAC) at the National Institutes of Health has been the lead Federal agency in genetic engineering. Its guidelines for laboratory research have evolved over the past seven years in response to changes in scientific attitudes and knowledge about the risks of different types of genetic engineering. The time has now come to broaden the area under scrutiny to include issues raised by the intended uses of the technique rather than solely the unintended exposure from laboratory experiments.

- It would also be desirable for this "next generation" RAC to be independent of Federal funding bodies such as NIH, which is the major Federal sponsor of gene splicing research, to avoid any real or perceived conflict of interest.

(8) The process of scrutiny should involve a range of participants with different backgrounds—not only the Congress and Executive Branch agencies but also scientific and academic associations, industrial and commercial groups, ethicists, lawyers, religious and educational leaders, and members of the general public.

- Several formats deserve consideration, including initial reliance on voluntary bodies of mixed public-private membership. Alternatively, the task could be assigned to this Commission's successor, as one among a variety of issues in medicine and research before such a body, or to a commission concerned solely with gene splicing.
- Whatever format is chosen, the group should be broadly based and not dominated by geneticists or other scientists, although it should be able to turn to experts to advise it on the laboratory, agricultural, environmental, industrial, pharmaceutical, and human uses of the technology as well as on international scientific and legal controls. Means for direct liaison with the government departments and agencies involved in this field will also be needed.

(9) The need for an appropriate oversight body is based upon the profound nature of the implications of gene splicing as applied to human beings, not upon any immediate threat of harm. Just as it is necessary to run risks and to accept change in order to reap the benefits of scientific progress, it is also desirable that society have means of providing its "informed consent," based upon reasonable assurances that risks have been minimized and that changes will occur within an acceptable range.

3. SOCIAL AND ETHICAL ISSUES

The preceding chapters have described the potential benefits of gene splicing, but they have also suggested the awesome and sometimes troubling implications that have shared this technology's spotlight. In this chapter, the Commission considers the social and ethical issues raised as society seeks ways to realize the benefits without incurring unacceptable risks. The Commission has found no ethical precepts that would preclude the initial clinical uses of gene splicing now being undertaken or planned or that would categorically prohibit the research procedures through which knowledge is currently being sought in this important field. But more distant possibilities—either in themselves or in conjunction with other scientific and social developments they may foster—could have less benign effects. Consequently, this Report recommends steps that can and should be taken to keep the social and ethical implications of gene splicing before the public and policymakers as these developments become feasible in the years ahead.

The Commission also believes, for several reasons, that balancing both present and future benefits and risks requires more than a simple arithmetical calculation. First, assessing this new technology through cost/benefit or risk/benefit analysis is complex because decisionmaking about gene splicing technology is characterized by several types and levels of uncertainty. The risks and benefits are poorly conceptualized and understood. Before they can be compared, they must be more clearly distinguished and articulated. Moreover, in many cases consensus—social or scientific—is lacking about whether a particular outcome is in fact a benefit or a detriment. For example, some people regard the prospect of eliminating a genetic disorder in future generations as laudable, while others worry about the unforeseeable consequences of making alterations in germ-line cells. Second, while some people focus on particular consequences of various applications of genetic engineering technology, others are concerned about the acceptability of genetic manipulation per se. In this context, balancing risks against benefits makes little sense because actions, not consequences, are at issue.

In the first part of this chapter, the Commission considers theological and secular attitudes toward the technology as such, rather than toward its possible consequences, and attempts to clarify the nature of these concerns. The Commission then turns to an examination of the types of risks at issue. Although the focus is on spelling out the meaning and significance of certain risks, the benefits being sought through genetic manipulations—and those foregone if progress is thwarted—are also part of the equation.

It should be emphasized that this discussion does not limit itself to concerns about gene splicing that the scientific community or the Commissioners view as valid. Moreover, this chapter is not a comprehensive survey of the social and ethical issues in genetic engineering. Since this Report addresses primarily the potential human uses of gene splicing, there is, for example, no detailed treatment of the subject of laboratory or industrial "biohazards" (that is, the danger of microorganisms to those involved in their creation or manufacture, or to the general public should they escape from a controlled environment). The problems of laboratory hazards and occupational safety have been scrutinized for almost a decade by the United States Congress (through hearings and through studies by the Office of Technology Assessment and the Library of Congress), by RAC, by various bodies at the Federal, state, and local level, and by numerous scientific organizations.[1]

Some of the doubts about the new technology may appear on close examination to be overly speculative or even fanciful. Nonetheless, they have been forcefully expressed in the popular press, by religious writers, and by members of the general public, and they represent important concerns about the responsible exercise of what may prove to be the means by which people achieve freedom from some of the dictates of their genetic inheritance.

The Commission believes it is important for society to address these concerns head-on. If some of these fears prove groundless, the clearing away of spurious issues will make it easier to focus on any problems of real concern. Without necessarily resolving the problems, the Commission tries to go beyond clarification of the issues to recommend concrete steps for dealing with them.

Concerns About "Playing God"

Hardly a popular article has been written about the social and ethical implications of genetic engineering that does not suggest a link between "God-like powers" and the ability to manipulate the basic material of life. Indeed, a popular book about gene splicing is entitled *Who Should Play God?*[2], and in their June 1980 letter to the President, the three religious leaders sounded a tocsin against the lack of a governmental policy concerning "[t]hose who would play God" through genetic engineering.[3]

Religious Viewpoints The Commission asked the General Secretaries of the three religious organizations to elaborate on any uniquely theological considerations underlying their concern about gene splicing in humans. The scholars appointed by the organizations to address this question were asked to draw specifically on their particular religious tradition to explain the basis of concerns about genetic engineering; further commentary was provided by other religious scholars.[4]

In the view of the theologians, contemporary developments in molecular biology raise issues of responsibility rather than being matters to be prohibited because they usurp powers that human beings should not possess. The Biblical religions teach that human beings are, in some sense, co-creators with the Supreme Creator.[5] Thus, as interpreted for the Commission by their representatives, these major religious faiths respect and encourage the enhancement of knowledge about nature, as well as responsible use of that knowledge.[6] Endorsement of genetic engineering, which is praised for its potential to improve the human estate, is linked with the recognition that the misuse of human freedom creates evil and that human knowledge and power can result in harm.

While religious leaders present theological bases for their concerns, essentially the same concerns have been raised—sometimes in slightly different words—by many thoughtful secular observers of contemporary science and technology. Concerns over unintended effects, over the morality of genetic manipulation in all its forms, and over the social and political consequences of new technologies are shared by religious and secular commentators. The examination of the various specific concerns need not be limited, therefore, to the religious format in which some of the issues have been raised.

Fully Understanding the Machinery of Life

Although it does not have a specific religious meaning, the objection to scientists "playing God" is assumed to be self-explanatory. On closer examination, however, it appears to the Commission that it conveys several rather different ideas, some describing the power of gene splicing itself and some relating merely to its consequences.

At its heart, the term represents a reaction to the realization that human beings are on the threshold of understanding how the fundamental machinery of life works.[7] A full understanding of what are now great mysteries, and the powers inherent in that understanding, would be so awesome as to justify the description "God-like." In this view, playing God is not actually an objection to the research but an expression of a sense of awe—and concern.

Since the Enlightenment, Western societies have exalted the search for greater knowledge, while recognizing its awesome implications. Some scientific discoveries reverberate with particular force because they not only open new avenues of research but also challenge people's entire understanding of the world and their place in it. Current discoveries in gene splicing—like the new knowledge associated with Copernicus and Darwin—further dethrone human beings as the unique center of the universe. By identifying DNA and learning how to manipulate it, science seems to have reduced people to a set of malleable molecules that can be interchanged with those of species that people regard as inferior. Yet unlike the earlier revolutionary discoveries, those in molecular biology are not merely descriptions; they give scientists vast powers for action.

Arrogant Interference with Nature By what standards are people to guide the exercise of this awesome new freedom if they want to act responsibly? In this context, the charge that human beings are playing God can mean that in "creating new life forms" scientists are abusing their learning by interfering with nature.

But in one sense *all* human activity that produces changes that otherwise would not have occurred interferes with nature. Medical activities as routine as the prescription of eyeglasses for myopia or as dramatic as the repair or replacement of a damaged heart are in this sense "unnatural." In another sense, human activity cannot interfere with nature—in the sense of contravening it—since all human activities, including gene splicing, proceed according to the scientific laws that describe natural processes. Ironically, to believe that "playing God" in this sense is even possible would itself be hubris according to some religious thought, which maintains that only God can interfere with the descriptive laws of nature (that is, perform miracles).

If, instead, what is meant is that gene splicing technology interferes with nature in the sense that it violates God's prescriptive natural law or goes against God's purposes as they are manifested in the natural order, then some reason must be given for this judgment. None of the scholars appointed to report their views by the three religious bodies that urged the Commission to undertake this study suggested that either natural reason or revelation imply that gene splicing technology as such is "unnatural" in this prescriptive sense. Although each scholar expressed concern over particular applications of gene splicing technology, they all also emphasized that human beings have not merely the right but the duty to employ their God-given powers to harness nature for human benefit. To turn away from gene splicing, which may provide a means of curing hereditary diseases, would itself raise serious ethical problems.[8]

Creating New Life Forms If "creating new life forms" is simply producing organisms with novel characteristics, then human beings create new life forms frequently and have done so since they first learned to cultivate new characteristics in plants and breed new traits in animals. Presumably the idea is that gene splicing creates new life forms, rather than merely modifying old ones, because it "breaches species barriers" by combining DNA from different species—groups of organisms that cannot mate to produce fertile offspring.

Genetic engineering is not the first exercise of humanity's ability to create new life forms through nonsexual reproduction. The creation of hybrid plants seems no more or no less natural than the development of a new strain of *E. coli* bacteria through gene splicing. Further, genetic engineering cannot accurately be called unique in that it involves the creation of new life forms through processes that do not occur in nature without human intervention. As described in Chapter Two, scientists have found that the transfer of DNA between organisms of different species occurs in nature without human intervention. Yet, as one eminent scientist in the field has pointed out, it would be unwarranted to assume that a dramatic increase in the frequency of such transfers through human intervention is not problematic simply because DNA transfer sometimes occurs naturally.[9]

In the absence of specific religious prohibitions, either revealed or derived by rational argument from religious premises, it is difficult to see why "breaching species barriers" as such is irreligious or otherwise objectionable. In fact, the very notion that there are barriers that must be breached prejudges the issue. The question is simply whether there is something intrinsically wrong with intentionally crossing species lines. Once the question is posed in this way the answer must be negative—unless one is willing to condemn the production of tangelos by hybridizing tangerines and grapefruits or the production of mules by the mating of asses with horses.

There may nonetheless be two distinct sources of concern about crossing species lines that deserve serious consideration. First, gene splicing affords the possibility of creating hybrids that can reproduce themselves (unlike mules, which are sterile). So the possibility of self-perpetuating "mistakes" adds a new dimension of concern, although here again, the point is not that crossing species lines is inherently wrong, but that it may have undesirable consequences and that these consequences may multiply beyond human control. As noted, the Commission's focus on the human applications of gene splicing has meant that it does not here address this important set of concerns, which lay behind the original self-imposed moratorium on certain categories of gene splicing research and which have been, and continue to be, addressed through various scientific and public mechanisms, such as RAC.[10]

Second, there is the issue of whether particular crossings of species—especially the mixing of human and nonhuman genes—might not be illicit. The moral revulsion at the creation of human-animal hybrids may be traced in part to the prohibition against sexual relations between human beings and lower animals. Sexual relations with lower animals are thought to degrade human beings and insult their God-given dignity as the highest of God's creatures. But unease at the prospect of human-animal hybrids goes beyond sexual prohibitions.

The possibility of creating such hybrids calls into question basic assumptions about the relationship of human beings to other living things. For example, those who believe that the current treatment of animals—in experimentation, food production, and sport—is morally suspect would not be alone in being troubled by the prospect of exploitive or insensitive treatment of creatures that possess even more human-like qualities than chimpanzees or porpoises do. Could genetic engineering be used to develop a group of virtual slaves—partly human, partly lower animal—to do people's bidding? Paradoxically, the very characteristics that would make such creatures more valuable than any existing animals (that is, their heightened cognitive powers and sensibilities) would also make the moral propriety of their subservient role more problematic. Dispassionate appraisal of the long history of gratuitous destruction and suffering that humanity has visited upon the other inhabitants of the earth indicates that such concerns should not be dismissed as fanciful.

Accordingly, the objection to the creation of new life forms by crossing species lines (whether through gene splicing or otherwise) reflects the concern that human beings lack the God-like knowledge and wisdom required for the exercise of these God-like powers. Specifically, people worry that interspecific hybrids that are partially human in their genetic makeup will be like Dr. Frankenstein's monster. A striking lesson of the Frankenstein story is the uncontrollability and uncertainty of the consequences of human interferences with the natural order. Like the tale of the Sorcerer's apprentice or the myth of the golem created from lifeless dust by the 16th century rabbi, Loew of Prague, the story of Dr. Frankenstein's monster serves as a reminder of the difficulty of restoring order if a creation intended to be helpful proves harmful instead. Indeed, each of these tales conveys a painful irony: in seeking to extend their control over the world, people may lessen it. The artifices they create to do their bidding may rebound destructively against them—the slave may become the master.

Suggesting that someone lacks sufficient knowledge or wisdom to engage in an activity the person knows how to perform thus means that the individual has insufficient knowledge of the consequences of that activity or insufficient wisdom to cope with those consequences. But if this is the rational kernel of the admonition against playing God, then the use of gene splicing technology is not claimed to be wrong as such but wrong because of its potential consequences. Understood in this way, the slogan that crossing species barriers is playing God does not end the debate, but it does make a point of fundamental importance.[11] It emphasizes that any realistic assessment of the potential consequences of the new technology must be founded upon a sober recognition of human fallibility and ignorance. At bottom, the warning not to play God is closely related to the Socratic injunction "know thyself": in this case, acknowledge the limits of understanding and prediction, rather than assuming that people can foresee all the consequences of their actions or plan adequately for every eventuality.[12]

Any further examination of the notion that the hybridization of species, at least when one of the species is human, is intrinsically wrong (and not merely wrong as a consequence of what is done with the hybrids) involves elaboration of two points. First, what characteristics are uniquely human, setting humanity apart from all other species? And second, does the wrong lie in bestowing some but not all of these characteristics on the new creation or does it stem from depriving the being that might otherwise have arisen from the human genetic material of the opportunity to have a totally human makeup? The Commission believes that these are important issues deserving of serious study.

It should be kept in mind, however, that the information available to the Commission suggests that the ability to create interspecific hybrids of the sort that would present intrinsic moral and religious concerns will not be available in the foreseeable future. The research currently being done on experimentation with recombinant DNA techniques through the use of single human genes (for example, the insertion of a particular human hemoglobin gene into mouse cells at the embryonic stage) or the study of cellular development through the combining of human genetic material with that of other species in a way that does not result in a mature organism (for example, *in vitro* fusion of human and mouse cells) does not, in the Commission's view, raise problems of an improper "breaching of the barriers."

Concerns About Consequences

To appreciate the complexity of the problem of assessing potential consequences and the individual and societal ability to cope with them, the several types of uncertainty . . . must be considered: the occurrence uncertainty that arises when it is not known whether a particular event will take place (or what sort of future it will take place in), the ethical uncertainty that follows from not knowing whether certain uses of a technology should be regarded as beneficial or harmful, and the conceptual uncertainty that attends new developments that challenge people's fundamental beliefs. The presence of any of these types of uncertainty complicates the task of estimating whether the potential benefits of genetic engineering outweigh the potential risks.

What Are the Likely Outcomes?

Medical applications. Two broad applications may be distinguished: the use of drugs produced by gene splicing (such as interferon or insulin) and the direct application of gene splicing to human beings through gene therapy or gene surgery.

The problems of personal safety involved in using drugs produced by gene splicing techniques do not appear to be radically different from those that accompany conventionally produced drugs. The basic scientific and ethical issues in this broad area are well known and need not be rehearsed here. The appropriate divisions within the Department of Health and Human Services (in particular, the relevant institutes of the NIH and the Office for Protection from Research Risks, regarding Federally supported research, and the Food and Drug Administration, regarding all drug and vaccine research) need to consider how to apply to genetically engineered drugs the existing mechanisms related to the margin of acceptable risk, the extent and type of animal and human studies required, the standards for manufacturers, and the decision to allow seriously ill patients to opt for more dangerous or less well tested experimental drugs.[13] According to the Department, appropriate steps are already being taken, especially by FDA, to resolve these issues, and the first product of gene splicing has already been approved.[14]

Some direct therapeutic applications of gene splicing technologies to human beings may present distinctive problems of uncertainty not ordinarily encountered in more conventional medical practice. Concern has been expressed that serious harm might result, for example, from a malfunctioning gene inserted by gene therapy. Yet even here the ethical and policy issues do not seem appreciably different from those involved in the development of any new diagnostic and therapeutic techniques. However, in the case of genetic interventions that involve alteration of germ cells, especially stringent animal testing and other precautions are appropriate, since any physical harms produced might extend to the subject's progeny.

Most experts agree there is a very small likelihood that inheritable changes in germ cells would inadvertently occur when the genetic material of somatic cells is being manipulated. However, the same animal tests and refinements of theoretical models that should precede the use of gene surgery in human beings may shed further light on whether such changes might produce inheritable changes in characteristic functions and whether they will influence germ cells. In both cases, the resolution of uncertainty depends upon increased understanding of how an inserted gene will perform its function.

Subjects of gene therapy or gene surgery might suffer psychological as well as physical harm. The revelation that a person has a genetic defect or is genetically predisposed to a disease may produce anxiety, fear, or loss of self-esteem —feelings that may be intensified by the belief that the defect is a part of a person's constitution, rather than an outside influence. Similarly, patients might regard alterations of their genes as a more profound change than a surgical procedure or the ingestion of a drug. Experience with genetic screening and counseling suggests that the special significance of a genetic condition to the individual may be accompanied by social stigma based on ignorance, but that efforts to educate individual patients and their families as well as the general public can minimize this problem.[15]

Evolutionary impact on human beings. Some critics warn against the dangers of attempting to control or interfere with the "wisdom of evolution" in order to satisfy scientific curiosity.[16] Those who hold this view object in particular to crossing species lines by gene splicing because they believe that the pervasive inability of different species to produce fertile offspring by sexual reproduction must be an adaptive feature, that is, it must confer some significant survival advantage. Thus they view species lines as natural protective barriers that human beings may circumvent only at their peril, although the harm such barriers are supposed to shield people from remains unspecified.

Most proponents of genetic engineering argue that the benefits it will bring are more tangible and important and will affect more people than those objecting suggest. Further, the notion of the "wisdom of evolution" that apparently underlies this consequentialist version of the objection to crossing species lines is not well founded. As the scientific theory of evolution does not postulate a plan that the process of evolution is to achieve, evolutionary changes cannot be said to promote such a plan, wisely or unwisely. Moreover, evolutionary theory recognizes (and natural history confirms) that a "wise" adaptation at one time or place can become a lethal flaw when circumstances change. So even if it could be shown that species barriers have thus far played an important adaptive role, it would not follow that this will continue. An evolutionary explanation of any inherited characteristic can at most show that having that characteristic gave an organism's ancestors some advantage in enabling them to live long enough to reproduce and that the characteristic has not yet proved maladaptive for the offspring.

Furthermore, as a philosopher concerned with assessing the risks of genetic engineering has recently noted, the ability to manipulate genes, both within and across species lines, may become a crucial asset for survival.

> There may . . . come a time when, because of natural or man-induced climatic change, the capacity to alter quickly the genetic composition of agricultural plants will be required to forestall catastrophic famine.[17]

The consequentialist version of the warning against crossing species lines seems, then, to be no more a conclusive argument against genetic engineering than the admonition that to cross species lines is wrong because it is playing God. But it does serve the vital purpose of urging that, so far as this is possible, the evolutionary effects of any interventions are taken into account.

One effect that is of particular concern to some observers is the loss of "heterozygote advantage"—the strength (in terms of individual health and species survival) engendered when members of a species have a variety of gene variants rather than all having the same gene. This advantage has two aspects. The first is the protection that varied genes offer for survival of a species in case of a radical change in environment or, more particularly, the occurrence of a novel pathogen. Of course, it would be virtually impossible to know which particular rare gene variant would prove to be valuable under such circumstances. This consideration would favor preserving as much genetic variation as possible, but it would be difficult to weigh this against the benefit to offspring of the variant gene in its homozygous form.

The second aspect is the advantage that may be conferred by a particular gene in past (and present) environments, perhaps accounting for its prevalence in a population. Although the existence of such an advantage could be construed as an argument against making inheritable gene changes, very little is actually known about the existence and nature of such advantages for most genes. The only instance that is widely acknowledged is the advantage, in terms of longevity and reproduction, possessed by sickle-cell carriers in tropical regions where malaria has been endemic.[18]

The possible beneficial effects of most gene variants are typically too small to be detected by current research methods—that is, other genetic and environmental effects on the health, longevity, and reproductive history of a population make it difficult to detect whether a particular gene confers any advantage on those who possess it. If it becomes feasible to remove an apparently deleterious gene from a population through routine use of gene surgery, the possible loss of heterozygote advantage will deserve careful evaluation.[19] Population geneticists tend to regard the loss of even minute advantages as serious, since such advantages can confer marked benefits on a species over a great many generations. Medical geneticists, on the other hand, are much less bothered by such losses because they believe that it should be possible to make up, through environmental manipulation (including medical treatment) for the loss of any advantage provided by a variant in any probable future environment.

Will Benefit or Harm Occur?

Parental rights and responsibilities. Current attitudes toward human reproductive activity are founded, in part, on several important assumptions, among them that becoming a parent requires a willingness, within very broad limits, to accept the child a woman gives birth to, that parents' basic duties to children are more or less clear and settled, and that reproduction and parenting are and should remain largely private and autonomous spheres of people's lives. The doors that genetic engineering can open challenge all three of these assumptions.

Genetic counseling and screening have already undercut the first assumption by enabling parents to make an informed decision to prevent the occurrence of some genetic defects by terminating pregnancy, by artificial insemination, or by avoiding conception. If gene therapy or gene surgery become available, parents could have more control over their children's characteristics. They will no longer face the stark alternatives of either playing the hand their child has been dealt by the "natural lottery" or avoiding birth or conception. Instead, they could prevent some genetic defects through gene surgery on the zygote and remedy others through gene therapy before the genetic defect produces irreversible changes in the child.

With this increased ability to act for the well-being of the child would come an expansion of parental responsibility. The boundaries of this responsibility—and hence people's conception of what it is to be a good parent—may shift rapidly. It seems safe to say that one important duty of a parent is to prevent or ameliorate serious defects (if it can be done safely) and that the duty to enhance favorable characteristics is less stringent and clear. Yet the new technological capabilities may change people's view of what counts as a defect. For example, if what is now regarded as the normal development of important cognitive skills could be significantly augmented by genetic engineering, then today's "normal" level might be considered deficient tomorrow. Thus ethical uncertainty about the scope of a parent's obligation is linked to conceptual uncertainty about what counts as a defect.

The problem of shifting conceptions of parental responsibility becomes even more complicated when the effects of parents' present actions on descendants beyond their immediate offspring are considered. Deciding whether to engineer a profound change in an expected or newborn child is difficult enough; if the change is inheritable, the burden of responsibility could be truly awesome.

Gene splicing technology may also change people's sense of family and kinship. On the one hand, the possibility of promoting significant inheritable changes through gene surgery may encourage people to think of their family as extending further into the future than they now do. On the other hand, knowing that future generations may employ an even more advanced technology to alter or replace the characteristics passed on to them may weaken people's sense of genetic continuity.

Traditional views of family and kinship associate reproduction with genetic contribution. If genetic engineering makes use of reproductive technologies such as artificial insemination and *in vitro* fertilization, it will increase the strains on this concept of lineage. Whether or not they are accurate, people's beliefs that they are linked to other members of their family by constitutional similarities may play an important role in a family's sense of solidarity and group identity. Knowledge that the genetic link between parents and children is only partial or nonexistent could attenuate these feelings of kinship and family and the sense of continuity and support that they foster. Experience with adoption illustrates successful integration of family members who are not biologically linked, but also demonstrates the importance some individuals place on an association with biological parents. Here, too, there may be as much uncertainty about whether such changes would be beneficial or harmful as there is about whether they are likely to occur.

Societal obligations. The concept of society's obligation to protect or enhance the health of children and future generations often rests on some notion of an adequate minimum of health care. This benchmark, in turn, depends upon assumptions about what counts as a serious defect or disability, on the one hand, and what constitutes normal functioning or adequate health, on the other. As technological capabilities grow, the boundary between these criteria will blur and shift, and with this will come changes in people's views about what society owes to children and to future generations.

As new technological capabilities raise the standard of normal functioning or adequate health, the scarcity of societal resources may raise anew a very difficult question that theorists of distributive justice have strongly disagreed about: where does justice to future generations end and generosity begin? This question is of vital practical import, for the demands of justice are characteristically thought of as valid claims or entitlements to be enforced by the coercive power of the state, while generosity is usually regarded as a private virtue.

Yet society has traditionally been reluctant to interfere with reproductive choice, at least in the case of competent adults. Even with the advent of genetic counseling and screening, social policy has for the most part scrupulously avoided restricting reproductive choice, either as a matter of justice or on any other grounds.[20] So long as the only alternatives are termination of pregnancy or avoidance of conception, any attempt to enforce a public policy designed to prevent genetic defects constitutes a severe infringement on freedom of reproductive choice. If genetic engineering and related reproductive technologies enable a marked reduction of genetic defects and the burden they impose on their victims and on societal resources, however, mandatory genetic treatments may be advocated. Involuntary blood transfusions of pregnant women have been ordered by courts when physicians conclude this is necessary to prevent serious harm to fetuses. Future developments in gene surgery or gene therapy may lead to further departures from the principle that a competent adult may always refuse medical procedures in nonemergency situations and from the assumption that parenting and reproduction are largely private and autonomous activities.

The commitment to equality of opportunity. Since the application of the burgeoning recombinant DNA technology will bring benefits as well as costs and since it will be funded at least in part by public resources, it is essential to ask several questions. Who will benefit from the new technology? And will the benefits and costs be distributed equitably?[21] Indeed, what sort of distribution would count as "fair" when the very thing that is being distributed (such as cognitive ability) is itself often the basis for distributing other things of value in society?[22]

The possibilities presented by gene therapy and gene surgery may in fact call into question the scope and limits of a central element of democratic political theory and practice: the commitment to equality of opportunity. One root idea behind the modern concept of equality of opportunity is the belief that because the social assets a person is born with are in no way earned or merited, it is unfair for someone's luck in the "social lottery" to determine that person's most basic prospects in life. Until recently, those who have sought to ground the commitment to equality of opportunity on this belief have only urged that social institutions be designed so as to minimize or compensate for the influence that the "social lottery" exerts on a person's opportunities.[23] Genetic engineering raises the question of whether equality of opportunity requires intervention in the "natural lottery" as well, for people's initial genetic assets, like their initial social assets, are unearned and yet exert a profound influence on opportunities in life. Even to ask this question challenges a fundamental assumption about the scope of principles of distributive justice, namely that they deal only with inequalities in social goods and play no role in regulating natural inequalities.

Genetic malleability and the sense of personal identity. The manipulation of genes that play an important role in regulating processes of growth and aging or that contribute significantly to personality or intelligence—if it ever becomes possible—could have considerable impact on the way people think of themselves. The current tendency is to think of a person as an individual of a certain character and personality that, following the normal stages of physical, social, and psychological development, is relatively fixed within certain parameters. But this concept—and the sense of predictability and stability in interpersonal relations that it confers—could quickly become outmoded if people use gene splicing to make basic changes in themselves over the course of a lifetime. People can already be changed profoundly through psychosurgery, behavior modification, or the therapeutic use of psychoactive drugs. But genetic engineering might possibly provide quicker, more selective, and easier means. Here again, uncertainty about possible shifts in some of people's most basic concepts brings with it evaluative and ethical uncertainty because the concepts in question are intimately tied to values and ethical assumptions. It is not likely that anything so profound as a change in the notion of personal identity or of normal stages of development over a lifetime is something to which people would have clear value responses in advance.

Changing the meaning of being human. Some geneticists have seen in their field the possibility of benefit through improving human traits.[24] Human beings have the chance to "rise above [their] nature" for "the first time in all time," as one leader in the field has observed:

> It has long been apparent that you and I do not enter this world as unformed clay compliant to any mold. Rather, we have in our beginnings some bent of mind, some shade of character. The origin of this structure—of the fiber in this clay—was for centuries mysterious. . . . Today . . . we know to look within. We seek not in the stars but in our genes for the herald of our fate.[25]

Will gene splicing actually make possible such changes in "human nature" for the first time? In some ways this question is unanswerable since there is great disagreement about which particular characteristics make up "human nature." For some people, the concept encompasses those characteristics that are uniquely human. Yet most human genes are actually found in other mammals as well; moreover, recent work by ethologists and other biologists on animal behavior and capacities is demonstrating that many characteristics once regarded as unique to human beings are actually shared by other animals, particularly by the higher primates, although an ability to record and study the past and to plan beyond the immediate future appears to be a singularly human trait.

Other people regard the critical qualities as those natural characteristics that are common to all human beings, or at least all who fall within a certain "normal range." "Natural" here means characteristics that people are born with as opposed to those that result from social convention, education, or acculturation.

To consider whether gene splicing would allow the changing of human nature thus breaks down into two questions. Which characteristics found in all human beings are inborn or have a large inborn basis? And will gene splicing techniques be able to alter or replace some of the genetic bases of those characteristics? As to the first, the history of religious, philosophical, and scientific thought abounds with fundamental disputes over human nature. Without a consensus on that issue the second question could only be answered affirmatively if it were clear that gene splicing will eventually allow the alteration of all natural characteristics of human beings.

As it is by no means certain that it will ever be possible to change the genetic basis of all natural characteristics, it seems premature to assume that gene splicing will enable changes in human nature. At most, it can perhaps be said that this technology may eventually allow some aspects of what it means to be human to be changed. Yet even that possibility rightly evokes profound concern and burdens everyone with an awesome and inescapable responsibility—either to develop and employ this capability for the good of humanity or to reject it in order to avoid potential undesirable consequences.

The possibility of changing human nature must, however, be kept in perspective. First, within the limits imposed by human beings' genetic endowment, there is already considerable scope by means other than gene splicing for changing some acquired characteristics that are distinctively human. For example, people's desires, values, and the way they live can be changed significantly through alterations in social and economic institutions and through mass education, indoctrination, and various forms of behavior control. Thus, even if gene splicing had the power that some people are concerned about, it would not be unique in its ability to produce major changes in what it means to be human—although it would be unusual in acting on the inheritable foundation of thoughts and actions. If the technology can ever be used in this way, the heritability of the changes ought probably to be regarded as significantly different from any changes now possible.[26]

Second, according to the theory of evolution, the genetic basis of what is distinctively human continually changes through the interplay of random mutation and natural selection. The concern, then, is that gene splicing will for the first time allow deliberate, selective, and rapid alterations to be made in the human genetic constitution.

Finally, concern about changing human nature may at bottom be still more narrowly focused upon those characteristics of human beings—whether unique to the species or not—that are especially valued or cherished. Here, too, there may be disagreement as to which characteristics are most valuable and the value of a given characteristic may depend upon the social or natural environment in which it is manifested.

In sum, the question of whether gene splicing will enable changes in human nature—and the ethical, social, and philosophical significance of such changes—cannot be determined until much more is known about human genetics, specifically the exact contribution of heredity to many human physical and, more important, behavioral traits. Indeed, one of the most important contributions genetic engineering could make to the science of behavioral genetics may be that it will help resolve the age-old controversy of nature versus nurture. If designed changes were possible, society would have to confront whether such changes should be made, and, if they should, which ones. The problems created by uncertainty are particularly notable here since any decision about what characteristics are "desirable" would depend on the world that people will be living in, which is itself unknowable in advance.

Unacceptable uses of gene splicing. A recent National Science Foundation survey indicates that though Americans are generally against restrictions on scientific research, "a notable exception was the opposition to scientists creating new life forms." The survey notes that

> Almost two thirds of the public believe that studies in this area should not be pursued. Fear of the unknown and of possible misuse of the discoveries by some malevolent dictator are among the reasons that could be given for opposition to such genetic engineering.[27]

Given the excesses of the eugenics movement in the United States and elsewhere in the early decades of this century and the role of eugenic theory in mass atrocities perpetrated by the Nazis, these fears cannot be dismissed as groundless. Some comfort may be drawn from the fact that although the possibility of directing human inheritance through simple breeding techniques has existed for centuries, it has not, with relatively minor exceptions, been attempted. Furthermore, the peculiar social and political circumstances that led to these attempts to control human reproduction through the coercive power of the state are not present in this country and are unlikely to occur in the foreseeable future.

Reassuring though they are, these answers are far from conclusive. Government control of sexual reproduction on a broad scale—through an enforced scheme for mating human beings—would require enormous repressive power and social control over individuals over an extended period of time. What might prove more tempting to a dictator or authoritarian ruling elite is the possibility of scientists rapidly making major changes in the genetic composition of a small group in the privacy of the laboratory.

Though there appears at present to be no evidence that the government of this or any other country is attempting to use gene splicing for unacceptable political purposes, the Commission believes that the appropriate posture for the public and the scientific community is one of vigilance. The best safeguards against such abuses are a continued support of democratic institutions and a commitment to individual rights combined with public education about the actual and potential uses of gene splicing technology. Of course, such efforts in this country would not avoid undesirable uses of genetic engineering by totalitarian governments, unless they led to effective international restrictions.[28]

A more subtle danger is that if genetically engineered changes ever become relatively easy to make, there may be a tendency to identify what are in fact social problems as genetic deficiencies of individuals or to assume that the appropriate solution to a given problem, whether social or individual, is genetic manipulation.[29] The relative ease of genetic methods (if gene therapy becomes an accepted medical technique) should most certainly not draw attention away from the underlying social causes of such problems.

Distributing the power to control gene splicing. Beyond any fear of the malevolent use of gene splicing, attention must be paid to a more basic question about the distribution of power: who should decide which lines of genetic engineering research ought to be pursued and which applications of the technology ought to be promoted?

This question is not ordinarily raised about medical technology in general. When it is, the assumption is that for the most part the key decisions are to be made by the relevant experts, the research community, and the medical profession, guided by the availability of research funds (which come predominately from Federal agencies) and by the dictates of medical malpractice law and of state and Federal regulatory agencies designed to protect the public from very tangible, unambiguous harms. Yet genetic engineering is more than a new medical technology. Its potential uses, as discussed, extend far beyond intervention to cure or prevent disease or to restore functioning. This more expansive nature makes it unlikely that decisions about the development of gene splicing technology can be made appropriately within institutions that have evolved to control medical technology and the practice of medicine.

Clearly, adequate institutional arrangements for decisionmaking about the further development of gene splicing technology must assign a substantial role to experts in the field. Yet it is important to understand the unavoidable limitations of technical expertise. On the one hand, there are the limitations of the experts' knowledge; on the other, there are the limitations of technical knowledge itself, no matter how thorough. Experts in genetic engineering can provide the most accurate available data, from which probability statements can be formulated. But neither geneticists nor scientists experienced in risk assessment have any special expertise about evaluative and conceptual uncertainties. An expert might conclude that there is a 5% probability that a certain harmful outcome will occur, but that knowledge is not sufficient for deciding whether such a probability is an acceptable degree of risk. Nor can scientific expertise answer the question of whether the burdens of risk would fall disproportionately upon some people, for this is a moral, not a scientific, question. This is not to say, of course, that scientific experts should not make moral judgments or that if they do they ought to be ignored. But the limitations of expertise must be clearly understood.

In general the public can reasonably rely on the judgments of experts in the field to the extent that at least three conditions are satisfied: (1) there is a strong consensus among the experts, (2) the process by which individuals come to be identified as experts is not unduly influenced by political factors or other forces unrelated to their qualifications as experts, and (3) the experts are not subject to serious conflicts of interest that are likely to distort their judgments or to make their advice unreliable.[30] Whether, or to what extent, these conditions are satisfied cannot be answered once and for all. Instead, they must be viewed as useful rules-of-thumb for assessing and reassessing the role of experts in the formation of responsible public policy.

Commercial-academic relations. Concern over the latter two points—unacceptable uses of the technology and the power to control it—have contributed to a growing public debate about the increased commercial involvement with university-based research on gene splicing. Constraints on support for basic science research by the Federal government in the past decade have been compounded by economic problems that have reduced both state budgets for higher education and the grants of philanthropic foundations. Consequently, academic research scientists are turning increasingly to industry,[31] forming ties that have raised concern about how to accommodate the divergent goals and norms of science and industry.

Universities have historically been dedicated to increasing the general fund of knowledge through basic research, the open exchange of information and ideas, and the training of new researchers and scholars. These goals may run headlong into those of industry—the development of marketable products and techniques through applied research by maintaining a competitive posture, protecting trade secrets, and seeking patent protection.

The conflicts occasioned by these developments are not unique to genetic engineering; indeed, at the beginning of this century a number of expanding universities shifted their focus from the traditional arts and sciences as they became allied with the burgeoning electrical and chemical industries. Medicine, agriculture, econometrics, solid state physics, and computer science have all been advanced in part because of combined forces of industry and universities. Yet the recent similar developments in biotechnology present these issues in sharper relief for several reasons.

First, commercialization of biotechnology seems to be proceeding more rapidly than in chemistry and physics. And in gene splicing, the gap between theory and application—between a graduate student's work in the lab and a highly lucrative product—is often quite small. Finally, the range of potential applications of the research is very broad.

Increased private funding for bioengineering research has therefore sparked questions about conflicts of interest and about the impact of commercialization on academe more generally.[32] Some see these issues as private concerns relating only to the particular universities and firms contracting with each other, a view reflected at a recent conference at Pajaro Dunes when university officials and industry representatives met in private to discuss concerns about commercialization. The participants at this privately funded conference of 5 leading universities and 11 corporations issued a statement intended to "get some general principles on the record" and "set an agenda for further discussion of the issues." The document raised questions of contract review and disclosure, exclusive licensure, and conflicts of interest encountered by university and faculty. It encouraged university faculties to continue examination of these issues over which commentators have noted that "[p]luralism and a certain measure of confusion prevail."[33]

Other issues are also at stake: Can professional virtue be maintained in the face of considerable financial temptations? How will private funding change professors' outlooks?[34] Will fewer be interested in teaching undergraduates? Will they encourage graduate students to focus on projects with maximum commercial potential, instead of those that would foster a more well rounded background? Will commercialization effect a shift from basic to applied research and, if so, with what consequences? Will the secrecy required by industry impede the free exchange of scientific information? What about conflicts of interest when the same academic department includes owners or employees of competitive bioengineering ventures? Will academic appointments and promotions be skewed to favor those who can attract private research funds to the university?

The Association of American Universities has recently suggested that it become a clearinghouse for information on commercialization.[35] These and related questions have also been the subject of debate in the press and before Congressional committees. Undoubtedly, such concerns spill over into the public arena when the question is whether the new agreements are "skimming off the cream produced by decades of taxpayer funded work," as Rep. Albert Gore, Jr., put it in opening Congressional hearings on the subject.[36] Only a continuing public debate over these as-yet-unresolved questions on the commercialization of biotechnology can ensure that the public's interests are being met—its interest in the integrity and credibility of scientific research, in a sound and balanced research agenda, and in the wise expenditure of Federal research dollars.

Continuing Concerns

A distinction has been drawn in this Report between two views: (1) that gene splicing technology is intrinsically wrong or contrary to important values and (2) that, while the technology is not inherently wrong, certain of its applications or consequences are undesirable. Regarding the latter, it has also been noted that genetic engineering involves an array of uncertainties beyond those usually found in technological developments. Not only is the occurrence of specific desirable or undesirable consequences impossible to predict but the application of gene splicing could have far-reaching consequences that could alter basic individual and social values.

The Commission could find no ground for concluding that any current or planned forms of genetic engineering, whether using human or nonhuman material, are intrinsically wrong or irreligious per se. The Commission does not see in the rapid development of gene splicing the "fundamental danger" to world safety or to human values that concerned the leaders of the three religious organizations.[37] Rather, the issue that deserves careful thought is: by what standards, and toward what objectives, should the great new powers of genetic engineering be guided?

Even though the many issues raised by gene splicing in human beings need to be considered one by one if their potential consequences are to be clearly assessed, it would be a mistake to compartmentalize the issues.[38] Although the Commission has not found any ethical, social, or legal barriers to continued research in this field, there remains an important concern expressed by the warning against "playing God." It not only reminds human beings that they are only human and will some day have to pay if they underestimate their own ignorance and fallibility; it also points to the weighty and unusual nature of this activity, which stirs elusive fears that are not easily calmed.

At this point in the development of genetic engineering no reasons have been found for abandoning the entire enterprise—indeed, it would probably be naive to assume that it could be. Given the great scientific, medical, and commercial interest in this technology, it is doubtful that efforts to foreclose important lines of investigation would succeed. If, for example, the United States were to attempt such a step, researchers and investment capital would probably shift to other countries where such prohibitions did not exist. To expect humanity to turn its back on what may be one of the greatest technological revolutions may itself betray a failure to recognize the limits of individual and social self-restraint. Even if important lines of research in this country or elsewhere could be halted, to do so would be to run a different sort of risk: that of depriving humanity of the great benefits genetic engineering may bring.

Assuming that research will continue somewhere, it seems more prudent to encourage its development and control under the sophisticated and responsive regulatory arrangements of this country, subject to the scrutiny of a free press and within the general framework of democratic institutions. In light of the potential benefits and risks—uncertain though they may be at this point—a responsible social policy on genetic engineering requires the cooperation of many institutions and organizations.

Efficient regulation and oversight will require considerable division of responsibility among different bodies and agencies. Legal controls will necessarily focus on the prevention of tangible harms to individuals and the environment. Nonetheless, the Commission believes it is crucial that those entrusted with such oversight and regulation do not lose sight of the more elusive, but equally important, concerns about the human significance of genetic engineering or neglect such concerns because they do not fit neatly into existing institutional jurisdictions. The continued development of gene splicing approved in this Report will require periodic reassessment as greater knowledge is gained about the ethical and social, as well as the technical, aspects of the subject.

NOTES TO CHAPTER 3

1. Office of Technology Assessment, U.S. Congress, *Impacts of Applied Genetics—Micro-organisms, Plants, and Animals*, U.S. Government Printing Office, Washington (1981); Congressional Research Service, Library of Congress, *Genetic Engineering, Human Genetics, and Cell Biology—Evolution of Technological Issues*, Report Prepared for the Subcomm. on Science, Research and Tech. of the House Comm. on Science and Tech., U.S. Government Printing Office, Washington (1976)...
2. Ted Howard and Jeremy Rifkin, *Who Should Play God?*, Dell Publishing Co., Inc., New York (1977).
3. *See* Appendix B . . . [of this report; not reprinted in this volume].
4. *See* Appendix D . . . [not reprinted in this volume], the religious commentators.
5. Seymour Siegel, "Genetic Engineering," in *Proc. of the Rabbinical Assembly of America*, New York (1978) at 164.
6. In the Biblical tradition of the major Western religions, the universe and all that exists in it is God's creation. In pagan religion, the gods inhabit nature, which is thus seen as sacrosanct, but the Biblical God transcends nature. However, since God created the world, it has meaning and purpose. God has placed a special being on earth—humans—formed in the image of God and endowed with creative powers of intelligence and freedom. Human beings must accept responsibility for the effects brought about by the use of the great powers with which they have been endowed—for the betterment of the world—to uncover nature's secrets.
7. As science journalist Nicholas Wade has observed: "We are about to enter an explosive phase of discovery in which we are going to reach close to the great goal of Western inquiry: the complete understanding of man as a physical-chemical system" ("Life," an episode of *Nova*, Boston: WGBH Transcripts, 1982 at 24).
8. Pope John Paul II, who had earlier been critical of genetic engineering, recently told a convocation on biological experimentation . . . of his approval and support for gene splicing when its aim is to "ameliorate the conditions of those who are affected by chromosomic diseases" because [it] offers "hope for the great number of people affected by those maladies":

   > I have no reason to be apprehensive for those experiments in biology that are performed by scientists who, like you, have a profound respect for the human person, since I am sure that they will contribute to the integral well-being of man. On the other hand, I condemn, in the most explicit and formal way, experimental manipulations of the human embryo, since the human being, from conception to death, cannot be exploited for any purpose whatsoever. . . . I praise those who have endeavoured to establish, with full respect for man's dignity and freedom, guidelines and limits for experiments concerning man.

   Pope John Paul II, "La sperimentozione in biologia deve contribuire al bene integrale dell'uomo," *L'Osservatore Romano*, Rome, Oct. 24, 1982, at 2.
9. Robert L. Sinsheimer, "Genetic Research: The Importance of Maximum Safety and Forethought" (Letter), *N.Y. Times*, May 30, 1977, at A14.
10. Despite the great attention paid to the "biohazards" of the research with, and products of, gene splicing, the Environmental Impact Statement filed by NIH on its RAC guidelines focuses on the health effects on humans, plants, and animals and does not deal with ecosystems as entities. Subsequently, however, the Environmental Protection Agency has supported research on the effects of introducing recombinant organisms on the stability of various ecosystems.
11. See, for example, the testimony of Dr. French Anderson, transcript of 22nd meeting of the President's Commission (July 10, 1982) at 115–16:

    > [W]hat made the Gallilean and the other major scientific revolutions disturbing is the reductionism, that we become less than what we are. [T]hat is what is so uncertain about

> gene therapy, because it gets back to a very fundamental question. . . . "Is there anything unique about humans?"
>
> And if there isn't anything unique about humans, there's nothing wrong with doing gene manipulation. But if there is something unique about humans, then it is wrong to pass over the barrier, wherever the barrier is—but we don't know where the barrier is.
>
> But as soon as you ask, "Where is the barrier?" you ask, "Is there a barrier?" And that's frightening. If there's nothing unique about humans—that's not a theological question but a very real one.

12. As one physician-scientist has remarked, "We must all get used to the idea that biomedical technology makes possible many things we should never do." Leon Kass, "The New Biology: What Price Reducing Man's Estate?," 174 *Science* 779 (1971). *See also*, "Ethical Issues in Experiments with Hybrids of Different Species," Appendix I, in Church and Society Office, *Manipulating life*, World Council of Churches, Geneva (1982) at 28.
13. If there is any special concern in the evaluation of the products of gene splicing, it is only that in the initial stages of any new process there are uncertainties about some effects of the process. For example, bacterial contaminants are a unique by-product of gene splicing and in testing human insulin it was important to determine whether these contaminants induced deleterious antibodies in humans.
14. *See* note 10, Chapter Two . . . [not reprinted in this volume].
15. President's Commission for the Study of Ethical Problems in Medicine and Biomedical and Behavioral Research, *Screening and Counseling for Genetic Conditions*, U.S. Government Printing Office, Washington (1983).
16. "Have we the right to counteract, irreversibly, the evolutionary wisdom of millions of years, in order to satisfy the curiosity of a few scientists? The future will curse us for it." Liebe F. Cavalieri, "New Strains of Life—Or Death," *N.Y. Times*, Aug. 22, 1976 (Magazine), at 8, 68 (quoting Erwin Chargaff).
17. Stephen Stitch, "The Recombinant DNA Debate," 7 *Phil. & Pub. Aff.* 187 (1978).
18. . . . Carriers of recessive diseases are people who possess one normal and one variant gene; they usually show no deleterious effects and may, as in the case of sickle-cell, have an advantage. The sickle-cell advantage is, however, dependent on time and place. In a temperate, nonmalarial area, or in a tropical climate from which the malaria parasite has been eliminated, carrying the sickle-cell gene would not confer an advantage.
19. A.M. Capron, "The Law of Genetic Therapy," in Michael P. Hamilton, ed., *The New Genetics and the Future of Man*, William B. Eerdmans Pub. Co., Grand Rapids, Mich. (1972) at 133, 140 (raising question of a need for a living "genes savings bank").
20. *Screening and Counseling for Genetic Conditions, supra* note 15, at second section of Chapter Two.
21. More specifically, it is important to ask whether the further development of gene splicing will reinforce or perhaps exacerbate existing social, cultural, and economic inequalities. This factor explains part of the concern that has been expressed about who will control this technology. Although objections have focused on corporations controlling access (through trade secrets and patents), Howard and Rifkin, *supra* note 2, at 189–207, the greatest abuses of genetics have involved governmental decision-making. Kenneth M. Ludmerer, *Genetics and American Society: A Historical Appraisal*, Johns Hopkins Univ. Press, Baltimore (1972) at 121–34.
22. "Suppose, for example, a society distributes certain scarce resources on the basis of merit—*e.g.*, intelligence, diligence, physical abilities. What if intelligence could be engineered upward? Who would merit this increase in merit? The very oddity of the inquiry calls into question the continued use of intelligence as a basis for resolving competing claims—say, for admission to educational institutions or for access to the intelligence-raising technology itself. We could resort to the other coexisting merit attributes—unless they too were alterable by design. Under these conditions, how could we retain our system of merit distribution? If we could not, how would we then distribute the resources? By resort to a standard of efficiency? By leaving matters to a market? Or by designing a lottery?" Michael H. Shapiro, "Introduction to the Issue: Some Dilemmas of Biotechnology Research," 51 *S. Cal. L. Rev.* 987, 1001–02 (1978) (citations omitted).
23. John Rawls, *A Theory of Justice*, Harvard Univ. Press, Cambridge, Mass. (1973) at 83.
24. Herman J. Muller is the scientist most associated with this view. In the mid-1960s he viewed selective breeding as a method for "a much greater, speedier, and more significant improvement of the population" than any direct rearrangement of genetic material possible in the 21st century. He advocated giving women "germinal choice" through artificial insemination of them with the genes for superior traits. Herman J. Muller, "Means and Aims in Human Genetic Betterment," in T.M. Sonneborn, ed., *Control of Human Heredity and Evolution*, Macmillan Co., New York (1965) at 100. The list of the traits found desirable by Professor Muller changed dramatically over time, as did the types of individuals whose sperm should be used—Lenin appeared on the first list but disappeared during the Cold War. Garland E. Allen, "Science and Society in the Eugenic Thought of H.J. Muller," 20 *BioScience* 346 (1970).
25. Robert L. Sinsheimer, "The Prospect of Designed Genetic Change," 32 *Engineering and Science* 8, 13 (April 1969). Prof. Sinsheimer took a different view from Prof. Muller. He contrasted the "older eugenics" of breeding, which would require a "massive social program," with the new eugenics that could permit "conversion of all the unfit to the highest genetic level" and "could, at least in principle, be implemented on a quite individual basis, in one generation, and subject to no existing social restrictions." *Id.* Prof. Sinsheimer subsequently became very doubtful about the wisdom of changing genes. . . .
26. "If any one age really attains, by eugenics and scientific education, the power to make its descendants what it pleases, all men who live after it are patients of that power. They are weaker, not stronger: for though we may have put wonderful machines in their hands we have pre-ordained how they are to use them. . . . The real picture is that of one dominant age . . . which resists all previous ages most successfully and dominates all subsequent ages most irresist-

ibly, and thus is the real master of the human species. But even within this master generation (itself an infinitesimal minority of the species) the power will be exercised by a minority smaller still. Man's conquest of Nature, if the dreams of the scientific planners are realized, means the rule of a few hundreds of men over billions upon billions of men." C.S. Lewis, *The Abolition of Man*, Collier-Macmillan, New York (1965) at 70–71.

27. John Walsh, "Public Attitude Toward Science Is Yes, but–", 215 *Science* 270 (1982) (quoting National Science Foundation, Science Indicators 1980).
28. Another misuse of gene splicing with international ramifications, described by the World Council of Churches as a "grave hazard," is "the deliberate production of pathogenic micro-organisms for biological warfare or terrorism." Paul Abrecht, ed., 2 *Faith and Science in an Unjust World: Report of the World Council of Churches' Conference on Faith, Science and the Future*, Fortress Press, Philadelphia (1980) at 53.
29. "In discussing the use of any science, including genetics, to solve social problems, it . . . becomes important to demarcate clearly the *limit* that scientific technique may be expected to contribute to an effective solution." Ludmerer, *supra* note 21, at 180. To take an extreme example, in a society in which gene surgery was widely used and accepted, it might be tempting to "solve" the problem of racial discrimination by making genetic changes to eliminate dark skin. A less fanciful example would be the decision to make genetic alterations in certain groups of workers who are exposed to dangerous chemicals in the workplace rather than to eliminate the dangers. *See also*, Marc Lappé and Patricia Archbold Martin, "The Place of the Public in the Conduct of Science":

> Moreover, genetic research may denigrate the value that society has perceived in the moral and autonomous aspects of human conduct by forcing society to question the limits of free will and self-determination. Thus, genetic research has the power to reorder society's priorities and restructure its values; fundamentally, it can change the structures of human thought and the social construction of reality (52 *S. Cal. L. Rev.* 1535, 1537 [1978] [citations omitted]).

30. *See* Stitch, *supra* note 17.
31. Estimates have put industry support of academic research at about $200 million per year. Although this represents only about 4% of what government contributes, it is a growing proportion. The formation in the past decade of about 200 new private ventures to pursue research and development in genetic engineering has been paralleled by increased interest on the part of existing industrial firms in universities that have strong programs in molecular biology. This interest has been capped by several well publicized multimillion dollar agreements.
32. *See* Wade, *supra* note 7:

> That journey of discovery can only be undertaken once, and it would be better undertaken by people who have no interest in anything other than discovering the truth, whose hands are clean, whose motives can never be criticized. That's in the public's interest; that is in science's true interest. And if the commercialization, if this secondary goal of getting rich, ever starts to influence a scientist's primary goal, a university's primary goal of discovering the truth, then the scientists themselves, I hope, will have the sense to put a halt to it. [at 24–25].

33. Barbara J. Culliton, "Pajaro Dunes: The Search for Consensus," 216 *Science* 155 (1982); Draft Statement Pajaro Dunes Conference (March 25–27, 1982).
34. One physician-scientist who formerly held high budgetary and science advisory positions in the Federal government and who is presently the Dean of a school of public health has suggested that the financial agreements between universities and medical school faculty in the clinical departments could be "at least partially relevant" in finding a means of protecting the research and educational commitments of the basic-science faculties while generating added income. Gilbert S. Omenn, "Taking University Research into the Marketplace," 307 *New Eng. J. Med.* 694, 699–700 (1982).
35. Letter from Robert M. Rosenzweig, chairman of the Association of American Universities Committee on University/Industry Relations, to Reps. Don Fuqua and Albert Gore, Jr. (Oct. 28, 1982) (on report of AAU study group).
36. *Commercialization of Academic Biomedical Research*, Hearings before the Subcomm. on Invest. and Oversight and the Subcomm. on Science, Research and Tech. of the House Comm. on Science and Tech., 97th Cong., 1st Sess., June 8, 1981, at 2.
37. *See* Appendix B [not reprinted in this volume].
38. [*See, e.g.,*] Halsted R. Holman and Diana B. Dutton, "A Case for Public Participation in Science Policy Formation and Practice," 51 *S. Cal. L. Rev.* 1505: at 1513–14 (1978) (citation omitted):

> The predominant methodological strategy of biological research is reductionism: the isolation of the phenomenon under study from its usual circumstances, thereby reducing the number of variables that affect the analysis. This allows a clearer understanding of the "basic" processes, and has led to important discoveries.
>
> The strength of reductionism is the principle of isolation. This principle, however, is also inherently limiting: the circumstances of the investigation are necessarily "unreal" in everyday terms. Of course, it may be that the isolated phenomena behave similarly under natural circumstances. This assumption, however, is often uncertain and may frequently be untrue. Moreover, the characteristics of those natural circumstances are rarely fully known. In some cases, knowledge of the multiple external influences upon biological processes could lead to a perception of those processes quite different from those obtained in the isolation of laboratory study. A critical understanding of present biological knowledge requires recognition of those methodological weaknesses. Public participation in science, by broadening the range of factors considered at each stage of investigation, provides a means of counteracting biases resulting from reductionist strategy.

NIH "POINTS TO CONSIDER" FOR GENE THERAPY RESEARCHERS

INTRODUCTION. *A direct line runs from Splicing Life, the report of the President's Commission on the social and ethical issues of genetic engineering and the two reports on gene therapy that follow. In April 1983, the chairman of the Recombinant DNA Advisory Committee (RAC), the attorney Robert Mitchell, asked RAC members whether they wished to respond to "Splicing Life." The committee appointed a working group and asked the group to review the report and make recommendations to the full committee. An incremental process followed in 1983 and 1984, during the course of which the RAC agreed to review gene-therapy protocols when researchers were ready to submit them. The review mechanism chosen by the RAC was the appointment of an interdisciplinary Working Group on Human Gene Therapy. The Working Group held its first meeting in October 1984 and immediately set to work on a series of questions or "Points to Consider" for researchers who were considering the submission of gene-therapy protocols. An initial version of the "Points to Consider" document was published in the Federal Register on January 22, 1985, but it was later revised in response to numerous public comments. The excerpt reprinted in this volume is from the revised version.*

Applicability

These "Points to Consider" apply only to research conducted at or sponsored by an institution that receives any support for recombinant DNA research from the National Institutes of Health (NIH). This includes research performed by NIH directly.

Introduction

(1) Experiments in which recombinant DNA is introduced into cells of a human subject with the intent of stably modifying the subject's genome are covered by Section III-A-4 of the NIH Guidelines for Research Involving Recombinant DNA Molecules (49 FR 46266). Section III-A-4 requires such experiments to be reviewed by the NIH Recombinant DNA Advisory Committee (RAC) and approved by the NIH. RAC consideration of each proposal will be on a case-by-case basis and will follow publication of a precis of the proposal in the *Federal Register*, an opportunity for public comment, and a review of the proposal by the working group of the RAC. RAC recommendations on each proposal will be forwarded to the NIH Director for a decision which will then be published in the Federal Register. In accordance with Section IV-C-1-b of the NIH Guidelines, the NIH Director may approve proposals only if he finds that they present "no significant risk to health or the environment." [Note that Section III-A-4 applies to both recombinant DNA and DNA derived from recombinant DNA.]

(2) In general, It is expected that somatic-cell gene therapy protocols will not present a risk to the environment as the recombinant DNA is expected to be confined to the human subject. Nevertheless, Section I-B-4-b of the "Points to Consider" document asks the researchers to address specifically this point.

(3) This document is intended to provide guidance in preparing proposals for NIH consideration under Section IIIA-4 of the NIH Guidelines for Research Involving Recombinant DNA Molecules. Not every point mentioned in the "Points to Consider" document will necessarily require attention in every proposal. It is expected that the

Excerpts from the U.S. National Institutes of Health, Recombinant DNA Advisory Committee, "Points to Consider in the Design and Submission of Human Somatic-Cell Gene Therapy Protocols," 50 *Federal Register* 160, August 19, 1985, pp. 33463–33464. Footnotes have been modified and appear within the text in square brackets.

document will be considered for revision at least annually as experience in evaluating proposals accumulates and as new scientific developments occur.

(4) A proposal will be considered by the RAC only after the protocol has been approved by the local Institutional Biosafety Committee (IBC) and by the local Institutional Review Board (IRB) in accordance with Department of Health and Human Services (DHHS) Regulations for the Protection of Human Subjects (45 CFR Part 46). If a proposal involves children, special attention should paid to subpart D of these DHHS regulations. The IRB and IBC may, at their discretion condition their approval on further specific deliberation by the RAC and its working group. Consideration of gene therapy proposals by the RAC may proceed simultaneously with review by any other involved federal agencies [e.g., the Food Administration (footnote omitted)] provided that the RAC is notified of the simultaneous review. Meetings of the committee will be open to the public except where trade secrets or proprietary information will be disclosed. The committee would prefer that the first proposal submitted for RAC review contain no proprietary information or trade secrets, enabling all aspects of the review to be open to the public. The public review of these protocols will serve to inform the public not only on the technical aspects of the proposals but also on the meaning and significance of the research.

(5) The clinical application of recombinant DNA techniques to human gene therapy raises two general kinds of questions: (1) The questions usually discussed by IRBs in their review of *any* proposed research involving human subjects; and (2) broader social issues. The first type of question is addressed principally in Part I of this document. Several of the broader social issues surrounding human gene therapy are discussed later in this Introduction and in Part II below.

(6) Following the Introduction, this document is divided into four parts. Part I deals with the short-term risks and benefits of the proposed research to the patient, to other people, as well as with issues of fairness in the selection of patients, informed consent, and privacy and confidentiality ["patient" and its variants refer to the patient-subject]. In Part II, investigators are requested to address special issues pertaining to the free flow of information about clinical trials of gene therapy. These issues lie outside the usual purview of IRBs and reflect general public concerns about biomedical research. Part III summarizes other requested documentation that will assist the RAC and its working group in their review of gene therapy proposals. Part IV specifies reporting requirements,

(7) A distinction should be drawn between making genetic changes in somatic cells and in germ line cells. The purpose of somatic cell gene therapy is to treat an individual patient, e.g., by inserting a properly functioning gene into a patient's bone marrow cells *in vitro* and then reintroducing the cells into the patient's body. In germ line alterations, a specific attempt is made to introduce genetic changes into the germ (reproductive) cells of an individual, with the aim of changing the set of genes passed on to the individual's offspring. The RAC and its working group will not at present entertain proposals for germ line alterations but will consider for approval protocols involving somatic-cell gene therapy.

(8) The acceptability of human somatic-cell gene therapy has been addressed in several recent documents as well as in numerous academic studies. The November 1982 report of the President's Commission for the Study of Ethical Problems in Medicine and Biomedical and Behavioral Research, *Splicing Life*, resulted from a two-year process of public deliberations and hearings; upon release of that report, a House subcommittee held three days of public hearings with witnesses from a wide range of fields from the biomedical and social sciences to theology, philosophy, and law. In December 1984, the Office of Technology Assessment released a background paper, *Human Gene Therapy*, which brought these earlier documents up-to-date. As the latter report concluded:

> Civic, religious, scientific, and medical groups have all accepted, in principle, the appropriateness of gene therapy of somatic cells in humans for specific genetic diseases. Somatic cell gene therapy is seen as an extension of present methods of therapy that might be preferable to other technologies.

(9) Concurring with this judgment, the RAC and its working group are prepared to consider for approval somatic-cell therapy protocols, provided that the design of such experiments offers adequate assurance that their *consequences* will not go beyond their *purpose*, which is the same as the traditional purpose of all clinical investigations, namely, to benefit the health and well-being of the individual being treated while at the same time gathering generalizable knowledge.

(10) The two possible undesirable consequences of somatic-cell therapy would be unintentional (1) vertical transmission of genetic changes from an individual to his or her offspring or (2) horizontal transmission of viral infection to other persons with whom the individual comes in contact. Accordingly, this document requests information that will enable the RAC and its working group to assess the likelihood that the proposed somatic-cell gene therapy will inadvertently affect reproductive cells or lead to infection of other people (e.g., treatment personnel or relatives).

(11) In recognition of the social concern that surrounds the general discussion of human gene therapy, the working group will continue to consider the possible long-range effects of applying knowledge gained from these and related experiments. While research in molecular biology could lead to the development of techniques for germ line intervention or for the use of genetic means to enhance human capabilities rather than to correct defects in patients, the working group does not believe that these effects will follow immediately or inevitably from experi-

ments with somatic-cell gene therapy. The working group will cooperate with other groups in assessing the possible long-term consequences of somatic-cell gene therapy and related laboratory and animal experiments in order to define appropriate human applications of this emerging technology.

(12) Responses to the questions raised in these "Points to Consider" should be provided in the form of either written answers or references to specific sections of the protocol or its appendices.

GENE THERAPY FOR HUMAN PATIENTS: INFORMATION FOR THE GENERAL PUBLIC

INTRODUCTION. *As the Working Group, now renamed the Human Gene Therapy Subcommittee, began reviewing protocols in 1988, it also considered how the technique of gene therapy and the mission of the RAC and its subcommittee could be explained to laypeople. The outcome of these deliberations was the decision to publish a brief, simply written description of gene therapy and the national public review process for gene-therapy protocols. An excerpt from Gene Therapy for Human Patients: Information for the General Public follows.*

Part 3: NIH "Points to Consider" for Gene Therapy Researchers

In anticipation of the first request to perform a human gene therapy experiment, the Human Gene Therapy Subcommittee prepared a document called *Points to Consider in the Design and Submission of Protocols for the Transfer of Recombinant DNA into the Genome of Human Subjects*. This document was approved by the NIH Recombinant DNA Advisory Committee and the Director of the NIH in 1986. The "Points to Consider" document provides guidance to physicians and scientists who are planning to submit proposals to the NIH for gene therapy treatment of patients. It describes the considerations that have been identified in the studies and hearings mentioned previously as the most important in evaluating this new mode of treatment.

In the "Points to Consider," researchers are first asked:

- What disease do you intend to treat with gene therapy?
- Why do you consider this disease to be an appropriate candidate for treatment with this new method?

In answering these questions, the researcher will discuss the seriousness of the disease, any alternative therapies, and the possible advantages of gene therapy for at least some patients.

Another part of the "Points to Consider" asks:

- What laboratory studies have been done, with cells and live animals, that make researchers hopeful that gene therapy will help patients rather than harming them?

Here the researcher will provide the results of studies performed in his/her laboratory or in other laboratories around the world. Especially important will be studies demonstrating that gene therapy does not harm laboratory animals and in fact demonstrates that the desired biological effects occur.

Even if the preceding questions are satisfactorily answered, important questions about the proposed use of gene therapy in patients will remain. The "Points to Consider" ask the following four questions:

- What are the probable benefits and harms of the proposed treatment, both to the patient and to others?
- If there are several patients who need gene therapy but only one of them can be treated initially, how will selection be made in a way that treats all patients fairly?
- How will patients—or, in the case of young children, the parents of patients—be properly informed about the possible benefits and risks of gene therapy?
- What steps will be taken to protect the privacy of the patient and the patient's family, while at the same time informing the public about the results of gene therapy?

In the Introduction to the "Points to Consider," reference is made to two possible undesirable or unintentional consequences of somatic cell gene therapy transmission of altered genes to a patient's offspring, and viral infection of persons who come in contact with the patient. The subcommittee requests that researchers describe what actions will be taken to prevent either event from occurring.

The "Points to Consider" acknowledge the public concern about some aspects of human gene therapy. It reads: "In recognition of the social concern that surrounds the general discussion of human gene therapy, the [subcom-

Excerpt from the U.S. National Institutes of Health, Recombinant DNA Advisory Committee and Human Gene Therapy Subcommittee, *Gene Therapy for Human Patients: Information for the General Public*, NIH Publication 90-2885, Bethesda, MD., April 1990.

mittee] will continue to consider the possible long-range effects of applying knowledge gained from these and related experiments." For the moment, the subcommittee agrees with the conclusion in the Office of Technology Assessment's report *Human Gene Therapy* that:

> Civic, religious, scientific, and medical groups have all accepted, in principle, the appropriateness of gene therapy of somatic cells in humans for specific genetic diseases. Somatic cell gene therapy is seen as an extension of present methods of therapy that might be preferable to other technologies.

While the RAC and its subcommittee believe that gene therapy for nonreproductive, or somatic, cells holds promise for patients suffering from certain genetic and other diseases, they will seek to ensure that patients are not subjected to unreasonable risk of harm, excessive discomfort, or unwanted invasion of privacy and that they will receive special care, monitoring, and consideration. The public will be informed about every step that is taken with this new technique.

Gene Therapy in Man: Recommendations of European Medical Research Councils

INTRODUCTION. *The following document represents an important step in the ongoing European discussion of human gene therapy. As noted previously, the Parliamentary Assembly of the Council of Europe had adopted a recommendation regarding gene therapy in January 1982. This pioneering effort was followed by reports from national advisory committees in Denmark (1984), Sweden (1984), and the Federal Republic of Germany (1985 and 1987). In June 1988, the medical research councils of these three countries joined the councils of eight other Western European countries in a consensus statement. The medical research councils agreed with earlier policy statements in Europe and North America that somatic-cell gene therapy is not qualitatively different from other types of clinical research. The councils recommended national guidelines for gene therapy and expert national bodies for the review of gene-therapy proposals.*

OVER THE PAST DECADE there have been major advances in the understanding at the molecular level of the structure and organisation of the genetic material of living organisms, including man. These advances have been driven by the application of recombinant DNA technology which, despite early concerns, has been used safely in laboratories throughout the world under the regulation of simple guidelines. Animal and human genes have been isolated and characterised; and the appropriate gene products, such as proteins or hormones, have been expressed following the introduction of genes into cultured cells in the laboratory. A further advance—the expression of specific genes after their introduction into laboratory animals—has raised the possibility that certain genetic defects in man might be corrected by applying similar techniques. Discussion of this possibility is well advanced in the USA, and the European Medical Research Councils (EMRC) consider it timely to formulate guidelines for the conduct of research on gene therapy in man and member countries.

"Gene Therapy in Man: Recommendations of European Medical Research Councils." Joint statement by the Medical Research Councils of Austria, Denmark, Finland, France, The Netherlands, Norway, Spain, Sweden, Switzerland, United Kingdom, and West Germany. June 1988. Reprinted from the Lancet, June 4, 1988.

General Considerations

SCOPE OF GENE THERAPY

The central consideration in this document is the correction of specific genetic defects in individual patients. This consideration should be distinguished from the application of gene therapy for the enhancement of general human characteristics such as physical appearance or intelligence, which raises profound ethical problems and should not be contemplated.

Distinction between Somatic and Germline Gene Therapy Foreign genes may be inserted either into somatic cells (i.e., any body cell except a germ cell) or into germ cells or cells that give rise to germ cells (e.g., early embryonic cells). Insertion of genetic material into somatic cells and their subsequent transplantation is not fundamentally different from any form of organ transplantation or blood transfusion. The insertion of genes into fertilised eggs or very early embryos is fundamentally different because these genes would be passed on to the offspring in subsequent generations. Germline gene therapy should not be contemplated.

Experience with Experimental Systems Somatic gene cell therapy in animals has given disappointing results and no successful "cures" can be claimed.[1] This has been due mainly to the inefficiency of methods for inserting genes into somatic cells, such as marrow stem cells, and to the low level of expression after transfection. More encouraging results have been achieved in dogs,[2] but further success in experimental systems will be necessary before trials in man can be justified.

Candidate Genetic Diseases and Target Tissues for Somatic Gene Therapy

Genetic diseases occur with an estimated frequency of 40–50 per 1000 population. They may be due to defects in single genes or to the interactions of a number of genes. Other diseases may have a genetic component but may also be influenced significantly by contributions from environmental factors. Single-gene defects, such as phenylketonuria (1 per 10 000 births) and muscular dystrophy (1 per 5000 births) affect 1–2% of newborn babies.

For the foreseeable future, diseases which might be treated with gene therapy will be exclusively single-gene disorders. Diseases in which the affected gene has not been identified or in which regulation of the expression of the normal gene is very complex would not be appropriate for investigation in the near future. Candidates for gene therapy would be diseases which are invariably fatal or severely disabling and for which current possible therapies, such as bone marrow transplantation, are not always feasible or carry a high level of risk.

Bone marrow disorders are appropriate targets for early investigation because there is substantial experience of removal, treatment, and replacement of marrow cells in patients. Disorders such as adenosine deaminase deficiency and purine nucleoside phosphorylase deficiency, both of which result in immunodeficiency, would be suitable targets although they are rare Although globin gene expression is tightly regulated, the haemoglobinopathies might also be suitable for study, since much is known about the mechanisms of regulation at the molecular level. The ability of transfected marrow cells to correct genetic defects in other tissues, such as the brain in Lesch-Nyhan disease, is less certain and should be accorded a lower priority. The possibility of implantation of modified fibroblasts or epidermal cells might also be considered in the future.

Technology and Safety of Introduction of Genes into Cells

In principle, genes may be introduced into human cells outside the body for later reimplantation, or cells may be treated in situ. There are several possible techniques for the introduction of normal genes into human cells. Although direct transfection of DNA is currently an inefficient means of modifying the large numbers of cells required for therapy, improved techniques may be developed in the future. Techniques of site-directed recombination, involving the simple exchange of the defective gene with a normal copy, are also currently inefficient, and the production of mutations following application of this method has been reported. However, this method is attractive in principle, and advances during the next few years may increase its practical value for therapy in man.

Most attention has been focused on the viral vectors, retroviruses in particular, for the introduction of genes into cells. The vector virus must be disabled so that it does not subsequently replicate, and there must be no active "helper" virus (used to package the disabled vector) in the vector preparations. Both these dangers can be avoided with modern production techniques. Vectors specific for particular tissues and cells are being developed, and vectors that occur naturally in the species to be treated are likely to be the most useful.

Safety is a major consideration in the introduction of genes into cells. There must be no possibility of producing active, possibly cancer-inducing, helper or vector viruses through recombination between disabled vector and helper viruses. It is also possible that insertion of a gene into the genetic material of the treated cell might (through "promoter insertion") activate the expression of genes involved in the induction of cancer or cause other harmful disturbances of cell regulation or function. In addition, the insertion might lead to rearrangement or relocation of particular host genes known to be involved in the induction of cancer (oncogenes). It should be noted, however, that certain current medical treatments, such as cancer chemotherapy, immunosuppression, and radiation, also carry a risk of predisposition to cancer. Finally, it will be necessary to ensure that the expression of an introduced gene is stable and sufficient to achieve a therapeutic effect.

The techniques for the introduction of genes into the cells, whether inside or initially outside the body, should not allow the spread of such genes or of any vectors to other cells, in particular germ cells, within the body or to people in contact with the patient. In this respect, great caution should be exercised with methods designed to target the introduction of genes into specific tissues within the body.

Manipulations in vitro must ensure that normal gene is introduced into a high proportion of stem cells and that such cells are given a proliferative advantage by procedures that specifically select for cells containing the gene. It seems that cells in the division cycle are more susceptible to the successful introduction of genes in retroviral vectors, and special methods, such as the use of growth factors, may be required to ensure that all the cells to be treated are in cycle. Techniques to select for, and therefore ensure the survival of, treated cells after transplantation into the patient will need investigation and may require the use of toxic drugs, with the possible complication of drug resistance, particularly if the selective therapies have to be applied for long periods.

Ethical Considerations

Somatic gene cell therapy by reimplantation of the patient's own cells is in principle similar to current routine therapies such as organ transplantation and therefore raises no new ethical issues. Judgments on the ethics of gene therapy in man will initially apply to individual cases and will require assessment of factors such as safety, efficacy, alternative treatments, and prognosis—in other words, the balance of risk and benefit for the patient. In the near future treatment by gene therapy might be justified in cases of invariably fatal or life-threatening diseases for which no alternative treatment is available. The patient should understand the issues involved and normally be asked to give informed consent to the treatment, although legal issues associated with "consent" by parents on behalf of a child may present difficulties. If damage caused by the genetic disorder in a particular patient is irreversible, then there may be no case for intervention through gene therapy. In the future, consideration might be given in particular disorders to treatment of the fetus before birth in order to prevent damage caused by early expression of the defect.

Regulation

National guidelines for the conduct of human gene therapy are essential. There should therefore be an expert national body to consider and approve proposals for such therapy in order to ensure public confidence in the introduction of a new and sophisticated treatment. In addition local ethical committees should subsequently consider and approve proposals. The assessment of early trials of human gene therapy should be monitored by a central body.

Summary

1. The purpose of gene therapy currently under consideration is the correction of genetic defects; attempts to enhance general human characteristics should not be contemplated. Only somatic cell gene therapy, resulting in non-heritable changes to particular body tissues, should be contemplated. Germline therapy, for introduction of heritable genetic modifications, is not acceptable. Further technical improvements in the expression of transferred genes in somatic cells will be necessary before successful gene therapy can be achieved even in animal models; in the meantime trials in man are not justified.

2. The most appropriate "candidate" genetic diseases for early investigation of treatment by gene therapy are single-gene disorders for which the affected gene and its regulation have been characterised.

3. In the near future, it is likely that success in the introduction of normal genes into human cells will be achieved through the use of disabled retrovirus vectors, although other techniques may advance rapidly. Much further work is required in the development of safe species-specific and tissue-specific retrovirus vectors. The methods of gene introduction should not result in the spread of gene or vector to other tissues within the body or to people in contact with the patient. The possibility of a significant increase in the predisposition of the patient to cancer should be evaluated in considering the risks and benefits of the treatment. In addition, the expression and regulation of the gene inserted should be stable and sufficient to ensure a therapeutic effect.

4. General ethical considerations applicable to any new clinical treatment apply to human gene therapy and, in the first instance, will require assessment in individual cases. In the near future it is likely that such therapy will be clinically justified in particular patients with invariably fatal or life-threatening diseases, provided informed consent is obtained and no alternative treatment is available.

5. A national body should consider all proposals for human gene therapy and ensure the application of agreed national guidelines. Early trials should be monitored by a central body.

NOTES

1. Williams DA, Orkin SH. Somatic gene therapy: Current status and future prospects. *J Clin Invest* 1986; 77: 1053–56.
2. Kwok WW, Scheuning F, Stead RB, Miller AD. Retroviral transfer of genes into canine hemopoietic progenital cells in culture: A model of human gene therapy. *Proc Natl Acad Sci* 1986; 83:4552–55.

THE DECLARATION OF INUYAMA

INTRODUCTION. *The following statement represents a remarkable consensus among an interdisciplinary group of participants from 24 countries and all continents. After dividing into three working groups on human genome mapping, genetic screening and testing, and human gene therapy, the participants came together to share their findings and adopt a declaration. A striking feature of the Declaration of Inuyama is its openness to the possibility of germ-line genetic intervention for therapeutic or preventive purposes. While acknowledging the technical difficulties involved in any germ-line intervention, the Declaration noted that such intervention might be the only means of treating certain conditions. The Declaration did stipulate that the safety of any germ-line studies in humans "must be very well established," presumably through extensive preclinical research.*

The Declaration

I. Discussion of human genetics is dominated today by the efforts now under way on an international basis to map and sequence the human genome. Such attention is warranted by the scale of the undertaking and its expected contribution to knowledge about human biology and disease. At the same time, the nature of the undertaking, concerned as it is with the basic elements of life, and the potential for abuse of the new knowledge which the project will generate, are giving rise to anxiety. The Conference agrees that efforts to map the human genome present no inherent ethical problems but are eminently worthwhile, especially as the knowledge revealed will be universally applicable to benefit human health. In terms of ethics and human values, what must be assured are that the manner in which gene mapping efforts are implemented adheres to ethical standards of research and that the knowledge gained will be used appropriately, particularly in genetic screening and gene therapy.

II. Public concern about the growth of genetic knowledge stems in part from the misconception that while the knowledge reveals an essential aspect of humanness it also diminishes human beings by reducing them to mere base pairs of deoxyribonucleic acid (DNA). This misconception can be corrected by education of the public and open discussion, which should reassure the public that plans for the medical use of genetic findings and techniques will be made openly and responsibly.

III. Some types of genetic testing or treatment not yet in prospect could raise novel issues—for example, whether limits should be placed on DNA alterations in human germ cells, because such changes would affect future generations, whose consent cannot be obtained and whose best interests would be difficult to calculate. The Conference concludes, however, that for the most part present genetic research and services do not raise unique or even novel issues, although their connection to private matters such as reproduction and personal health and life prospects, and the rapidity of advances in genetic knowledge and technology, accentuate the need for ethical sensitivity in policy-making.

IV. It is primarily in regard to genetic testing that the human genome project gives rise to concern about ethics and human values. The identification, cloning and sequencing of new genes without first needing to know their protein products greatly expand the possible scope for screening and diagnostic tests. The central objective of genetic screening and diagnosis should always be to safeguard the welfare of the person tested: test results must always be protected against unconsented disclosure, confidentiality must be ensured at all costs, and adequate counselling must be provided. Physicians and others who counsel should endeavor to ensure that all those concerned understand the difference between being the carrier of a defective gene and having the corresponding genetic disease. In autosomal recessive conditions, the health of carriers (heterozygotes) is usually not affected by their having a single copy of the disease gene; in dominant disorders,

Reprinted from the Council for International Organizations of Medical Sciences, "The Declaration of Inuyama." Twenty-Fourth Round Table Conference, Tokyo and Inuyama City, Japan: CIOMS, July 1990.

what is of concern is the manifestation of the disease, not the mere presence of the defective gene, especially when years may elapse between the results of a genetic test and the manifestation of the disease.

V. The genome project will produce knowledge of relevance to human gene therapy, which will very soon be clinically applicable to a few rare but very burdensome recessive disorders. Alterations in somatic cells, which will affect only the DNA of the treated individual, should be evaluated like other innovative therapies. Particular attention by independent ethical review committees is necessary, especially when gene therapy involves children, as it will for many of the disorders in question. Interventions should be limited to conditions that cause significant disability and not employed merely to enhance or suppress cosmetic, behavioural or cognitive characteristics unrelated to any recognized human disease.

VI. The modification of human germ cells for therapeutic or preventive purposes would be technically much more difficult than that of somatic cells and is not at present in prospect. Such therapy might, however, be the only means of treating certain conditions, so continued discussion of both its technical and its ethical aspects is essential. Before germ-line therapy is undertaken, its safety must be very well established, for changes in germ cells would affect the descendants of patients.

VII. Genetic researchers and therapists have a strong responsibility to ensure that the techniques they develop are used ethically. By insisting on truly voluntary programmes designed to benefit directly those involved, they can ensure that no precedents are set for eugenic programmes or other misuse of the techniques by the State or by private parties. One means of ensuring the setting and observance of ethical standards is continuous multidisciplinary and transcultural dialogue.

VIII. The needs of developing countries should receive special attention, to ensure that they obtain their due share of the benefits that ensue from the human genome project. In particular, methods and techniques of testing and therapy that are affordable and easily accessible to the populations of such countries should be developed and disseminated whenever possible. ¨

MAPPING AND SEQUENCING THE HUMAN GENOME

INTRODUCTION. *In 1986 an international debate began over the feasibility and utility of attempting to map and sequence the human genome—that is, to specify the approximately three million base pairs that make up the genes and intervening DNA in a typical human being. In the United States this debate led to the launching of two parallel studies, the one conducted by biomedical scientists under the aegis of the National Research Council, the other conducted by the Congressional Office of Technology Assessment, with background papers from an interdisciplinary group of contractors and periodic meetings of an advisory panel. The National Research Council study was completed first and published in February 1988. Its eighth and final chapter, reprinted here, represents a very early attempt to grapple with the ethical, legal, and social implications of the proposed human genome project. Albert Jonsen and Eric Juengst contributed heavily to the writing of this chapter.*

8. Implications for Society

The applications and implications for biology and medicine of a project to map and sequence the human genome have been mentioned often in this report. In this final chapter we discuss some of the other issues for society, including the commercial, legal, and ethical implications of such a project.

COMMERCIAL AND LEGAL IMPLICATIONS

Mapping and sequencing the human genome will result in new information and materials of potential commercial value, for example, clones that encode previously undiscovered hormones, growth factors, or mediators of immunity. The commercial value of these resources raises questions concerning possible copyright protection of the data and ownership of the intellectual property and materials generated by participants in the human genome project. Should it be possible to copyright sequences from the human genome and, if so, by whom? Should a central agency of the government own the patents for new materials, such as DNA clones generated by this project? What are the implications for international collaboration? Because these are complex issues requiring study by scientists, lawyers, and policymakers, the committee believes that they should be given prompt study by an independent body. It is important to resolve the legal issues concerning the conduct of the human genome project. Absolutely essential to the success of the project will be cooperation between laboratories and centers—within the United States and internationally—and the ready availability of data and materials to all participants. This committee believes that human genome sequences should be a public trust and therefore should not be subject to copyright.

ETHICAL AND SOCIAL IMPLICATIONS

Whatever its scientific merits, a concerted effort to map and sequence the human genome would have profound social significance. Human beings are fascinated with the reasons we are what we are, both for what those reasons tell us about ourselves and for the insights they give us into those around us. In this context, the prospect of a complete biological book on humankind provokes both excitement and concern and raises philosophical and ethical questions. Three sorts of questions seem particularly important to reflect upon in advance of any genome mapping and sequencing effort: How should the project proceed? How should the information be interpreted? To what use should the resulting information be applied? None of these are

National Research Council, Committee on Mapping and Sequencing the Human Genome, *Mapping and Sequencing the Human Genome*, Washington, D.C.: National Academy Press, 1988.

new questions for human geneticists. In fact, the ethical and social challenges presented by a human genome mapping and sequencing project are largely the same as those already addressed by scientists, clinicians, patients, and policymakers in other settings (Macklin, 1985). Still, the scale and significance of this project require that these questions be carefully assessed in this context.

Conducting a Genome Mapping and Sequencing Project The ethical considerations involved in conducting this project are shared by those conducting any biomedical analysis of human tissue. One consideration concerns privacy and confidentiality. The privacy and autonomy of the individuals who contribute the material studied must be protected. For most research in this project, this goal is easily accomplished: The isolated cell lines and genetic materials analyzed will come from a wide variety of sources, through standard channels designed to preserve the confidentiality of the contributors and ensure that their participation is voluntary (U.S. Congress, House Committee on Science and Technology, 1986). However, where family histories are studied to produce genetic linkage maps, geneticists will sometimes face ethical dilemmas over maintaining confidentiality or disclosing research findings to a relative discovered to be at risk for genetic disease. Again, this is not a new problem for human geneticists (Capron, 1979). As the mapping research proceeds, it will become increasingly important to reconfirm the geneticist's traditional willingness to take on the burden of responsibility in decisions to break confidentiality and to consider such a breach only when the probability is high that serious, avoidable harm would otherwise come to identifiable individuals (President's Commission, 1983).

Interpreting the Medical Implications of Genetic Information Mapping and sequencing the human genome could provide a great deal of new knowledge about the genetic basis of human disease. However, the effects of that knowledge will be highly colored by the way its practical implications are interpreted. Without careful interpretation, information that links particular genes with disease can have harmful consequences for the people who carry those genes, quite apart from the disease itself.

For example, without clear guidance it would be easy for people to misinterpret statistical correlations between clinical diseases and particular genetic markers, so that they take the discovery of the marker to be diagnostic of the disease. Genetic susceptibilities, predispositions, or risks for disease are variable and sometimes ambiguous concepts (Lappé, 1979a). If interpreted too strongly, preventive efforts could force certain groups or individuals to assume the social and psychological burdens of the afflicted unnecessarily. For example, only 0.10 percent of those who have the HLA B 27 marker associated with ankylosing spondylitis will ever develop the disease (Lappé, 1979b). That association, however, could heighten the anxieties and affect the plans of many more people if it is misunderstood or overstressed.

These misinterpretations can also affect our social policies. Because of the connection we make between our genetic constitutions and our identities as individuals, diagnoses that trace diseases to our genes can also convey stigma and set the stage for social prejudice (Ablon, 1981). It will be the burden of the researchers to interpret the correlations they draw as clearly as possible, to avoid simplistic associations between genetic markers and clinical conditions, and to educate clinicians and the public about the actual implications of their findings for individuals.

Moreover, even where prognostic information about disease is interpreted correctly, it may still be clinically problematic. Where there is no effective therapy, new abilities to detect diseases in advance of their onset create harder choices for clinicians and patients. As we explore the human genome, more people will be faced with the dilemma that now faces those at risk from Huntington's disease: Is it better or not to know one's fate when it is out of one's control? At the same time, the very discoveries that exacerbate those dilemmas will also be crucial steps in developing of the new therapies that can help resolve them. It will be important as the project proceeds to pursue those steps and attempt to narrow, rather than widen, the gap between our abilities to diagnose and treat disease (Fletcher and Jonsen, 1984).

The Use and Abuse of a Complete Genome Map Probably the most contentious set of social problems resulting from a human genome project would be in the use of its findings. As a byproduct of the project, a great number of new diagnostic tests for specific traits and conditions will become available. The scientific and medical communities will receive an increasing variety of screening requests, ranging between those from couples making reproductive decisions to those from employers planning personnel policies. The issues they will face in considering those requests again return to the very personal nature of the information the screening tests yield: Is it ever appropriate to screen an individual for the benefit or profit of some other person or institution?

The most controversial applications of the new genetic screen would be their use by industries and insurance companies to identify individuals who might be occupational or insurance risks (Murray, 1983). As the human genome project proceeds, the ongoing discussion of these practices, and the need for sound social policy about them, will only intensify. Questions about protecting individual autonomy, the ownership of genetic information, and the interpretation of map-based medical prognoses will figure heavily in this discussion. To a large extent, any changes in social policy will reflect the ways those same questions are addressed by the scientific community in conducting the project.

Ethical questions about the appropriate use of genetic information may also be raised within the more intimate circle of the nuclear family. For example, are there limits on the traits that parents may decide their children must have? Traditionally, these limits have been set at the boundaries of the pathological conditions; screening requests for traits that have no pathological import, such as the sex of the child, are usually denied (Juengst, 1987). Yet the boundaries of conditions that might be regarded as pathological are vague. As genetic markers become available for an increasing range of traits, the ability to identify those markers prenatally will present difficult decisions for clinical geneticists: What levels of disease susceptibility or risk warrant prenatal diagnosis? Are prenatal tests for somatically correctable genetic defects, diseases with late onset, or minor defects appropriate?

Once again, these questions are not unique to the effort to map and sequence the human genome. They are all questions already presented to clinicians, geneticists, and prospective parents by current diagnostic techniques. By making an increasingly wide range of screening tests available, however, the human genome project is likely to increase the frequency with which these questions arise and the need for settled professional and social approaches to them. Fortunately, in the development of social policy and professional ethics with regard to these questions, it is already possible to draw on the resources of a large literature base and lively public discussion (for example, see Milunsky and Annas, 1985). Important steps toward social consensus on the issues have even taken place at the national level. For example, the reports of the President's Commission for the Study of Ethical Problems in Medicine and Biomedical and Behavioral Research (1982, 1983) already offer a useful orientation that can help meet the ethical challenges that mapping and sequencing the human genome would present.

Finally, it should be noted that RFLPs will continue to be developed, maps will be made, and genetic counseling will occur even without a concerted effort to map and sequence the human genome. The greater coordination and quality control that will result from a concerted effort will in fact benefit the public by reducing the chance of misuse of poorly organized information.

REFERENCES

Ablon, J. 1981. Stigmatized health conditions. Soc. Sci. Med. 15B:5–9.

Capron, A. M. 1979. Autonomy, confidentiality and quality care in genetic counseling. In A. M. Capron *et al.*, eds. Genetic Counseling: Facts, Values, and Norms (Birth Defects: Original Article Series, vol. 15). Alan R. Liss, New York. Pp. 307–340.

Fletcher, J., and A. Jonsen. 1984. Ethical considerations in prenatal diagnosis and treatment. In M. R. Harrison, M. S. Golbus, and R. A. Filly, eds. The Unborn Patient: Prenatal Diagnosis and Treatment. Grune and Stratton, New York. Pp. 159–167.

Juengst, E. 1987. Prenatal diagnosis and the ethics of uncertainty. In J. F. Monagle, and D. C. Thomasa, eds. Medical Ethics: A Guide for Health Care Professionals. Aspen, Rockville, Md. Pp. 23–32.

Lappé, M. 1979a. Theories of genetic causation in human disease. In A. M. Capron *et al.*, eds. Genetic Counseling: Facts, Values, and Norms (Birth Defects: Original Article Series, volume 15). Alan R. Liss, New York. Pp. 3–47.

Lappé, M. 1979b. Genetic Politics: The Limits of Biological Control. Simon and Schuster, New York.

Macklin, R. 1985. Mapping the human genome: Problems of privacy and free choice. In A. Milunsky and G. J. Annas, eds. Genetics and the Law III. Plenum, New York. Pp. 107–115

Milunsky, A., and G. J. Annas, eds. 1985. Genetics and the Law III. Plenum, New York.

Murray, T. H. 1983. Genetic screening in the workplace: Ethical issues. J. Occup. Med. 25:451–454.

President's Commission for the Study of Ethical Problems in Medicine and Biomedical and Behavioral Research. 1982. Splicing Life: The Social and Ethical Issues of Genetic Engineering with Human Beings. Government Printing Office, Washington, D.C.

President's Commission for the Study of Ethical Problems in Medicine and Biomedical and Behavioral Research. 1983. Screening and Counseling for Genetic Conditions: The Ethical, Social and Legal Implications of Genetic Screening, Counseling, and Education Programs. Government Printing Office, Washington, D.C.

U.S. Congress, House Committee on Science and Technology, Subcommittee on Investigations and Oversight. 1986. The Use of Human Biological Materials in the Development of Biomedical Products. 99th Cong., 1st sess. Government Printing Office, Washington, D.C.

MAPPING OUR GENES: THE GENOME PROJECTS—HOW BIG, HOW FAST?

INTRODUCTION. *In parallel with the National Research Council's investigation, the Congressional Office of Technology Assessment (OTA) conducted its own evaluation of the proposed human genome projects, as well as other genome projects in nonhuman species. Because OTA performed assessments at the request of Congress, it generally avoided making recommendations in its reports. It preferred to analyze the major issues involved in a topic, then to suggest a range of policy options for Congress. Chapter Four of this report follows. It represents the second attempt to survey the variety of ethical, legal, and social issues raised by the human genome project in a nationally circulated report. Several of the questions identified in this chapter later featured prominently in the research agenda of the Ethical, Legal, and Social Issues (ELSI) program at the National Center for Human Genome Research.*

4. Social and Ethical Considerations

INTRODUCTION

As projects to map and sequence the human genome are undertaken, their long-range social and ethical implications need to be considered as part of policy analysis, yet further knowledge is needed before many of these implications emerge. Some will arise in the course of deciding what priority to give genome projects and what level of resolution (coarse genetic linkage map, complete DNA sequence) is most appropriate. More profound ethical questions are posed by possible applications of genetic data for altering the basis of human disease, human talents, and social behavior. Questions about personal freedom, privacy, and societal versus individual rights of access to genetic information are among the most important. A full picture of the human genome will of necessity raise questions about the desirability of using genetic information to control and shape the future of human society. The complexity and urgency of these issues will increase in proportion to advances in mapping and sequencing.

Part of the reason for studying genomes is to see how *variations* in genes account for differences among people. Some of the issues raised in this chapter relate specifically to these variations: What will be the impact of discovering that, in their genetic endowment, human beings are either more equal or more unequal than we now suppose? Other problems do not concern genetic differences, but rather the impact of discovering the extent to which genes do or do not limit the options of human beings in general. One commentator has argued that scientists bear a responsibility for using "moral imagination" to anticipate the full range of uses and consequences of their work, especially when that work is in the basic sciences (2).

The social considerations raised by genome projects include ethical issues. Ethical issues often arise in the context of debates about values, principles, or human actions that have had particular merit in the past. Such debates about what *ought* to be done often cannot be resolved by empirical inquiry. Specific genetic information such as the location of a gene along a chromosome or the sequence of nucleotide bases composing a specific gene is value-neutral and as such is not ethically troublesome. However, questions about private investment versus the allocation of Federal resources or about the proper use and availability of genetic information are ethical questions because they involve choices among actions based upon competing notions about what is good, right, or desirable.

Competing ideas about the desirable course of human action are developed from considerations about the greater good, personal freedom, benefiting others, avoiding harm, and fairness and equality. It is important to note that the ethical issues surrounding the use of and access to genetic

U.S. Congress, Office of Technology Assessment, *Mapping Our Genes: The Genome Projects—How Big, How Fast?* OTA-BA-373. Washington, D.C.: U.S. Government Printing Office, April 1988.

information are not unique to the enterprise of mapping and sequencing the human genome (10). The existing uses of genetic screening, which in most cases are based on incomplete information about the location of a specific gene, already raise ethical questions. In addition, some general ethical questions are moot because of contemporary realities, for example, the question of whether there should be any human genome mapping and sequencing activities at all. This question is moot because mapping and sequencing projects have been underway for over a decade and there has been no concerted effort to prohibit them. The more immediate questions, therefore, are how these projects should best proceed from now on and what use should be made of new genetic information.

Each of the following sections begins with a list of important social and ethical questions, followed by a short general discussion establishing the context of these issues and, in some cases, outlining opposing arguments. Decisions about mapping and sequencing rest in part on arguments about appropriate allocation of resources. Arguments about access to versus control of knowledge turn on debates about the relative importance of ethical principles such as autonomy (that is, self-determination or personal freedom of action) and beneficence (the duty to act in ways that benefit and do not inflict harm on others). There is general concern about the ways in which personal freedom of action might be either enhanced or diminished by increased knowledge about human genetics. Finally, there is significant concern about the possibility of *eugenics*, that is, that new and existing information will be used in attempts to improve hereditary qualities. The social and ethical arguments relevant to mapping and sequencing the human genome reveal the tension between an attempt to arrive at some clear insight about duties and obligations and an attempt to weigh benefits versus harms. The purpose of this chapter is to describe and clarify important points of social and ethical controversy, not to resolve them.

Basic Research

- How should the conduct of research in the basic sciences, such as genome mapping and sequencing, be influenced by a concern for the social good?
- What are the considerations when basic research in the biological sciences seems to take resources away from areas of research that might have more immediate social benefit?

A genetic linkage map of the human genome already exists and progress has been made in the development of a physical map. Practical debate, therefore, centers on questions about the most efficient and effective way to develop the complete physical map, that is, whether the whole human genome should be sequenced in a systematic way and how new genetic information should be applied.

How these questions are answered depends upon the values attached to scientific progress and the relationship between scientific progress and human good. There is a strong argument that basic scientific research is valuable in and of itself and should be pursued for its own sake. Coordinated, systematic mapping of the human genome is consistent with this view, and proponents argue for resources and against constraints in the name of conducting *good science*. Others argue that scientists need to be responsive to and sometimes even constrained by the public interest (7).

Levels of Resolution

- What level of resolution of the physical map is really needed, and for what purposes?

While even a rough genetic map, permitting the identification of markers linked with major diseases, might prove useful to insurers or others bent on identifying high-risk individuals, it would have less value for basic researchers than a more precise map. From an ethical standpoint, the key arguments about levels of resolution, or molecular detail, are based on the distribution of costs and benefits involved. If the public is asked to pay an appreciable portion of the cost, then it deserves to participate in the political debate about embarking on an expensive, full-scale project. Scientific and technical factors being equal, chromosomal regions in which greater clarity would benefit many people (e.g., those associated with prevalent genetic diseases) might be addressed first. If the largest share of the costs is borne by the private sector, then few, if any, questions of priority will be posed, other than those chosen by the persons investing in the projects.

Access and Ownership

- What are the ethical considerations pertaining to control of knowledge and access to information generated by mapping and sequencing efforts?
- Who should have access to map and sequence information in data banks?
- Do scientists have a duty to share information; what are the practical extent and limits of such an obligation?
- Who owns genetic information?
- Do property rights to individuals' genetic identities adhere to them or to the human species (14)?
- Is genetic information merely a more detailed account of an individual's vital statistics, or should this information be treated as intrinsically private, not to be sought or disclosed without the individual's express consent (10)?

There is a method in scientific research that allows investigators to pursue their hunches, test their hypotheses, replicate their results, and publish their findings in roughly that order. Careful adherence to this process ensures accuracy and the orderly development of knowledge. The time lag between discovery of new information and communication of it, however, has caused some commentators to question whether scientists have the right to withhold information about genetic markers that might be of great interest to the public at large.

From an ethical perspective, it may be argued that genetic information is by definition in the public domain: The human genome is a collective property that should be held in common among all persons of human heritage (8). An opposing argument is that, since gene sequences are not commonly knowable and understanding them requires the use of expensive and often patentable machinery, discovery of sequences and the fruits that derive from them belong to the person who uncovered them. By this reasoning, it does not matter whether the sequences are unique or how they might be used; it is the labor and inventiveness associated with the discovery of them that makes them valid intellectual property. Current patent law takes the latter tack but limits patentability by preventing the patenting of a person or an idea.

One prominent scientist has acknowledged the public's special claim to the genome but argues that a public enterprise may not be the best way to satisfy this claim and that delay on so urgent a project serves no one (5). A significant portion of the value of the genetic information gathered through human genome projects will not be fully realized until some decades after the projects are completed, but there is little doubt that it will help elucidate the function and physical location of genes that cause or predispose to illness and disease. For this reason alone, the sequences will have substantial commercial value.

Commercialization

- What facets, if any, of human genome mapping and sequencing activities should be commercialized?

The commercial value of genome sequences has already been recognized by companies that have applied for patents on a number of specific materials and techniques. At least one company has argued that it has the right to copyright and control the materials and maps that it develops (5).

The selective forces of the marketplace have generated a database network, some portions of which are in the public domain and others of which are held by individual companies. The ethical issues of privatization of this knowledge turn on the importance of sequences lost to others by academic communities or corporations which have restricted the use of them. On one level, the problem is largely academic, since the data needed for a complete map and sequence could be assembled by the public sector, with duplication or purchase of the data held by private parties. On another level, however, the potential loss of critical data, the duplication of effort, and the control of knowledge raise serious questions about a combined scheme of public versus proprietary holding of fundamental knowledge. There is a strong argument that parts of research that are funded publicly should yield public information, while allowing scientists and others to retain the benefits of commercial exploitation of inventions.

Diagnostic/Therapeutic Gap

- What are the ethical implications of the growing gap between diagnostic and therapeutic capabilities?
- Should diagnostic information about genetic disorders for which there is no therapeutic remedy be handled differently from that about disorders for which there *are* therapeutic interventions?

There is no doubt that continuing scientific advances in mapping and sequencing the human genome accelerate diagnostic applications. One philosopher has noted that the ability to map the human genome yields information about susceptibility that is more precise, more certain, and potentially more threatening to individual freedom and privacy than earlier methods of presymptomatic diagnosis and vague hypotheses about familial traits (10). A related issue is the need to protect information that may be available to or sought by third parties such as insurance companies or employers. Progress to date indicates that the ability to diagnose a genetic abnormality precedes the development of therapeutic interventions and that this gap may be growing. This is true for many genetic diseases, an important example being Huntington's disease.

Physician Practice

- Do physicians and other health care providers face a conflict between an increasingly reductive approach to medical science and a focus on holistic patient care (17)?

Increased information about human genetics changes attitudes and alters the knowledge that serves as a basis for health care interventions. Physicians and other health care providers must constantly alter their views and understanding of human behavior, health, and disease. There are many examples of diseases that were once thought to be amenable to preventive health care that are now known to have a genetic component or cause. On a practical level this presents obvious difficulties, as health care providers are increasingly uncertain whether they are dealing with patterns of health and illness in individuals that can be ameliorated by changes in life style and medical treatment or if such patterns are in large part a matter of genetic destiny. In addition, the ethical principle of respect for persons indicates that individuals must be treated with care, compassion, and hope because they are persons and not merely the embodiments of a genetic formula or code.

Reproductive Choices

- What ethical considerations arise from the increased ability of parents to determine the genetic endowment of their children (through such practices as selective termination of pregnancy, selective discarding of human embryos created in vitro, or selection of X- or Y-bearing sperm to determine the sex of the child)?

The ethical question of one generation's duties and obligations to another becomes more evident as genome mapping generates data pointing to the serious consequences of certain cultural practices or mating patterns. For example, it has been demonstrated that, if it were possible to choose the sex of their children, many individuals and couples would prefer that their firstborn be male (18). It has also been demonstrated that firstborn children benefit from their early period of exclusive parental attention. If firstborn boys became the norm, it might further compromise equality of opportunity between men and women (16). In such circumstances, the conflicts among values and ethical principles such as autonomy, justice, and beneficence will be strong. Human mating that proceeds without the use of genetic data about the risks of transmitting diseases will produce greater mortality and medical costs than if carriers of potentially deleterious genes are alerted to their status and encouraged to mate with noncarriers or to use artificial insemination or other reproductive strategies (3).

On a practical level, the availability of information that couples might use to select embryos created in vitro has been hampered by an absence of federally funded research concerning many aspects of human fertilization. There has been a de facto moratorium on such research since 1980 (13).

Eugenic Implications

- What ethical concerns arise from possible eugenic applications of mapping and sequencing data?

The possibility of mastery and control over human DNA once again raises the highly charged issue of genetic selection. One major difference between current and previous attempts at eugenic manipulation is that any potential eugenicist will have substantially more powerful techniques to effect desired ends and more data with which to muster support. With even the modest knowledge achieved in their first century, genetic techniques have become sophisticated enough to permit the use of selective breeding to produce animals with desired qualities.

When Francis Galton defined eugenics in 1883 as the science of improving the "stock," he intended the concept to extend to any techniques that might serve to increase the representation of those with "good genes." Thus, he indicated that eugenics was "by no means confined to questions of judicious mating, but takes cognisance of all the influences that tend, in however remote a degree, to give the more suitable races or strains of blood a better chance of prevailing speedily over the less suitable than they otherwise would have had" (4). Prior to the development of recombinant DNA technology, eugenic aims were primarily achieved by attempting to control social practices such as marriage. New technologies for identifying traits and altering genes make it possible for eugenic goals to be achieved through technological as opposed to social control.

Knowledge of human genetics will amplify the power to intervene in the diagnosis and treatment of disease. Each time a person who would otherwise have died of a disease caused or influenced by a gene is treated successfully by genetic or nongenetic means, the frequency of that gene in the population increases. Human genome projects will intensify and accelerate the already difficult debates about who should have access to one's genetic information by providing faster and cheaper methods of testing for genetic variations, by making much more information available, and by increasing the specificity of genetic information (15). The ethical debate about eugenic applications more properly focuses on *how to use* new information rather than on *whether to discover* it. Eugenic programs are offensive because they single out particular people and therefore can be socially coercive and threatening to the ideas that human beings have dignity and are free agents.

Positive Eugenics Beginning with Plato, philosophers have recognized that eugenic ends could be achieved through subtle or direct incentives to bring together presumptively fit human beings. Positive eugenics is defined here as the achievement of systematic or planned genetic changes in individuals or their offspring that improve overall human life and health and that can be achieved by programs that do not require direct manipulation of genetic material.

Most commentators have rejected or cast doubt on any uses of genetic engineering to enhance or directly improve the human condition. The President's Commission for the Study of Ethical Problems in Medicine and Biomedical and Behavioral Research declared that efforts to improve or enhance normal people, as opposed to ameliorating the deleterious effects of genes, are at best problematic (11).

It may well be that the problem with positive eugenics has more to do with the means than with the ends. The basic objective of improving the human condition is generally supported, although debates about just what constitutes such improvement continue. Many concerns about eugenic policies in the past focused on the methods used to attain them, such as sterilization, rather than on the ends themselves.

Negative Eugenics Negative eugenics refers to policies and programs that are intended to reduce the occurrence of genetically determined disease. It implies the selective elimination of gametes (ova or sperm) and fetuses that carry deleterious genes, as well as the discouraging of carriers of markers for genetic disease from procreation. There are few technical obstacles to karyotyping human beings for eugenic reasons. Verbal genetic histories of sperm donors, for example, are designed to exclude donors carrying some genetic diseases. Such a screening process, accompanied by a physical examination and laboratory tests, has already been recommended by the Ethics Committee of the American Fertility Society (1). The development of specific genetic tests could make gamete screening easier and more specific and will also expand existing capabilities to conduct prenatal tests.

Eugenics of Normalcy The third eugenic use of genetic information would be to ensure not merely that a person lacks severe incapacitating genetic conditions, but that each individual has at least a modicum of normal genes. One commentator has argued that individuals have a paramount right to be born with a normal, adequate hereditary endowment (6). This argument is based on the idea that there can be some consensus about the nature of a normal genetic endowment for different groups of the human species. The idea of genetic normalcy, once far-fetched, is drawing closer with the development of a full genetic map and sequence; however, concepts of what is normal will always be influenced by cultural variations and subject to considerable debate.

Attitudes

- How will a complete map and sequence of the human genome transform attitudes and perceptions of ourselves and others?

One of the strongest arguments for supporting human genome projects is that they will provide knowledge about the determinants of the human condition. One group of scientists has urged support of human genome projects because sequencing the human genome will provide one of the most powerful tools humankind has ever had for deciphering the mysteries of its own existence (12).

The relevance of this proposition will depend on the degree to which complex human behaviors are determined by understandable genetic factors. It will also depend on how important human genome projects are to understanding genetic factors for complex traits. Whether higher human attributes are reducible to molecular constructs is a topic of considerable debate in the philosophy of biology, and human genome projects would doubtless enlarge and intensify this debate. A reasonable hypothesis is that, while little information of direct or immediate value regarding complex behaviors is likely to result from human genome projects, insights into the possible construction of control regions for the development of the human embryo, the genetic basis for organizing neuronal pathways, and the genetic control of sexual differentiation will all be significantly enhanced. In the long run, knowledge of human genetics will make scientific understanding of human life more sophisticated.

A greatly increased understanding of how genes shape characteristics could influence human beings' attitudes toward themselves and others. Such increased understanding might highlight the degree to which genetic factors are equal or unequal for traits that confer social advantage. This information might reveal that human beings have fewer options than they suppose and could thereby encourage a determinist view of human choices, or it could reveal just the opposite. A general increase in genetic information might also alter social customs based on erroneous scientific assumptions.

Many individuals have general beliefs about their genetic potential for achievement in certain spheres of activity, about the limits of possible improvement through effort or environmental change. These intuitive beliefs are often vague and inaccurate. Often, it is only in regard to a few skills or characteristics that individuals have pushed against the limits of their potential. When science makes it possible to trace the actual limits of individuals, intuitive perceptions may turn out to be wrong. This has the potential of both enhancing and limiting personal liberty.

Role of Government

- What is the proper role of government in mapping and sequencing the human genome?
- Specifically, does the government have a role in deciding what data should be collected in gene mapping and sequencing? How should this information be disseminated and guarded from abuse?

The lines of power, coercion, and authority in the public and private scientific sectors are blurred because the first genetic maps are being made in corporations (e.g., Collaborative Research, Inc.) and in private philanthropies based in universities (e.g., the Howard Hughes Medical Institute at the University of Utah).

The ethical arguments for involving the Federal Government in the process of genome mapping, whether by shaping, constraining, blocking, or doing nothing, center on the public interest in making resources available in ways that are consistent with the considerations of beneficence, justice, and autonomy. These issues encompass academic freedom or freedom of scientific inquiry because the projects have universal and lasting implications. Once the human genome is mapped and sequenced, the resulting data will have widespread implications for generations to come.

The precise boundary between basic and applied science is hard to draw, but there is enough understanding of where it lies to be able to use it as a basis for policy. A case might very well be made for a government policy that would leave basic research unrestricted but that would place some stringent controls on applied research and technological applications, for example, by ensuring that genetic testing is voluntary and access to data is controlled.

All research carries with it the likelihood of changing one's conception of the world and so of changing one's attitudes. For these reasons, there is a strong case against government intervention to stop research. There are four main arguments:

1. Stopping research might be opting for comfortable ignorance or illusion rather than uncomfortable truth. The growth of science has rested on the preference for uncomfortable truth. Those who view science as one of mankind's finest creations will be dismayed at any wholesale repudiation of this preference.
2. It is unlikely that existing world views, beliefs, and attitudes can be protected by shutting down basic research. The knowledge that such protection was needed might itself start to undermine existing views.
3. As a practical matter, it may be that government cannot stop basic research. It is not easy to monitor what goes on in laboratories, and what is stopped in one country may take place in another.
4. Stopping research blocks both possible benefits and risks. The belief that research can be performed to permit benefits while coping with and occasionally avoiding risks is a matter of historical precedent.

Duties Beyond Borders

- What, if any, ethical issues are raised when considerations of international competitiveness influence basic scientific research?
- What, if any, are the duties and obligations of the United States to disseminate mapping and sequencing information abroad?
- What are the implications of shared information for international competitiveness?
- What are the international implications of sharing technological applications of mapping and sequencing information?
- What issues are involved when applications of genetic information or biotechnology that are of great use to Third World countries are not developed or fully exploited because they are less profitable for industrialized countries?

The United States has recently proposed an international framework of rules for science. The purpose of this framework is to see that all nations do their fair share of basic research and that all the results of such research be made public, except for those with strategic implications (9). The increased protection of intellectual property and patent rights for technological innovations formed the basis of this proposal; these rights were also central to recent international trade talks. There is some sentiment that barriers to the transfer of technology would continue even if there were no reward for intellectual property. One commentator has noted that, unless products are protected by a set of principles now, basic scientific results could become increasingly restricted; some nations might do less basic research and instead emphasize applying other nations' results (9).

The most common single-gene defects, disorders of the hemoglobin molecules that carry oxygen in red blood cells, are highly prevalent in many nations in Southern Europe, Africa, the Middle East, and Asia. Such nations would benefit most if research tools became widely available as they were developed and if priorities for which chromosomal regions are mapped first took world prevalence of disorders into account. Use of map and sequence information by developing nations may also require special attention to devising screening tests that are cheap and simple, and might entail access to services (e.g., sequencing or mapping) located in developed nations.

Conclusion

All human beings have a vital interest in the social and ethical implications of mapping and sequencing the human genome. It is not surprising, therefore, that there are debates about how genome projects should proceed. These extend beyond considerations of scientific efficacy and involve the interests of patients, research subjects, physicians, academicians, lawyers, entrepreneurs, and politicians. Mapping the human genome accelerates our rate of understanding—and the distance between increased understanding and direct intervention to alter the human genome is shrinking. Add to this the development of scientific tools such as gene probes, and immediate practical questions are posed: How should basic research be conducted? What level of resolution in mapping is necessary? Who should have access to and ownership of data banks and clone repositories? How should thorny questions surrounding commercialization be handled? Long-range questions about eugenics; reproductive choices, the role of government, and possible duties and obligations beyond national borders also arise. These questions are complex and are not likely to be resolved in the near future. It will therefore be necessary to ensure that some means for explicitly addressing ethical issues attends scientific work.

REFERENCES

1. American Fertility Society, Ethics Committee, "Ethical Considerations of the New Reproductive Technologies," *Fertility and Sterility* 46:1S-94S, 1986.
2. Callahan, D., "Ethical Responsibility in Science in the Face of Uncertain Consequences," *Annals of the New York Academy of Sciences* 265:1–12, 1976.
3. Campbell, R.B., "The Effects of Genetic Screening and Assortative Mating on Lethal Recessive-Allele Frequencies and Homozygote Incidence," *American Journal of Human Genetics* 41:671–677, 1987.
4. Galton, F., *Inquiries Into Human Faculty* (London: Macmillan, 1883).
5. Gilbert, W., quoted in Roberts, L., "Who Owns the Human Genome?" *Science* 237:358–361, 1987.
6. Glass, B., "Ethical Problems Raised by Genetics," in *Genetics and the Quality of Life*, Charles Birch and Paul Abrecht (eds.) (New York, NY: Pergamon Press, 1974), pp. 51–57.
7. Institute of Medicine, *Responding to Health Needs and Scientific Opportunity: The Organizational Structure of the National Institutes of Health* (Washington, DC: National Academy Press, 1984).
8. Issues of Collaboration for Human Genome Projects, OTA workshop, June 26, 1987.
9. MacKenzie, D., "US Advocates a 'World Code' for Science," *New Scientist* 5 (November): 245, 1987.
10. Macklin, R., "Mapping the Human Genome: Problems of Privacy and Free Choice," *Genetics and the Law III*, A. Milunsky and G.J. Annas (eds.) (New York, NY: Plenum Press, 1985), pp. 107–114.
11. President's Commission for the Study of Ethical Problems in Medicine and Biomedical and Behavioral Research, *Screening and Counseling for Genetic Conditions: A Report on the Ethical, Social, and Legal Implications for Genetic Screening, Counseling and Education Programs* (Washington, DC: U.S. Government Printing Office, 1983).
12. Smith, L., and Hood, L., "Mapping and Sequencing the Human Genome: How To Proceed," *BioTechnology* 5:933–939, 1987.
13. U.S. Congress, Office of Technology Assessment, *Infertility: Medical and Social Choices*, OTA-BA-358 (Washington, DC: U.S. Government Printing Office, May 1988).
14. U.S. Congress, Office of Technology Assessment, *New Developments in Biotechnology: Ownership of Human Tissues and Cells*, OTA-BA-337 (Washington, DC: U.S. Government Printing Office, March 1987).
15. U.S. Congress, Office of Technology Assessment, *Human Gene Therapy*, OTA-BP-BA-32 (Washington, DC: U.S. Government Printing Office, December, 1984), App. B.
16. Walters, L., "Is Sex Selection a Frivolous Practice? Yes," *Washington Post*, Apr. 7, 1987, p. 11.
17. Weatherall, D., "Molecules and Man," *Nature* 328: 771–772, 1987.
18. Westoff, C.F., "Sex Preselection in the United States, Some Implications," *Science* 184:633–636, 1974.

Part IV

ETHICAL ISSUES ARISING FROM HUMAN REPRODUCTIVE TECHNOLOGIES AND ARRANGEMENTS

READINGS ON HUMAN REPRODUCTION: INTRODUCTION

LeRoy Walters

PART FOUR CONTAINS readings on older and newer techniques for assisting human reproduction. It does not cover the topic of abortion or include readings on human embryo research or fetal research (for the latter, see part 1). The three primary techniques covered in this chapter are assisted insemination, in vitro (test-tube) fertilization, and surrogate parenting arrangements.

Principal Reproductive Technologies and Arrangements

Artificial Insemination Of three principal reproductive technologies and arrangements, artificial insemination is the oldest technique of assisted reproduction. Already in 1779 an Italian priest and physiologist, Lazaro Spallanzani, had unequivocally demonstrated assisted insemination in toads. The next step was taken in 1790 by John Hunter, a Scottish anatomist and surgeon. Hunter inseminated the wife of a linen draper, using her husband's sperm (Corea, 1985). Assisted insemination with donor sperm was not undertaken until almost a century later. In the late 1800s William Panacost, a medical professor in Philadelphia, agreed to help a wealthy couple overcome their infertility. Panacost asked the best-looking student of the current medical-school class to volunteer as a semen donor. He then performed the insemination in his office, with the wife under general anesthesia. Neither the husband nor the wife was informed about the precise method employed to initiate the pregnancy (Andrews, 1985).

A survey by the Congressional Office of Technology Assessment (OTA) provides rather detailed information about the practice of assisted insemination in the late 1980s. Based on a cross-sectional sample, OTA estimated that approximately 172,000 women underwent assisted insemination during a twelve-month period in 1986 to 1987. As a result of these inseminations approximately 65,000 infants were born—35,000 after insemination with the husband's sperm (AIH), and 30,000 after insemination with donor sperm (AID). About 92 percent of the inseminated women were married, and another 2 percent were living with male partners.

Approximately half the donor semen was derived from sperm banks; the other half was provided by physician-selected donors. In 1986–1987, 22 percent of practitioners used fresh semen exclusively in their donor inseminations. However, by early 1988 the American Fertility Society, the Center for Disease Control, and the Food and Drug Administration all recommended that only frozen semen be used for donor insemination, so that donor sperm could be quarantined for six months and the donor retested for antibody to the virus that causes AIDS. It is therefore likely that most donor inseminations in the United States are currently performed with frozen sperm (Office of Technology Assessment, 1988a).

In the selections that follow, assisted insemination is a subsidiary theme, in part because many of the issues it raises are also raised by egg donation and in vitro fertilization. Nevertheless, documents from the Vatican's Congregation for the Doctrine of the Faith, the Office of Technology Assessment, the Glover Commission, and the Canadian Royal Commission all consider the question of assisted insemination.

In Vitro Fertilization The first documented success with in vitro fertilization (IVF) in the laboratory occurred in 1959. In a paper published in *Nature*, M.C. Chang of the Worcester Foundation in Massachusetts reported that he had used sperm from male rabbits to fertilize eggs taken from female rabbits. The fact that the offspring had characteristics that were present in the males but absent in the females demonstrated that in vitro fertilization had in fact occurred (Chang, 1959).

The next step in the development of IVF occurred in 1970, when R.G. Edwards, P.C. Steptoe, and J.M. Purdy reported a successful fertilization in vitro using human sperm and egg cells (Edwards et al., 1970). Attempts at embryo transfer after IVF followed in 1973 (de Kretzer et al., 1973) and 1976 (Steptoe and Edwards, 1976). Finally, in 1978 Steptoe and Edwards reported the first human birth following in vitro fertilization (Steptoe and Edwards, 1978).

The birth of Louise Brown in Lancashire, England, on July 25, 1978, inaugurated a new era in the history of the reproductive technologies. Her birth was followed by similar successes in Australia and the United States. By the early 1990s there were so many births after IVF in so many parts of the world that it was difficult for anyone to keep to maintain a global record. The best estimates were that, worldwide, more than 25,000 infants had been born with the assistance of this new technique.

The most common situation for the use of IVF involved sperm from the husband and eggs from the wife and immediate embryo transfer; however, this situation was gradually supplemented by more complex variations. Many centers began to administer hormones to women, in order to stimulate the production of multiple eggs per cycle. The goal of this intervention was to reduce the number of egg retrieval procedures women would need to undergo. Gradually, infertility centers also developed the capacity to freeze early embryos after IVF, thus allowing the deferral of embryo transfer to a later ovarian cycle, or, if a pregnancy was established, to a later stage in the couple's life. Sperm and egg donation also became part of the IVF picture in cases where one or both members of the couple were unable to provide viable reproductive cells.

More than any other reproductive technique, the practice of IVF has captured public attention since the late 1970s. All but two of the documents reprinted in this chapter discuss in vitro fertilization.

Surrogate Parenting Arrangements Surrogate parenting arrangements usually involve a commissioning couple and a woman who gestates and delivers the child for the couple. The reproductive techniques employed are either artificial insemination of the surrogate mother with sperm from the commissioning father, or in vitro fertilization using sperm and eggs from the commissioning couple and subsequent embryo transfer to the uterus of the surrogate. The novel reproductive arrangement is that the surrogate mother is the gestational mother for the commissioning couple.

The first documented attempt to employ a surrogate motherhood arrangement in the United States occurred in 1976 under the direction of Michigan attorney Noel Keane (Keane and Breo, 1981). In 1985 the first instance of surrogate motherhood following in vitro fertilization was reported (Utian et al., 1985). While surrogate parenthood in the United States has usually involved an intermediary who formalizes an agreement, or contract, between the surrogate mother and the commissioning parents, as well as arranging for the payment of a fee, a formal and commercial relationship is not a necessary part of surrogate motherhood. In some subcultures a fertile wife readily conceives and bears an extra child for her sister if the sister is infertile. Further, there have been anecdotal reports of noncommercial surrogacy arrangements in which a fertile woman bore a child for an infertile friend or coworker.

What distinguishes surrogate parenting arrangements from other types of third-party involvement in reproduction is the duration and intensity of the third party's involvement. Whereas semen donation requires only minutes and egg donation only days, a surrogate mother is pregnant for approximately nine months, interacts physically with the fetus, gives birth to a child, may interact with the future social parents, and sometimes develops an emotional attachment to the fetus or child. Thus, it is not surprising that conflicts have sometimes occurred between commissioning parents and surrogate mothers. A few of these conflicts have had to be resolved by the courts.

In terms of its frequency, surrogate motherhood pales by comparison with assisted insemination and in vitro fertilization. There are probably no more than 100 paid surrogate motherhood arrangements in the United States in any given year. However, the questions that surrogacy has raised about the meaning of parenthood are profound. Eight of the excerpts reprinted in this section discuss the topic.

Ethical and General Issues Arising from Assisted Reproduction

Each of the reproductive techniques surveyed here raises unique ethical issues, but some important general questions are also raised by assisted reproduction. A first question is whether it is somehow unnatural for would-be parents to seek professional assistance in reproduction and for health professionals to provide such assistance. Common to all three assisted techniques is the collection of reproductive cells or early human embryos and the placement of those cells or embryos into the body of the woman by some means other than sexual intercourse. For some critics of assisted reproduction—for example, Leon Kass and the Congregation for the Doctrine of the Faith—this separation of reproduction from sexual intercourse, in and of itself, renders the entire approach ethically dubious. On the other hand, proponents of assisted reproduction point to what they consider to be the rational and even natural desire of infertile couples to have children that are as closely related to them as possible.

A second issue that relates especially to in vitro fertilization and gestational surrogacy (surrogate motherhood in conjunction with IVF) is the moral status of the early human embryo. As in the research context, some commentators regard the early human embryo in the clinical context as a human being in the strong sense of that term. Thus, they criticize the discarding of early embryos that are not needed by a couple or that are diagnosed to have a genetic or chromosomal abnormality. Even the freezing and long-term cryopreservation of early embryos raises difficult metaphysical and ethical questions. Proponents of assisted reproduction argue that the early human embryo deserves respect because of its potential to become a person; nonetheless, it does not deserve the full measure of respect accorded to persons precisely because it is not yet a person.

A third issue raised by reproductive technologies and arrangements is the role of genetic lineage. Some ethical commentators favor the use of assisted reproduction when the sperm cells and egg cells originate with the couple that intends to raise the child—usually a husband and wife. These commentators thus approve of assisted insemination with the husband's sperm and of in vitro fertilization using the husband's sperm and the wife's egg. However, they regard as ethically unacceptable the introduction of extramarital reproductive cells into the marital relationship. Proponents of this "intramarital" position sometimes urge couples who cannot have a child with their own reproductive cells to consider the alternative of adoption.

Other ethical commentators disagree with the intramarital position, arguing that some couples may have no other alternative if they wish to have a child who is genetically related to either one of them. Proponents of the "extramarital" position also note that couples may resort to assisted reproduction with donor sperm or eggs in order to avoid passing on a genetic trait or disease to their children. According to supporters of donation, even in the most extreme case—two infertile spouses and the transfer of a donor embryo into the uterus of the wife—the experience of gestation and birth allows both husband and wife to participate in reproduction as fully as possible.

A fourth and final issue raised by these technologies is the role of payment or commercial motivation in assisted reproduction. This issue can be confronted at several levels. The first question is whether the providers of sperm, eggs, or early embryos should be paid and, if so, for what they are being paid—their time, the risks to their physical health, or the reproductive cells or embryos themselves. Second, in surrogate parenting arrangements most surrogate mothers are paid a fee for the gestation and delivery of a child. Some ethical commentators have asked whether this payment is for the risks to the surrogate's health and her service of carrying and delivering the child or whether the payment is for the infant itself.

Third, in the case of donor sperm and eggs, as well as in the case of surrogacy, there are often third parties who serve as intermediaries between prospective parents and donors or surrogates. Sperm banks and surrogate parenting agencies are examples of such intermediaries. Some commentators have questioned whether such intermediaries should be commercial firms seeking to make a profit from reproduction. More recently, a fourth question has been raised about commercial motivation—namely, whether assisted reproduction, and especially in vitro fertilization, has been oversold by infertility clinics, some of which may have engaged in deceptive advertising about success rates.

Social and Public-Policy Responses to the New Reproductive Techniques

During the early 1970s, sporadic discussion of the new reproductive techniques, especially in vitro fertilization, occurred in the public domain. Commentators like Paul Ramsey and Leon Kass expressed serious reservations about IVF (Ramsey, 1972; Kass, 1971 and 1972). In contrast, Joseph Fletcher celebrated the liberation of human reproduction from the throes of what he termed "reproductive roulette" (Fletcher, 1971 and 1974). However, it was 1978 before an official public-policy group—the Ethics Advisory Board of the U.S. Department of Health, Education, and Welfare (DHEW)—undertook a detailed study of IVF. Published in May 1979, this study initiated what might be called the golden age of public reports on the reproductive technologies. Between 1979 and 1987, no fewer than 16 reports on this topic were available from countries as diverse as Spain, the Netherlands, Australia, and the United Kingdom (Walters, 1987; Institute of Medicine, 1989). The first three excerpts in this chapter represent this golden age.

The technology of IVF diffused from the United Kingdom to Australia to the United States. However, in the United States, public policy on assisted reproduction was stymied in the late 1970s and early 1980s. The dismissal of Secretary Joseph Califano before he could respond to the Ethics Advisory Board report was an initial setback. The Board itself was dissolved in 1980, following the establishment of the President's Commission on Bioethics in 1979. In the 1980s, neither Democratic nor Republican administrations saw fit to respond to the Ethics Advisory Board report or to lift a de facto moratorium on federal funding for research on IVF that had existed since 1975. Moreover, the mandate of the President's Commission on Bioethics did not include any of the reproductive technologies and arrangements.

Since 1983, public responsibility for evaluating the clinical uses of assisted reproductive techniques has been divided among three groups in the United States. First, professional organizations like the American College of Obstetricians and Gynecologists (ACOG) and the American Fertility Society (AFS) have published ethical analyses and guidelines—for their members, of course, but also for the broader society. Excerpts from an AFS report and the entire text of an ACOG committee statement are reprinted in this volume. Second, in the absence of any action by the President, the Congressional Office of Technology Assessment undertook important studies of assisted insemination (1988a) and infertility (1988b). The ethics chapter of the infertility report is reprinted below. Third, the states became involved with the reproductive technologies, both in the courts and in reports by state-level bioethics commissions or task forces (New York, 1988; New Jersey, 1992). Excerpts from the best-known court decision on reproduction—*In the Matter of Baby M*—are included in this section. Other important court decisions were handed down by the state supreme courts of Tennessee and California (Tennessee, 1992; California, 1993).

Three recent perspectives from outside the United States are also represented in this section. The first is the official position of the Roman Catholic Church, as represented by the *Instruction on Respect for Human Life.* According to the Instruction, most of the assisted reproductive technologies and arrangements are incompatible with the Church's teaching on sexuality and respect for the early forms of human life. Assisted insemination with the husband's sperm, when performed in conjunction with sexual intercourse, and possibly the placement of a couple's sperm and egg cells at the distal end of the Fallopian tube—a procedure called gamete intrafallopian transfer (GIFT)—are the only modes of assisted reproduction that are deemed to be ethically acceptable.

The second perspective comes from an international consortium of Europeans led by British philosopher Jonathan Glover. This group sought to achieve a moderate consensus that could then be recommended for adoption by the European Commission. The final perspective is provided by a well-financed and comprehensive Canadian study, the report of the Royal Commission on New Reproductive Technologies. In this report a growing skepticism is evident concerning the value of assisted reproduction, at least in many cases, and a willingness to have government actively involved in regulating some activities and prohibiting others.

REFERENCES

Andrews, Lori B. *New Conceptions: A Consumer's Guide to the Newest Infertility Treatments.* New York: Ballantine Books, 1985.

California, State Department of Health Services, Genetic Disease Branch. The California Alpha Fetoprotein Screening Program. Berkeley: Genetic Disease Branch, 1994.

Chang, M.C. "Fertilization of Rabbit Ova 'in vitro'." *Nature* 184(4684): 466–467; 8 August 1959.

Corea, Gena. *The Mother Machine: From Artificial Insemination to Artificial Wombs.* New York: Harper & Row, 1985.

de Kretzer, D., et al. "Transfer of a Human Zygote." *Lancet* 2(7831): 728–729; 29 September 1973.

Edwards R.G., et al. "Fertilization and Cleavage in vitro of Preovulator Human Oocytes." *Nature* 227(5265): 1307–1309; 26 September 1970.

Fletcher, Joseph. "Ethical Aspects of Genetic Controls: Designed Genetic Changes in Man." *New England Journal of Medicine* 285(14): 776–783; 30 September 1971.

———. *The Ethics of Genetic Control.* Garden City, NY: Anchor Books, 1974.

Institute of Medicine, Division of Health Sciences Policy, and National Research Council, Board on Agriculture, Committee on the Basic Science Foundations of Medically Assisted Conception. *Medically Assisted Conception: An Agenda for Research.* Washington, DC: National Academy Press, 1989.

Kass, Leon R. "Babies by Means of In Vitro Fertilization: Unethical Experiments on the Unborn?" *New England Journal of Medicine* 285(21): 1174–1179; 18 November 1971.

———. "Making Babies—The New Biology and the 'Old' Morality." *Public Interest* No. 26: 18–56; Winter 1972.

Keane, Noel P., and Dennis L. Breo. *The Surrogate Mother.* New York: Dodd, Mead, 1981.

New Jersey Commission on Legal and Ethical Problems in the Delivery of Health Care. *After Baby M: The Legal, Ethical and Social Dimensions of Surrogacy.* Trenton, New Jersey: the Commission, September 1992.

New York State Task Force on Life and the Law. *Surrogate Parenting: Analysis and Recommendations for Public Policy.* New York: the Task Force, May 1988.

Ramsey, Paul. "Shall We 'Reproduce'?" *Journal of the American Medical Association* 220(10): 1346–1350; 5 June 1972 and 220(11): 1480–1485; 12 June 1972.

Steptoe, P.C., and Edwards, R.G. "Preimplantation of a Human Embryo with Subsequent Tubal Pregnancy." *Lancet* 1(7965): 880–882; 24 April 1976.

———. "Birth after the Reimplantation of a Human Embryo" [Letter]. *Lancet* 2(8085): 366; 12 August 1978.

Tennessee Supreme Court at Knoxville. *Davis v. Davis.* Decided. June 1, 1992. South Western Reporter, 2d Series, 842: 588–604.

U.S. Congress, Office of Technology Assessment. *Artificial Insemination: Practice in the United States.* Washington, D.C.: U.S. Government Printing Office, 1988a.

———. *Infertility: Medical and Social Choices.* Washington, D.C.: U.S. Government Printing Office, 1988b.

Utian, Wulf H., et al. "Successful Pregnancy after In Vitro Fertilization and Embryo Transfer from an Infertile Woman to a Surrogate" [Letter]. *New England Journal of Medicine* 313(21): 1351–1352; 21 November 1985.

Walters, LeRoy. "Ethics and New Reproductive Technologies: An International Review of Committee Statements." *Hastings Center Report* 17(3, Supplement): S3-S9; June 1987.

HEW SUPPORT OF RESEARCH INVOLVING *IN VITRO* FERTILIZATION AND EMBRYO TRANSFER

INTRODUCTION. *In May 1978, the newly created Ethics Advisory Board (EAB) agreed to review a research proposal that involved in vitro fertilization and to forward its recommendations to the Secretary of Health, Education, and Welfare. The birth of Louise Brown in Lancashire, England, on July 25 of that year led to a dramatic increase of public interest in this topic. While the primary focus of the May 1977 report was on research, several of its recommendations were also relevant to clinical practice—particularly the recommendation that embryo transfer be attempted only when the gametes had been obtained from "lawfully married couples." The EAB report was the first extended treatment of the new reproductive technology by a national advisory commission or committee. (A more extended excerpt from this report appears in the research section [part one] of this volume.)*

Conclusion 1

The department should consider support of carefully designed research involving *in vitro* fertilization and embryo transfer in animals, including nonhuman primates, in order to obtain a better understanding of the process of fertilization, implantation and embryo development, to assess the risks to both mother and offspring associated with such procedures, and to improve the efficacy of the procedure.

* * *

Conclusion 2

The ethics advisory board finds that it is acceptable from an ethical standpoint to undertake research involving human *in vitro* fertilization and embryo transfer provided that:

A. If the research involves human *in vitro* fertilization without embryo transfer, the following conditions are satisfied:

1. The research complies with all appropriate provisions of the regulations governing research with human subjects (45 CFR 46);
2. The research is designed primarily: (a) to establish the safety and efficacy of embryo transfer and (b) to obtain important scientific information toward that end not reasonably attainable by other means;
3. Human gametes used in such research will be obtained exclusively from persons who have been informed of the nature and purpose of the research in which such materials will be used and have specifically consented to such use;
4. No embryos will be sustained *in vitro* beyond the stage normally associated with the completion of implantation (14 days after fertilization); and
5. All interested parties and the general public will be advised if evidence begins to show that the procedure entails risks of abnormal offspring higher than those associated with natural human reproduction.

B. In addition, if the research involves embryo transfer following human *in vitro* fertilization, embryo transfer will be attempted only with gametes obtained from lawfully married couples.

* * *

U.S. Department of Health, Education, and Welfare, Ethics Advisory Board, *Report and Conclusions: HEW Support of Research Involving In Vitro Fertilization and Embryo Transfer*, Washington, D.C.: U.S. Government Printing Office, May 4, 1979.

Conclusion 3

The board finds it acceptable from an ethical standpoint for the department to support or conduct research involving human *in vitro* fertilization and embryo transfer, provided that the applicable conditions set forth in conclusion 2 are met. However, the board has decided not to address the question of the level of funding, if any, which such research might be given.

* * *

Conclusion 4

The National Institute of Child Health and Human Development (NICHD) and other appropriate agencies should work with professional societies, foreign governments and international organizations to collect, analyze and disseminate information derived from research (in both animals and humans) and clinical experience throughout the world involving *in vitro* fertilization and embryo transfer.

* * *

Conclusion 5

The secretary should encourage the development of a uniform or model law to clarify the legal status of children born as a result of *in vitro* fertilization and embryo transfer. To the extent that funds may be necessary to develop such legislation, the department should consider providing appropriate support.

COMMITTEE TO CONSIDER THE SOCIAL, ETHICAL AND LEGAL ISSUES ARISING FROM *IN VITRO* FERTILIZATION—FIRST INTERIM REPORT OF THE WALLER COMMITTEE, VICTORIA, AUSTRALIA

INTRODUCTION. *In 1979 the first Australian clinical pregnancy after in vitro fertilization (IVF) was initiated at the Royal Women's Hospital in the state of Victoria. During the next two years, additional IVF pregnancies at this hospital and the Queen Victoria Medical Center established Victoria as one of the world's leading centers for the new reproductive technologies. Not surprisingly, questions began to be raised about coverage for this expensive technology under the state's public health insurance program, about criteria for the selection of participants in IVF programs, and about research involving early human embryos. In response, in May 1982 the state government of Victoria appointed an interdisciplinary advisory committee to study IVF and to make recommendations to public policymakers. The following pages are excerpts from the first of three reports issued by the Waller Committee between 1982 and 1984.*

Establishment of the Committee

On 11 March, 1982 the then Attorney-General and the Minister of Health jointly announced the Government's intention to establish a Committee to investigate the social, ethical and legal issues surrounding the procedure of in vitro fertilization (IVF) as conducted in Victoria. . . . The Attorney-General and the Minister of Health finalized the Committee's terms of reference and its membership, which were announced on 24 May, 1982.

The Committee is of an interdisciplinary nature with nine members. The Chairman of the Committee is Professor Louis Waller, Sir Leo Cussen Professor of Law, Monash University, and Law Reform Commissioner, and the other members are Reverend Dr. Francis Harman, moral theologian of the Catholic Church; Mrs. Jasna Hay, former teacher with interests in migrant welfare and education; the Reverend Dr. John Henley, Lecturer in Christian Ethics and Dean of the Melbourne College of Divinity; Ms. Eva Learner, Social Worker and Director of the Human Resource Centre of La Trobe University and the Lincoln Institute of Health Sciences; Dr. James McDonald, general practitioner with a substantial practice in obstetrics and gynaecology; Miss Lynnette Opas, senior Counsel practising in family law; Professor Priscilla Kincaid-Smith, Professor of Medicine, University of Melbourne, Director, Department of Nephrology, Royal Melbourne Hospital and Professor Roger Pepperell, Professor of Obstetrics and Gynaecology, University of Melbourne.

1. The Committee's Terms of Reference

To consider whether the process of in vitro fertilization (IVF) should be conducted in Victoria and, if so, the procedures and guidelines that should be implemented in respect of such processes in legislative form or otherwise.

In relation to this issue, particular consideration should be given to

Committee to Consider the Social, Ethical and Legal Issues Arising from *In Vitro* Fertilization, Interim Report. Victoria, Australia, September, 1982.

- whether the process and practice of IVF (whereby conception occurs outside normal physiological, emotional and social conditions and relationships) give rise to undesirable social and moral practices.

To consider whether the community and the parties (that is, the donors, the embryo and the medical and scientific personnel) involved in the process of IVF have any rights and/or obligations and, if so, whether such rights and/or obligations should be enforced, in legislative form or otherwise.

In relation to this issue, consideration should be included of the following aspects:

- the rights of infertile persons to take advantage of IVF processes.
- the criteria and selection procedures to be applied in determining persons who are to participate in these processes and the conditions to which such selection will be subject.
- the manner of determining who should make the decision of selection.
- the methods of selection, treatment and protection of embryos prior to and after implantation and, if implantation does not proceed, the destruction or use of embryos for other purpose.

To make recommendations upon such related matters as the Committee considers appropriate. . . .

To make an interim report to the Attorney-General within three months of the Committee first convening.

* * *

5. The Most Common Situation

The history and present practice of IVF in Victoria constitute the context in which the Committee has begun its work. It has considered a large number of papers and submissions dealing with IVF. It is aware that there is strong support for and substantial opposition to the process.

In its Interim Report the Committee has not considered a number of issues relating to IVF which it has identified, which it believes deserve careful attention and about which it expects to make particular recommendations.

Some of these issues are of great urgency, in that they involve parts of IVF programmes which are already being carried out or have been plainly foreshadowed in Victoria. These are freezing and storage of embryos and the use of donor ova and donor sperm. Other issues have been raised.

- These include surrogate motherhood, that is, implantation of an embryo in the uterus of a woman who is not the contributor of the ovum or oocyte.
- Fertilization of embryos specifically for research and experimentation or for therapeutic use.

Other issues, which may be described as more contentious include cloning, development of hybrids and other genetic engineering techniques—either for research and experimentation or therapeutic use. Finally, there is the possibility of IVF followed by laboratory nurture and birth—the 'test-tube baby' complete.

In its Interim Report the Committee has concentrated its attention solely on the most common situation in which IVF is employed in Victoria. This involves a husband and wife supplying their own genetic material for the production of an embryo or embryos which will be inserted into the uterus of the wife with the aim of implantation occurring and a successful pregnancy ensuing.

The Committee considers this form of the procedure to be acceptable to the Victorian community and accordingly recommends that it be recognized in those terms.

In reaching this conclusion, the Committee acknowledges that, in the Victorian community, there are several groups who, while expressing strong support and sympathy for infertile couples, reject IVF as unnatural conception. Others reject it because of inadequate prior research on animals, of the inherent experimentation on and risk of damage to the embryos produced, and of the possible risk of personality traumas in the children as they develop through childhood and adolescence to adulthood.

While developments since the first successful IVF birth have tended to diminish but not dispel some of these concerns, the first remains. Associated with this is a deeply held philosophical view that the embryo is, immediately after fertilization, a form of human life to which both protection and respect must be accorded. (The level and strength of that recognition and protection, in terms of legal rules conferring it, is itself a matter of debate.) The Committee recognizes, therefore, that some groups in the Victorian community will not participate in or countenance IVF. Their views deserve respect, in line with the views of members of the community who oppose other lawful procedures well established in current medical practice. But, nonetheless, the practice of IVF in the most common situation does, in the Committee's view, command substantial support in the Victorian community.

Safeguards

Even in what it believes to be the most common situation in which IVF is employed it is the Committee's view that the abovementioned matters require safeguards to protect the interests of the community and the individuals involved in the programme, including the embryo formed in the laboratory.

Centres Conducting IVF and Embryo Transfer It will be apparent from the contents of section 4 [not reprinted] of this report that the process of IVF is a complicated one requiring skilled doctors, technicians and support staff. The procedure is a relatively expensive one. The Committee has concluded, therefore, that IVF should only be conducted in hospitals authorized to do so by, and responsible to, the Health Commission of Victoria. It recommends that legislation to give effect to this recommendation be enacted as soon as possible. The terms of any authorization should encompass some of the matters considered in succeeding paragraphs.

Counselling The Committee is concerned about the needs and the wishes of infertile couples who seek to resolve the problems that may ensue from their infertility. In this connection it notes that it is misleading to describe IVF and ET as a cure or even a treatment of infertility. It is rather a *means* of circumventing infertility and, for this reason, may even tend to discourage couples involved in a programme from facing up to the anger, guilt, despair and isolation that, to a greater or lesser degree, go together with the knowledge that they are infertile. For this reason the Committee believes that counselling must be available in any IVF programme.

The Committee further believes that counsellors should be specifically trained to deal with the problems of infertility. Counselling available in any IVF programme shall include:

- provision of general information about an IVF programme and what it may involve for the couple;
- support for the couple while on the waiting list, when involved in the programme, and, if pregnancy is not achieved, for 12 months after leaving the programme; and
- infertility counselling which may, if necessary and mutually agreed, take the form of therapeutic counselling.

Adoption of this recommendation should help to ensure that infertile couples arrive at a position from which they can determine for themselves whether or not to become and remain involved in an IVF programme. A counselling programme should from the outset provide information about self-help groups.

Information and Consent

The Committee believes that each couple seeking admission to an IVF programme must be provided with clear and comprehensive information about the programme. Each couple must be advised of any risks involved in the programme and of its likely duration and given the most accurate information about the prospects of success. This will then permit each couple to express in writing their free and informed consent to participate in the programme.

Community Education

Some of the problems encountered by infertile couples stem in part from community ignorance concerning the extent and nature of infertility. The Committee has therefore decided that provision should be made for appropriate forms of education in secondary schools and in other suitable contexts, including the media, with the aim of increasing the awareness and the understanding of infertility in the Victorian community. This should include information about the causes of infertility, about methods to prevent its occurrence, about treatments which may be available, about adoption, and about marriage without children. The Committee has been impressed by the work done and the publications produced on this subject by the Institute of Family Studies and the Citizens Welfare Service of Victoria.

Selection of Participants

In the context of the Interim Report the Committee is of the view that the procedure should be available, at present, only to married couples. While there is increasing tolerance of and some recognition of de facto relationships in the community, it is in the context of a husband/wife relationship and the framework of the traditional family that the community in general approves of IVF.

The Committee believes that the selection of couples for the IVF programme should not be solely made on the basis of first in line or the capacity to pay, but should be made on the basis of defined priorities relating to individual needs. In view of the cost of the programme, the complexity of the techniques used, and the large number of patients seeking treatment, each couple should have attempted other appropriate means of treatment prior to selection for the IVF programme. Where infertility has proven unresponsive to other means of treatment or the couple has sought alternative treatment for a period in excess of 12 months then such couple shall be entitled to be selected to join the IVF programme if they are otherwise suitable candidates for treatment. Information relating to alternative means of treatment should be widely disseminated.

Surplus Embryos

The Committee appreciates the deep concern of a section of the Victorian community which considers that from the moment of fertilization an embryo is a human being to be accorded a substantial measure of respect and rights (some would say at the same level as persons born alive). At the same time the Committee is aware that not all sections of the community share this philosophical view of personhood and the attitude towards embryonic life that derives from it. In these circumstances, and for the purposes of the Interim Report, the Committee is of the view that in the Victorian community IVF and ET are acceptable if *all* fertilized oocytes are transferred to the uterus of the mother.

A majority of the Committee also believes that where a couple requests that attempts be made to fertilize all oocytes recovered, and where too many embryos are produced for all to be transferred, the wishes of the couple concerning handling of such excess embryos should be respected. The majority opinion takes into account data indicating a higher rate of successful pregnancies when all oocytes recovered are fertilized. This view is not held by the Chairman, the Reverend Dr. Harman and Mrs. Hay, who are of the view that the problem of surplus embryos needs to be further considered in depth.

Three members of the Committee, the Chairman, Reverend Dr. Harman and Mrs. Hay, believe that until the Committee has had time to consider fully the implications of alternatives such as freeze thawing of embryos, donation of embryos, and surrogate motherhood, that these procedures should not be employed in IVF programmes in Victoria. The remaining members believe the process of freeze thawing should be allowed to continue while this is being considered.

Legal Implications in the Most Common Situation

The Committee considers that in the most common situation there are no questions of status which arise specifically out of IVF procedures. The Committee believes that the legal status of the child born as a result of IVF in that situation is clear; it is the legitimate issue of the marriage.

The Committee has not considered questions of criminal responsibility or civil liability which may arise in the context of IVF.

The Committee is aware that the Standing Committee of Attorneys-General has been considering the preparation of legislation in relation to the legal status of children born as a result of artificial insemination by donor (AID) and IVF. The Committee supports the view that there should be uniform legislation on this subject, and would value the opportunity to examine the draft legislation, with a view to considering its substance and its form in connection with its further work.

Recommendations

In view of the matters considered above, the Committee recommends that, pending its further report or reports, the Government should

- institute a campaign of public education on the nature, causes and treatment of infertility.
- enact legislation to authorize hospitals as centres in which IVF programmes may be conducted. The terms of the authorization should provide that
  - before a couple is admitted to the IVF programme they must have undertaken all other medical procedures during a period in excess of 12 months which may, in their particular circumstances, overcome their infertility;
  - the IVF programme be limited to cases in which the gametes are obtained from husband and wife and the embryos are transferred into the uterus of the wife;
  - admission to the IVF programme is preceded, accompanied and followed by appropriate counselling.

REPORT OF THE COMMITTEE OF INQUIRY INTO HUMAN FERTILISATION AND EMBRYOLOGY: THE WARNOCK COMMITTEE, LONDON

INTRODUCTION. *In July 1982 an interdisciplinary committee was established in the United Kingdom. The group was called the Committee of Inquiry into Human Fertilisation and Embryology; its chair was philosopher Mary Warnock. The committee's charge was to "examine the social, ethical and legal implications of recent, and potential developments in the field of human assisted reproduction" (Report, p. iv). This clearly written and influential report provided a synthesis of ethical analysis from the early 1980s, when the central questions seemed to be, "Which of the new reproductive technologies and arrangements are ethically acceptable?" and "Which technologies or arrangements, if any, should be legally discouraged or even prohibited?" The principal focus in the following excerpts is on IVF and surrogate parenting arrangements.*

1. The General Approach

BACKGROUND TO THE INQUIRY

1.1 The birth of the first child resulting from the technique of *in vitro*[1] fertilisation in July 1978 was a considerable achievement. The technique, long sought, at last successful, opened up new horizons in the alleviation of infertility and in the science of embryology. It was now possible to observe the very earliest stages of human development, and with these discoveries came the hope of remedying defects at this very early stage. However, there were also anxieties. There was a sense that events were moving too fast for their implications to be assimilated. Society's views on the new techniques were divided between pride in the technological achievement, pleasure at the newfound means to relieve, at least for some, the unhappiness of infertility, and unease at the apparently uncontrolled advance of science, bringing with it new possibilities for manipulating the early stages of human development.

1.2 Against this background of public excitement and concern, this Inquiry was established in July 1982, with the following terms of reference:

> To consider recent and potential developments in medicine and science related to human fertilisation and embryology; to consider what policies and safeguards should be applied, including consideration of the social, ethical and legal implications of these developments; and to make recommendations.

SCOPE OF THE INQUIRY

1.3 In considering our terms of reference, we recognised that we were being asked to examine a sphere of activity still developing, and rapidly changing. A common factor linking all the developments, recent or potential, medical or scientific, was the anxiety which they generated in the public mind. We have therefore looked at the new processes of assisted reproduction, including surrogacy, which can cause public concern. We have also considered artificial insemination, which, though practised in this country for many years, is not universally accepted ethically, nor indeed regulated by law. There were, however,

---

Department of Health and Social Security, *Report of the Committee of Inquiry into Human Fertilisation and Embryology*, London, England: Her Majesty's Stationery Office, July, 1984. Footnotes have been numbered consecutively, and appear at the end of the report. Recommendations in the original were set in bold type.

some matters which, though in some sense related, fell outside our terms of reference. Chief among these were abortion and contraception. We have not concerned ourselves directly with these, although the present state of the law in relation to them has been a necessary point of reference in discussions.

1.4 Within the terms of reference we were given two words that had to be clarified. The first of these was *embryology*. While the term "embryo" has been variously defined in considering human embryology, we have taken as our starting point the meeting of egg and sperm at fertilisation. We have regarded the embryonic stage to be the six weeks immediately following fertilisation which usually corresponds with the first eight weeks of gestation counted from the first day of the woman's last menstrual period.

1.5 The second word in need of clarification was *potential*. The pace of scientific discovery is unpredictable. Indeed, a number of major developments has taken place during the lifetime of the Inquiry. The changes which take place in society itself are also difficult to predict. The impact of scientific discoveries on the society of the future is therefore doubly hard to predict. We took the pragmatic view that we could react only to what we knew, and what we could realistically foresee. This meant that we must react to the ways in which people now see childlessness and the process of family formation, taking into account the range of views encompassed by our pluralistic society, the nature and value of clinical and scientific advances, and the benefits of research.

METHODS OF WORKING

1.6 We found it convenient to divide our task into two parts. The first concerned processes designed to benefit the individual within society who faced a particular problem, namely infertility; the second concerned the pursuit of knowledge, much of it designed to benefit society at large rather than the individual. The distinction is not absolute. One cannot divorce pursuit of an individual's goals from the goals of society as a whole and, moreover, policies undertaken for the public good while they may well also benefit individuals can, on the other hand, impose limitations on them. Nonetheless, we found it a useful division, and the report thus deals first with the alleviation of infertility, and second with scientific developments.

1.7 We recognised that within society there is a multiplicity of views on the issues before the Inquiry. We therefore decided to seek evidence from as many organisations, reflecting as many different perspectives, as possible. . . . We are particularly grateful for all the time and trouble taken by those who prepared submissions and for the insight they gave us into the problems we were asked to consider. But even with submissions from so many organisations we have to record with regret that we did not receive evidence from as wide a range of minority and special interest groups as we would have liked, despite our best endeavours.

THE INTERNATIONAL DIMENSION

1.8 Anxiety about the implications of the new developments in assisted reproduction is not confined to the United Kingdom. While there is an obvious attraction in a unity of approach to difficult ethical issues, and we have tried as far as possible to keep in touch with developments around the world, there are, in our view, sound reasons for not pursuing this unity of approach at the present time. Different countries are at different stages in the development both of services and of a policy response. They have different cultural, moral and legal traditions, influencing the way in which a problem is tackled and the ways in which it might be resolved. We have therefore made recommendations which we believe to be appropriate specifically in the United Kingdom.

Nonetheless, we hope that others may find our proposals of value, just as we have benefitted from the experience of other countries. We accept that there is a case for an international approach. This approach will be best formulated, however, when individual countries have formed their own views, and are ready to pool knowledge and experience.

THE ROLE OF THE INQUIRY

1.9 We have confined our recommendations to certain practical proposals, capable of implementation. We have tried to frame these recommendations in general terms, leaving matters of detail to be worked out by Government and other appropriate organisations. We have also indicated what we consider should be matters of good practice. We have clearly indicated where our formal recommendations, if accepted, would require legislative change. The development of science and medical technology in the field of human fertilisation opens up many new issues for the law. *In vitro* fertilisation, for example, has brought about situations not previously contemplated, in relation to which there is either no law at all, or such law as exists was designed for entirely different circumstances. We believe that new laws will be necessary to cope with the new techniques for alleviating infertility and their consequences, and to deal with the developments in research in the field of embryology. But we foresee real dangers in the law intervening too fast and too extensively in areas where there is no clear public consensus. Furthermore both medical science and opinion within society may advance with startling rapidity.

1.10 We do not discuss in the following chapters every situation which might arise and then relate it to all existing law. We have had neither the time nor the resources to do this; nor, in our view, would such a course have been appropriate. Rather we have considered the fundamental questions there raised in relation to any existing law and confined ourselves to what we regard as essential legislative changes. We wish to stress our view that the changes which we propose should apply equally throughout the United Kingdom of Great Britain and Northern Ireland.

* * *

5. Techniques for the Alleviation of Infertility [*cont'd*]

II. IN VITRO FERTILISATION

5.1 Unlike AID [artificial insemination with donor sperm], *in vitro* fertilisation (IVF) is very much a new development. Of those women who are infertile a small proportion can produce healthy eggs but, although they have a normal uterus, have damaged or diseased fallopian tubes which prevent the egg passing from the ovary to the uterus. A certain proportion of these women can be helped by tubal surgery. Until IVF became a reality, the possibility of achieving a pregnancy for women with tubal problems was not great. IVF may be appropriate perhaps for 5% of infertile couples. Recently claims have been made for IVF as a treatment for other forms of infertility including its use in the treatment of oligospermia[2] and unexplained infertility.

5.2 The concept of IVF is simple. A ripe human egg is extracted from the ovary, shortly before it would have been released naturally. Next, the egg is mixed with the semen of the husband or partner, so that fertilisation can occur. The fertilised egg, once it has started to divide, is then transferred back to the mother's uterus. In practice the technique for recovery of the eggs, their culture outside the mother's body, and the transfer of the developing embryo to the uterus has to be carried out under very carefully controlled conditions. The development of laparoscopic[3] techniques during the 1960s made the collection of the egg, in cases where the ovaries were accessible, relatively easy. (Another technique for egg recovery based on ultrasound identification[4] has now been developed.) It was not particularly difficult to fertilise the human egg *in vitro*. The real difficulty related to the implantation of the embryo in the uterus after transfer. A pregnancy achieved in this way must not only survive the normal hazards of implantation of *in vivo* conception, but also the additional problems of IVF and embryo transfer. More is now known about how best to replicate the natural sequence of events, but undoubtedly achieving a successful implantation is still the most uncertain part of the procedure.

5.3 Because of these difficulties it is common practice to transfer more than one embryo to the potential mother whenever possible, and for this reason several eggs need to be recovered. This is achieved by artificial stimulation, known as superovulation, of the woman's ovaries to ensure that she produces several eggs in one cycle. After an appropriate course of drugs, as many ripe eggs as are accessible are harvested just before the time of ovulation. Each egg is then mixed with semen to achieve fertilisation. Assuming there is no abnormality in the semen, the success rate of fertilisation is usually at least 75%. Some embryos may however show signs of poor or abnormal development; when the time comes to transfer the embryos to the woman, it may be that there is only one embryo suitable for transfer, or there may be several.

5.4 The case for transferring more than one embryo is that this should give the woman a better chance of achieving a pregnancy. There is also an argument that if two or more embryos are transferred each helps the other towards implantation. However, if too many embryos are transferred and they all implant this may result in a multiple pregnancy with all the added risks of such a pregnancy including the risks of miscarriage, premature delivery and resulting immaturity at birth. There are differences of opinion about how many embryos should be transferred, given these risks. This is a field where constant reassessment is needed as new evidence becomes available. We have considered arguments that a limit should be imposed on the total number of embryos that should be transferred on each occasion, but we believe that in each individual case the number of embryos to be transferred must be a matter of clinical judgment on the part of the practitioner responsible for the woman's care. This responsibility should be made clear in the consent form. In addition to the technical arguments we have outlined, a practitioner must also give very serious consideration to the social problems for the family that may follow the birth of more than twins, problems that may affect the continuing health and wellbeing of the mother in looking after the children and may adversely affect the children themselves.

5.5 Despite the technical difficulties of IVF, at the time we write, there have been some hundreds of such births throughout the world. These births continue to exercise considerable fascination. At the same time, this public interest creates, in itself, difficulties, adding to the pressure on doctors practising in this field who are not only trying to provide a new treatment for their patients, but are also constantly working in the public eye.

ARGUMENTS AGAINST IVF AND RESPONSES

5.6 Although many people regard IVF as an exciting new possibility for helping the childless, there are those who are deeply worried by its development. This opposition can be categorised as opposition either based on fundamental principles, or based on the consequences of the practice of IVF. The fundamental arguments against IVF are the same as those against AIH [artificial insemination with the husband's sperm]—that this practice represents a deviation from normal intercourse and that the unitive and procreative aspects of sexual intercourse should not be separated. Those who hold this view believe that this is an absolute moral principle which must be upheld without exception. This view is sincerely and strongly held. As a question of individual conscience, there will be those who will not wish to receive this form of treatment nor participate in its practice, but we would not rely on those arguments for the formulation of a public policy.

5.7 The arguments against IVF based on a consideration of the consequences are more varied; but those who put forward such arguments may take as their starting point the acceptance of IVF as a legitimate form of treatment for infertility. Their reservations start when IVF results in more embryos being brought into existence than will be transferred to the mother's uterus. They argue that it is not acceptable deliberately to produce embryos which have potential for human life when that potential will never be realised. As we have noted above, the opinion of the medical profession on the whole is that in the present state of knowledge superovulation is very desirable. But if more embryos are brought into existence than are transferred, it is held to be morally unacceptable to allow them to die.

5.8 Another argument against IVF is that which draws an analogy between IVF and heart transplants, or other forms of "high technology" medical care, and asks whether the country can afford such expensive treatment which benefits only a few, and whether money could not be "better" spent, that is, with beneficial effects for more people, elsewhere. While we accept that questions about the uses of resources are proper questions, deserving serious consideration, essentially they relate to the extent of provision, not to whether there should be any provision at all. Further, without some provision of a service there can be no opportunity to evaluate the real costs and benefits of a technique, nor can the technique be refined and developed so as to become more cost-effective. The priorities argument is, in our view, an argument for controlled development, not an argument against the technique itself.

ARGUMENTS FOR IVF

5.9 The positive argument in favour of IVF is simple: the technique will increase the chances for some infertile couples to have a child. For some couples this will be the only method by which they may have a child that is genetically entirely theirs.

THE INQUIRY'S VIEW

5.10 We have reached the conclusion that IVF is an acceptable means of treating infertility and we therefore recommend that the service of IVF should continue to be available subject to the same type of licensing and inspection as we have recommended with regard to the regulation of AID (see Chapter Four [not reprinted in this volume]). For the protection and reassurance of the public this recommendation must apply equally to IVF within the NHS (National Health Service) and in the private medical sector. At the present time IVF is available on a limited scale within the NHS and we recommend that IVF should continue to be available within the NHS. One member of the Inquiry would not like to see any expansion of NHS IVF services until the results obtained in using this technique are more satisfactory. IVF requires a concentration of skilled medical and scientific expertise, and it is appropriate for only a small proportion of infertile couples. Therefore we would not argue that it should be available at all district general hospitals, or even at all university teaching hospitals. However in order to minimise travelling and other inconvenience to patients, we believe that ultimately NHS centres should be distributed throughout the UK. We recognise that there will be those who will press for at least one in every region.

5.11 We are conscious that such specialised units with their distinctive organisational features, would have considerable cost implications, and we are mindful of the priorities argument mentioned above. We are also mindful that IVF is only one of a range of treatments for infertility and, . . . that there is scope for improvement in the provision of infertility services generally. We would not want to see IVF, with its present relatively low success rate, cream off all the resources available for the treatment of infertility just because it has the glamour of novelty. Details of the financing of the service are outside our terms of reference, but these factors make it desirable that the early development of the service within the NHS be carefully monitored. We recommend that one of the first tasks of the working group, whose establishment we recommend[ed] in 2.17 [not reprinted here] should be to consider how best an IVF service can be organised within the NHS. There will be continuing development of private IVF clinics alongside those within the NHS, but we believe it is important that there should be a sufficient level of NHS provision for childless couples not to feel that their only recourse is to the private sector.

5.12 In order to put IVF into perspective we are particularly concerned that an accurate estimate of success is given, because childless couples develop high expectations of the technique. We do not want the unhappiness and disappointment they may have already experienced to be exacerbated by false or unrealistic hopes. It is now very difficult to give an estimate of the success of the technique because of differing methods of measuring success and also because rates vary between centres. However we have been given permission by Mr Steptoe and Dr Edwards to quote the following figures on the outcome of IVF treatment carried out at Bourn Hall Clinic, as an illustration. During the period October 1980 (when the clinic opened) to the end of December 1983, 2,388 laparoscopies were carried out for 1,234 women, of whom 690 were admitted for treatment on two or more occasions. These resulted in a total of 362 pregnancies, of which 105 ended in miscarriage and four in an ectopic pregnancy. Of these 362 pregnancies, in 271 treatment was undertaken because of diseased or absent fallopian tubes without associated semen problems. The majority of the remainder were undertaken either because of a combination of semen problems and diseased fallopian tubes or because of semen problems alone.

5.13 In 1983 there were 967 laparoscopies performed for 579 women. In 934 of these laparoscopies one or more eggs was recovered, and in 762 one or more eggs was fertilised. In all these cases one or more embryos was transferred to the woman and in 192 a pregnancy occurred which ended in birth or a clinically recognisable miscarriage.[5]

5.14 By May 1984 the clinic knew of 439 pregnancies, of which 131 were ongoing. 215 children had been born since it had opened, including 18 sets of twins and one set of triplets. Among these infants there had been no major congenital malformations.

5.15 It seems to us that the technique has now passed the research stage and can be regarded as an established form of treatment for infertility.

* * *

6. Techniques for the Alleviation of Infertility [*cont'd*]

III. EGG DONATION

6.1 Egg donation has been attempted in the United States of America and in Australia, where there has been one live birth. This procedure may help those women who cannot themselves produce an egg. It may also help those who would be candidates for IVF except that in their case egg collection is impossible because their ovaries are inaccessible. About 5% of infertile couples might benefit from the technique. A mature egg is recovered from a fertile woman donor, for example during sterilisation, and is fertilised *in vitro*, using the semen of the husband of the infertile woman. The resulting embryo is then transferred to the patient's uterus. If it implants she may then carry the pregnancy to term. There are other situations where eggs might be donated. When a woman is herself undergoing infertility treatment and several eggs have been recovered from her, she may be prepared to donate one or more eggs to another woman whose infertility can be treated only by egg donation.

6.2 A major feature of the technique is timing. It is essential to monitor closely the donor's menstrual cycle so that egg recovery takes place at the correct time, shortly before the ripe egg would have been released naturally from the ovary. This means that for donors who are giving an egg while undergoing some other treatment, the main operation has to take place at the time dictated by the decision to collect the egg. Such monitoring is complicated and time-consuming, and at present would necessitate the donor attending hospital more frequently than the main operation itself would require. Experience with IVF has shown that reliance on the natural cycle to produce eggs results in a lower success rate than when superovulation is used to stimulate egg production. For egg donation to have much chance of success it would similarly be necessary to induce superovulation in the donor.

6.3 At the present time human eggs cannot be successfully used after freezing and thawing, which means they must be used soon after collection. And so it is necessary not only to time egg collection at the right point in the donor's cycle, but also to have a suitable recipient immediately ready to receive the fertilised egg. The practical problems thus presented limit the applicability of the technique. The problems would be substantially reduced if it became possible to store eggs by freezing. . . . Just as the use of frozen semen in AID permits a greater flexibility, the same would be true for egg donation. The freezing, storing and thawing of eggs is likely to become feasible within a few years. In the future it may be possible to mature eggs *in vitro* that have been recovered at an immature stage.

ARGUMENTS AGAINST EGG DONATION

6.4 Egg donation is open to the same kinds of objection as AID. There is the same objection to the introduction of a third party into the marriage. There is also concern about the possible impact on the child and the possible harmful effects on society in general. In addition, egg donation involves a considerable degree of intervention in the normal process of fertilisation. In this respect it is similar to IVF. We have examined these views elsewhere. Moreover, egg donation can be opposed on grounds of the physical risks involved for the donor, for there is some risk, as there is in any invasive procedure, to the egg donor from the actual removal of eggs.

ARGUMENTS FOR EGG DONATION

6.5 For some couples egg donation provides the only chance of their having a child which the woman can carry to term, and which is the genetic child of her husband. The couple, it is argued, experience the pregnancy as other couples do, and for this reason egg donation has an advantage over AID, in that both partners contribute to the birth of the child.

THE INQUIRY'S VIEW

6.6 In weighing up the arguments for and against egg donation we have concluded that since we have accepted AID and IVF it would be illogical not to accept egg donation, notwithstanding the relatively minor surgical risks to the donor inherent in egg recovery. We consider that egg donation is ethically acceptable where the donor has been properly counselled and is fully aware of the risks. It is both logical and consistent that the law should treat egg donation in the same way as AID and that the same principles of practice . . . should apply to both. However, there is an important practical difference between the two procedures. Egg donation requires an invasive procedure to obtain the egg and the whole process necessitates the active assistance of the medical profession. Nonetheless, so far as possible, similar principles should apply in relation to the anonymity of the donor, screening, donor profiles, the child's right to know the facts of the donation and access for the couples to information about the donor's ethnic origin and genetic health and, similarly, access for the child to this information on reaching the age of majority. We recommend that egg donation be accepted as a recognised technique in the treatment of infertility subject to the same type of licensing and controls as we have recommended for the regulation of AID and IVF. The principles of good practice we have already considered in relation to these other techniques should apply, including the anonymity of the donor, limitation of the number of children born from the eggs of any one donor to ten, openness with the child about his genetic origins, the availability of counselling for all parties and informed consent.

6.7 Despite our desire to maintain the anonymity of the donor we recognise that because of the present practicalities of egg donation, particularly the fact that eggs cannot be successfully stored, it may not always at present be possible to achieve this. An exception to the principle of anonymity would occur where the egg was donated by a sister or close friend. In such cases particularly careful counselling for all concerned would be necessary and thought would have to be given as to how and at what stage the child should be told about its parentage.

6.8 Egg donation produces for the first time circumstances in which the genetic mother (the woman who donates the egg), is a different person from the woman who gives birth to the child, the carrying mother. The law has never, till now, had to face this problem. There are inevitably going to be instances where the stark issue arises of who is the mother. In order to achieve some certainty in this situation it is our view that where a woman donates an egg for transfer to another, the donation should be treated as absolute and that, like a male donor, she should have no rights or duties with regard to any resulting child. We recommend that legislation should provide that when a child is born to a woman following donation of another's egg the woman giving birth should, for all purposes, be regarded in law as the mother of that child, and that the egg donor should have no rights or obligations in respect of the child. We also consider that as with AID . . . , if the parents so wish, the mother's name may be followed in the birth register by the words "by donation."

7. Techniques for the Alleviation of Infertility [*cont'd*]

IV. EMBRYO DONATION

7.1 Embryo donation would help the same groups of women who might benefit from egg donation and, more particularly, the even smaller number whose husbands are also infertile. Embryo donation may take two forms. One involves the donation of both egg and semen. The donated egg is fertilised *in vitro* with donated semen and the resulting embryo transferred to a woman who is unable to produce an egg herself and whose husband is infertile. The second method, known as lavage, does not involve removing the egg by surgical intervention. Instead the egg is released naturally from the ovary at the normal time in the donor's menstrual cycle. At the predicted time of ovulation she is artificially inseminated with semen from the husband of the infertile woman (or from a donor if the husband is also infertile). Some three to four days later, before the start of implantation, the donor's uterus is "washed out" and any embryo retrieved is then transferred to the uterus of the infertile woman. If the embryo implants successfully the recipient carries the pregnancy to term. Embryo donation by lavage is, according to its advocates, much safer for the donor as it does not require general anaesthesia, and a simple and safer procedure is involved; moreover, for the embryo, there is the advantage of a shorter interval *in vitro* during which time it might deteriorate. When semen from the husband is used, the child is genetically his though not his wife's.

ARGUMENTS AGAINST EMBRYO DONATION

7.2 The objections that are raised in relation to egg donation and AID can also be made to embryo donation, that is, the introduction of a third party into an exclusive relationship, and the possible impact on the child and on society in general. Again, where a surgical procedure is used to recover the egg there is some risk to the donor. Further, where lavage is used, there is a risk of pregnancy in the donor, since the embryo may not be washed out; and of the introduction of infection to the uterus or other problems. A further objection to embryo donation where a semen donor is used is that neither of the nurturing parents has contributed genetically to the child.

ARGUMENTS FOR EMBRYO DONATION

7.3 In the evidence it was suggested that embryo donation constituted a form of pre-natal adoption, with the advantage over normal adoption that the couple share the experience of pregnancy and childbirth, and, it is further argued, the mother and child experience bonding during pregnancy.

THE INQUIRY'S VIEW

7.4 Embryo donation is probably the least satisfactory form of donation. There is, however, likely to be a very limited number of cases where a donated egg is fertilised by donated semen *in vitro* and the resultant embryo transferred to the uterus of a woman who would otherwise be unable to have a child. We therefore recommend that the form of embryo donation involving donated semen and egg which are brought together *in vitro* be accepted as a treatment for infertility, subject to the same type of licensing and controls as we have recommended with regard to the regulation of AID, IVF and egg donation.

7.5 We do, however, have some reservations about the use of lavage because of the risk to the egg donor. We recommend that the technique of embryo donation by lavage should not be used at the present time.

7.6 It is entirely consistent with our view that donation should lead to negation of all rights and duties that such an embryo once transferred should be regarded for all purposes as that of the carrying mother. Should the risks of donation by lavage be overcome and that technique become acceptable any embryo donated in this way should likewise be treated as that of the woman who carries the pregnancy. We recommend that the legislation proposed in 4.25 and 6.8 should cover children born following embryo donation. These recommendations mean that a child born following embryo donation to a married couple will, in the eyes of the law, have that couple as parents. In a case where the carrying mother is unmarried she will, in any event, in the eyes of the law be regarded as the mother of the child. The changes in the law we have earlier proposed would make it possible for the child to be registered, without making a false declaration, in the name of the nurturing parents, thus ensuring the child's legitimacy, assuming they had given informed consent. We also suggest that their names could be followed by the words "by donation" in the birth register, if the parents so wish.

7.7 As with donation and AID there is a number of principles which should underlie the provision of embryo donation—the anonymity of the donor; openness about the treatment, especially with the child; the provision of a full explanation of what is involved to those taking part, including donors, screening and donor profiles, and access for the parents and the child (on reaching the age of majority) to information about the donor's genetic health. . . .

8. Techniques for the Alleviation of Infertility [*cont'd*]

WHAT IS SURROGACY?

8.1 Surrogacy is the practice whereby one woman carries a child for another with the intention that the child should be handed over after birth. The use of artificial insemination and the recent development of *in vitro* fertilisation have eliminated the necessity for sexual intercourse in order to establish a surrogate pregnancy. Surrogacy can take a number of forms. The commissioning mother may be the genetic mother, in that she provides the egg, or she may make no contribution to the establishment of the pregnancy. The genetic father may be the husband of the commissioning mother, or of the carrying mother; or he may be an anonymous donor. There are thus many possible combinations of persons who are relevant to the child's conception, birth and early environment. Of these various forms perhaps the most likely are surrogacy involving artificial insemination, where the carrying mother is the genetic mother inseminated with semen from the male partner of the commissioning couple, and surrogacy using *in vitro* fertilisation where both egg and semen come from the commissioning couple, and the resultant embryo is transferred to and implants in the carrying mother.

8.2 There are certain circumstances in which surrogacy would be an option for the alleviation of infertility. Examples are where a woman has a severe pelvic disease which cannot be remedied surgically, or has no uterus. The practice might also be used to help those women who have suffered repeated miscarriages. There are also perhaps circumstances where the genetic mother, although not infertile, could benefit from the pregnancy being carried by another woman. An example is where the genetic mother is fit to care for a child after it is born, but suffers from a condition making pregnancy medically undesirable.

8.3 If surrogacy takes place, it generally involves some payment to the carrying mother. Payment may vary between reimbursement of expenses, and a substantial fee. There may, however, be some instances where no money is involved, for example, where one sister carries the pregnancy for another.

THE PRESENT POSITION

8.4 There is at present no provision for a surrogacy service within the NHS. Private agencies exist in certain other countries, and in the UK one agency is said to have started to operate. The practice is not in itself unlawful. None of the parties to a surrogacy arrangement, including any agency operating on a commercial basis, contravenes existing criminal law, unless the terms of the agreement contravene the provisions of adoption law, which prohibit payments in connection with adoption.[6]

8.5 Any surrogacy arrangement would necessarily involve some form of agreement between the parties concerned, however informal. Although it may be assumed that in the majority of cases the agreement would be kept and the matter never brought before a court, it is likely that grave difficulties of enforcement would ensue in the event of a dispute over such an agreement. There is little doubt that the Courts would treat most, if not all, surrogacy agreements as contrary to public policy and therefore unenforceable. Where one party broke the agreement the other party could not expect to invoke the court's assistance. Thus, if the carrying mother changed her mind and decided she wished to keep the child it is most unlikely that a court would order her, because she had previously agreed to do so, to hand over the child against her will. Nor in such a case would a court order the surrogate mother to repay any fee paid to her under the terms of the agreement.

8.6 The Courts do, however, have jurisdiction over children which is quite separate from and independent of the law of contract. Where a court has to consider the future of a child born following a surrogacy agreement, it must do so in accordance with the child's best interests in all the circumstances of the case, and not according to the terms of any agreement between the various adults. The child's interests being the first and paramount consideration, it seems likely that only in very exceptional circumstances would a court direct a surrogate mother to hand over the child to the commissioning couple. The present state of the law makes any surrogacy agreement a risky undertaking for those involved.

8.7 Many unforeseen events may occur between the moment of entering into the surrogacy agreement and the time for handing over the child, and these may alter the whole picture. Apart from the most obvious one of the surrogate mother changing her mind, it may, for example, be discovered that the child is handicapped or the commissioning mother may die or become disabled.

8.8 Embryo transfer makes possible for the first time a situation where the carrying mother is not the genetic mother. Where there has been a donation of egg or embryo to the carrying mother we have recommended that the woman who gives birth should, for all purposes in law, be regarded as the mother. The position following surrogacy is far less straightforward. It is not difficult to envisage circumstances where serious arguments could develop as to whether the genetic mother or the carrying mother ought in truth to be regarded as the mother of the child. The resolution of this issue could be of great importance in questions such as inheritance, citizenship or a claim for wrongful death.

THE FATHER'S POSITION

8.9 We have also considered the case of the commissioning father. In most cases the genetic father will be the husband of the commissioning mother. As regards enforcing any surrogacy agreement to which he is party, the commissioning father faces the difficulties described in 8.5. He may also be vulnerable to a claim by the carrying mother for an affiliation order if she keeps the child and the court might or might not make such an order according to the facts of the particular case. Unless he is married to the carrying mother he will, in the eyes of the law, be treated as an "unmarried" father with all the consequences that ordinarily flow from that.

ARGUMENTS AGAINST SURROGACY

8.10 There are strongly held objections to the concept of surrogacy, and it seems from the evidence submitted to us that the weight of public opinion is against the practice. The objections turn essentially on the view that to introduce a third party into the process of procreation which should be confined to the loving partnership between two people, is an attack on the value of the marital relationship. . . . Further, the intrusion is worse than in the case of AID, since the contribution of the carrying mother is greater, more intimate and personal, than the contribution of a semen donor. It is also argued that it is inconsistent with human dignity that a woman should use her uterus for financial profit and treat it as an incubator for someone else's child. The objection is not diminished, indeed it is strengthened, where the woman entered an agreement to conceive a child, with the sole purpose of handing the child over to the commissioning couple after birth.

8.11 Again, it is argued that the relationship between mother and child is itself distorted by surrogacy. For in such an arrangement a woman deliberately allows herself to become pregnant with the intention of giving up the child to which she will give birth, and this is the wrong way to approach pregnancy. It is also potentially damaging to the child, whose bonds with the carrying mother, regardless of genetic connections, are held to be strong, and whose welfare must be considered to be of paramount importance. Further it is felt that a surrogacy agreement is degrading to the child who is to be the outcome of it, since, for all practical purposes, the child will have been bought for money.

8.12 It is also argued that since there are some risks attached to pregnancy, no woman ought to be asked to undertake pregnancy for another, in order to earn money. Nor, it is argued, should a woman be forced by legal sanctions to part with a child, to which she has recently given birth, against her will.

ARGUMENTS FOR SURROGACY

8.13 If infertility is a condition which should, where possible, be remedied, it is argued that surrogacy must not be ruled out, since it offers to some couples their only chance of having a child genetically related to one or both of them. In particular, it may well be the only way that the husband of an infertile woman can have a child. Moreover, the bearing of a child for another can be seen, not as an undertaking that trivialises or commercialises pregnancy, but, on the contrary, as a deliberate and thoughtful act of generosity on the part of one woman to another. If there are risks attached to pregnancy, then the generosity is all the greater.

8.14 There is no reason, it is argued, to suppose that carrying mothers will enter into agreements lightly, and they have a perfect right to enter into such agreements if they so wish, just as they have a right to use their own bodies in other ways, according to their own decision. Where agreements are genuinely voluntary, there can be no question of exploitation, nor does the fact that surrogates will be paid for their pregnancy of itself entail exploitation of either party to the agreement.

8.15 As for intrusion into the marriage relationship, it is argued that those who feel strongly about this need not seek such treatment, but they should not seek to prevent others from having access to it.

8.16 On the question of bonding, it is argued that as very little is actually known about the extent to which bonding occurs when the child is *in utero*, no great claims should be made in this respect. In any case the breaking of such bonds, even if less than ideal, is not held to be an overriding argument against placing a child for adoption, where the mother wants this.

THE INQUIRY'S VIEW

8.17 The question of surrogacy presented us with some of the most difficult problems we encountered. The evidence submitted to us contained a range of strongly held views and this was reflected in our own views. The moral and social objections to surrogacy have weighed heavily with us. In the first place we are all agreed that surrogacy for convenience alone, that is, where a woman is physically capable of bearing a child but does not wish to undergo pregnancy, is totally ethically unacceptable. Even in compelling medical circumstances the danger of exploitation of one human being by another appears to the majority of us far to outweigh the potential benefits, in almost every case. That people should treat others as a means to their own ends, however desirable the consequences, must always be liable to moral objection. Such treatment of one person by another becomes positively exploitative when financial interests are involved. It is therefore with the commercial exploitation of surrogacy that we have been primarily, but by no means exclusively, concerned.

8.18 We have considered whether the criminal law should have any part to play in the control of surrogacy and have concluded that it should. We recognise that there is a serious risk of commercial exploitation of surrogacy and that this would be difficult to prevent without the assistance of the criminal law.[7] We have considered whether a limited, non-profit making surrogacy service, subject to licensing and inspection, could have any useful part to play but the majority agreed that the existence of such a service would in itself encourage the growth of surrogacy. We recommend that legislation be introduced to render criminal the creation or the operation in the United Kingdom of agencies whose purposes include the recruitment of women for surrogate pregnancy or making arrangements for individuals or couples who wish to utilise the services of a carrying mother; such legislation should be wide enough to include both profit and non-profit making organisations. We further recommend that the legislation be sufficiently wide to render criminally liable the actions of professionals and others who knowingly assist in the establishment of a surrogate pregnancy.

8.19 We do not envisage that this legislation would render private persons entering into surrogacy arrangements liable to criminal prosection, as we are anxious to avoid children being born to mothers subject to the taint of criminality. We nonetheless recognise that there will continue to be privately arranged surrogacy agreements. While we consider that most, if not all, surrogacy arrangements would be legally unenforceable in any of their terms, we feel that the position should be put beyond any possible doubt in law. We recommend that it be provided by statute that all surrogacy agreements are illegal contracts and therefore unenforceable in the courts.

8.20 We are conscious that surrogacy like egg and embryo donation may raise the question as to whether the genetic or the carrying mother is the true mother. Our recommendations in 6.8 and 7.6 cover cases where eggs or embryos have been donated. There remains however the possible case where the egg or embryo has not been donated but has been provided by the commissioning mother or parents with the intention that they should bring up the resultant child. If our recommendation in 8.18 is accepted, such cases are unlikely to occur because of the probability that the practitioner administering the treatment would be committing an offence. However, for the avoidance of doubt, we consider that the legislation proposed in 6.8 and 7.6 should be sufficiently widely drawn to cover any such case. If experience shows that this gives rise to an injustice for children who live with their genetic mother rather than the mother who bore them, then in our view the remedy is to make the adoption laws more flexible so as to enable the genetic mother to adopt.

* * *

10. The Freezing and Storage of Human Semen, Eggs and Embryos

10.1 The freezing, storage and thawing of human semen and embryos for subsequent use in artificial insemination or IVF are already practical realities, but a safe and reliable method of freezing and thawing human eggs has not yet been developed, although this is probably not far in the future. First, we see no objection in principle to the use of freezing in the treatment of infertility. There are however practical problems which may cause concern. There is anxiety that the process of freezing could induce damage in the gametes or embryos in a way which might lead to the birth of a child with an abnormality of structure or function. Nevertheless the experience of using frozen human semen for artificial insemination is reassuring, and so are animal studies in which semen has been used for AI after long-term frozen storage. We therefore recommend that the use of frozen semen in artificial insemination should continue.

10.2 This situation is not however paralleled in the case of eggs which have been fertilised after frozen storage. At present human eggs fertilised after freezing and thawing do not develop successfully. In addition, if this difficulty were overcome, the problem of whether the resulting embryo would develop normally would still remain to be resolved. So far there is insufficient evidence on which to base a judgement that the freezing and thawing of human eggs will not result in abnormalities. We therefore recommend that the use of frozen eggs in therapeutic procedures should not be undertaken until research has shown that no unacceptable risk is involved. This will be a matter for review by the licensing body. . . .

10.3 At the time of writing a small number of pregnancies has been achieved after frozen storage of human embryos, of which at least one has led to a live birth. Animal studies suggest that any damage caused by freezing is more likely to kill the embryo entirely than to impair its development, and it is not thought likely that freezing of human embryos will cause abnormalities. Nevertheless, as a matter of good clinical practice, checks should be made after thawing, to ensure so far as possible, that any frozen human embryo which is to be transferred to a woman is developing normally. We recommend that the clinical use of frozen embryos may continue to be developed under review by the licensing body. . . .

10.4 The other problem centres on the possibility of storage for prolonged periods. Human semen is now routinely frozen and stored for future use; there appears to be no upper limit to the length of time for which it is safe for frozen storage to continue before use. However the evidence presented to us drew attention to non-medical problems that may arise if frozen gametes or embryos are used after prolonged storage. Serious legal complications may well arise, for example in relation to inheritance and the use or disposal of frozen semen, eggs and embryos. We discuss these problems in the following paragraphs.

10.5 If our recommendations (see 4.22 and 6.8) are accepted, donors will have no rights or obligations with regard to their donations when semen or eggs are donated to benefit some other person. The same will apply when semen or eggs are donated for research. The question of ultimate disposal is therefore the responsibility of those storing the material, bearing in mind so far as possible the donor's wishes, if any have been expressed.

10.6 Disposal problems mainly arise when people have stored semen, eggs or embryos for their own personal use. We first consider the case of stored semen and eggs; secondly the position where a couple have stored an embryo. In both, there are good practical reasons for those responsible for the frozen storage of gametes or embryos to keep in regular touch with the man, woman or couple for whom this has been undertaken.

10.7 It seems to us that the only motive for storage would be to make possible the birth of a child at a subsequent date. For example a man might wish to store semen before undergoing surgery, chemotherapy or radiotherapy that is likely to make him sterile, or because he has sustained a spinal cord injury, in the hope that he may father a child by artificial insemination at a later date. Similarly, in the future, a woman might, for example, wish to store healthy eggs if these could be collected before undergoing surgery that might result in the removal of her ovaries. Her hope would be that she might have a child at a future date by IVF. Such men and women might well be only in their teens when their gametes are first stored. Therefore we feel it is unreasonable to put an absolute limit on the length of time for which eggs or semen can be stored. On the other hand it would also be unreasonable and impractical to expect those responsible for storage to maintain all eggs and semen stored indefinitely.

10.8 We believe there should be a system of five yearly reviews. When the reviews are carried out, men and women who have stored semen or eggs can indicate whether they wish storage to continue or whether they have no further use for the gametes and wish them to be destroyed or donated. As a matter of good practice we also suggest that those responsible for storage should consult the individuals who have deposited semen or eggs to ascertain their wishes well in advance of the expiry of the five years. We recommend that there should be automatic five-yearly reviews of semen and egg deposits. We recommend that legislation provide that where a person dies during the storage period or cannot be traced at a review date the right of use or disposal of his or her frozen gametes should pass to the storage authority. In this latter situation, as a matter of good practice the storage authority should, in disposing of them, bear in mind any previously expressed wishes in relation to disposal.

10.9 The use by a widow of her dead husband's semen for AIH is a practice which we feel should be actively discouraged. Despite our own views in this matter, . . . we realise that such requests may occasionally be made. It is obviously essential that there should be some finality for those administering estates of deceased persons since, in such cases posthumous fertilisation could cause real problems of inheritance and succession. Account would have to be taken of issue who might be born years after the death. We recommend that legislation be introduced to provide that any child born by AIH who was not *in utero* at the date of the death of its father shall be disregarded for the purposes of succession to and inheritance from the latter.

10.10 We also considered the case where a couple had stored an embryo for their own future use. Such an embryo might exist as a result of IVF when more eggs had been successfully fertilised than were needed for immediate embryo transfer. In this situation embryo storage might be undertaken so that further transfers might be made if the initial IVF treatment proved unsuccessful, or for a subsequent pregnancy, without the need for the woman to undergo further egg recovery. In such cases the couple might very well wish to have more than one child, and we had therefore to bear in mind their need to space pregnancies. At the same time there should in our opinion be a definite time limit set to the storage of embryos both because of the current ignorance of the possible effects of long storage and because of the legal and ethical complications that might arise over disposal of embryos whose parents have died or divorced or otherwise been separated. We believe that, as in the case of semen and eggs, there should be a review after five years of all embryos held and that the maximum time for storage of an embryo should be ten years. We recommend a maximum of ten years for storage of embryos after which time the right to use or disposal should pass to the storage authority.

10.11 Until now the law has never had to consider the existence of embryos outside the mother's uterus. The existence of such embryos raises potentially difficult problems as to ownership. The concept of ownership of human embryos seems to us to be undesirable. We recommend that legislation be enacted to ensure there is no right of ownership in a human embryo. Nevertheless, the couple who have stored an embryo for their use should be recognised as having rights to the use and disposal of the embryo, although these rights ought to be subject to limitation. The precise nature of that limitation will obviously require careful consideration. We hope the couple will recognise that they have a responsibility to make a firm decision as to the disposal and use of the embryo.

10.12 We consider that the position that may arise in the event of the death of one or both of a couple who have stored an embryo should be clarified. We therefore recommend that when one of a couple dies the right to use or dispose or any embryo stored by that couple should pass to the survivor. We make this recommendation notwithstanding our reservations about the possibility of posthumous pregnancies. We recommend that if both die that right should pass to the storage authority.

10.13 Problems might also arise when, whether in cases of marital breakdown or not, the couple fail to agree how the shared embryo should be used. We recommend that where there is no agreement between the couple the right to determine the use or disposal of an embryo should pass to the storage authority as though the ten year period had expired. This recommendation and those in the previous paragraph will require legislation.

10.14 On the question of inheritance and succession we hold that the order in which fertilisation *in vitro* took place should not alter the principle that the first born among siblings in a multiple pregnancy is deemed to be the eldest. The same principle should apply to embryos that have been stored. We recommend, therefore, that for the purposes of establishing primogeniture the date and time of birth, and not the date of fertilisation, shall be the determining factor.

10.15 With regard to the possibility of a frozen embryo being transferred to the mother after the death of the father we consider that a similar situation to that which we have recommended in the case of posthumous AIH should apply (see 10.9). We therefore recommend that legislation be introduced to provide that any child born following IVF, using an embryo that had been frozen and stored, who was not *in utero* at the date of the death of the father, shall be disregarded for the purposes of succession to and inheritance from the latter.

NOTES

1. This report distinguishes between *in vitro* meaning "in a glass," and *in vivo* meaning "in the body."
2. Oligospermia is the term used to describe semen in which the number of sperm present is reduced or markedly reduced compared with the number of sperm present in normal semen.
3. The laparoscope is an optical surgical instrument which is used to inspect the internal abdominal and pelvic organs so that minor surgical procedures can be performed including the recovery of one or more eggs from those ovarian follicles that are ripe. Laparoscopy usually requires a general anaesthetic but does not usually involve an overnight stay in hospital.
4. Ultrasound can now be used to identify the position of a ripe follicle containing an egg. A needle is then passed through the woman's abdominal wall and other organs and is guided to the follicle by use of ultrasound. The egg is then withdrawn through the needle. This technique can be used under local anaesthetic and can be used to recover more than one egg at a time.
5. This total does not include "biochemical pregnancies" where early tests following embryo transfer suggest that implantation might have occurred, but there is no subsequent clinical evidence of pregnancy.
6. Section 50 of the Adoption Act 1958.
7. [From this view Dr Greengross and Dr Davies dissent.]

ETHICAL CONSIDERATIONS OF THE NEW REPRODUCTIVE TECHNOLOGIES: AMERICAN FERTILITY SOCIETY, 1986

INTRODUCTION. *By 1984 it was clear that the U.S. Department of Health and Human Services would neither respond to the 1979 Ethics Advisory Board report nor establish a new Ethics Advisory Board to confront emerging issues in the reproductive sphere. Further, the President's Commission on Bioethics had completed its work in March 1983, without having devoted major attention to reproductive questions. Into this vacuum stepped two private-sector organizations, the American College of Obstetricians and Gynecologists (with its already-established Committee on Ethics) and the American Fertility Society.*

In November 1984, the President of the American Fertility Society (since renamed the American Society for Reproductive Medicine) appointed Howard W. Jones, Jr., M.D., to be the chair of a new Ethics Committee and asked him and the committee to help the Society "take a leadership position in addressing ethical issues in reproduction." This interdisciplinary group worked for 18 months on a survey of ethical and legal issues surrounding the new reproductive technologies and arrangements. The following excerpts illustrate the committee's approach to the ethical and legal issues, generally, and its evaluation of specific reproductive alternatives.

8. ETHICS AND THE NEW REPRODUCTIVE TECHNOLOGIES

Many ethical questions have been raised about specific cases involving the new reproductive technologies. This chapter seeks to survey some of the generic issues under discussion and to examine the ethical principles and theories that inform the current debate.

Issues

The Naturalness or Artificiality of the New Technologies If one believes that nothing artificial should intrude into the sexual relations between human beings, that belief will have profound implications for one's attitude toward contraceptive techniques and the new reproductive technologies. One critic of these technologies has formulated his objection as follows:

> Is there possibly some wisdom in that mystery of nature which joins the pleasure of sex, the communication of love, and the desire for children in the very activity by which we continue the chain of human existence? . . . My point is simply this: there are more and less human ways of bringing a child into the world. I am arguing that the laboratory production of human beings is no longer *human* procreation, that making babies in laboratories—even "perfect" babies—means a degradation of parenthood (Kass, 1972).

Diametrically opposed to this antitechnologic viewpoint is the perspective of those who regard the rational control of nature as one of the major achievements of human beings. According to this view, liberation from some of the unpredictable aspects of human reproduction is a major boon to the human species.

> Should we leave the fruits of human reproduction to take shape at random, keeping our children dependent upon the accidents of romance and genetic endowment, of (the) sexual lottery, or what one physician calls 'the meiotic roulette of his parents' chromosomes'? Or should we be responsible about this, that is, exercise

Ethics Committee, American Fertility Society, "Ethical Considerations of the New Reproductive Technologies," *Fertility and Sterility* 46(3) Supplement, 1986. Notes omitted.

> our rational and human choice, no longer submissively trusting to the blind worship of raw nature? (Fletcher, 1974).

A third position tends to mediate between these radically divergent views. In agreement with the first, this third position accepts reproduction without technologic assistance as natural and good. However, this position also argues that the development and use of new methods of contraception or reproduction can be morally justifiable, depending on the circumstances and on the reasons adduced. According to this view, it is natural for human beings to create a social structure in an effort to cope with the uncertainties and inconveniences of the "natural" world; technology is an important part of that structure (Callahan, 1972). The Committee accepts this third position, as evidenced especially in chapter 13.

The Moral Status of the Human Preembryo To speak of the moral status of anything is to use a shorthand expression for more complex formulations, such as "What are our moral obligations to X?" or "What moral rights does X possess?" Analogously, one can speak of the legal status of an adult, a newborn infant, or a human preembryo.

There are three principal viewpoints on the moral status of the human preembryo. The first viewpoint asserts that human preembryos are entitled to protection as human beings from the time of fertilization forward. According to this view, any research or other manipulation, such as freezing, that may damage a preembryo or interfere with its prospects for transfer to a uterus and its subsequent development is ethically unacceptable. This perspective on preembryonic status cites two kinds of factual evidence. First, a new genotype is established during fertilization. Second, given the appropriate environment, some preembryos have the potential to become full-term fetuses, children, and adults.

A second viewpoint denies that human preembryos have any moral status. According to this viewpoint, we have no moral obligations to human preembryos. This position also appeals to scientific evidence, especially the fact that only 30% to 40% of preembryos produced through human sexual intercourse develop to maturity in utero and are delivered as live infants (Leridon, 1973). It also notes that the biologic individuality of the preembryo is assured only toward the end of the first 14 days of development; before that time, one preembryo can divide into twins; or, experimentally, multiple preembryos with different genotypes can be combined into a single preembryo. Finally, this position argues that an undifferentiated entity like the preembryo—which has no organs, limbs, or sentience—cannot have moral status.

Again on this issue there is an intermediate position. This viewpoint accords some moral status to the preembryo on grounds both of its unique genotype and its potential. The potential to become an adult differentiates the preembryo from nonembryonic human tissues or cells. However, this third viewpoint acknowledges that our prima facie moral obligations to human preembryos can be outweighed by other moral duties, for example, the duty to develop new and better methods of providing care to infertile couples or pregnant women. (Not reprinted in this volume.)

The Role of Family or Genetic Lineage The modern techniques of artificial insemination (AID, AIH), in vitro fertilization (IVF), and—to a lesser extent—uterine lavage have made the notion of "parenthood" more complex. In some contexts of medically assisted reproduction, one must distinguish among the genetic, gestational, and rearing mothers and between the genetic and rearing fathers. Table 1 illustrates the major ways in which third parties can become participants in the reproductive process (Walters, 1985a).

The practice of donating gametes or preembryos has occasioned debate among commentators on the new reproductive technologies. One view is that these technologies should be employed only within the family unit. Proponents of this view conclude that if the couple cannot conceive a child by means of their own gametes, even with medical assistance, they should accept their infertility and explore alternatives such as adoption. According to this viewpoint, adoption is qualitatively different from the deliberate and premeditated introduction of "foreign" gametes or preembryos into the family unit, because adopting parents rescue an already existing child from a situation of homelessness.

The opposing viewpoint on gamete and preembryo donation is that these practices are morally justified when employed by a couple for good reasons, such as untreatable infertility or the presence of a genetic defect in one or both partners. The use of the new reproductive technologies is therefore seen as a useful adjunct that allows couples to approximate, as closely as possible, the usual experience of reproduction.

In chapters 15 through 19 and 25, the Committee discusses various types of gamete or preembryo donation [not reprinted in this volume]. The conclusion of the Committee in most of the donation scenarios is that the alleviation of infertility or the prevention of the transmission of known genetic defects provides a sufficient rationale for donation. On the other hand, the Committee finds that the use of donation for nonmedical reasons, such as the desire to produce a "superbaby," is ethically unacceptable.

A second controversial issue is the meaning of the term *family*. The traditional understanding of family was that it included a husband, a wife, and one or more children. This traditional understanding has been challenged not primarily by the new reproductive technologies but rather by several social developments of the 20th century, especially divorce rates approaching 50% in the United States and the

TABLE 1. Alternative Reproductive Methods[a,b]

	Source of Gametes				Site of Fertilization			Site of Pregnancy		Notes
	Male		Female							
1	H		W		W			W		Customary, AIH
2		S	W		W			W		AID
3	H		W			L		W		IVF
4		S	W			L		W		IVF with donated sperm
5	H			S		L		W		IVF with donated egg
6		S		S		L		W		IVF with both gametes donated (or donated embryo)
7	H			S			S	W		AIH with donor woman plus uterine lavage (semidonated embryo)
8		S		S			S	W		AID with donor woman plus uterine lavage (donated embryo)
9	H		W		W				S	Surrogate motherhood (rows 9–16)
10		S	W		W				S	
11	H		W			L			S	
12		S	W			L			S	
13	H			S		L			S	
14		S		S		L			S	
15	H			S			S		S	
16[c]		S		S			S		S	

[a]Chart developed by William B. Weil, Jr., and LeRoy Walters.
[b]H, husband; W, wife; S, third-party substitute, or surrogate; and L, laboratory.
[c]Planned procreation for placement; traditional adoption is not part of the schematic.

increasing number of children born to single women. The general debate about the meaning of family, however, will be carried over into discussions of the new reproductive technologies as members of nontraditional families—unmarried heterosexual couples, homosexual couples, single men or women—request technical assistance in reproduction.

The Committee considers parenthood by a heterosexual couple to be the most appropriate arrangement, other things being equal. However, the Committee discusses (particularly in chapter 9, not reprinted) the moral right to reproduce in terms that allow a role for other patterns of parenthood. The Committee is opposed to the legal prohibition of medically assisted reproduction by nontraditional families [footnote omitted].

A third controversial issue is whether or not the donors of gametes or preembryos should be known to members of the rearing family. In other words, should donors be regarded as part of an extended family? If donations are made by relatives or close friends, they will automatically be known to the recipient couple. In other donation situations, practice has varied, with artificial insemination donor (AID) usually remaining anonymous; surrogate mothers, however, are often known to the rearing couple. The Committee viewpoint is that practice in this area should be governed by the results of careful empiric research on the effects of the arrangements on the participants, which includes the children, and by the wishes of the principals involved. However, the Committee considers it an ethical obligation of the health professionals involved to retain some means for recontacting donors and providing medical follow-up. . . . This information link with donors becomes especially critical if offspring are born with genetic defects.

The Appropriate Role of Government To philosophers like Plato, the classical Western view of the proper role of government was that it should promote virtue in its citizens, who were viewed as parts of an organic whole, the state. In modern times, this view has been rejected by most Western political philosophers. The closest modern parallel to the Platonic viewpoint is that a government should ensure that its citizens act in accordance with the principles of morality. According to this view, governments are justified in intervening to prevent even private immoral behavior, such as illicit sexual activity, because in the long run such behavior undermines the public good (Devlin, 1965).

A second viewpoint sees the primary role of government as protecting individual liberties and preventing persons from inflicting harm on others. This view often includes the "clear and present danger" test, namely, that only serious, imminent harms are of sufficient importance to warrant government intrusion (Feinberg, 1973). According to this view, government would not normally intervene in the private sexual activities or reproductive efforts of consenting adults except perhaps to prevent tangible, highly probable physical harm to potential offspring.

A third view limits individual liberty, not only to protect citizens from harm, but also to ensure that every citizen enjoys at least a certain minimum of welfare—income, food, clothing, shelter, and health care (Rawls, 1971; Daniels, 1985). Applied to the new reproductive technologies, this view of government might include infertility treatment within the scope of guaranteed minimum health services.

The Committee is aware that the general role of government in the delivery of health care services differs among the countries that have devoted the most detailed discussion to the new reproductive technologies. The Committee clearly subscribes to the view that government should intervene to prevent substantial harm to offspring, for example, by requiring donor screening if such screening is not voluntarily practiced by sperm banks or health practitioners involved in the donation process. . . .

Principles

Contemporary moral philosophers have identified three ethical principles that underlie particular moral judgments: respect for autonomy, beneficence, and justice (Beauchamp, 1983).

Respect for Autonomy The principle of respect for autonomy acknowledges a sphere in which the individual should be free to exert control. One classic formulation of this principle, in John Stuart Mill's *On Liberty,* is that individuals should be able to choose freely what they will do, unless or until their actions cause serious harm to others or seriously limit others' liberty. This principle is closely related to the liberty rights discussed in chapters 6 and 9. It is also clearly pertinent to the notion of informed consent, for only well-informed and uncoerced persons can make autonomous choices (chapter 7). The principle of autonomy provides the basis for our concern about protecting confidentiality, particularly in the context of gamete or preembryo donation.

Beneficence Beneficence includes two distinct aspects. Positively, it refers to promoting the welfare of others. Negatively, it refers to "doing no harm" to other persons. The principle of beneficence has traditionally faced at least two major problems. The first is identifying whose welfare or harm is to be taken into account. In discussions of the new reproductive technologies, especially of research with human preembryos, a critical question will therefore be whether preembryos can be the objects of either benefit or harm (chapter 23). A second problem is the relative weight to be assigned to different kinds of benefits or harms. In the reproductive context, for example, physical harm to the wife must sometimes be compared with psychological benefits for her and her spouse.

In the following chapters on specific technologies, the Committee sometimes recommends measures for minimizing the possible harms associated with a specific reproductive technology (for example, chapters 15 and 25). In other cases, the Committee judges the potential harm of a technique to be so uncertain that it recommends the conduct of a clinical experiment or trial, rather than the immediate adoption of a technique into clinical practice (chapters 19 and 22). In still other cases, the Committee concludes, on the basis of extensive experience, that the risks of a new technique are minimal (chapter 13).

Justice Justice governs the distribution of liberties on the one hand, and harms and benefits on the other hand. Most people can agree on the formal principle of justice: "to everyone his or her due." What is more controversial is the answer to the question, "What is due to various individuals and on what basis is it due?" Several answers to this question have been proposed, including the following:

a. To everyone according to his or her merit
b. To everyone according to his or her need
c. To everyone an equal share
d. To everyone what he or she has acquired by proper means.

Because justice is concerned in part with the distribution of benefits and harms, the question of who is included or excluded recurs again with this principle. Further, viewpoints of "what is due" will determine, in part, whether or not the inability of some members of society to afford the new reproductive technologies is regarded as an ethical problem. If one accepts answer *a* or *d* above, the de facto lack of access may not be seen as an injustice. However, if one accepts answer *b* or *c,* then economic exclusion from access may be viewed as unjust (chapter 9).

Ethical Theories

Some ethical theories give precedence to one of the above three principles in any case of conflict among the principles. In a sense, one principle always takes precedence over the other two. For utilitarians, the principle of beneficence is always uppermost; for libertarians, the principle of respect for autonomy; for egalitarians, a particular understanding of the principle of justice.

In this report, the Committee has been unwilling to assign universal precedence to any of the three principles. Concern for the potential harms and the long-term social impact of the new reproductive technologies looms large in the Committee's thinking, but so does respect for the autonomy of persons making reproductive decisions and the autonomy of researchers and clinicians who develop or offer these new technologies. The principle of justice informs the Committee's efforts to avoid discriminating against particular groups and the Committee's interest in the problem of access. Thus, the Committee is pluralistic in its ethical theory, holding the three ethical principles in tension and regarding each of the three as fundamentally important. Each informs the Committee's consideration of what is due to the person integrally and adequately considered (chapter 5).

* * *

13. *IN VITRO* FERTILIZATION

Background

The extracorporeal fertilization of eggs and the transfer of preembryos in a mammalian system was first reported over 20 years ago. Since then there have been more and more reports of successful human in vitro fertilization (IVF) in Europe, Australia, the United States, and elsewhere (Lopata, 1983; Jones, 1984; Marrs, 1985). Most IVF centers use ovarian stimulation to produce multiple eggs, because pregnancy rates are higher with transfer of more than one preembryo. Various agents are used for ovarian stimulation, such as clomiphene citrate, human menopausal gonadotropin, and combinations of these agents. After stimulation, the response is monitored by measurement of urinary or serum estrogens and by ultrasound visualization of follicle growth. At the appropriate time, egg recovery is performed, either by laparoscopy and follicle aspiration or, more recently, one of several other ultrasound-directed methods now in clinical trial (Wikland, 1983). The laboratory culture conditions for culturing eggs and sperm have been refined extensively in the past few years. Sperm and eggs are coincubated for approximately 12 to 18 hours so that fertilization can occur; then, after an additional 48 or 72 hours, the resulting preembryo(s) is transferred to the uterine cavity by means of a small catheter placed transcervically. Implantation of the preembryo should begin in the next 2 to 3 days, and detection of pregnancy should be possible within 2 weeks after the transfer. Success rates with human IVF techniques have steadily improved since the first birth in 1978. Currently, the success rates vary but have been reported to be up to 25% per cycle of treatment.

The term IVF is used to refer to the procedure as such, without any of its possible variants (e.g., donor semen, donor eggs, surrogate wombs, etc.) or accompaniments (e.g., experimentation on the preembryo). It is therefore meant to refer to the process of IVF (of gametes from husband and wife) with embryo transfer, as a substitute for tubal fertilization and natural implantation. It is this basic IVF that was approved by the Ethics Advisory Board (of the then United States Department of Health, Education and Welfare) as "ethically acceptable."

Medical Indications

The primary medical indication for human IVF is failure of conventional therapy to provide a pregnancy for the infertile couple. The most common indication for the use of human IVF procedures is irreconcilable tubal damage or destruction, which exists in patients who have undergone surgical removal of the fallopian tubes because of inflammatory disease or tubal ectopic pregnancy. Certain other pelvic factors that are indications for IVF include pelvic endometriosis that has failed conservative surgical and medical therapy, and pelvic adhesive disease that has similarly failed conventional surgical therapy. Such female pelvic factors are the second most common diagnosis in the patient population undergoing IVF. Anomalies of the uterus and/or reproductive tract, whether due to a congenital factor or drug exposure in vivo (diethylstilbestrol), are also accepted indications for IVF.

Another very strong indication for IVF stems from the male factor. The partner of an oligospermic man is also a candidate for IVF, because fertilization in vitro has been demonstrated with very low sperm concentrations.

In either partner, immunologic disorders unresponsive to conventional therapy are another indication for IVF. Also, an increasing percentage of couples are entering IVF with the diagnosis of unexplained or idiopathic infertility. Whether this will remain a primary indication for IVF after all conventional therapy has failed is somewhat dependent on relative success of intrafallopian gamete transfer in producing ongoing clinical pregnancies (Asch, personal communication, 1985).

Reservations

Several objections have been raised against the procedure. The first is that it separates procreation from sexual union, life-giving from love-making. The assumption of the objection is that, for the good of the child and the couple, the child should be conceived in an act of sexual love-making.

A second objection is speculative in character. It argues that the standard procedure involves the possibility that it might produce some deformed or retarded children and is therefore an immoral means, for it involves exposing others to potential risk without their consent. It is a procedure to benefit the parents, with the risks borne by the unconsenting child.

A third objection underlines the problem of containment; if the standard procedure is approved, we will be on a "slippery slope" and will inevitably proceed to the variants and accompaniments of IVF, some or all of which would be rejected by large numbers of people.

Fourth, it has been objected that infertility is not a life-threatening disorder. Use of IVF as a therapeutic modality for a condition that is not medically harmful tends to medicalize other basic human problems. Furthermore, if IVF is not a corrective procedure and if it basically bypasses the disorder that cannot be corrected by therapeutic modalities, then there are likely to be reservations from those concerned about health care costs.

The fifth concern is that IVF involves the use of expertise and resources to produce more offspring in an already overpopulated world.

Rationale

The overall basic rationale for the IVF procedure is that the benefits provided outweigh the risks both to the couple and to the offspring produced. From the facts currently available, the procedure produces normal, healthy offspring with a success rate that approaches the natural one. There is no known increased risk to the parents or to the offspring (Seppala, 1985). Therefore, IVF has become an accepted therapy for intractable infertility.

Deliberations

The Committee could find no persuasive evidence that the child and/or married couple suffer harm (the personal criterion) when IVF is used as a last resort. The analysis insisting on the inseparability of the life-giving and love-making dimensions is built on an excessively biologic notion of what is morally right and wrong. Furthermore, numerous commentators see IVF not as a substitute for sexual intimacy, but as an extension of it, and therefore as not involving the radical separation of procreation and sexual intimacy. (For an extended discussion of these reservations and objections, please see McCormick, 1984.)

As for risks, similar risks are run by couples in their ordinary sexual lives. Therefore, if the risks in IVF are not notably greater than those involved in sexual intercourse, the argument loses force. Factually, on the basis of experience so far, IVF involves no greater risk to the child.

The extension of reproductive technology into suspect areas is a legitimate concern. Yet, the response to such a concern is that possible abuse does not invalidate appropriate use. Furthermore, there is likely to be sharp pluralism about what constitutes abuse.

Finally, the Committee argued that the infertile couple should not be held responsible for the population problems of the world. Realistically, IVF would not affect such problems one way or another.

Recommendations

The Committee unanimously finds that basic IVF is ethically acceptable.

* * *

25. SURROGATE MOTHERS

Background

A surrogate mother is a woman who is artificially inseminated with the sperm of a man who is not her husband; she carries the pregnancy and then turns the resulting child over to the man to rear. In almost all instances, the man has chosen to use a surrogate mother because his wife is infertile. After the birth, the wife will adopt the child.

Unlike surrogate gestational motherhood, which involves an embryo transfer after in vivo or in vitro fertilization (IVF), surrogate motherhood depends only on the technology of artificial insemination. The primary reason for the use of surrogate motherhood as a reproductive option is to produce a child with a genetic link to the husband.

The use of the term "surrogate" for the woman who is the genetic and gestational mother of the child appears a misnomer to some people, who argue that the adoptive mother is actually the "surrogate" for the biologic mother, who has given up the child. Nevertheless, a contrary position can be articulated, because the adoptive woman will be performing the major mothering role by rearing the child, with the biologic mother serving as a surrogate for her in providing the component for reproduction that she lacks. Although the term "surrogate mother" is, in any case, ambiguous and not a medical term, it has nevertheless received widespread public recognition and will be used in this report to mean a woman who conceives and gestates a child to be reared by the biologic father and his wife. The use of a surrogate mother, who provides the egg and the womb for the child, is currently much more common than the use of a surrogate gestational mother, who provides only the womb.

In comparison with the other reproductive technologies discussed in this report, surrogate motherhood has received scant attention in the medical literature. Although it has produced many more babies than have been born after cryopreservation of a preembryo or by preembryo donation after in vivo fertilization, there have been no medical articles published about the procedure, its success rate, or the mental or physical health of the children produced.

There are only a few studies of the psychological ramifications of surrogate motherhood. These studies include speculation about the potential effects on the participants (Andrews, 1985b) and preliminary research on the selection of surrogate mothers and their responses to the pregnancy and subsequent relinquishment of the child (Franks, 1981; Parker, 1983).

One reason for the lack of scientific attention to the medical aspects of surrogate motherhood is that it has developed in an entrepreneurial setting, generally apart from medical institutions. Although the founders of some surrogate mother programs are physicians, the majority are lawyers, social workers, or persons with no professional training. However, most programs do use the services of a physician to perform a physical examination of the surrogate mother and to perform the artificial insemination. The extent to which these programs undertake an independent assessment of the infertility of the wife is unclear. Some couples who have infertility problems that could be helped by drugs, surgery, IVF, or other alternatives may be employing a surrogate at a substantial fee because they do not undergo medical screening as part of the surrogate program and thus do not realize that they have other options. Existing surrogate mother programs generally perform medical screening on the surrogate, and some perform a physical on the man who will provide the sperm (Andrews, 1985).

Some women serve as surrogate mothers for an infertile friend or relative and charge no fee. In other instances, the surrogate mother is a stranger who receives compensation for her services.

The demographic studies of surrogate mothers, which deal mainly with potential paid surrogates, have found that their average age is 25. Over one-half of the women are married, one-fifth divorced, and about one-fourth single. Over one-half (57%) are Protestant and 42% are Catholic (Parker, 1983). Over one-half are high school graduates and over one-fourth have schooling beyond high school.

Polls show that the public is less favorably disposed toward surrogate motherhood as an infertility solution than it is toward IVF, artificial insemination donor (AID), embryo donation, or adoption (Brodsky, 1983). However, surveys of the public and of child welfare professionals regarding how the law should handle surrogate motherhood indicate that most people feel that the procedure should not be banned but rather should be regulated (Child Welfare League, 1983).

Indications

When a woman is infertile, she and her husband may need the assistance of a surrogate mother to conceive and carry a child for her. Sperm from the husband of the infertile woman is used to inseminate the surrogate mother, who will carry the pregnancy and then turn the resulting child over to the couple.

The primary medical indication for use of a surrogate mother is the inability of a woman to provide either the genetic or the gestational component for childbearing, for example, a woman who has had a hysterectomy combined with removal of the ovaries. This is the only situation in which surrogate motherhood provides the sole medical solution. For other indications, other medical options are possible, although they may not be readily available.

A second indication for surrogate motherhood is the inability to provide the genetic component, for example, because of premature menopause or the desire not to risk passing on a genetic defect. Under these circumstances, the woman could alternatively have the genetic component provided through egg or embryo donation, but donors might be more difficult to find than surrogate mothers.

A third indication for the use of a surrogate mother is the inability to gestate. A woman with severe hypertension, a uterine malformation, or the absence of a uterus after hysterectomy may use the services of a surrogate mother. If that woman wanted to provide the genetic component for her child, she and her husband could create an embryo either in vitro or in vivo, then have it transferred to a surrogate gestational mother.

The use of a surrogate mother is also available as a secondary approach for women with any other type of infertility; essentially, it eliminates the need for the social mother to play any biologic role in reproduction.

Reservations about Surrogate Motherhood

The reservations about surrogate motherhood, like reservations about other reproductive technologies, focus on the potential effects on the surrogate, the couple, the potential child, and society. Because of the dearth of research on the subject, most of the potential risks are highly speculative. There is concern that it is improper to ask a surrogate to put herself through the physical hazards of a pregnancy to benefit other persons. There is also concern that the surrogate might be psychologically harmed by giving up her genetic child. There are some surrogates who go through a period of grief and mourning after giving up the child (*Psychiatric News*, 1984).

There is also a risk that, because of the uncertain legal status of the procedure, the surrogate will be required to keep (or put up for general adoption) a child for whom she did not intend to have parental responsibility. This situation might occur if a paternity test revealed that the child was not the offspring of the man who contracted with the surrogate or if the child were born with a defect so that the couple refused to take custody of the child.

In addition to the potential harm to the surrogate, there is concern that the couple might be harmed by the procedure. The woman might be harmed by not having access to medical advice to help her resolve her infertility in other ways. The couple might be at risk of harassment from the surrogate in those rare instances in which she learns the couple's identities and seeks them out after relinquishing the child. Or, if the surrogate is a friend or relative, her continued involvement with the couple may cause tension in their marital relationship. Also, the couple are financially and emotionally at risk because of the uncertain legal status of the procedure. If the surrogate keeps the child, the contracting husband might nevertheless have to pay child support because he is the biologic father. The couple who pay a surrogate might be prosecuted under criminal law in those states that prohibit payment beyond certain enumerated medical and legal expenses of a woman in connection with her giving up her child for adoption (Andrews, 1986).

The potential physical and psychological effects on the child are cause for concern as well. The child might be physically harmed if the surrogate mother passes on a genetic defect. This possibility is similar to the risk involved in using sperm donors, and it merits similar handling by appropriate screening. The surrogate mother has the responsibility not only of providing the gamete for conception but also of gestating. A surrogate mother who knows that she will not have the responsibility of rearing a child might not be sufficiently careful during the pregnancy. Moreover, the surrogate might be less likely than a woman planning to rear the child to give priority to the fetus in situations in which there is a conflict between maternal and fetal needs. For these reasons, screening of potential surrogate mothers is necessary to determine what gestational risks they present.

In addition, there are concerns about the psychological development of the child, who may feel a need for information about the surrogate mother or may want to learn her identity. If the surrogate mother is a friend or relative who maintains contact with the child, it is unclear what effect a connection with two mothers will have on the child's development or identity.

As with donation of sperm, eggs, or embryos, the use of a surrogate mother who provides an egg, as well as gestational services, raises questions about the ethics of donor involvement in procreation. There is concern that the involvement of a surrogate mother in childbearing will weaken the marital bond and undermine the integrity of the institution of the family. To some, third-party involvement in procreation is considered to be threatening to the sanctity of the marital relationship, whether or not there is provable physical or psychological harm to the participants in the process.

Some commentators have voiced the further concern that if surrogates are paid for their services, human reproduction will become commercialized, and children might come to be perceived as a "consumer item" (Hellegers, 1978).

A final reservation is that surrogate motherhood might be used for convenience when the potential rearing mother does not wish to undergo pregnancy. However, it is less likely that a woman would use a surrogate mother, rather than a surrogate gestational mother, for those purposes. With a surrogate mother, the woman gives up not only the gestational inconvenience but also the chance to be the genetic mother for the child.

Rationale for the Use of a Surrogate Mother

For some couples, of whom the wife has no uterus or ovaries, the use of a surrogate mother is the only means to have a child genetically related to one of them. In all of its applications, the use of a surrogate mother allows the infertile woman who wishes to rear a child the opportunity to adopt an infant more rapidly than by waiting several years for a traditional adoption. In addition, it allows her to rear her husband's genetic child.

For the husband of an infertile woman, the use of a surrogate may be the only way in which he can conceive and rear a child with a biologic tie to himself, short of divorcing his wife and remarrying only for that reason or of having an adulterous union. Certainly, the use of a surrogate mother under the auspices of a medical practitioner seems far less destructive of the institution of the family than the latter two options.

For the child, the use of a surrogate mother gives him or her an opportunity that would not otherwise be available: the opportunity to exist. Furthermore, the child would be reared by a couple who so wanted him or her that they were willing to participate in a novel process with potential legal and other risks.

The process offers potential benefits for the surrogates as well. As in the case of organ transplantation, it offers them the chance to be altruistic. In addition, some surrogate mothers enjoy being pregnant. Moreover, one preliminary study found that about one-third of surrogate mothers may be using the process to help themselves psychologically. These are women who in the past have voluntarily aborted or given up a child through adoption and have then become surrogate mothers in order to relive the experience of pregnancy in a psychologically satisfactory way (Parker, 1983). Those women who become surrogate mothers for a fee are benefited by having another income option. For example, some divorced women with young children have chosen to be surrogates in order to support their children and to remain at home to care for them.

Although there are potential risks to surrogacy, those risks can be understood by the prospective participants. Thus informed, they can engage in competent decision making about whether or not to pursue this reproductive option. Initial data indicate that the couples and surrogates can understand in advance how they will react to the procedure. "Preliminary evidence indicates that only a few surrogates and the parental couple felt surprised by their own psychological responses after the relinquishment or by the other party's response" (Parker, 1984).

Committee Considerations

Surrogate motherhood has received extensive media attention and has raised a panoply of emotional reactions and ethical concerns. Unlike AID, which was developed in a shroud of secrecy, surrogate motherhood was thrust before the public eye, often for the pragmatic reason of needing high visibility in order to recruit potential surrogates. The use of a surrogate mother has raised a range of issues about third-party involvement in procreation, such as whether that involvement is destructive to the marital bond or psychologically harmful to the third party and whether the child has a right to learn about the history or identity of the third party. Unfortunately, there is little precedent for answering these questions; the policy of secrecy surrounding sperm donation has served to limit studies in that context that might have served as a basis for understanding the psychological implications of using third parties in reproduction generally. Nevertheless, large segments of our society view as permissible the donation of sperm to compensate for a male infertility problem. The use of a surrogate mother to compensate for a female infertility problem could similarly be viewed as permissible, unless it can be demonstrated to be significantly more risky to the participants or to society than AID or other activities that our society condones.

The Committee's main concerns about surrogate motherhood are threefold. First, there appear to be potential risks to all participants that need to be considered. There is concern that a woman who becomes a surrogate mother may be subjecting herself to too many physical and psychological risks. There is some sentiment that it is improper to ask a woman to be a surrogate mother, because she will be facing the potential physical risks of pregnancy and childbirth without receiving what seems to be a commensurate benefit. There are further concerns that a woman who is a friend or relative of the couple may be coerced into being a surrogate or that a paid surrogate may be exploited.

The perceived degree of involvement (duration, intensity, and medical risks) of the surrogate mother leads the Committee to see this third-party involvement as different from AID or egg donation. However, the Committee is mindful that society allows competent adults to take risks (for example, trying an experimental medical procedure, donating a kidney, engaging in a risky sports activity or occupation, or joining the armed services). In the medical realm, people are allowed to make risky choices as long as they have given voluntary, informed consent. With respect to surrogate motherhood, then, it is of the utmost importance to ensure that the potential surrogate mother is appropriately informed and has not been coerced into serving as a surrogate. It may be useful for the physician to interview the potential surrogate separately to ensure that she has not been coerced into participation; this may be especially important when the surrogate is a friend or relative of the couple and may have been subjected to personal pressures regarding participation.

Although the couple are not at physical risk, they may be at emotional or financial risk because the surrogate might decide to keep the child, which would require them to seek a court order to gain custody. Again, however, if voluntary, informed consent is obtained from the couple, it may be excessively paternalistic to deny them their chosen option on the speculation that it could be harmful to them.

Naturally, a prime ethical concern regarding the participants is focused on the child. A realistic assessment needs to be made of the potential physical and psychological risks to the child. Although there exists a potential for surrogates to risk harm to the child by failing to disclose a genetic defect that would disqualify them for surrogacy or by engaging in harmful behavior during pregnancy, such risk could be minimized by proper medical and psychological screening of surrogates. As is true with AID, there is little follow-up data on the health of the children born to surrogates. But the high visibility of the surrogate arrangements, as well as the fact that news about unhealthy children has been extremely rare, suggests that the potential physical risks have not frequently materialized under the current system.

As to potential psychological harm to the child, there is concern that the child's self-identity might be confused because of his or her blurred genealogy. The use of a surrogate mother does not have to have a "blurring" effect on the child's genealogy. Situations in which full disclosures are made to the child about the personal history of the surrogate (and perhaps even her identity) might provide clear knowledge of genealogy. However, it is true that any use of a third party may make the genealogy more complex and perhaps bothersome to the child. Even if there are psychological risks, most infertile couples who go through with a reproduction arrangement that involves a third party do so as a last resort. In some cases, their willingness to make sacrifices to have a child may testify to their worthiness as loving parents. A child conceived through surrogate motherhood may be born into a much healthier climate than a child whose birth was unplanned. For this reason, some of the risks caused by confused genealogy may be outweighed by possible benefits to the child of having parents who want him or her.

Concerns are also raised by payment to a surrogate. Some people may approve of voluntary surrogate motherhood but disapprove of surrogate motherhood for a fee. The ramifications of prohibiting payment are widespread, however, because there are not enough voluntary surrogates to meet the needs of infertile couples. Because a surrogate mother has a much greater involvement in reproduction than does a donor of sperm, eggs, or embryos, she usually requires remuneration. On the couple's side, spending money for childbearing does not in itself seem unethical. Even without the involvement of a surrogate, couples spend substantial sums to investigate and treat their infertility. This financial outlay does not seem to create unusually high expectations about the child that might lead to psychological problems for him or her.

Commercialization in connection with giving up a child for adoption has traditionally been banned on the grounds that it might force biologic mothers to give up children whom they do not wish to give up and that the mere willingness to pay for a child does not guarantee that the potential parent will treat the child well. Because the sperm donor is merely turning over a gamete, whereas the surrogate mother is turning over a child, the latter action may seem to fit more closely into traditional concerns about baby selling. Nevertheless, paying the surrogate a fee is readily distinguishable from paying an already pregnant woman for her child. The payment to a surrogate is made in exchange for her help in creating a child, not in exchange for possession of the child. Because the decision is made before the pregnancy ensues and the arrangement is entered into with the specific intention of relinquishing the child, the woman is less likely than an already-pregnant woman to be coerced into giving up a child whom she wishes to keep. Because the child will be reared by the genetic father and his wife, it may be more likely that the rearing father will have a greater sense of responsibility for the child than if the child were turned over to a stranger. Because the surrogate's responsibilities are set out in a contract before the conception occurs, she is more likely to understand and abide by them and less likely later to harass the couple with a change of heart.

A psychiatrist who has interviewed over 500 potential surrogates and who has followed several dozen surrogates through their pregnancies and beyond has written about surrogates' financial motivation, "There is no evidence that such a motivating factor results in more adverse psychological, medical, or legal consequences" (P. J. Parker, unpublished essay, 1982).

More troublesome is the commercialization and potential for exploitation of the couples and surrogates by professionals acting as brokers. The Committee is concerned that professionals who attempt to serve both the couple and the surrogate or who receive finder's fees for surrogates may have a conflict of interest or may exploit the parties.

As a final reservation, the lack of laws protecting couples who use a surrogate leads to a reluctance on the part of practitioners to recommend it (chapter 7). This, of course, could be solved by the enactment of laws clarifying the points that the contracting couple are the legal parents and that the surrogate mother has no parental rights or responsibilities with respect to the child after birth. Such laws are already being proposed in some states. Laws that take the opposite approach and attempt to prohibit the use of surrogate mothers would likely be struck down as unconstitutional for violating the couple's right to privacy in making procreative decisions (chapter 6).

Until favorable laws are passed, the rights and duties among the parties will likely be handled by a contract that includes an agreement by the surrogate to turn the child over to the couple for adoption. Of particular importance will be the provisions for human leukocyte antigen typing of the man providing the sperm and of the child, for assurance that the surrogate did not inadvertently become pregnant by her own partner rather than through the artificial insemination procedure.

Committee Recommendations

The Committee finds that surrogate motherhood is a matter that requires intense scrutiny. The Committee does not recommend the use of a surrogate mother for a nonmedical reason, such as the convenience of the rearing mother, because nonmedical reasons seem inadequate to justify using a surrogate to undertake the risks of pregnancy and delivery. As for surrogate motherhood for medical reasons, the Committee is dismayed by the scarcity of empiric evidence about how the surrogacy process works and how it affects those involved. Nevertheless, this process offers promise as the only medical solution to infertility in a couple of whom the woman has no uterus and who does not produce eggs or does not want to risk passing on a genetic defect that she carries.

There may be individual practitioners or medical groups asked to aid a surrogate mother arrangement who find that the reservations about the procedure outweigh the benefits, i.e., that the procedure is not in the best interests of the persons integrally and adequately considered. In that circumstance, the practitioner or group could ethically decline to participate in the arrangement.

The Committee does not recommend widespread clinical application of surrogate motherhood at this time. Because of the legal risks, ethical concerns, and potential physical and psychological effects of surrogate motherhood, it would seem to be more problematic than most of the other reproductive technologies discussed in this report. The Committee believes that there are not adequate reasons to recommend legal prohibition of surrogate motherhood, but the Committee has serious ethical reservations about surrogacy that cannot be fully resolved until appropriate data are available for assessment of the risks and possible benefits of this alternative.

The Committee recommends that if surrogate motherhood is pursued, it should be pursued as a clinical experiment. Among the issues to be addressed in the research on surrogate mothers are the following:

a. the psychological effects of the procedure on the surrogates, the couples, and the resulting children
b. the effects, if any, of bonding between the surrogate and the fetus in utero
c. the appropriate screening of the surrogate and the man who provides the sperm

d. the likelihood that the surrogate will exercise appropriate care during the pregnancy
e. the effects of having the couple and the surrogate meet or not meet
f. the effects on the surrogate's own family of her participation in the process
g. the effects of disclosing or not disclosing the use of a surrogate mother or her identity to the child
h. other issues that shed light on the effects of surrogacy on the welfare of the various persons involved and on society.

In the course of the clinical experiments on surrogate motherhood, special attention should be paid to whether the surrogate and the couple have given voluntary, informed consent. Both the surrogate and the man providing the sperm should be screened for infectious diseases, and the surrogate should be screened for genetic defects. . . .

So that potential conflicts of interest or exploitation by professionals can be avoided, the Committee recommends that professionals receive only their customary fees for services and receive no finder's fees for participation in surrogate motherhood. Although it would be preferable that surrogates not receive payment beyond compensation for expenses and their inconvenience, the Committee recognizes that in some cases payment will be necessary for surrogacy to occur [note omitted]. If surrogate motherhood turns out to be useful, a change in the law would be appropriate for assurance that the couple who contract with a surrogate mother are viewed as the legal parents [notes omitted].

REFERENCES

Andrews LB: New Conception: A Consumer's Guide to the Newest Infertility Treatments, Including In Vitro Fertilization, Artificial Insemination, and Surrogate Motherhood. New York, Ballentine Books, 1985

Andrews LB: Legal and ethical aspects of new reproductive technologies. Clin Obstet Gynecol 29:190, 1986

Beauchamp TL, Childress JF: Principles of Biomedical Ethics, 2nd ed. New York, Oxford University Press, 1983.

Brodsky AM, Martin DJ, Kelly AM, Bierman K: Survey of attitudes about reproductive technologies. Presentation to the American Psychological Association, Anaheim, CA 1983

Callahan D: New beginnings in life: a philosopher's response. In The New Genetics and the Future of Man, Edited by M Hamilton. Grand Rapids, MI, Eerdmans, 1972, p 100

Child Welfare League of America: Report of Agency Survey on Surrogate Parenting. New York, Child Welfare League, 1983

Daniels N: Just Health Care. New York, Cambridge University Press, 1985

Devlin P: The Enforcement of Morals. New York, Oxford University Press, 1965

Feinberg J: Social Philosophy. Englewood Cliffs, NJ, Prentice Hall, 1973, p 36

Fletcher J: The Ethics of Genetic Control. Garden City, NY, Anchor Books, 1974, p 36

Franks DD: Psychiatric evaluation of women in a surrogate mother program. Am J Psychiatry 138:1378, 1981

Hellegers AE, McCormick RA: Unanswered questions on test tube life. America 74:139, 1978

Jones HW Jr, Acosta AA, Andrews MC, Garcia JE, Jones GS, Mayer J, McDowell JS, Rosenwaks Z, Sandow BA, Veeck LL, Wilkes CA: Three years of in vitro fertilization at Norfolk. Fetil Steril 42:826, 1984

Kass LR: Making babies—the new biology and the 'old' morality. Public Interest 26:49, 1972

Leridon H: Démographie des échecs de la reproduction. In Les Accidents Chromosomiques de la Reproduction, Edited by A Boue, C Thibault. Paris, Centre International de l'Enfance, 1973, p 13

Lopata A: Concepts in human in vitro fertilization and embryo transfer. Fertil Steril 40:289, 1983

McCormick RA: Notes on moral theology. Theolog St 45:96, 1984

Marrs RP, Vargyas J, Hoffman D, Yee B: Use of various ovarian stimulation methods to improve oocyte and embryo production for human in vitro fertilization. Ann NY Acad Sci 442:112., 1985

Parker PJ: Motivation of surrogate mothers: initial findings. Am J Psychiat 140:117, 1983

Parker PJ: Surrogate motherhood, psychiatric screening and informed consent, baby selling, and public policy. Bull Am Acad Psychiat Law 12:21, 1984

Psychiatric News: Effects of surrogate motherhood, other childbearing options need closer study, says researcher. Psychiatric News, 19:10, 18 May 1984.

Rawls J: A Theory of Justice. Boston, Belknap Press, 1971, p 302

Seppala M: The world collaborative report on in vitro fertilization and embryo replacement: current state of the art in January 1984. Ann NY Acad Sci 442:558, 1985

Walters L: Editor's introduction. J Med Philos 10:210, 1985a

Wikland M, Nilsson L, Hansson R. Hamberger L, Jansen PO: Collection of human oocytes by the use of sonography. Fertil Steril 39:603, 1983

INSTRUCTION ON RESPECT FOR HUMAN LIFE BY THE CONGREGATION FOR THE DOCTRINE OF THE FAITH, 1987

INTRODUCTION. *In response to inquiries by bishops, theologians, physicians, and scientists, the leadership of the Catholic Church sought to clarify the Church's official position on several new reproductive options. A point of particular importance was relating the Church's teaching on new reproductive alternatives to Pope Paul VI's 1968 encyclical on birth control, an encyclical entitled Humanae Vitae. The central thesis that emerges from the following excerpts is that any technique that separates sexual intercourse from reproduction—either to avoid reproduction or to assist it—is morally wrong. This moral prohibition applies to situations involving sperm and egg cells from husband and wife and to situations involving donor gametes or a surrogate mother.*

II. INTERVENTIONS UPON HUMAN PROCREATION

By "artificial procreation" or " artificial fertilization" are understood here the different technical procedures directed towards obtaining a human conception in a manner other than the sexual union of man and woman. This Instruction deals with fertilization of an ovum in a test-tube (*in vitro* fertilization) and artificial insemination through transfer into the woman's genital tract of previously collected sperm.

A preliminary point for the moral evaluation of such technical procedures is constituted by the consideration of the circumstances and consequences which those procedures involve in relation to the respect due the human embryo. Development of the practice of *in vitro* fertilization has required innumerable fertilizations and destructions of human embryos. Even today, the usual practice presupposes a hyperovulation on the part of the woman: a number of ova are withdrawn, fertilized and then cultivated *in vitro* for some days. Usually not all are transferred into the genital tracts of the woman; some embryos, generally called "spare," are destroyed or frozen. On occasion, some of the implanted embryos are sacrificed for various eugenic, economic or psychological reasons. Such deliberate destruction of human beings or their utilization for different purposes to the detriment of their integrity and life is contrary to the doctrine on procured abortion already recalled.

The connection between *in vitro* fertilization and the voluntary destruction of human embryos occurs too often. This is significant: through these procedures, with apparently contrary purposes, life and death are subjected to the decision of man, who thus sets himself up as the giver of life and death by decree. This dynamic of violence and domination may remain unnoticed by those very individuals who, in wishing to utilize this procedure, become subject to it themselves. The facts recorded and the cold logic which links them must be taken into consideration for a moral judgment on IVF and ET (*in vitro* fertilization and embryo transfer): the abortion-mentality which has made this procedure possible thus leads, whether one wants it or not, to man's domination over the life and death of his fellow human beings and can lead to a system of radical eugenics.

Nevertheless, such abuses do not exempt one from a further and thorough ethical study of the techniques of artificial procreation considered in themselves, abstracting as far as possible from the destruction of embryos produced *in vitro*.

The present Instruction will therefore take into consideration in the first place the problems posed by heterolo-

Congregation for the Doctrine of the Faith, *Instruction on Respect for Human Life in its Origin and on the Dignity of Procreation: Replies to Certain Questions of the Day*. Rome, Vatican City, February 22, 1987. All notes have been renumbered consecutively and placed at the end of the text.

gous artificial fertilization . . . ,[1] and subsequently those linked with homologous artificial fertilization.[2]

Before formulating an ethical judgment on each of these procedures, the principles and values which determine the moral evaluation of each of them will be considered.

A. Heterologous Artificial Fertilization

1. WHY MUST HUMAN PROCREATION TAKE PLACE IN MARRIAGE?

Every human being is always to be accepted as a gift and blessing of God. However, from the moral point of view a truly responsible procreation vis-à-vis the unborn child must be the fruit of marriage.

For human procreation has specific characteristics by virtue of the personal dignity of the parents and of the children: the procreation of a new person, whereby the man and the woman collaborate with the power of the Creator, must be the fruit and the sign of the mutual self-giving of the spouses, of their love and of their fidelity.[3] *The fidelity of the spouses in the unity of marriage involves reciprocal respect of their right to become a father and a mother only through each other.*

The child has the right to be conceived, carried in the womb, brought into the world and brought up within marriage: it is through the secure and recognized relationship to his own parents that the child can discover his own identity and achieve his own proper human development.

The parents find in their child a confirmation and completion of their reciprocal self-giving: the child is the living image of their love, the permanent sign of their conjugal union, the living and indissoluble concrete expression of their paternity and maternity.[4]

By reason of the vocation and social responsibilities of the person, the good of the children and of the parents contributes to the good of civil society; the vitality and stability of society require that children come into the world within a family and that the family be firmly based on marriage.

The tradition of the Church and anthropological reflection recognize in marriage and in its indissoluble unity the only setting worthy of truly responsible procreation.

2. DOES HETEROLOGOUS ARTIFICIAL FERTILIZATION CONFORM TO THE DIGNITY OF THE COUPLE AND TO THE TRUTH OF MARRIAGE?

Through IVF and ET and heterologous artificial insemination, human conception is achieved through the fusion of gametes of at least one donor other than the spouses who are united in marriage. *Heterologous artificial fertilization is contrary to the unity of marriage, to the dignity of the spouses, to the vocation proper to parents, and to the child's right to be conceived and brought into the world in marriage and from marriage.*[5]

Respect for the unity of marriage and for conjugal fidelity demands that the child be conceived in marriage; the bond existing between husband and wife accords the spouses, in an objective and inalienable manner, the exclusive right to become father and mother solely through each other.[6] Recourse to the gametes of a third person, in order to have sperm or ovum available, constitutes a violation of the reciprocal commitment of the spouses and a grave lack in regard to that essential property of marriage which is its unity.

Heterologous artificial fertilization violates the rights of the child; it deprives him of his filial relationship with his parental origins and can hinder the maturing of his personal identity. Furthermore, it offends the common vocation of the spouses who are called to fatherhood and motherhood: it objectively deprives conjugal fruitfulness of its unity and integrity; it brings about and manifests a rupture between genetic parenthood, gestational parenthood and responsibility for upbringing. Such damage to the personal relationships within the family has repercussions on civil society: what threatens the unity and stability of the family is a source of dissension, disorder and injustice in the whole of social life.

These reasons lead to a negative moral judgment concerning heterologous artificial fertilization: consequently fertilization of a married woman with the sperm of a donor different from her husband and fertilization with the husband's sperm of an ovum not coming from his wife are morally illicit. Furthermore, the artificial fertilization of a woman who is unmarried or a widow, whoever the donor may be, cannot be morally justified.

The desire to have a child and the love between spouses who long to obviate a sterility which cannot be overcome in any other way constitute understandable motivations; but subjectively good intentions do not render heterologous artificial fertilization conformable to the objective and inalienable properties of marriage or respectful of the rights of the child and of the spouses.

3. IS "SURROGATE"[7] MOTHERHOOD MORALLY LICIT?

No, for the same reasons which lead one to reject heterologous artificial fertilization: for it is contrary to the unity of marriage and to the dignity of the procreation of the human person.

Surrogate motherhood represents an objective failure to meet the obligations of maternal love, of conjugal fidelity and of responsible motherhood; it offends the dignity and the right of the child to be conceived, carried in the womb, brought into the world and brought up by his own parents; it sets up, to the detriment of families, a division between the physical, psychological and moral elements which constitute those families.

B. Homologous Artificial Fertilization

Since heterologous artificial fertilization has been declared unacceptable, the question arises of how to evaluate morally the process of homologous artificial fertilization: IVF and ET and artificial insemination between husband and wife. First a question of principle must be clarified.

4. WHAT CONNECTION IS REQUIRED FROM THE MORAL POINT OF VIEW BETWEEN PROCREATION AND THE CONJUGAL ACT?

a) The Church's teaching on marriage and human procreation affirms the "inseparable connection, willed by God and unable to be broken by man on his own initiative, between the two meanings of the conjugal act: the unitive meaning and the procreative meaning. Indeed, by its intimate structure, the conjugal act, while most closely uniting husband and wife, capacitates them for the generation of new lives, according to laws inscribed in the very being of man and of woman."[8] This principle, which is based upon the nature of marriage and the intimate connection of the goods of marriage, has well-known consequences on the level of responsible fatherhood and motherhood. "By safeguarding both these essential aspects, the unitive and the procreative, the conjugal act preserves in its fullness the sense of true mutual love and its ordination towards man's exalted vocation to parenthood."[9]

The same doctrine concerning the link between the meanings of the conjugal act and between the goods of marriage throws light on the moral problem of homologous artificial fertilization, since "it is never permitted to separate these different aspects to such a degree as positively to exclude either the procreative intention or the conjugal relation."[10]

Contraception deliberately deprives the conjugal act of its openness to procreation and in this way brings about a voluntary dissociation of the ends of marriage. Homologous artificial fertilization, in seeking a procreation which is not the fruit of a specific act of conjugal union, objectively effects an analogous separation between the goods and the meanings of marriage.

Thus, *fertilization is licitly sought when it is the result of a "conjugal act which is per se suitable for the generation of children to which marriage is ordered by its nature and by which the spouses become one flesh."*[11] *But from the moral point of view procreation is deprived of its proper perfection when it is not desired as the fruit of the conjugal act, that is to say of the specific act of the spouses' union.*

b) The moral value of the intimate link between the goods of marriage and between the meanings of the conjugal act is based upon the unity of the human being, a unity involving body and spiritual soul.[12] Spouses mutually express their personal love in the "language of the body," which clearly involves both "sponsal meanings" and parental ones.[13] The conjugal act by which the couple mutually express their self-gift at the same time expresses openness to the gift of life. It is an act that is inseparably corporal and spiritual. It is in their bodies and through their bodies that the spouses consummate their marriage and are able to become father and mother. In order to respect the language of their bodies and their natural generosity, the conjugal union must take place with respect for its openness to procreation; and the procreation of a person must be the fruit and the result of married love. The origin of the human being thus follows from a procreation that is "linked to the union, not only biological but also spiritual, of the parents, made one by the bond of marriage."[14] Fertilization achieved outside the bodies of the couple remains by this very fact deprived of the meanings and the values which are expressed in the language of the body and in the union of human persons.

c) Only respect for the link between the meanings of the conjugal act and respect for the unity of the human being make possible procreation in conformity with the dignity of the person. In his unique and irrepeatable origin, the child must be respected and recognized as equal in personal dignity to those who give him life. The human person must be accepted in his parents' act of union and love; the generation of a child must therefore be the fruit of that mutual giving[15] which is realized in the conjugal act wherein the spouses cooperate as servants and not as masters in the work of the Creator who is Love.[16]

In reality, the origin of a human person is the result of an act of giving. The one conceived must be the fruit of his parents' love. He cannot be desired or conceived as the product of an intervention of medical or biological techniques; that would be equivalent to reducing him to an object of scientific technology. No one may subject the coming of a child into the world to conditions of technical efficiency which are to be evaluated according to standards of control and dominion.

The moral relevance of the link between the meanings of the conjugal act and between the goods of marriage, as well as the unity of the human being and the dignity of his origin, demand that the procreation of a human person be brought about as the fruit of the conjugal act specific to the love between spouses. The link between procreation and the conjugal act is thus shown to be of great importance on the anthropological and moral planes, and it throws light on the positions of the Magisterium with regard to homologous artificial fertilization.

5. IS HOMOLOGOUS 'IN VITRO' FERTILIZATION MORALLY LICIT?

The answer to this question is strictly dependent on the principles just mentioned. Certainly one cannot ignore the legitimate aspirations of sterile couples. For some, recourse to homologous IVF and ET appears to be the only way of fulfilling their sincere desire for a child. The question is asked whether the totality of conjugal life in such situations is not sufficient to ensure the dignity proper to human procreation. It is acknowledged that IVF and ET certainly cannot supply for the absence of sexual relations[17] and cannot be preferred to the specific acts of conjugal union, given the risks involved for the child and the difficulties of the procedure. But it is asked whether, when there is no other way of overcoming the sterility which is a source of suffering, homologous *in vitro* fertilization may not constitute an aid, if not a form of therapy, whereby its moral licitness could be admitted.

The desire for a child—or at the very least an openness to the transmission of life—is a necessary prerequisite from the moral point of view for responsible human procreation. But this good intention is not sufficient for making a positive moral evaluation of *in vitro* fertilization between spouses. The process of IVF and ET must be judged in itself and cannot borrow its definitive moral quality from the totality of conjugal life of which it becomes part nor from the conjugal acts which may precede or follow it.[18]

It has already been recalled that, in the circumstances in which it is regularly practised, IVF and ET involves the destruction of human beings, which is something contrary to the doctrine on the illicitness of abortion previously mentioned.[19] But even in a situation in which every precaution were taken to avoid the death of human embryos, homologous IVF and ET dissociates from the conjugal act the actions which are directed to human fertilization. For this reason the very nature of homologous IVF and ET also must be taken into account, even abstracting from the link with procured abortion.

Homologous IVF and ET is brought about outside the bodies of the couple through actions of third parties whose competence and technical activity determine the success of the procedure. Such fertilization entrusts the life and identity of the embryo into the power of doctors and biologists and establishes the domination of technology over the origin and destiny of the human person. Such a relationship of domination is in itself contrary to the dignity and equality that must be common to parents and children.

Conception *in vitro* is the result of the technical action which presides over fertilization. *Such fertilization is neither in fact achieved nor positively willed as the expression and fruit of a specific act of the conjugal union. In homologous IVF and ET, therefore, even if it is considered in the context of 'de facto' existing sexual relations, the generation of the human person is objectively deprived of its proper perfection: namely, that of being the result and fruit of a conjugal act* in which the spouses can become "cooperators with God for giving life to a new person."[20]

These reasons enable us to understand why the act of conjugal love is considered in the teaching of the Church as the only setting worthy of human procreation. For the same reasons the so-called "simple case," i.e. a homologous IVF and ET procedure that is free of any compromise with the abortive practice of destroying embryos and with masturbation, remains a technique which is morally illicit because it deprives human procreation of the dignity which is proper and connatural to it.

Certainly, homologous IVF and ET fertilization is not marked by all that ethical negativity found in extraconjugal procreation; the family and marriage continue to constitute the setting for the birth and upbringing of the children. Nevertheless, in conformity with the traditional doctrine relating to the goods of marriage and the dignity of the person, *the Church remains opposed from the moral point of view to homologous 'in vitro' fertilization. Such fertilization is in itself illicit and in opposition to the dignity of procreation and of the conjugal union, even when everything is done to avoid the death of the human embryo.*

Although the manner in which human conception is achieved with IVF and ET cannot be approved, every child which comes into the world must in any case be accepted as a living gift of the divine Goodness and must be brought up with love.

6. HOW IS HOMOLOGOUS ARTIFICIAL INSEMINATION TO BE EVALUATED FROM THE MORAL POINT OF VIEW?

Homologous artificial insemination within marriage cannot be admitted except for those cases in which the technical means is not a substitute for the conjugal act but serves to facilitate and to help so that the act attains its natural purpose.

The teaching of the Magisterium on this point has already been stated.[21] This teaching is not just an expression of particular historical circumstances but is based on the Church's doctrine concerning the connection between the conjugal union and procreation and on a consideration of the personal nature of the conjugal act and of human procreation. "In its natural structure, the conjugal act is a personal action, a simultaneous and immediate cooperation on the part of the husband and wife, which by the very nature of the agents and the proper nature of the act is the expression of the mutual gift which, according to the words of Scripture, brings about union 'in one flesh'."[22] Thus moral conscience "does not necessarily proscribe the use of certain artificial means destined solely either to the facilitating of the natural act or to ensuring that the natural act normally performed achieves its proper end."[23] If the technical means facilitates the conjugal act or helps it to reach its natural objectives, it can be morally acceptable. If, on the other hand, the procedure were to replace the conjugal act, it is morally illicit.

Artificial insemination as a substitute for the conjugal act is prohibited by reason of the voluntarily achieved dissociation of the two meanings of the conjugal act. Masturbation, through which the sperm is normally obtained, is another sign of this dissociation: even when it is done for the purpose of procreation, the act remains deprived of its unitive meaning: "It lacks the sexual relationship called for by the moral order, namely the relationship which realizes 'the full sense of mutual self-giving and human procreation in the context of true love.' "[24]

7. WHAT MORAL CRITERION CAN BE PROPOSED WITH REGARD TO MEDICAL INTERVENTION IN HUMAN PROCREATION?

The medical act must be evaluated not only with reference to its technical dimension but also and above all in relation to its goal which is the good of persons and their bodily and psychological health. The moral criteria for medical intervention in procreation are deduced from the dignity of human persons, of their sexuality and of their origin.

Medicine which seeks to be ordered to the integral good of the person must respect the specifically human values of sexuality.[25] *The doctor is at the service of persons and of human procreation. He does not have the authority to dispose of them or to decide their fate.* "A medical intervention respects the dignity of persons when it seeks to assist the conjugal act either in order to facilitate its performance or in order to enable it to achieve its objective once it has been normally performed."[26]

On the other hand, it sometimes happens that a medical procedure technologically replaces the conjugal act in order to obtain a procreation which is neither its result nor its fruit. In this case the medical act is not, as it should be, at the service of conjugal union but rather appropriates to itself the procreative function and thus contradicts the dignity and the inalienable rights of the spouses and of the child to be born.

The humanization of medicine, which is insisted upon today by everyone, requires respect for the integral dignity of the human person first of all in the act and at the moment in which the spouses transmit life to a new person. It is only logical therefore to address an urgent appeal to Catholic doctors and scientists that they bear exemplary witness to the respect due to the human embryo and to the dignity of procreation. The medical and nursing staff of Catholic hospitals and clinics are in a special way urged to do justice to the moral obligations which they have assumed, frequently also, as part of their contract. Those who are in charge of Catholic hospitals and clinics and who are often Religious will take special care to safeguard and promote a diligent observance of the moral norms recalled in the present Instruction.

8. THE SUFFERING CAUSED BY INFERTILITY IN MARRIAGE

The suffering of spouses who cannot have children or who are afraid of bringing a handicapped child into the world is a suffering that everyone must understand and properly evaluate.

On the part of the spouses, the desire for a child is natural: it expresses the vocation to fatherhood and motherhood inscribed in conjugal love. This desire can be even stronger if the couple is affected by sterility which appears incurable. Nevertheless, marriage does not confer upon the spouses the right to have a child, but only the right to perform those natural acts which are *per se* ordered to procreation.[27]

A true and proper right to a child would be contrary to the child's dignity and nature. The child is not an object to which one has a right, nor can he be considered as an object of ownership: rather, a child is a gift, "the supreme gift"[28] *and the most gratuitous gift of marriage, and is a living testimony of the mutual giving of his parents. For this reason, the child has the right, as already mentioned, to be the fruit of the specific act of the conjugal love of his parents; and he also has the right to be respected as a person from the moment of his conception.*

Nevertheless, whatever its cause or prognosis, sterility is certainly a difficult trial. The community of believers is called to shed light upon and support the suffering of those who are unable to fulfill their legitimate aspiration to motherhood and fatherhood. Spouses who find themselves in this sad situation are called to find in it an opportunity for sharing in a particular way in the Lord's Cross, the source of spiritual fruitfulness. Sterile couples must not forget that "even when procreation is not possible, conjugal life does not for this reason lose its value. Physical sterility in fact can be for spouses the occasion for other important services to the life of the human person, for example, adoption, various forms of educational work, and assistance to other families and to poor or handicapped children."[29]

Many researchers are engaged in the fight against sterility. While fully safeguarding the dignity of human procreation, some have achieved results which previously seemed unattainable. Scientists therefore are to be encouraged to continue their research with the aim of preventing the causes of sterility and of being able to remedy them so that sterile couples will be able to procreate in full respect for their own personal dignity and that of the child to be born.

NOTES

1. By the term *heterologous artificial fertilization* or *procreation,* the Instruction means techniques used to obtain a human conception artificially by the use of gametes coming from at least one donor other than the spouses who are joined in marriage. Such techniques can be of two types:

   a) Heterologous IVF and ET: the technique used to obtain a human conception through the meeting *in vitro* of gametes taken from at least one donor other than the two spouses joined in marriage.

b) Heterologous artificial insemination: the technique used to obtain a human conception through the transfer into the genital tracts of the woman of the sperm previously collected from a donor other than the husband.

2. By *artificial homologous fertilization or procreation,* the Instruction means the technique used to obtain a human conception using the gametes of the two spouses joined in marriage. Homologous artificial fertilization can be carried out by two different methods:

a) Homologous IVF and ET: the technique used to obtain a human conception through the meeting *in vitro* of the gametes of the spouses joined in marriage.

b) Homologous artificial insemination: the technique used to obtain a human conception through the transfer into the genital tracts of a married woman of the sperm previously collected from her husband.

3. Cf. Pastoral Constitution on the Church in the Modern World, *Gaudium et Spes,* 50.
4. Cf. Pope John Paul II, Apostolic Exhortation *Familiaris Consortio,* 14: *AAS* 74 (1982) 96.
5. Cf. Pope Pius XII, *Discourse to those taking part in the 4th International Congress of Catholic Doctors,* 29 September 1949: *AAS* 41 (1949) 559. According to the plan of the Creator, "A man leaves his father and his mother and cleaves to his wife, and they become one flesh" (*Gen* 2:24). The unity of marriage, bound to the order of creation, is a truth accessible to natural reason. The Church's Tradition and Magisterium frequently make reference to the Book of Genesis, both directly and through the passages of the New Testament that refer to it: *Mt* 19:4–6; *Mk* 10:5–8; *Eph* 5:31. Cf. Athenagoras, *Legatio pro christianis,* 33: *PG* 6, 965–967; St Chrysostom, *In Matthaeum homiliae,* LXII, 19, 1: *PG* 58 597; St Leo the Great, *Epist. ad Rusticum,* 4: *PL* 54, 1204; Innocent III, Epist. *Gaudemus in Domino: DS* 778; Council of Lyons II, *IV Session: DS* 860; Council of Trent, *XXIV Session: DS* 1798. 1802; Pope Leo XIII, Encyclical *Arcanum Divinae Sapientiae: ASS* 12 (1879/80) 388–391; Pope Pius XI, Encyclical *Casti Connubii: AAS* 22 (1930) 546–547; Second Vatican Council, *Gaudium et Spes,* 48; Pope John Paul II, Apostolic Exhortation *Familiaris Consortio,* 19: *AAS* 74 (1982) 101–102; *Code of Canon Law,* Can. 1056.
6. Cf. Pope Pius XII, *Discourse to those taking part in the 4th International Congress of Catholic Doctors,* 29 September 1949: *AAS* 41 (1949) 560; *Discourse to those taking part in the Congress of the Italian Catholic Union of Midwives,* 29 October 1951: *AAS* 43 (1951) 850; *Code of Canon Law,* Can. 1134.
7. By "surrogate mother" the Instruction means:

a) the woman who carries in pregnancy an embryo implanted in her uterus and who is genetically a stranger to the embryo because it has been obtained through the union of the gametes of "donors." She carries the pregnancy with a pledge to surrender the baby once it is born to the party who commissioned or made the agreement for the pregnancy.

b) the woman who carries in pregnancy an embryo to whose procreation she has contributed the donation of her own ovum, fertilized through insemination with the sperm of a man other than her husband. She carries the pregnancy with a pledge to surrender the child once it is born to the party who commissioned or made the agreement for the pregnancy.

8. Pope Paul VI, Encyclical Letter *Humanae Vitae,* 12: *AAS* 60 (1968) 488–489.
9. *Loc. cit., ibid.,* 489.
10. Pope Pius XII, *Discourse to those taking part in the Second Naples World Congress on Fertility and Human Sterility,* 19 May 1956: *AAS* 48 (1956) 470.
11. *Code of Canon Law,* Can. 1061. According to this Canon, the conjugal act is that by which the marriage is consummated if the couple "have performed (it) between themselves in a human manner."
12. Cf. Pastoral Constitution *Gaudium et Spes,* 14.
13. Cf. Pope John Paul II, *General Audience on 16 January 1980: Insegnamenti di Giovanni Paolo II,* III, 1 (1980) 148–152.
14. Pope John Paul II, *Discourse to those taking part in the 35th General Assembly of the World Medical Association,* 29 October 1983: *AAS* 76 (1984) 393.
15. Cf. Pastoral Constitution *Gaudium et Spes,* 51.
16. Cf. Pastoral Constitution *Gaudium et Spes,* 50.
17. Cf. Pope Pius XII, *Discourse to those taking part in the 4th International Congress of Catholic Doctors,* 29 September 1949: *AAS* 41 (1949) 560: "It would be erroneous . . . to think that the possibility of resorting to this means (artificial fertilization) might render valid a marriage between persons unable to contract it because of the *impedimentum impotentiae.*"
18. A similar question was dealt with by Pope Paul VI, Encyclical *Humanae Vitae,* 14: *AAS* 60 (1968) 490–491.
19. Cf. *supra:* I, 1 ff. (Not reprinted in this volume.)
20. Pope John Paul II, Apostolic Exhortation *Familiaris Consortio,* 14: *AAS* 74 (1982) 96.
21. Cf. *Response of the Holy Office,* 17 March 1897: *DS* 3323; Pope Pius XII, *Discourse to those taking part in the 4th International Congress of Catholic Doctors,* 29 September 1949: *AAS* 41 (1949) 560; *Discourse to the Italian Catholic Union of Midwives,* 29 October 1951: *AAS* 43 (1951) 850; *Discourse to those taking part in the Second Naples World Congress on Fertility and Human Sterility,* 19 May 1956: *AAS* 48 (1956) 471–473; *Discourse to those taking part in the 7th International Congress of the International Society of Haematology,* 12 September 1958: *AAS* 50 (1958) 733; Pope John XXIII, Encyclical *Mater et Magistra,* III: *AAS* 53 (1961) 447.
22. Pope Pius XII, *Discourse to the Italian Catholic Union of Midwives,* 29 October 1951: *AAS* 43 (1951) 850.
23. Pope Pius XII, *Discourse to those taking part in the 4th International Congress of Catholic Doctors,* 29 September 1949: *AAS* 41 (1949) 560.
24. Sacred Congregation for the Doctrine of the Faith, *Declaration on Certain Questions Concerning Sexual Ethics,* 9: *AAS* 68 (1976) 86, which quotes the Pastoral Constitution *Gaudium et Spes,* 51. Cf. *Decree of the Holy Office,* 2 August 1929: *AAS* 21 (1929) 490; Pope Pius XII, *Discourse to those taking part in the 26th Congress of*

the Italian Society of Urology, 8 October 1953: *AAS* 45 (1953) 678.

25. Cf. Pope John XXIII, Encyclical *Mater et Magistra*, III: *AAS* 53 (1961) 447.
26. Cf. Pope Pius XII, *Discourse to those taking part in the 4th International Congress of Catholic Doctors*, 29 September 1949: *AAS* 41 (1949), 560.
27. Cf. Pope Pius XII, *Discourse to the taking part in the Second Naples World Congress on Fertility and Human Sterility*, 19 May 1956: *AAS* 48 (1956) 471–473.
28. Pastoral Constitution *Gaudium et Spes*, 50.
29. Pope John Paul II, Apostolic Exhortation *Familiaris Consortio*, 14: *AAS* 74 (1982) 97.

IN THE MATTER OF BABY M, NEW JERSEY SUPREME COURT

INTRODUCTION. *The most celebrated case of surrogate motherhood to date involved attorney Noel Keane as arranger, Mary Beth Whitehead as surrogate mother, William Stern as genetic father and intended social father, and an infant, "Baby M," who became the object of an intense and protracted custody dispute. After a New Jersey trial court had declared the surrogacy contract valid and awarded sole custody of the child to Mr. Stern, Mrs. Whitehead appealed. In a carefully nuanced opinion, the New Jersey Supreme Court found the surrogacy contract to be invalid and unenforceable but argued that it would be in the best interests of Baby M if she were raised by the Sterns. The Supreme Court also concluded that, as the genetic and gestational mother of Baby M, Mrs. Whitehead should enjoy at least some visitation rights.*

In this matter the Court is asked to determine the validity of a contract that purports to provide a new way of bringing children into a family. For a fee of $10,000, a woman agrees to be artificially inseminated with the semen of another woman's husband; she is to conceive a child, carry it to term, and after its birth surrender it to the natural father and his wife. The intent of the contract is that the child's natural mother will thereafter be forever separated from her child. The wife is to adopt the child, and she and the natural father are to be regarded as its parents for all purposes. The contract providing for this is called a "surrogacy contract," the natural mother inappropriately called the "surrogate mother."

We invalidate the surrogacy contract because it conflicts with the law and public policy of this State. While we recognize the depth of the yearning of infertile couples to have their own children, we find the payment of money to a "surrogate" mother illegal, perhaps criminal, and potentially degrading to women. Although in this case we grant custody to the natural father, the evidence having clearly proved such custody to be in the best interests of the infant, we void both the termination of the surrogate mother's parental rights and the adoption of the child by the wife/stepparent. We thus restore the "surrogate" as the mother of the child. We remand the issue of the natural mother's visitation rights to the trial court, since that issue was not reached below and the record before us is not sufficient to permit us to decide it *de novo*.

We find no offense to our present laws where a woman voluntarily and without payment agrees to act as a "surrogate" mother, provided that she is not subject to a binding agreement to surrender her child. Moreover, our holding today does not preclude the Legislature from altering the current statutory scheme, within constitutional limits, so as to permit surrogacy contracts. Under current law, however, the surrogacy agreement before us is illegal and invalid.

I. Facts

In February 1985, William Stern and Mary Beth Whitehead entered into a surrogacy contract. It recited that Stern's wife, Elizabeth, was infertile, that they wanted a child, and that Mrs. Whitehead was willing to provide that child as the mother with Mr. Stern as the father.

The contract provided that through artificial insemination using Mr. Stern's sperm, Mrs. Whitehead would become pregnant, carry the child to term, bear it, deliver it to the Sterns, and thereafter do whatever was necessary to terminate her maternal rights so that Mrs. Stern could thereafter adopt the child. Mrs. Whitehead's husband, Richard,[1] was also a party to the contract; Mrs. Stern was not. Mr. Whitehead promised to do all acts necessary to rebut the presumption of paternity under the Parentage Act. *N.J.S.A.* 9:17-43a(1), -44a. Although Mrs. Stern was

Reprinted from New Jersey, Supreme Court, *In the Matter of Baby M* 537 A.2d 1227 (New Jersey, February 3, 1988). Opinion delivered by Wilentz, C.J.

not a party to the surrogacy agreement, the contract gave her sole custody of the child in the event of Mr. Stern's death. Mrs. Stern's status as a nonparty to the surrogate parenting agreement presumably was to avoid the application of the baby-selling statute to this arrangement. N.J.S.A. 9:3-54.

Mr. Stern, on his part, agreed to attempt the artificial insemination and to pay Mrs. Whitehead $10,000 after the child's birth, on its delivery to him. In a separate contract, Mr. Stern agreed to pay $7,500 to the Infertility Center of New York ("ICNY"). The Center's advertising campaigns solicit surrogate mothers and encourage infertile couples to consider surrogacy. ICNY arranged for the surrogacy contract by bringing the parties together, explaining the process to them, furnishing the contractual form . . . and providing legal counsel.

The history of the parties' involvement in this arrangement suggests their good faith. William and Elizabeth Stern were married in July 1974, having met at the University of Michigan, where both were Ph.D. candidates. Due to financial considerations and Mrs. Stern's pursuit of a medical degree and residency, they decided to defer starting a family until 1981. Before then, however, Mrs. Stern learned that she might have multiple sclerosis and that the disease in some cases renders pregnancy a serious health risk. Her anxiety appears to have exceeded the actual risk, which current medical authorities assess as minimal. Nonetheless that anxiety was evidently quite real, Mrs. Stern fearing that pregnancy might precipitate blindness, paraplegia, or other forms of debilitation. Based on the perceived risk, the Sterns decided to forego having their own children. The decision had a special significance for Mr. Stern. Most of his family had been destroyed in the Holocaust. As the family's only survivor, he very much wanted to continue his bloodline.

Initially the Sterns considered adoption, but were discouraged by the substantial delay apparently involved and by the potential problem they saw arising from their age and their differing religious backgrounds. They were most eager for some other means to start a family.

The paths of Mrs. Whitehead and the Sterns to surrogacy were similar. Both responded to advertising by ICNY. The Sterns' response, following their inquiries into adoption, was the result of their longstanding decision to have a child. Mrs. Whitehead's response apparently resulted from her sympathy with family members and others who could have no children (she stated that she wanted to give another couple the "gift of life"); she also wanted the $10,000 to help her family.

Both parties, undoubtedly because of their own self-interest, were less sensitive to the implications of the transaction than they might otherwise have been. Mrs. Whitehead, for instance, appears not to have been concerned about whether the Sterns would make good parents for her child; the Sterns, on their part, while conscious of the obvious possibility that surrendering the child might cause grief to Mrs. Whitehead, overcame their qualms because of their desire for a child. At any rate, both the Sterns and Mrs. Whitehead were committed to the arrangement; both thought it right and constructive.

Mrs. Whitehead had reached her decision concerning surrogacy before the Sterns, and had actually been involved as a potential surrogate mother with another couple. After numerous unsuccessful artificial inseminations, that effort was abandoned. Thereafter, the Sterns learned of the Infertility Center, the possibilities of surrogacy, and of Mary Beth Whitehead. The two couples met to discuss the surrogacy arrangement and decided to go forward. On February 6, 1985, Mr. Stern and Mr. and Mrs. Whitehead executed the surrogate parenting agreement. After several artificial inseminations over a period of months, Mrs. Whitehead became pregnant. The pregnancy was uneventful and on March 27, 1986, Baby M was born.

Not wishing anyone at the hospital to be aware of the surrogacy arrangement, Mr. and Mrs. Whitehead appeared to all as the proud parents of a healthy female child. Her birth certificate indicated her name to be Sara Elizabeth Whitehead and her father to be Richard Whitehead. In accordance with Mrs. Whitehead's request, the Sterns visited the hospital unobtrusively to see the newborn child.

Mrs. Whitehead realized, almost from the moment of birth, that she could not part with this child. She had felt a bond with it even during pregnancy. Some indication of the attachment was conveyed to the Sterns at the hospital when they told Mrs. Whitehead what they were going to name the baby. She apparently broke into tears and indicated that she did not know if she could give up the child. She talked about how the baby looked like her other daughter, and made it clear that she was experiencing great difficulty with the decision.

Nonetheless, Mrs. Whitehead was, for the moment, true to her word. Despite powerful inclinations to the contrary, she turned her child over to the Sterns on March 30 at the Whiteheads' home.

The Sterns were thrilled with their new child. They had planned extensively for its arrival, far beyond the practical furnishing of a room for her. It was a time of joyful celebration—not just for them but for their friends as well. The Sterns looked forward to raising their daughter, whom they named Melissa. While aware by then that Mrs. Whitehead was undergoing an emotional crisis, they were as yet not cognizant of the depth of that crisis and its implications for their newly-enlarged family.

Later in the evening of March 30, Mrs. Whitehead became deeply disturbed, disconsolate, stricken with unbearable sadness. She had to have her child. She could not eat, sleep, or concentrate on anything other than her need for her baby. The next day she went to the Sterns' home and told them how much she was suffering.

The depth of Mrs. Whitehead's despair surprised and frightened the Sterns. She told them that she could not live without her baby, that she must have her, even if only for one week, that thereafter she would surrender her child. The Sterns, concerned that Mrs. Whitehead might indeed commit suicide, not wanting under any circumstances to risk that, and in any event believing that Mrs. Whitehead would keep her word, turned the child over to her. It was not until four months later, after a series of attempts to regain possession of the child, that Melissa was returned to the Sterns, having been forcibly removed from the home where she was then living with Mr. and Mrs. Whitehead, the home in Florida owned by Mary Beth Whitehead's parents.

The struggle over Baby M began when it became apparent that Mrs. Whitehead could not return the child to Mr. Stern. Due to Mrs. Whitehead's refusal to relinquish the baby, Mr. Stern filed a complaint seeking enforcement of the surrogacy contract. He alleged, accurately, that Mrs. Whitehead had not only refused to comply with the surrogacy contract but had threatened to flee from New Jersey with the child in order to avoid even the possibility of his obtaining custody. The court papers asserted that if Mrs. Whitehead were to be given notice of the application for an order requiring her to relinquish custody, she would, prior to the hearing, leave the state with the baby. And that is precisely what she did. After the order was entered, *ex parte*, the process server, aided by the police, in the presence of the Sterns, entered Mrs. Whitehead's home to execute the order. Mr. Whitehead fled with the child, who had been handed to him through a window while those who came to enforce the order were thrown off balance by a dispute over the child's current name.

The Whiteheads immediately fled to Florida with Baby M. They stayed initially with Mrs. Whitehead's parents, where one of Mrs. Whitehead's children had been living. For the next three months, the Whiteheads and Melissa lived at roughly twenty different hotels, motels, and homes in order to avoid apprehension. From time to time Mrs. Whitehead would call Mr. Stern to discuss the matter; the conversations, recorded by Mr. Stern on advice of counsel, show an escalating dispute about rights, morality, and power, accompanied by threats of Mrs. Whitehead to kill herself, to kill the child, and falsely to accuse Mr. Stern of sexually molesting Mrs. Whitehead's other daughter.

Eventually the Sterns discovered where the Whiteheads were staying, commenced supplementary proceedings in Florida, and obtained an order requiring the Whiteheads to turn over the child. Police in Florida enforced the order, forcibly removing the child from her grandparents' home. She was soon thereafter brought to New Jersey and turned over to the Sterns. The prior order of the court, issued *ex parte*, awarding custody of the child to the Sterns *pendente lite*, was reaffirmed by the trial court after consideration of the certified representations of the parties (both represented by counsel) concerning the unusual sequence of events that had unfolded. Pending final judgment, Mrs. Whitehead was awarded limited visitation with Baby M.

The Sterns' complaint, in addition to seeking possession and ultimately custody of the child, sought enforcement of the surrogacy contract. Pursuant to the contract, it asked that the child be permanently placed in their custody, that Mrs. Whitehead's parental rights be terminated, and that Mrs. Stern be allowed to adopt the child, *i.e.*, that, for all purposes, Melissa become the Sterns' child.

The trial took thirty-two days over a period of more than two months. It included numerous interlocutory appeals and attempted interlocutory appeals. There were twenty-three witnesses to the facts recited above and fifteen expert witnesses, eleven testifying on the issue of custody and four on the subject of Mrs. Stern's multiple sclerosis; the bulk of the testimony was devoted to determining the parenting arrangement most compatible with the child's best interests. Soon after the conclusion of the trial, the trial court announced its opinion from the bench. 217 *N.J.Super*. 313, 525 *A*.2d 1128 (1987). It held that the surrogacy contract was valid; ordered that Mrs. Whitehead's parental rights be terminated and that sole custody of the child be granted to Mr. Stern; and, after hearing brief testimony from Mrs. Stern, immediately entered an order allowing the adoption of Melissa by Mrs. Stern, all in accordance with the surrogacy contract. Pending the outcome of the appeal, we granted a continuation of visitation to Mrs. Whitehead, although slightly more limited than the visitation allowed during the trial.

Although clearly expressing its view that the surrogacy contract was valid, the trial court devoted the major portion of its opinion to the question of the baby's best interests. The inconsistency is apparent. The surrogacy contract calls for the surrender of the child to the Sterns, permanent and sole custody in the Sterns, and termination of Mrs. Whitehead's parental rights, all without qualification, all regardless of any evaluation of the best interests of the child. As a matter of fact the contract recites (even before the child was conceived) that it is in the best interests of the child to be placed with Mr. Stern. In effect, the trial court awarded custody to Mr. Stern, the natural father, based on the same kind of evidence and analysis as might be expected had no surrogacy contract existed. Its rationalization, however, was that while the surrogacy contract was valid, specific performance would not be granted unless that remedy was in the best interests of the child. The factual issues confronted and decided by the trial court were the same as if Mr. Stern and Mrs. Whitehead had had the child out of wedlock, intended or unintended, and then disagreed about custody. The trial court's awareness of the irrelevance of the contract in the court's determination of custody is suggested by its remark that beyond the question of the child's best interests, "[a]ll other concerns raised by counsel constitute commentary." 217 *N.J.Super*. at 323, 525 *A*.2d 1128.

On the question of best interests—and we agree, but for different reasons, that custody was the critical issue—the court's analysis of the testimony was perceptive, demonstrating both its understanding of the case and its considerable experience in these matters. We agree substantially with both its analysis and conclusions on the matter of custody.

The court's review and analysis of the surrogacy contract, however, is not at all in accord with ours. The trial court concluded that the various statutes governing this matter, including those concerning adoption, termination of parental rights, and payment of money in connection with adoptions, do not apply to surrogacy contracts. . . . It reasoned that because the Legislature did not have surrogacy contracts in mind when it passed those laws, those laws were therefore irrelevant. Thus, assuming it was writing on a clean slate, the trial court analyzed the interests involved and the power of the court to accommodate them. It then held that surrogacy contracts are valid and should be enforced . . . and furthermore that Mr. Stern's rights under the surrogacy contract were constitutionally protected. . . .

Mrs. Whitehead appealed. This Court granted direct certification. . . . The briefs of the parties on appeal were joined by numerous briefs filed by *amici* expressing various interests and views on surrogacy and on this case. We have found many of them helpful in resolving the issues before us.

Mrs. Whitehead contends that the surrogacy contract, for a variety of reasons, is invalid. She contends that it conflicts with public policy since it guarantees that the child will not have the nurturing of both natural parents—presumably New Jersey's goal for families. She further argues that it deprives the mother of her constitutional right to the companionship of her child, and that it conflicts with statutes concerning termination of parental rights and adoption. With the contract thus void, Mrs. Whitehead claims primary custody (with visitation rights in Mr. Stern) both on a best interests basis (stressing the "tender years" doctrine) as well as on the policy basis of discouraging surrogacy contracts. She maintains that even if custody would ordinarily go to Mr. Stern, here it should be awarded to Mrs. Whitehead to deter future surrogacy arrangements.

In a brief filed after oral argument, counsel for Mrs. Whitehead suggests that the standard for determining best interests where the infant resulted from a surrogacy contract is that the child should be placed with the mother absent a showing of unfitness. All parties agree that no expert testified that Mary Beth Whitehead was unfit as a mother; the trial court expressly found that she was *not* "unfit," that, on the contrary, "she is a good mother for and to her older children," . . . and no one now claims anything to the contrary.

One of the repeated themes put forth by Mrs. Whitehead is that the court's initial *ex parte* order granting custody to the Sterns during the trial was a substantial factor in the ultimate "best interests" determination. That initial order, claimed to be erroneous by Mrs. Whitehead, not only established Melissa as part of the Stern family, but brought enormous pressure on Mrs. Whitehead. The order brought the resulting pressure, Mrs. Whitehead contends, caused her to act in ways that were atypical of her ordinary behavior when not under stress, and to act in ways that were thought to be inimical to the child's best interests in that they demonstrated a failure of character, maturity, and consistency. She claims that any mother who truly loved her child might so respond and that it is doubly unfair to judge her on the basis of her reaction to an extreme situation rarely faced by any mother, where that situation was itself caused by an erroneous order of the court. Therefore, according to Mrs. Whitehead, the erroneous *ex parte* order precipitated a series of events that proved instrumental in the final result.[2]

The Sterns claim that the surrogacy contract is valid and should be enforced, largely for the reasons given by the trial court. They claim a constitutional right of privacy, which includes the right of procreation, and the right of consenting adults to deal with matters of reproduction as they see fit. As for the child's best interests, their position is factual: given all of the circumstances, the child is better off in their custody with no residual parental rights reserved for Mrs. Whitehead.

Of considerable interest in this clash of views is the position of the child's guardian *ad litem*, wisely appointed by the court at the outset of the litigation. As the child's representative, her role in the litigation, as she viewed it, was solely to protect the child's best interests. She therefore took no position on the validity of the surrogacy contract, and instead devoted her energies to obtaining expert testimony uninfluenced by any interest other than the child's. We agree with the guardian's perception of her role in this litigation. She appropriately refrained from taking any position that might have appeared to compromise her role as the child's advocate. She first took the position, based on her experts' testimony, that the Sterns should have primary custody, and that while Mrs. Whitehead's parental rights should not be terminated, no visitation should be allowed for five years. As a result of subsequent developments, mentioned *infra*, her view has changed. She now recommends that no visitation be allowed at least until Baby M reaches maturity.

Although some of the experts' opinions touched on visitation, the major issue they addressed was whether custody should be reposed in the Sterns or in the Whiteheads. The trial court, consistent in this respect with its view that the surrogacy contract was valid, did not deal at all with the question of visitation. Having concluded that the best interests of the child called for custody in the Sterns, the trial court enforced the operative provisions of the surrogacy contract, terminated Mrs. Whitehead's parental rights, and granted an adoption to Mrs. Stern. Explicit in the ruling was the conclusion that the best interests determination removed whatever impediment might have existed in enforcing the surrogacy contract. This Court, therefore, is without guidance from the trial court on the visitation issue, an issue of considerable importance in any event, and especially important in view of our determination that the surrogacy contract is invalid.

II. Invalidity and Unenforceability of Surrogacy Contract

We have concluded that this surrogacy contract is invalid. Our conclusion has two bases: direct conflict with existing statutes and conflict with the public policies of this State, as expressed in its statutory and decisional law.

One of the surrogacy contract's basic purposes, to achieve the adoption of a child through private placement, though permitted in New Jersey "is very much disfavored." . . . Its use of money for this purpose—and we have no doubt whatsoever that the money is being paid to obtain an adoption and not, as the Sterns argue, for the personal services of Mary Beth Whitehead—is illegal and perhaps criminal. . . . In addition to the inducement of money, there is the coercion of contract: the natural mother's irrevocable agreement, prior to birth, even prior to conception, to surrender the child to the adoptive couple. Such an agreement is totally unenforceable in private placement adoption. . . . Even where the adoption is through an approved agency, the formal agreement to surrender occurs only *after* birth . . . , and then, by regulation, only after the birth mother has been counseled. . . . Integral to these invalid provisions of the surrogacy contract is the related agreement, equally invalid, on the part of the natural mother to cooperate with, and not to contest, proceedings to terminate her parental rights, as well as her contractual concession, in aid of the adoption, that the child's best interests would be served by awarding custody to the natural father and his wife—all of this before she has even conceived, and, in some cases, before she has the slightest idea of what the natural father and adoptive mother are like.

The foregoing provisions not only directly conflict with New Jersey statutes, but also offend long-established State policies. These critical terms, which are at the heart of the contract, are invalid and unenforceable; the conclusion therefore follows, without more, that the entire contract is unenforceable.

* * *

III. Termination

We have already noted that under our laws termination of parental rights cannot be based on contract, but may be granted only on proof of the statutory requirements. That conclusion was one of the bases for invalidating the surrogacy contract. Although excluding the contract as a basis for parental termination, we did not explicitly deal with the question of whether the statutory bases for termination existed. We do so here.

As noted before, if termination of Mrs. Whitehead's parental rights is justified, Mrs. Whitehead will have no further claim either to custody or to visitation, and adoption by Mrs. Stern may proceed pursuant to the private placement adoption statute. . . . If termination is not justified, Mrs. Whitehead remains the legal mother, and even if not entitled to custody, she would ordinarily be expected to have some rights of visitation. . . .

Nothing in this record justifies a finding that would allow a court to terminate Mary Beth Whitehead's parental rights under the statutory standard. It is not simply that obviously there was no "intentional abandonment or very substantial neglect of parental duties without a reasonable expectation of reversal of that conduct in the future," *N.J.S.A.* 9:3—48c(1), quite the contrary, but furthermore that the trial court never found Mrs. Whitehead an unfit mother and indeed affirmatively stated that Mary Beth Whitehead had been a good mother to her other children. . . .

There is simply no basis. . . to warrant termination of Mrs. Whitehead's parental rights. We therefore conclude that the natural mother is entitled to retain her rights as a mother.

IV. Constitutional Issues

Both parties argue that the Constitutions—state and federal—mandate approval of their basic claims. The source of their constitutional arguments is essentially the same: the right of privacy, the right to procreate, the right to the companionship of one's child, those rights flowing either directly from the fourteenth amendment or by its incorporation of the Bill of Rights, or from the ninth amendment, or through the penumbra surrounding all of the Bill of Rights. They are the rights of personal intimacy, of marriage, of sex, of family, of procreation. Whatever their source, it is clear that they are fundamental rights protected by both the federal and state Constitutions. . . . The right asserted by the Sterns is the right of procreation; that asserted by Mary Beth Whitehead is the right to the companionship of her child. We find that the right of procreation does not extend as far as claimed by the Sterns. As for the right asserted by Mrs. Whitehead, since we uphold it on other grounds (*i.e.*, we have restored her as mother and recognized her right, limited by the child's best interests, to her companionship), we need not decide that constitutional issue, and for reasons set forth below, we should not.

The right to procreate, as protected by the Constitution, has been ruled on directly only once by the United States Supreme Court. *See Skinner v. Oklahoma, 316 U.S.* 535, 62 *S.Ct.* 1110, 86 *L.Ed.* 1655 (forced sterilization of habitual criminals violates equal protection clause of fourteenth amendment). Although *Griswold v. Connecticut*, 381 *U.S.* 479, 85 *S.Ct.* 1678, 14 *L.Ed.*2d 510, is obviously of a similar class, strictly speaking it involves the right *not* to procreate. The right to procreate very simply is the right to have natural children, whether through sexual intercourse or artificial insemination. It is no more than that. Mr. Stern has not been deprived of that right. Through artificial insemination of Mrs. Whitehead, Baby M is his child. The custody, care, companionship, and nurturing that follow birth are not parts of the right to procreation; they are rights that may also be constitutionally protected, but that involve many considerations other than the right of procreation. To assert that Mr. Stern's right of procreation gives him the right to the custody of Baby M would be to assert that Mrs. Whitehead's right of procreation does *not* give her the right to the custody of Baby M; it would be to assert that the constitutional right of procreation includes within it a constitutionally protected contractual right to destroy someone else's right of procreation.

We conclude that the right of procreation is best understood and protected if confined to its essentials, and that when dealing with rights concerning the resulting child, different interests come into play. There is nothing in our culture or society that even begins to suggest a fundamental right on the part of the father to the custody of the child as part of his right to procreate when opposed by the claim of the mother to the same child. We therefore disagree with the trial court: there is no constitutional basis whatsoever requiring that Mr. Stern's claim to the custody of Baby M be sustained. Our conclusion may thus be understood as illustrating that a person's rights of privacy and self-determination are qualified by the effect on innocent third persons of the exercise of those rights.[3]

Mr. Stern also contends that he has been denied equal protection of the laws by the State's statute granting full parental rights to a husband in relation to the child produced, with his consent, by the union of his wife with a sperm donor. . . . The claim really is that of Mrs. Stern. It is that she is in precisely the same position as the husband in the statute: she is presumably infertile, as is the husband in the statute; her spouse by agreement with a third party procreates with the understanding that the child will be the couple's child. The alleged unequal protection is that the understanding is honored in the statute when the husband is the infertile party, but no similar understanding is honored when it is the wife who is infertile.

It is quite obvious that the situations are not parallel. A sperm donor simply cannot be equated with a surrogate mother. The State has more than a sufficient basis to distinguish the two situations—even if the only difference is between the time it takes to provide sperm for artificial insemination and the time invested in a nine-month pregnancy—so as to justify automatically divesting the sperm donor of his parental rights without automatically divesting a surrogate mother. Some basis for an equal protection argument might exist if Mary Beth Whitehead had contributed her egg to be implanted, fertilized or otherwise, in Mrs. Stern, resulting in the latter's pregnancy. That is not the case here, however.

Mrs. Whitehead, on the other hand, asserts a claim that falls within the scope of a recognized fundamental interest protected by the Constitution. As a mother, she claims the right to the companionship of her child. This is a fundamental interest, constitutionally protected. Furthermore, it was taken away from her by the action of the court below. Whether that action under these circumstances would constitute a constitutional deprivation, however, we need not and do not decide. By virtue of our decision Mrs. Whitehead's constitutional complaint—that her parental rights have been unconstitutionally terminated—is moot. We have decided that both the statutes and public policy of this state require that that termination be voided and that her parental rights be restored. It therefore becomes unnecessary to decide whether that same result would be required by virtue of the federal or state Constitutions. . . .

V. Custody

Having decided that the surrogacy contract is illegal and unenforceable, we now must decide the custody question without regard to the provisions of the surrogacy contract that would give Mr. Stern sole and permanent custody. (That does not mean that the existence of the contract and the circumstances under which it was entered may not be considered to the extent deemed relevant to the child's best interests.) With the surrogacy contract disposed of, the legal framework becomes a dispute between two couples over the custody of a child produced by the artificial insemination of one couple's wife by the other's husband. Under the Parentage Act the claims of the natural father and the natural mother are entitled to equal weight, *i.e.*, one is not preferred over the other solely because it is the father or the mother. *N.J.S.A.* 9:17-40.[4] The applicable rule given these circumstances is clear: the child's best interests determine custody. . . .

We are not concerned at this point with the question of termination of parental rights, either those of Mrs. Whitehead or of Mr. Stern. As noted in various places in this opinion, such termination, in the absence of abandonment or a valid surrender, generally depends on a showing that the particular parent is unfit. The question of custody in this case, as in practically all cases, assumes the fitness of both parents, and no serious contention is made in this case that either is unfit. The issue here is which life would be better *for Baby M, one with primary custody in the Whiteheads or one with primary custody in the Sterns.*

The circumstances of this custody dispute are unusual and they have provoked some unusual contentions. The Whiteheads claim that even if the child's best interests would be served by our awarding custody to the Sterns, we should not do so, since that will encourage surrogacy contracts—contracts claimed by the Whiteheads, and we agree, to be violative of important legislatively-stated public policies. Their position is that in order that surrogacy contracts be deterred, custody should remain in the surrogate mother unless she is unfit, regardless of the best interests of the child. We disagree. Our declaration that this surrogacy contract is unenforceable and illegal is sufficient to deter similar agreements. We need not sacrifice the child's interests in order to make that point sharper. . . .

The Whiteheads also contend that the award of custody to the Sterns *pendente lite* was erroneous and that the error should not be allowed to affect the final custody decision. As noted above, at the very commencement of this action the court issued an ex parte order requiring Mrs. Whitehead to turn over the baby to the Sterns; Mrs. Whitehead did not comply but rather took the child to Florida. Thereafter, a similar order was enforced by the Florida authorities resulting in the transfer of possession of Baby M to the Sterns. The Sterns retained custody of the child throughout the litigation. The Whiteheads' point, assuming the *pendente* award of custody *was* erroneous, is that most of the factors arguing for awarding permanent custody to the Sterns resulted from that initial *pendente lite* order. Some of Mrs. Whitehead's alleged character failings, as testified to by experts and concurred in by the trial court, were demonstrated by her actions brought on by the custody crisis. For instance, in order to demonstrate her impulsiveness, those experts stressed the Whiteheads' flight to Florida with Baby M; to show her willingness to use her children for her own aims, they noted the telephone threats to kill Baby M and to accuse Mr. Stern of sexual abuse of her daughter; in order to show Mrs. Whitehead's manipulativeness, they pointed to her threat to kill herself; and in order to show her unsettled family life, they noted the innumerable moves from one hotel or motel to another in Florida. Furthermore, the argument continues, one of the most important factors, whether mentioned or not, in favor of custody in the Sterns is their continuing custody during the litigation, now having lasted for one-and-a-half years. The Whiteheads' conclusion is that had the trial court not given initial custody to the Sterns during the litigation, Mrs. Whitehead not only would have demonstrated her perfectly acceptable personality—the general tenor of the opinion of experts was that her personality problems surfaced primarily in crises—but would also have been able to prove better her parental skills along with an even stronger bond than may now exist between her and Baby M. Had she not been limited to custody for four months, she could have proved all of these things much more persuasively through almost two years of custody.

The argument has considerable force. It is of course possible that the trial court was wrong in its initial award of custody. It is also possible that such error, if that is what it was, may have affected the outcome. We disagree with the premise, however, that in determining custody a court should decide what the child's best interests *would be* if some hypothetical state of facts had existed. Rather, we must look to what those best interests *are, today,* even if some of the facts may have resulted in part from legal error. The child's interests come first: we will not punish it for judicial errors, assuming any were made. . . . The custody decision must be based on all circumstances, on everything that *actually* has occurred, on everything that is relevant to the child's best interests. Those circumstances include the trip to Florida, the telephone calls and threats, the substantial period of successful custody with the Sterns, and all other relevant circumstances. . . .

There were eleven experts who testified concerning the child's best interests, either directly or in connection with matters related to that issue. Our reading of the record persuades us that the trial court's decision awarding custody to the Sterns (technically to Mr. Stern) should be affirmed since "its findings. . . could reasonably have been reached on sufficient credible evidence present in the record." . . . More than that, on this record we find little room for any different conclusion. The trial court's treatment of this issue . . . is both comprehensive and, in most respects, perceptive. We agree substantially with its analysis with but few exceptions that, although important, do not change our ultimate views.

Our custody conclusion is based on strongly persuasive testimony contrasting both the family life of the Whiteheads and the Sterns and the personalities and characters of the individuals. The stability of the Whitehead family life was doubtful at the time of trial. Their finances were in serious trouble (foreclosure by Mrs. Whitehead's sister on a second mortgage was in process). Mr. Whitehead's employment, though relatively steady, was always at risk because of his alcoholism, a condition that he seems not to have been able to confront effectively. Mrs. Whitehead had not worked for quite some time, her last two employments having been part-time. One of the Whiteheads' positive attributes was their ability to bring up two children, and apparently well, even in so vulnerable a household. Yet substantial question was raised even about that aspect of their home life. The expert testimony contained criticism of Mrs. Whitehead's handling of her son's educational difficulties. Certain of the experts noted that Mrs. Whitehead perceived herself as omnipotent and omniscient concerning her children. She knew what they were thinking, what they wanted, and she spoke for them. As to Melissa, Mrs. Whitehead expressed the view that she alone knew what that child's cries and sounds meant. Her inconsistent stories about various things engendered grave doubts about her ability to explain honestly and sensitively to Baby M—and at the right time—the nature of her origin. Although faith in professional counseling is not a *sine qua non* of parenting, several experts believed that Mrs. Whitehead's contempt for professional help, especially professional psychological help, coincided with her feelings of omnipotence in a way that could be devastating to a child who most likely will need such help. In short, while love and affection there would be, Baby M's life with the Whiteheads promised to be too closely controlled by Mrs. Whitehead. The prospects for a wholesome independent psychological growth and development would be at serious risk.

The Sterns have no other children, but all indications are that their household and their personalities promise a much more likely foundation for Melissa to grow and thrive. There *is* a track record of sorts—during the one-and-a-half years of custody Baby M has done very well, and the relationship between both Mr. and Mrs. Stern and the baby has become very strong. The household is stable, and likely to remain so. Their finances are more than adequate, their circle of friends supportive, and their marriage happy. Most important, they are loving, giving, nurturing, and open-minded people. They have demonstrated the wish and ability to nurture and protect Melissa, yet at the same time to encourage her independence. Their lack of experience is more than made up for by a willingness to learn and to listen, a willingness that is enhanced by their professional training, especially Mrs. Stern's experience as a pediatrician. They are honest; they can recognize error, deal with it, and learn from it. They will try to determine rationally the best way to cope with problems in their relationship with Melissa. When the time comes to tell her about her origins, they will probably have found a means of doing so that accords with the best interests of Baby M. All in all, Melissa's future appears solid, happy, and promising with them.

Based on all of this we have concluded, independent of the trial court's identical conclusion, that Melissa's best interests call for custody in the Sterns. Our above-mentioned disagreements with the trial court do not, as we have noted, in any way diminish our concurrence with its conclusions. We feel, however, that those disagreements are important enough to be stated. They are disagreements about the evaluation of conduct. They also may provide some insight about the potential consequences of surrogacy.

It seems to us that given her predicament, Mrs. Whitehead was rather harshly judged—both by the trial court and by some of the experts. She was guilty of a breach of contract, and indeed, she did break a very important promise, but we think it is expecting something well beyond normal human capabilities to suggest that this mother should have parted with her newly born infant without a struggle. Other than survival, what stronger force is there? We do not know of, and cannot conceive of, any other case where a perfectly fit mother was expected to surrender her newly born infant, perhaps forever, and was then told she was a bad mother because she did not. We know of no authority suggesting that the moral quality of her act in those circumstances should be judged by referring to a contract made before she became pregnant. We do not countenance, and would never countenance, violating a court order as Mrs. Whitehead did, even a court order that is wrong; but her resistance to an order that she surrender her infant, possibly forever, merits a measure of understanding. We do not find it so clear that her efforts to keep her infant, when measured against the Sterns' efforts to take her away, make one, rather than the other, the wrongdoer. The Sterns suffered, but so did she. And if we go beyond suffering to an evaluation of the human stakes involved in the struggle, how much weight should be given to her nine months of pregnancy, the labor of childbirth, the risk to her life, compared to the payment of money, the anticipation of a child and the donation of sperm?

There has emerged a portrait of Mrs. Whitehead, exposing her children to the media, engaging in negotiations to sell a book, granting interviews that seemed helpful to her, whether hurtful to Baby M or not, that suggests a selfish, grasping woman ready to sacrifice the interests of Baby M and her other children for fame and wealth. That portrait is a half-truth, for while it may accurately reflect what ultimately occurred, its implication, that this is what Mary Beth Whitehead wanted, is totally inaccurate, at least insofar as the record before us is concerned. There is not one word in that record to support a claim that had she been allowed to continue her possession of her newly born infant, Mrs. Whitehead would have ever been heard of again; not one word in the record suggests that her change of mind and her subsequent fight for her child was motivated by anything other than love—whatever complex underlying psychological motivations may have existed.

We have a further concern regarding the trial court's emphasis on the Sterns' interest in Melissa's education as compared to the Whiteheads'. That this difference is a legitimate factor to be considered we have no doubt. But it should not be overlooked that a best-interests test is designed to create not a new member of the intelligentsia but rather a well-integrated person who might reasonably be expected to be happy with life. "Best interests" does not contain within it any idealized lifestyle; the question boils down to a judgment, consisting of many factors, about the likely future happiness of a human being. . . . Stability, love, family happiness, tolerance, and, ultimately, support of independence—all rank much higher in predicting future happiness than the likelihood of a college education. We do not mean to suggest that the trial court would disagree. We simply want to dispel any possible misunderstanding on the issue.

Even allowing for these differences, the facts, the experts' opinions, and the trial court's analysis of both argue strongly in favor of custody in the Sterns. Mary Beth Whitehead's family life, into which Baby M would be placed, was anything but secure—the quality Melissa needs most. And today it may be even less so.[5] Furthermore, the evidence and expert opinion based on it reveal personality characteristics, mentioned above, that might threaten the child's best development. The Sterns promise a secure home, with an understanding relationship that allows nurturing and independent growth to develop together. Although there is no substitute for reading the entire record, including the review of every word of each expert's testimony and reports, a summary of their conclusions is revealing. Six experts testified for Mrs. Whitehead: one favored joint custody, clearly unwarranted in this case; one simply rebutted an opposing expert's claim that Mary Beth Whitehead had a recognized personality disorder; one testified to the adverse impact of separation on *Mrs. Whitehead;* one testified about the evils of adoption and, to him, the probable analogous evils of surrogacy; one spoke only on the question of whether Mrs. Whitehead's consent in the surrogacy agreement was "informed consent"; and one spelled out the strong bond between mother and child. None of them unequivocally stated, or even necessarily implied, an opinion that custody in the Whiteheads was in the best interests of Melissa—the ultimate issue. The Sterns' experts, both well qualified—as were the Whiteheads'—concluded that the best interests of Melissa required custody in Mr. Stern. Most convincingly, the three experts chosen by the court-appointed guardian *ad litem* of Baby M, each clearly free of all bias and interest, unanimously and persuasively recommended custody in the Sterns.

* * *

VI. Visitation

The trial court's decision to terminate Mrs. Whitehead's parental rights precluded it from making any determination on visitation. 217 *N.J.Super.* at 399, 408, 525 *A.*2d 1128. Our reversal of the trial court's order, however, requires delineation of Mrs. Whitehead's rights to visitation. It is apparent to us that this factually sensitive issue, which was never addressed below, should not be determined *de novo* by this Court. We therefore remand the visitation issue to the trial court for an abbreviated hearing and determination as set forth below. . . .

We also note the following for the trial court's consideration: First, this is not a divorce case where visitation is almost invariably granted to the non-custodial spouse. To some extent the facts here resemble cases where the non-custodial spouse has had practically no relationship with the child; . . . but it only "resembles" those cases. In the instant case, Mrs. Whitehead spent the first four months of this child's life as her mother and has regularly visited the child since then. Second, she is not only the natural mother, but also the legal mother, and is not to be penalized one iota because of the surrogacy contract. Mrs. Whitehead, as the mother (indeed, as a mother who nurtured her child for its first four months—unquestionably a relevant consideration), is entitled to have her own interest in visitation considered. Visitation cannot be determined without considering the parents' interests along with those of the child.

In all of this, the trial court should recall the touchstones of visitation: that it is desirable for the child to have contact with both parents; that besides the child's interests, the parents' interests also must be considered; but that when all is said and done, the best interests of the child are paramount.

We have decided that Mrs. Whitehead is entitled to visitation at some point, and that question is not open to the trial court on this remand. The trial court will determine what kind of visitation shall be granted to her, with or without conditions, and when and under what circumstances it should commence. It also should be noted that the guardian's recommendation of a five-year delay is most unusual—one might argue that it begins to border on termination. Nevertheless, if the circumstances as further developed by appropriate proofs or as reconsidered on remand clearly call for that suspension under applicable legal principles of visitation, it should be so ordered.

In order that the matter be determined as expeditiously as possible, we grant to the trial court the broadest powers to reach its determination. A decision shall be rendered in no more than ninety days from the date of this opinion. . . .

Conclusion

This case affords some insight into a new reproductive arrangement: the artificial insemination of a surrogate mother. The unfortunate events that have unfolded illustrate that its unregulated use can bring suffering to all involved. Potential victims include the surrogate mother and her family, the natural father and his wife, and most importantly, the child. Although surrogacy has apparently provided positive results for some infertile couples, it can also, as this case demonstrates, cause suffering to participants, here essentially innocent and well-intended.

We have found that our present laws do not permit the surrogacy contract used in this case. Nowhere, however, do we find any legal prohibition against surrogacy when the surrogate mother volunteers, without any payment, to act as a surrogate and is given the right to change her mind and to assert her parental rights. Moreover, the Legislature remains free to deal with this most sensitive issue as it sees fit, subject only to constitutional constraints.

If the Legislature decides to address surrogacy, consideration of this case will highlight many of its potential harms. We do not underestimate the difficulties of legislating on this subject. In addition to the inevitable confrontation with the ethical and moral issues involved, there is the question of the wisdom and effectiveness of regulating a matter so private, yet of such public interest. Legislative consideration of surrogacy may also provide the opportunity to begin to focus on the overall implications of the new reproductive biotechnology—*in vitro* fertilization, preservation of sperm and eggs, embryo implantation and the like. The problem is how to enjoy the benefits of the technology—especially for infertile couples—while minimizing the risk of abuse. The problem can be addressed only when society decides what its values and objectives are in this troubling, yet promising, area.

The judgment is affirmed in part, reversed in part, and remanded for further proceedings consistent with this opinion.

For affirmance in part, reversal in part and remandment —Chief Justice Wilentz and Justices Clifford, Handler, Pollock, O'Hern, Garibaldi and Stein—7.

Opposed—None.

NOTES

1. Subsequent to the trial court proceedings, Mr. and Mrs. Whitehead were divorced, and soon thereafter Mrs. Whitehead remarried. Nevertheless, in the course of this opinion we will make reference almost exclusively to the facts as they existed at the time of trial, the facts on which the decision we now review was reached. We note moreover that Mr. Whitehead remains a party to this dispute. For these reasons, we continue to refer to appellants as Mr. and Mrs. Whitehead.
2. Another argument advanced by Mrs. Whitehead is that the surrogacy agreement violates state wage regulations, *N.J.S.A.* 34:11-4.7, and the Minimum Wage Standard Act, *N.J.S.A.* 34:1156a to -56a30. Given our disposition of the matter, we need not reach those issues.
3. As a general rule, a person should be accorded the right to make decisions affecting his or her own body, health, and life, unless that choice adversely affects others. Thus, the United States Supreme Court, while recognizing the right of women to control their own bodies, has rejected the view that the federal constitution vests a pregnant woman with an absolute right to terminate her pregnancy. Instead the court declared that the right was "not absolute" so that "at some point the protection of health, medical standards, and prenatal life, become dominant. . . . The balance struck in *Roe v. Wade* recognizes increasing rights of the mother as the pregnancy progresses. Similarly, in the termination-of-treatment cases, courts generally have viewed a patient's right to terminate or refuse life-sustaining treatment as constrained by other considerations including the rights of innocent third parties, such as the patient's children. . . .

   In the present case, the parties' right to procreate by methods of their own choosing cannot be enforced without consideration of the state's interest in protecting the resulting child, just as the right to the companionship of one's child cannot be enforced without consideration of that crucial state interest.
4. At common law the rights of women were so fragile that the husband generally had the paramount right to the custody of children upon separation or divorce. *State v. Baird*, 21 *N.J.Eq.* 384, 388 (E. & A. 1869). In 1860 a statute concerning separation provided that children "within the age of seven years" be placed with the mother "unless said mother shall be of such character and habits as to render her an improper guardian." *L.* 1860, *c.* 167. The inequities of the common-law rule and the 1860 statute were redressed by an 1871 statute, providing that "the rights of both parents, in the absence of misconduct, shall be held to be equal." *L.* 1871, *c.* 48, § 6 (currently codified at *N.J.S.A.* 9:2–4). Under this statute the father's superior right to the children was abolished and the mother's right to custody of children of tender years was also eliminated. Under the 1871 statute, "the happiness and welfare of the children" were to determine custody, *L.* 1871, *c.* 48, § 6, a rule that remains law to this day. *N.J.S.A.* 9:2–4.
5. Subsequent to trial, and by the time of oral argument, Mr. and Mrs. Whitehead had separated, and the representation was that there was no likelihood of change. Thereafter Mrs. Whitehead became pregnant by another man, divorced Mr. Whitehead, and remarried the other man. Both children are living with Mrs. Whitehead and her new husband. Both the former and present husband continue to assert the desire to have whatever parental relationship with Melissa that the law allows, Mrs. Whitehead continuing to maintain her claim for custody.

   We refer to this development only because it suggests less stability in the Whiteheads' lives. It does not necessarily suggest that Mrs. Whitehead's conduct renders her any less a fit parent. In any event, this new development has not affected our decision.

INFERTILITY: MEDICAL AND SOCIAL CHOICES—U.S. CONGRESS, OFFICE OF TECHNOLOGY ASSESSMENT, 1988

INTRODUCTION. *Given the absence of an Ethics Advisory Board for the U.S. Department of Health and Human Services and the lack of a national advisory commission on bioethics in the mid-1980s, two congressional committees asked the Office of Technology Assessment, the research arm of the U.S. Congress to undertake a study of infertility and the assisted reproductive technologies. The Office of Technology Assessment (OTA) was the research arm of the U.S. Congress. The following excerpts from its report, written by staff members with substantial input from outside contractors and an advisory panel, summarizes attitudes toward the new reproductive technologies and surveys the major ethical issues discussed in policy statements and academic commentary. The principal author of this chapter was Gladys B. White.*

11. ETHICAL CONSIDERATIONS

Ethical issues raised by the use of reproductive technologies can be examined in a variety of ways. One method is to study the arguments for and against the use of such technologies, with special emphasis on impacts that are unintended, indirect, and delayed. Another way is to list novel questions raised by the use of reproductive technologies. New ethical questions arise, for example, when third parties are involved in procreative interactions, when sperm and ova are banked for indefinite periods of time, and when surplus human embryos are created. A third method is to list the human values that are generally at stake in the diagnosis and treatment of infertility.

This chapter analyzes ethical arguments, raises novel ethical questions, and surveys relevant human values through discussion of six basic themes that pertain to specific reproductive technologies:

- the right to procreate or reproduce,
- the moral status of the embryo,
- parenthood and parent-child bonding,
- research initiatives and the rights of patients and research subjects,
- truth-telling and confidentiality, and
- intergenerational responsibilities.

Context of the Ethical Debate

Professional, public, religious, and personal opinions infuse ethical debates about the use of reproductive technologies. The concerns expressed by health care personnel are important, since these individuals are among those most intimately involved in the development and application of such techniques. Position statements have been prepared by relevant committees of the American Medical Association, the American College of Obstetricians and Gynecologists, and the American Fertility Society (1,2,4).

All these professional groups consider at least some, if not all, of the existing reproductive technologies to be morally licit, and all advocate their use in carefully circumscribed situations. Yet all share certain concerns and maintain that the use of these techniques requires careful monitoring. Seen to be especially central are the issues of confidentiality; informed consent; minimization of risk to the pregnant woman, the fetus, or the future child; adequate screening of donors; appropriate handling of embryos; and ongoing evaluation of data obtained through the use of these techniques.

U.S. Congress, Office of Technology Assessment, *Infertility: Medical and Social Choices*, OTA-BA-358 (Washington, D.C.: U.S. Government Printing Office, May, 1988.)

Public opinion is reflected in the many responses of public commissions and groups in this country and throughout the world, particularly since the 1970s. . . . Several themes emerge from such reports:

- support for artificial insemination by husband, artificial insemination by donor, and in vitro fertilization (IVF) as treatments for infertility;
- support for ova and sperm donation (with the exception of the U.S. Ethics Advisory Board, which barred the use of Federal funding, and the French National Ethics Committee);
- support for embryo donation (with the exception of the U.S. Ethics Advisory Board, the French National Ethics Committee, and the Working Party in South Australia);
- the imposition of guidelines and procedural regulations on the use of these techniques, such as restrictions on their use to stable couples and to physicians practicing in appropriate facilities, restrictions for donors of gametes, guidelines on the disclosure of information to protect confidentiality, and provisions to ensure informed consent and to clarify the legal status of children born as a result; and
- great controversy surrounding issues of surrogate motherhood (regardless of whether a fee is paid), the treatment of embryos not transferred, and the use of these techniques by single women.

Many religious and secular communities emphasize the moral significance of parenthood in a general way, with several variations on this theme. One variation emphasizes the ways in which parenthood enriches the life of individual couples; a second focuses on the importance of parenthood for the social order. These two approaches are best viewed as instances of the appeal to consequences or outcomes of actions. A third emphasizes a theological dimension to parenthood, which is viewed as fulfilling a divine commitment to procreate or as a way of human participation in the divine activity of creating and sustaining life.

Religious traditions offer widespread support for traditional infertility workups and medical and surgical interventions. . . . The Protestant, Jewish, and Muslim traditions affirm artificial insemination by husband. The Roman Catholic tradition has special reasons for officially opposing artificial insemination by husband, although some theologians dissent (8,23). Most religious traditions find donation of sperm, eggs, or embryos to be problematic. The Roman Catholic, Orthodox Jewish, Muslim, and some Protestant traditions oppose it, while other Protestant and Conservative and Reform Jewish traditions allow it. Surrogate motherhood in any form is generally opposed by religious traditions. A few religious thinkers, notably biblical theologians (influenced by Old Testament patriarchal accounts about the importance of preserving male lineage) give guarded approval, but these are exceptions. It is important to note that not all members of a particular religious background adhere to the official tradition of their church.

Arguments about the use of reproductive technologies are generally expressed in terms of rights and responsibilities. There are two types of moral rights—liberty rights (negative or noninterference rights) and welfare rights (positive or correlative rights). Responsibilities are also described and sometimes referred to as duties and obligations. These terms are chosen because contemporary ethical discussion, whether it is based on intuition, ethical principles, or faith, is often couched in terms of rights and responsibilities.

A liberty right is defined as a natural right based on human freedom such that any human adult capable of choice has the right to forbearance on the part of all others from the use of coercion or restraint except to hinder coercion or restraint itself, and is at liberty to take any action that is not coercing or restraining or designed to injure other persons (16). In addition, liberty rights indicate the limits of the plausible authority of others, including government. Many people would extend to adolescents, children, and the unborn liberty rights in the form of a right to life (25). A liberty right is a kind of free assertion that requires only noninterference on the part of others, which is why it is characterized as a negative right. Exercising such a right does not require any positive response from others—only that they do not interfere. A liberty right does not claim aid from others in pursuit of a person's own goal. This is unrelated to the issue of whether the aid of others can be paid for or not. The exercise of a liberty right simply does not require such assistance.

A welfare right is a claim asserted by an individual that requires a corresponding response, obligation, or duty on the part of others. Welfare rights depend on a social consensus about the value of the goal. The right to be educated is a welfare right because it involves the assistance, contributions, and resources of others. The United States, for example, has a system of public as well as private education. The right to be educated, particularly at the public expense, is a kind of welfare right because it of necessity involves the talents, energies, and resources of others. It is important to note that the assertion of a *welfare right* does not necessarily indicate the presence or need for what is commonly called a *welfare system*. The claims made by infertile individuals or couples may or may not be something for which they can pay.

The infertile couple or individual must make decisions and come to terms with the problem of infertility in the midst of this professional, public, and religious debate about the ethics of reproductive technologies. The personal experience of infertility diagnosis and treatment may either reinforce or come into conflict with deeply held values. In addition, there are special problems in establishing a definitive resolution of many of these issues because of the plurality of moral viewpoints. In such circumstances, it becomes more difficult to restrict the informed and free collaboration of various parties in achieving conception.

The Right to Reproduce

A fundamental aspect of much modern moral thinking is the significance of free and autonomous choices. The exact definitions of freedom and autonomy are controversial, but basically considerable moral significance is attached to a person's freedom to make voluntary, uncoerced choices based on self-legislated principles and values. When applied to an evaluation of techniques for preventing and treating infertility, the result is an emphasis on the moral significance of couples and individuals freely choosing to act in accordance with their own values.

A second aspect of modern moral thought is the recognition of duties, obligations, or responsibilities that may limit or constrain human actions. The performance of some types of actions is morally illicit, however valuable the consequences and however much the people involved want to perform them. The exact nature of these constraints and the conditions under which they may be overridden are matters of great controversy, but the basic idea that they exist and do impose limitations on choices is relatively straightforward. In terms of preventing and treating infertility, the emphasis is on examining whether particular techniques do or do not violate any of these constraints.

The right to reproduce appears to be linked to freedom and autonomy in the most basic way: the desire to have children and create a family is a natural expression of generative urges and commitments to religious, ethnic, and familial values that have characterized the human race from its beginning. At present, the right to reproduce is a natural as well as a necessary aspect of human existence for at least some human beings if the species is to continue. The right to reproduce is most often a liberty right in that it demands only that others not interfere. When infertility is not a factor, individuals can exercise their right to reproduce in a way that minimizes claims on the goods, services, and resources of others.

Even as a liberty right, some argue that it is and should be constrained by inordinate population growth. The right does not exist in a vacuum but is tempered by societal circumstances in which people live. China, for example, has a policy limiting to one the number of children married couples in most of the country may have. This public policy is inconsistent with American values and probably would never be adopted in this country, although some have urged that considerations of world population growth should influence the size of American families (21).

The right to reproduce, then, as a liberty right is not particularly controversial, especially when it is asserted by a fertile couple or an individual. When a man or a woman is infertile, however, this right involves claims on others for responses, actions, and services. Such claims, even when those exercising the right have a full ability to pay, must be balanced against a host of other health care needs and priorities. Obviously the right to reproduce can more easily be exercised by those who can pay for needed medical service or intervention. Whether such services *ought* to be for sale is an important question, as is the question of when, if ever, others in society should subsidize or defray the costs of infertility diagnosis and treatment for those who cannot afford needed services. The use of tax dollars for infertility treatment services is also problematic to those members of society who think that some or all reproductive technologies are immoral.

Because it is desirable that procreation be achieved without the direct contributions of third parties or the services of health care providers, it would be better if the condition of infertility did not exist. The reality of infertility makes this a moot point, and it is the basis of a strong ethical argument for a heavy emphasis on preventive measures. For example, based on the ethical principle of respect for persons, it is important that factors that could contribute to infertility, such as a high incidence of sexually transmitted disease resulting in tubal disorders . . . be minimized. When attempts to prevent infertility are not initiated early or have failed, some assistance is required for individuals or couples to satisfy their desire to procreate.

When artificial insemination, gamete intrafallopian transfer, sperm and ovum banking, IVF, or surrogacy are needed, exercising the right to procreate makes extensive and in some cases troublesome claims on the interests and resources of others.

In the cases of drug therapy for ovulatory failure and surgical intervention for mechanical failure, the right to procreate can be exercised by infertile couples as long as they are able to procure the necessary expertise and pay for it either directly or through a third party. These technologies are widely available and the provision of them would not compromise the interests of any third party. In fact, infertile couples, health care professionals, and pharmaceutical companies all appear to benefit when such services are appropriately sought.

With artificial insemination, the ethical considerations become more complex. In the case of insemination with the husband's sperm, there is often no compelling objection as long as both partners are fully informed and choose to engage freely in this practice. In rare cases in which the husband is deceased, any harms to the child that might be born associated with not having a living biological father must be weighed against the mother's right to procreate using the stored sperm of a deceased spouse. This right has indeed been claimed by a widow for the use of sperm from her deceased husband (11).

The right to procreate when it involves insemination with a donor's sperm is least problematic when it is asserted by the couple because the husband's desire to see his wife become pregnant has obviously transcended his thwarted desire to be the genetic father. The desires of single women to be artificially inseminated by a donor do not cause any apparent harm to the donor but are most often evaluated with some consideration of the abilities to competently raise a child as a single parent and to the societal consequences of individuals conceiving with the explicit intention of raising a child alone, notwithstanding a trend toward single-parent adoption in this country.

Surrogates and donors of sperm and ova are not necessarily exercising a right to procreate but are contributing their human biological materials for a variety of motives, ranging from pure altruism to a desire to make money. Ethical considerations concerning these transactions center on issues of confidentiality, truth-telling, and the moral status of contracts.

Do infertile couples have a right to financial assistance if they are unable to pay for the cost of diagnosing and treating infertility? The American Fertility Society has noted that if techniques of assisted reproduction are included in the notion of an adequate level of health care, then it is consistent with the work of the President's Commission for the Study of Ethical Problems in Medicine and Biomedical and Behavioral Research that all citizens be provided with infertility services (2,28). A variation of this position is the view that individuals have a positive right only to a fair share of what may fulfill true human needs (15). It can also be said that infertile individuals and couples are entitled to diagnosis and treatment for infertility if they have had the foresight to select and supplement insurance coverage in a way that such services are included (9).

Providing Federal funds either through a possible extension of Medicaid benefits or by means of a separate enactment is one of the most controversial aspects of complete support of the right to procreate for all infertile couples. Some Americans view selected reproductive technologies as immoral. Spending Federal dollars always raises questions about the allocation of scarce resources. The principal arguments in such debates are:

- *utilitarianism*, that resources should be allocated in a way that promotes the greatest good for the greatest number (24);
- *libertarianism*, that individuals are entitled to whatever resources they possess provided they acquired such resources fairly, that resources may be exchanged commercially or as gifts, and that inequalities in the distribution of resources may be unfortunate but they are not inherently unfair (27);
- *maximin*, that as a matter of first principle, individuals are entitled to equal shares of resources and, as a matter of second principle, inequalities (either excess or scarce resources) should be distributed to benefit the least advantaged provided there is fair equality of opportunity (29); and
- *egalitarianism*, that resources should always be distributed equally (26).

The utilitarian argument can be used to support funding for infertility services by demonstrating how such support would contribute to the greater good. The libertarian argument is largely consistent with the status quo, in which infertility services are available on a limited basis to those who can pay for them. The maximin position could be used to justify some special consideration for infertility services if it could be demonstrated that such services are generally available and that the infertile have the special status of a *least advantaged* group. Finally, an egalitarian argument about the availability of infertility services would support only those services it is feasible to provide to everyone in need. Thus, the arguments about just distribution and the allocation of scarce resources suggest a variety of ethical responses on access to and provision of infertility services for those who cannot currently afford them.

Moral Status of the Embryo

Human fertilization creates a biological entity that is commonly regarded as more than and different from the precursor germ cells of human sperm and ovum. This new entity may develop into a fetus and, eventually, an infant. A number of human embryos are naturally lost when the embryo does not implant in the lining of the womb. . . .

There is no societal consensus about the earliest point, if any, at which a human embryo should be considered to be a person. At least two important moral or ethical questions are raised about embryos. First, how should we regard or value embryos? Second, what actions are morally acceptable and morally unacceptable with respect to embryos?

These questions are directly relevant to two of the reproductive technologies examined in this report—IVF and embryo banking. In addition, the freezing of embryos, research using embryos, and in vitro embryo culture are influenced by the way in which the embryo is regarded. In the process of IVF . . . , it is standard practice to mix several ova with sperm in order to increase the likelihood that several fertilizations will take place. The desired result is the development of embryos. Although the precise moment of fertilization and activation of the new genome may be as late as the four-to eight-cell stage of cell division, ethical questions do arise when more embryos develop than are needed for transfer to the womb or when embryos are created for purposes other than transfer, such as research (19).

It has been suggested that decisions about the use of human embryos can be made depending on the neurological development of the embryo at a given point in time (14,33). The Waller Committee in Victoria, Australia, the Warnock Committee in Great Britain . . . , and the 1979 report of the Ethics Advisory Board in the United States all approve of research involving human embryos fertilized in vitro, with varying restrictions but with agreement on a time limit of 14 days after fertilization (35).

There are at least three major philosophical positions on the moral status or meaning of the human embryo. The first is that the embryo is no different from other human biological material and that it has meaning only in terms of the goals and aspirations of others regarding its use and possible maturation. Adherents of this position point out that a large portion of all human embryos are naturally cast off when implantation fails to occur and, further, that an intrauterine device results in the loss of embryos that are even more developed than those that might be discarded in the course of IVF (10, 20).

A second position proposes that the embryo, while not a person and while not necessarily requiring the respect and rights due to fully functioning persons in society, is not an objective product or thing, and that it serves as a powerful symbol of respect for life (30,31,34). The embryo, in this scheme, is a "transient identity" and should be accorded "transient rights." These rights are not derived from the values others place on its existence, but from the nature of the potentiality of existence the embryo possesses. Still, while couples have the primary obligation to respect the life of the conceptus, however early its human form, respect for that life may itself lead some to consider abortion on genetic or other grounds. These grounds are open to some public scrutiny and control. When the embryo is at risk—during transfers, freezings, transplants, and future genetic manipulations—public scrutiny may also include public controls. It may be inappropriate to sell such material for research purposes, because that would violate the inherent transient rights of such entities (34).

A third position, which is held by the Roman Catholic church and others, is that the human being must be respected—as a person—from the very first instant of existence (8). From the time an ovum is fertilized, a new life is begun that is of neither the father nor the mother; it is rather the life of a new human being with an individual growth. It would never be made human if it were not human already. "Right from fertilization is begun the adventure of a human life" (32). This position has important implications for any use or treatment of the human embryo that would be different from or less than that afforded to a human person.

In practice, the issue of the use of surplus embryos in IVF is sometimes avoided by implanting all the eggs that are fertilized, increasing the probability of multiple births. One commentator, however, has argued that the deontological (duty-based) problem of the moral status of the embryo in this case gives way to the teleological (outcome-based) problem of how to care for more than one newborn (18). In addition, the presence of multiple fetuses in utero is correlated with lower birth weight per child and greater risks to the mother and to fetal health.

A recent Australian case demonstrates some of the problems and issues associated with the moral and legal status of unimplanted embryos. . . . From an ethical standpoint, the Rios case illustrates why it is important to discern the moral status of the embryo. Aside from the intents of the parents, who in this case are no longer living, it is difficult to ascertain what duties and obligations are owed the frozen embryos.

The extent to which a human embryo should be respected was addressed in 1986 by the American Fertility Society in its recommendations that:

- cryopreservation should be continued only as long as the normal reproductive span of the egg donor or as long as the original objective of the storage is in force;
- transfer of embryos from one generation to another is unacceptable; and
- formal discussion with the couple should take place in advance to decide whether excess embryos can be transferred to other couples, used for approved research, examined, or discarded (2).

Parenthood and Parent-Child Bonding

Opinion differs on the extent to which the genetic, gestational, and social functions of parenting can be separated and yet preserve the welfare of parents and children. Some who contend that new reproductive technologies are ethically acceptable regard parenthood as a relationship defined by acts of nurturing as opposed to acts of conceiving and giving birth. Others, although recognizing that acts of nurturing and generating life are distinct and that acts of nurturing are included in the meaning of parenthood, affirm that acts of generating life are parental in nature (22).

Bonding between a human infant and an adult is a prerequisite to the physical and psychological growth of the child and creates and sustains the abilities of the parents to nurture the child. Do parents and children possess a possible welfare right to at least the minimum conditions necessary for human bonding to take place? Now that it is possible for a child to have a total of five "parents"—three types of mothers (genetic, gestational, and rearing) and two types of fathers (genetic and rearing)—which of these parents has the right to form a parent-child bond? Now that it is possible through surrogacy arrangements and artificial insemination by donor for individuals to plan to create a single-parent family, does this violate a possible right of the child to bond to more than one parent? These questions have important implications for the way in which parent-child bonding takes place and for possible new variations in the developing identities of some children.

Any one of these variations on the theme of the moral significance of parenthood and the importance of parent-child bonding has considerable relevance to an ethical assessment of techniques for preventing and treating infertility. Depending on a number of factors (e.g., the way in which a particular variation views parenthood and the particular treatment used), the importance of the parent-child bond may lead to a positive ethical evaluation of techniques for preventing and treating infertility (6).

Research Initiatives and the Rights of Patients and Research Subjects

In the process of diagnosis and treatment for infertility, individuals or couples may find themselves in the role of research subjects as well as patients. Typically they start out as patients and are presumably informed about and give consent to each step of the diagnostic process. Couples are asserting a right to be treated for their infertility using medical therapy.

To expand and improve on the scientific basis of diagnosis and treatment for infertility, information about patients and their problems must be gathered and recorded in a systematic way. This is an aspect of medical treatment that can result in descriptive research about the course and outcome of medical therapy. As long as patients are informed that facts about them are being collected, in part for research purposes, and that their anonymity will be preserved, the benefits of this accumulating database seem to outweigh any possible harms or inconveniences to the infertile couples. These couples are now, in addition to being patients, also serving as research subjects although they may always choose to exercise their right to not participate. This pattern is not substantially different from that conducted in other areas of human health and disease.

A more troubling research aspect of infertility diagnosis and treatment (as well as the diagnosis and treatment of many other conditions) is how to make appropriate use of new technologies that have not yet entered the realm of tried and true medical therapy. Which reproductive technologies, if any, are more experimental than therapeutic? Do infertile couples become research subjects as a result of the experimental nature of the technologies that may be used in their treatment? Is there a subtle pressure occasionally present that the development of new knowledge can sometimes justify placing a human subject at a disproportionate risk or engaging in research with inadequate informed consent procedures?

All the parties interested in effective infertility diagnosis and treatment share a concern about how to distinguish properly among medical therapies, clinical trials, and clinical experiments. A specific reproductive technology may be *used* in a standard way in one instance and in a novel or experimental way another time. So it is not only the technologies themselves, but the way in which they are used, that determines whether a patient receives care that is more experimental than therapeutic (7).

Clinicians and researchers note that the problem of consistently developing medical therapies is particularly acute in the treatment of infertility because a de facto moratorium since 1980 on Federal funding for many forms of research involving fertilization of human egg and sperm has impeded the development of knowledge about fertility, infertility, and contraception. . . .

Although research initiatives may result in the steady transition of reproductive technologies from the domain of experimental to that of standard medical therapy, the rights of patients who are being treated for infertility to be appropriately informed about the research aspects of their treatment persist. In the course of diagnosing and treating infertility, the liberty or noninterference rights of scientists to pursue research and of physicians to practice medicine are constrained by the correlative right of infertile couples to be informed about the experimental nature of selected reproductive technologies.

Individuals and couples with problems of infertility are an extremely vulnerable population group. Because of their strong desire to exhaust all possibly successful avenues of treatment, an attitude they share with those who are considering participation in research under the pressure of severe illness, their ability to give free and informed consent is to some extent always compromised. For this reason, it is particularly important that care be taken to carefully inform infertile couples when new reproductive technologies are suggested as possible methods of treatment. The special vulnerability of this group makes quality control of reproductive technologies a vital societal concern. . . .

Truth-Telling and Confidentiality

Infertility prevention, diagnosis, and treatment are interactive processes in which the infertile individuals, physicians, and others exchange information, make evaluations, and even offer predictions. All parties to these interactions have a right to know the truth. At least two moral arguments for telling the truth can be cited: Truth-telling is a general requirement for an action to be moral, and truth-telling generally has the best consequences in the realms of personal interaction (37). A common counterargument is that the truth might result in some harm, such as increased personal suffering or a denial of access to a desired service. Using the language of moral rights mentioned earlier in the chapter, the right to be told the truth is a claim right involving the full disclosure of otherwise unknown or unavailable information. The liberty right to be left alone, or free from harm, might be best exercised with or without the truth.

Infertile individuals and couples who seek diagnosis and treatment are not asking merely to be left alone. In their quest for a solution to their infertility, truthful information is an important basis for accurate diagnosis. It is important for the physician to know, for example, about any occurrence of sexually transmitted disease in order to make an accurate diagnosis and to devise an appropriate treatment. It is also important for the physician to know the extent of previous diagnostic workups and treatment failures.

By the same token, it is important for the patient to know the truth about a specific treatment and the likelihood of success of a given effort. A common criterion used in evaluating various IVF programs is the pregnancy rate achieved by a specific program. There is considerable variation, however, in the way that this rate is reported. The variations include reporting in terms of pregnancies per ovarian stimulation cycle, and pregnancies per embryo transfer. . . . A group of prominent clinicians has noted that what constitutes pregnancy is confusing to the lay public. Couples who seek treatment for infertility are really interested in taking home babies, and a claim to a high pregnancy rate based on a limited number of chemical pregnancies, for example, is misleading (5). One commentator makes the point that technically accurate statements that convey misleading messages are no less a violation of the principle of truth-telling because their content happens to be technically true (36).

One area in which physicians have made judgments that truth-telling may not ultimately be of benefit to the patients they are trying to treat is in filing insurance claims on behalf of patients. The great variation in coverage among third-party payers may lead to physician subterfuge about the actual services provided and the goals of treatment. . . . This is a case in which the physician may knowingly compromise his or her own integrity in order to assist patients in acquiring reimbursement. Physicians who do this have made the judgment that the negative consequences of telling the truth in a way that corresponds to insurance reimbursement categories outweigh the general moral requirement to tell the truth.

A major feature of the physician-patient relationship is the expectation that the highly charged personal information pertaining to the diagnosis and treatment of infertility will be held in confidence. This is true for most of the interactions that take place between physicians and patients but is particularly pressing in an area of medical practice where problems are of such an intimate nature and strike at the heart of personal and family relationships. The fundamental statement concerning medical confidentiality appears in the Hippocratic oath:

> What I may see or hear in the course of the treatment or even outside of the treatment in regard to the life of men, which on no account one must spread abroad, I will keep to myself, holding such things to be shameful to be spoken about (12).

This principle has been reiterated in modern times by many groups and in numerous codes of professional ethics. It has been maintained, for example, that a doctor owes a patient absolute secrecy on all that has been confided or that the doctor knows because of the confidence entrusted in him or her, and that the patient has the right to expect that all communications and records pertaining to care should be treated as confidential (3,4).

The use of reproductive technologies can place a strain on maintaining confidentiality in several important ways. The use of donor ova or sperm involves the transfer of relevant information about the donor although the anonymity of the donor can be maintained. It may be impossible to treat the problem of infertility as a problem of the couple if one partner holds the physician to a principle of confidentiality, for example, with respect to past sexual practices. The maintenance of confidentiality is also linked to the reestablishment of privacy concerning sexual matters that may be essential to the well-being of the couple after the crisis of infertility has been resolved.

Intergenerational Responsibilities

One important aspect of ethical arguments for and against specific reproductive technologies is the significance of considering the consequences of individual actions and social practices for all those affected. These individuals can include those who perform the actions or participate in the practices, or they may be other members of society. Any evaluation must consider the consequences of these techniques for the infertile couples, for their prospective children, and for the rest of society (6).

Some argue that the use of reproductive technologies carries with it the duty of not harming either the infertile patient or the resulting embryo, fetus, and child. The ethical principle of nonmaleficence has a long tradition in medical ethics that many trace back to the Hippocratic oath (36). In addition, others would argue that there is a strong obligation to circumvent or treat the problem of infertility in ways that do not harm future generations in general. Does one generation have obligations to another and, if so, how are these duties weighed against individual needs and desires?

These questions are particularly relevant to issues of confidentiality and truth-telling in the context of donor gametes (ova or sperm) and surrogate motherhood. Should a child be told that his or her rearing parent is not the child's genetic and/or gestational parent, and also how he or she was conceived? Should information about a child's biological origin be kept on file? Should a child who is not living with his or her father or mother be entitled to at least some information about this genetic parent? Should a child be entitled to know the identity of the genetic father or mother and thus be afforded the opportunity to contact this parent?

In his book *The Philosophy of Right,* G.W.F. Hegel stated:

> Children are potentially free and their life directly embodies nothing save potential freedom. Consequently they are not things and cannot be the property either of their parents or others (17).

Children are ends in themselves and not merely the means or objects of the goals of their parents. If this is true, then it would be unacceptable to utilize a reproductive technology that would impinge on the freedom or autonomy of children. One philosopher argues that duties to future generations must be much weaker than duties to contemporaries, for contemporaries are actual persons who can have actual views about what is important (13). Even so, there is an important argument that it is prudent to support those practices that are least likely to be harmful to the next generation.

Reproductive technologies also raise intergenerational concerns about the use of resources. Increased funding for infertility research can have important benefits for humanity but this claim for the research dollar has to compete with other research interests. In addition, any general shift in the reproductive years of the population as a whole has important economic and demographic implications for the generations that follow.

Summary and Conclusions

For individuals and couples with problems of infertility, the right to procreate may be exercised as a simple liberty right involving the noninterference or forbearance of others or as a welfare right that makes significant claims on technology and the expertise and resources of others. The right to reproduce becomes problematic when it involves large financial resources extending beyond those available to an infertile individual or couple. Given the fundamental nature of the desire to procreate, however, it seems desirable that individuals from a variety of backgrounds have some access to reproductive technologies.

The right to reproduce becomes more difficult to justify when it begins to compromise the interests of a third party. There is a strong moral sentiment that the exercise of the right to procreate by some individuals should not result in the exploitation of women, for example, in surrogate mother arrangements. Alternatively, some moral support exists for the view that in a free society it is possible and should be legal to give the gift of genetic or gestational surrogacy to an infertile couple.

A strong ethical argument can be made that resources and support should be devoted to the prevention of infertility in order that the right to procreate can most often be expressed as a liberty right. Individuals have an interest in avoiding any curtailment of their reproductive capacity when they wish to reproduce. This places a heavy emphasis on the eradication of factors that lead to infertility.

The moral status of the human embryo is a subject of considerable debate. Many people have made judgments about whether the embryo has the status and meaning of a person. In addition, cryopreservation of embryos presents legal and ethical questions about the rights of such entities and any duties and obligations owed to them. The unresolved debate about appropriate uses of human embryos and the de facto moratorium on Federal support for IVF research have impeded the growth of new knowledge about fertility, infertility, and contraception.

Reproductive technologies make it technically possible for a child to have a total of five "parents" —three types of mothers (genetic, gestational, and rearing) and two types of fathers (genetic and rearing). These possibilities change the nature of parenting and may have implications for the ways in which parent-child bonding takes place. Such bonding has important psychological benefits for parents and is essential to the developing personalities of children.

The right to conduct research is a noninterference or liberty right as well as a welfare or correlative right. The right to pursue research is always balanced against other societal goods, and the resources to conduct research are always limited. Infertile patients have a right to know when their treatment is in the realm of proven medical therapy or is essentially experimental.

Telling the truth and maintaining confidentiality are important aspects of the physician-patient relationship. The intimate nature of the diagnosis and treatment of infertility and the special features of reproductive technologies that make use of donor ova or sperm complicate simple ethical imperatives to tell the truth and to hold personal information in confidence. A strong argument can be made that individuals have a duty to refrain from utilizing reproductive technologies in ways that could possibly harm future generations or make disproportionate claims on the resources of existing generations.

Most religious traditions in the United States:

- support the treatment of infertility when such treatment involves traditional drug therapy or surgical intervention, and accept the moral licitness of such treatments;
- accept the moral licitness of artificial insemination by husband, have considerable hesitation about artificial insemination by donor, and show even less support for artificial insemination of single women with donor sperm;
- support IVF as long as only spousal gametes (ova and sperm) are used and as long as no embryos are wasted, though support lessens to some degree when there is early embryo wastage and to a much greater degree when donor gametes are used; and
- oppose surrogate motherhood in both its genetic and gestational forms.

REFERENCES

1. American College of Obstetricians and Gynecologists, *Ethical Issues in Human In Vitro Fertilization and Embryo Placement* (Washington, DC: 1986).
2. American Fertility Society, Ethics Committee, "Ethical Considerations of the New Reproductive Technologies," *Fertility and Sterility* 46:1S-94S, 1986.
3. American Hospital Association, "Statement on a Patient's Bill of Rights," *Hospitals* 47:41, 1973.

4. American Medical Association, Judicial Council, *Opinions and Reports* (Chicago, IL: 1968).
5. Blackwell, R.E., Carr, B.R., Chang, R.J., et al., "Are We Exploiting the Infertile Couple?" *Fertility and Sterility* 48:735–739, 1987.
6. Brody, B.A., "Religious and Secular Perspectives About Infertility Prevention and Treatment," prepared for the Office of Technology Assessment, U.S. Congress, Washington, DC, June 1987.
7. Caplan, A.L., "The New Technologies in Reproduction—New Ethical Problems," *Annals of the New York Academy of Sciences,* in press, 1988.
8. Congregation for the Doctrine of the Faith, *Instruction on Respect for Human Life in its Origin and on the Dignity of Procreation* (Vatican City: 1987).
9. Daniels, N., "Am I My Parents' Keeper?" *Midwest Studies in Philosophy* 7:517–520, 1982.
10. Dickens, B.M., Faculty of Law, University of Toronto, Toronto, Canada, personal communication, Aug. 28, 1987.
11. Dionne, E.J., "Paris Widow Wins Suit To Use Sperm; Court Decides Against Sperm Bank in Plea From Wife of Man Who Died in 1983," *New York Times,* Aug. 2, 1984.
12. Edelstein, L., "The Hippocratic Oath: Text, Translation and Interpretation," *Ancient Medicine: Selected Papers of Ludwig Edelstein,* O. Tempkin and C. Tempkin (eds.) (Baltimore, MD: Johns Hopkins University Press, 1967).
13. Engelhardt, H.T., Jr., Center for Ethics, Medicine and Public Issues, Baylor College of Medicine, Houston, TX, personal communication, June 24, 1987.
14. Flower, M.J., "The Neuromaturation of the Fetus," *Journal of Medicine and Philosophy* 10:237–251, 1985.
15. Fried, C., *Right and Wrong* (Cambridge, MA: Harvard University Press, 1978).
16. Hart, H.L.A., "Are There Any Natural Rights?" *Rights,* D. Lyons (ed.) (Belmont, CA: Wadsworth Publishing Co., 1979).
17. Hegel, G.W.F., *The Philosophy of Right,* Trans. T.M. Knox (Oxford, UK: Clarendon Press, 1952).
18. Jansen, R., "Ethics in Infertility Treatment," *The Infertile Couple,* R. Pepperell, C. Wood, and B. Hudson (eds.) (New York, NY: Churchill Livingstone, in press).
19. Jones, H.W., and Schrader, C., "The Process of Human Fertilization: Implications for Moral Status," *Fertility and Sterility* 48:189–192, 1987.
20. Kuhse, H., and Singer, P., "The Moral Status of the Embryo," *Test-Tube Babies,* W. Walters and P. Singer (eds.) (Melbourne, Australia: Oxford University Press, 1982).
21. Mann, D., "Growth Means Doom," *Science Digest* 4:79–81, 1983.
22. McCormick, R.A., "Reproductive Technologies: Ethical Issues," *Encyclopedia of Bioethics,* W.T. Reich (ed.) (New York, NY: Macmillan/Free Press, 1978).
23. McCormick, R.A., "Vatican Asks Governments To Curb Birth Technology and To Outlaw Surrogates," *New York Times,* Mar. 11, 1987.
24. Mill, J.S., *Utilitarianism and Other Writings* (New York, NY: The New American Library, Inc., 1962).
25. Moraczewski, A.S., Regional Director, Pope John XXIII Medical-Moral Research and Education Center, Houston, TX, personal communication, Aug. 28, 1987.
26. Nielsen, K., "Radical Egalitarian Justice: Justice as Equality," *Social Theory and Practice* 5:209–226, 1979.
27. Nozick, R., *Anarchy, State and Utopia* (New York, NY: Basic Books, 1974).
28. President's Commission for the Study of Ethical Problems in Medicine and Biomedical and Behavioral Research, *Securing Access to Health Care* (Washington, DC: U.S. Government Printing Office, 1983).
29. Rawls, J., *A Theory of Justice* (Cambridge, MA: Belknap Press of Harvard University Press, 1971).
30. Robertson, J.A., "Embryos, Families and Procreative Liberty: The Legal Structure of the New Reproduction," *Southern California Law Review* 59: 971–987, 1986.
31. Robertson, J.A., "Ethical and Legal Issues in Cryopreservation of Human Embryos," *Fertility and Sterility* 47:371–381, 1987.
32. Sacred Congregation for the Doctrine of the Faith, *Declaration on Procured Abortion* (AAS) 66:12–13, 1974.
33. Tauer, C.A., "Personhood and Human Embryos and Fetuses," *Journal of Medicine and Philosophy* 10: 253–266, 1985.
34. Thomasma, D.C., Director, Medical Humanities Program, Loyola University Stritch School of Medicine, Chicago, IL, personal communication, Mar. 16, 1987.
35. U.S. Department of Health, Education, and Welfare, Ethics Advisory Board, *HEW Support of Research Involving Human In Vitro Fertilization and Embryo Transfer,* May 4, 1979.
36. Veatch, R.M., *A Theory of Medical Ethics* (New York, NY: Basic Books, 1981).
37. Walters, L., "Ethical Aspects of Medical Confidentiality," *Contemporary Issues in Bioethics,* T. Beauchamp and L. Walters (eds.) (Belmont, CA: Wadsworth Publishing Co., 1982).

ETHICS OF NEW REPRODUCTIVE TECHNOLOGIES: THE GLOVER REPORT TO THE EUROPEAN COMMISSION, 1989

INTRODUCTION. *The Glover Report represents an attempt by an interdisciplinary, international committee to formulate a distinctly European approach to the new reproductive technologies and arrangements. Oxford philosopher Jonathan Glover chaired the committee. Building on the prior work of several national advisory committees or commissions—in Sweden, the United Kingdom, Italy, West Germany, and France—as well as the Vatican's* Instruction, *the committee focused particular attention on artificial insemination and in vitro fertilization. The following excerpt summarizes the committee's conclusions.*

Summary of Conclusions

Since this report deals with ethics at least as much as with public policy, there is something dogmatic about a bald list of assertions to the effect that this is right and that is wrong. Before listing our conclusions, we wish to stress that their force can only be assessed in the context of the argument which has led to them. A report of this kind makes more of a contribution when people are encouraged to think more deeply, and probably to disagree, than when they uncritically accept the conclusions.

1. PARENTS, DONORS AND CHILDREN

1. We think there should be a *presumption* that those born as a result of semen donation should ultimately have access to knowledge of the identity of their biological father, but that this presumption could be overridden by evidence that it drastically reduced the supply of donors.

There is a case for an *experiment* on Swedish lines, where for a trial period:

(a) the child is given a legal right to know the father's identity on reaching maturity.
and
(b) legal paternity is assigned to the married woman's husband, and donors are given protection against any legal claims.

A severe and continuing shortage of donors would be a good reason for reversing the policy after the trial period.

2. We think that there should be no general presumption for or against related donors. But, in the interests of donation being fully voluntary, daughters should not normally donate eggs to their mothers.

3. In the case of related donors, the child should not be deceived about the relationship.

4. We are divided on whether reproductive technology should be made available to people other than infertile heterosexual couples. But we agree that the birth of a child should not be associated with criminality; and consequently we agree that no use of these techniques by individuals or couples should be illegal.

2. SURROGACY

1. We favour a restrictive approach to surrogacy, in the interests of protecting the surrogate mother from exploitation, and in the interests of protecting the child from harmfully prolonged battles between the surrogate and the prospective parents.

From Jonathan Glover et al., *Ethics of New Reproductive Technologies: The Glover Report to the European Commission*, DeKalb, Illinois: Northern Illinois University Press, 1989. Note that Dr. Simone Novaes's reservations (originally in an unnumbered note after the first paragraph) appear at the end of the selection.

2. Commercial agencies should not be permitted.

3. Any public agencies set up should help people to find a surrogate mother only when there is a clear medical reason for doing so.

4. To avoid criminalizing the birth of a child, private surrogacy arrangements between individuals should not be illegal.

5. If a surrogate makes a contract, it should in certain respects not be enforceable: whether or not she has an abortion, and whether or not she hands over the child, should not be matters over which she is legally compelled.

6. If the surrogate does hand over the child, she should have no right to claim the child back.

7. Except where the surrogate is in the same family, the normal practice should be for relations between her and the child to be severed.

8. Agencies should screen potential surrogate mothers, on medical and on psychological grounds.

9. We are not enthusiastic about payment to the surrogate mother, beyond the meeting of her expenses. But we are agreed that such payment should not be illegal.

3. RESEARCH

1. We value the benefits which research on pre-embryos may bring.

2. Despite having differing views on the moral claims of the pre-embryo and embryo, we agree that they are not strong enough to exclude all research, or even to exclude all research which destroys the life of an embryo.

3. We agree that research is easier to justify at early stages of development than at later stages.

4. The stage of development at which research should no longer be permitted should be decided by a regulatory authority with powers to vary the boundary in the light of new evidence.

5. No research causing foetal pain should be carried out.

6. Where an embryo or pre-embryo will eventually become a child, to avoid the risk of harm to that child no research on the pre-embryo or embryo should be carried out.

7. We see no objection to the use of material from aborted foetuses for medical purposes such as transplants. But such material should not be used for non-medical purposes.

8. Transplants should be obtained from foetuses aborted on other grounds, and the beneficiary should normally be unknown to the woman having the abortion.

9. We see no objection to cultivating cells of a particular kind (e.g. blood cells) for medical purposes, nor to this cultivation going beyond the time-limit set for research on the whole embryo.

10. Research should be regulated by a statutory body, to which ethics committees would refer any decisions involving major new issues of principle. This body should be independent of government, and among those well represented on it should be women and those who are neither doctors nor scientists. It should make public the reasoning behind its decisions.

We recommend that, if the scope of the activities of the body is broader than research, and includes the whole field of new reproductive technology, it should commission a large-scale study of the children resulting from these kinds of intervention. This should include investigation of the psychological effects on children of having a donor in the family as against the donor being unknown.

At many points, we have been struck by the high ratio of assertion to evidence on these matters. A substantial study would enable people a generation from now to make far better based decisions than ours.

(An unavoidable dilemma is that often we cannot be sure what the right policy is without evidence, but the evidence only comes from trying out policies. The best response is to go carefully, choosing what looks the best policy, but following up the consequences and being prepared to change as a result. The same dilemma is familiar to doctors trying out treatments for illness. Doctors sometimes say that the *only* ethical form of medicine is experimental. This may be true of social policies too.)

11. Each country should have its own regulatory body. There should not be an imposed European policy.

4. DECIDING WHO IS BORN

1. It is desirable that donors should be screened to reduce the risk of the birth of a severely handicapped child.

2. We accept that abortion in cases of serious handicap is justifiable.

3. The objection to gene therapy of somatic cells is its high level of risk. If this could be overcome, we see no objection to its use.

4. If 'positive' genetic engineering becomes possible, it should not be permitted until it becomes clear (if it ever does) that the problems it raises can be overcome.

5. Clinics should not be permitted to offer sex selection of children, except on medical grounds.

6. 'Do it yourself' sex selection should not be illegal.

[Note:] Dr. Simone Novaes, while not dissenting from the report as a whole, has two reservations:

1. The report does not sufficiently discuss the role of physicians and other medical intermediaries in the way these new reproductive technologies are used. Because of the role of the medical profession, there is a tendency to see these technologies in terms of a medical model: as ways of 'treating' infertility. However, the medical profession is making available, for procreative purposes, a medical alternative to sexual relations. In AID this is particularly clear. This is what, in

the long run, makes reproductive technology such an explosive issue. It automatically transforms reproduction into something more than an intimate family matter. The role of the medical intermediary in this transformation deserves fuller treatment.

2. The list of conclusions may induce a false sense of security, at least among those inclined to agree with them. They seem too reductionist to do justice to the complex arguments of the report. It would have been preferable to have had conclusions along more general lines, summarizing the different groups of problems, as well as new questions and lines of thought, with less suggestion that we might have solved some of them. This might have been more helpful in stimulating reflection.

ETHICAL ISSUES IN SURROGATE MOTHERHOOD: AMERICAN COLLEGE OF OBSTETRICIANS AND GYNECOLOGISTS, 1990

INTRODUCTION. *In parallel with the American Fertility Society's Ethics Committee, the ACOG Committee on Ethics worked behind the scenes and in the private sector to formulate guidelines for the appropriate use of the new reproductive technologies and arrangements. The products of its work usually appeared as statements on specific issues. The following statement revisits an issue that the Committee on Ethics had already considered in 1983. In the earlier statement the committee had expressed serious reservations about surrogate parenting arrangements and especially about the potential for financial exploitation of participants in those arrangements. In its 1990 statement the committee made an explicit decision to favor the birth mother over the commissioning couple in any custody dispute that might arise after the birth of a child. This position represents an acceptance of family law, not contract law, as the branch of law most relevant to surrogate parenting.*

Ethical Issues in Surrogate Motherhood

This statement is intended to update and replace the May 1983 ACOG statement of policy entitled "Ethical Issues in Surrogate Motherhood." A revised statement is required because there is now more experience with surrogate parenthood arrangements, because there has been further ethical discussion in the meantime, and because there have been intervening legal developments, both in the courts and in state legislatures.

The statement is divided into two major parts. In the first part, general ethical and social issues surrounding surrogate parenthood are addressed, and a way of approaching the topic is proposed. In the second part, issues of particular concern to obstetricians and gynecologists are outlined and discussed.

American College of Obstetricians and Gynecologists, Committee on Ethics, *Ethical Issues in Surrogate Motherhood.* ACOG Opinion 88. Washington, D.C.: American College of Obstetricians and Gynecologists, 1990. In this reprint, unnumbered notes and references appear as endnotes.

GENERAL ISSUES

Surrogate parenthood is a highly controversial and emotionally charged topic that both reflects and has implications for our notions of parenthood and family. After extensive deliberation and debate, the Committee on Ethics has adopted an analytical framework and reached a conclusion which it now puts forward for public discussion and critical evaluation. The committee's general view is that the surrogate mother, who both carries the fetus and delivers the infant, 1) should be the sole source of consent for all questions regarding prenatal care and delivery and 2) should have a specified time period after the birth of the infant during which she can decide whether or not to carry out her original intention to place the infant for adoption. Thus, in all relevant respects the position of the surrogate mother should be the same as the position of any other woman who, either prenatally or postnatally, has expressed the intention of placing an infant for adoption.

The major differences between the usual adoptive situation and surrogate parenting arrangements are, first, that in surrogacy there is an intention to undertake an adoption *before* the initiation of pregnancy and, second, that in most surrogacy arrangements the semen donor is the would-be adoptive father. Thus, the analogy between surrogate parenthood and adoption is by no means perfect. However, in the committee's view, the adoption analogy is the one that most nearly corresponds to the actual situation in surrogate parenting arrangements. The analogy takes seriously the central role of the gestational mother as the person who carries the pregnancy and delivers the infant. Thus, the adoption analogy is much more satisfactory than other possible analogies, for example, artificial insemination by donor or in vitro fertilization with donor gametes.

Major Types of Surrogacy

In the most frequent arrangement the would-be parents are a husband and wife (who will be called "the commissioning couple"). The couple reaches an agreement with a woman (who will be called "the surrogate mother") whereby the surrogate mother will be artificially inseminated with sperm provided by the husband of the commissioning couple. Thus, the genetic and gestational mother of any resultant child is the surrogate mother. The genetic father is the husband of the commissioning couple. The members of the commissioning couple plan to be the social parents of the child.

Less frequently, in vitro fertilization and embryo transfer are combined with surrogate parenting arrangements. In this case it is possible for both the husband and the wife of the commissioning couple to be the genetic parents of the child, while the surrogate fulfills only the role of gestational mother. This type of arrangement is often called "surrogate gestational motherhood."

In the committee's view, the genetic link between the commissioning parent(s) and the resulting infant, while important, is less weighty than the link between surrogate mother and fetus or infant that is created through gestation and birth. Thus, in the analysis and recommendations that follow no distinction will be drawn between the usual pattern of surrogate parenting and surrogate gestational motherhood.

A Preliminary Question: Medical Need or Convenience?

In most cases, commissioning couples resort to surrogate parenting arrangements because of their own involuntary infertility. Frequently the wife either has no uterus or has a uterus incapable of carrying a pregnancy to term. In other cases the wife has a medical condition that makes pregnancy a genuine threat to her health. These cases of medical need can be distinguished from a hypothetical case in which a commissioning couple might choose surrogate parenting arrangements because the couple does not want to experience the usual burdens of pregnancy. The latter case can fairly be described as surrogacy for convenience.

As will become clear in the following analysis, surrogate parenting arrangements are inherently complicated, even under the best of circumstances. This caution is not intended to invoke a prohibition of such arrangements. It merely acknowledges that adoptions can be complicated and that a pregnancy undertaken with the prior intent to enter into an adoption agreement can add further complexity. Therefore, the committee recommends that surrogate parenthood arrangements be considered at present only in cases of medical need. The remainder of this statement will focus on such cases.

Major Arguments For and Against Surrogate Parenting Arrangements (in the Absence of Financial Considerations)

The principal argument in favor of surrogate parenthood arrangements is precisely that they open another way for couples to become parents. This argument focuses on the benefits to the commissioning couples of such arrangements. The discovery that they are unable to have a child, or in some cases another child, is a severe blow to the life-plans of some couples who plan to have a child. They belong to the large and apparently growing group of couples that are described as "involuntarily infertile."[1]

A possible alternative to surrogate parenting arrangements for the couples under discussion is adoption. However, in adoption the couple would give up the possibility of having any genetic link to their child. Further, the number of infants available for adoption in the United States is exceeded by the number of couples seeking to adopt.[2]

Surrogate parenthood arrangements may also benefit the surrogate mother herself in nonfinancial ways. (The financial question will be considered below.) Many women enjoy the experience of pregnancy. Further, some women may derive satisfaction from being able to help others who need their help, just as the donors of blood or bone marrow do.

Benefits can also be postulated for the children who are born as a result of surrogate parenthood arrangements. These particular children would not have come into existence had it not been for the cooperative efforts of the commissioning couple and the surrogate mother. Existence is the precondition for enjoying the positive experiences of life. Further, such children are almost always intensely wanted by commissioning couples.

There are also important liberty-based arguments in favor of surrogate parenting arrangements. Within both ethics and the law there has been a gradual trend toward acknowledging the freedom of consenting adults to decide whether and how to bear or beget children. One aspect of this freedom is the liberty to purchase and use contraception when couples wish to enjoy sexual intercourse but seek to avoid pregnancy. Similarly, one could argue for the freedom of commissioning couples and surrogate mothers, at least in cases of medical need, to agree to cooperate in procreation. This moral right to reproduce is, of course, constrained by moral obligations to avoid harming other affected parties, including any child that may result from the agreement.

The primary arguments against surrogate motherhood are based on the harms that the practice is thought to produce—harms to the child that is born, harms to the surrogate herself, harms to her existing children if she has children, and harms to society. It is surely harmful to any child to be the object of a custody dispute, especially if the dispute is highly publicized. In addition, the rejection of an infant—for example, a handicapped infant's rejection by both commissioning parents and surrogate mother—is not in any infant's best interests. If an existing relationship is used to coerce relatives or close friends to become surrogate mothers, that coercion is a harm resulting from the practice of surrogate parenthood. And if the already-existing children of surrogate mothers are made to fear that they too may be given away, their fear is a tangible harm of the surrogate parenting relationship. Further, insofar as the practice of surrogate parenthood contributes to the trivializing of reproduction or to a tendency to regard women or infants as commodities, it causes social harm.

Some distinctions need to be drawn here. Children are much more vulnerable than adults, and harms to children who have no choice in a matter are much more serious, from an ethical standpoint, than harms to adults who make a choice that they later come to regret. Further, a distinction should be drawn between harms that are inevitably or almost invariably associated with a practice and harms that could in most cases be avoided through advance planning, appropriate counseling, or oversight mechanisms.

Thus, there are weighty arguments both for and against the practice of surrogate parenthood. After lengthy deliberation, the committee has concluded that the harms caused by the practice can be outweighed by the benefits that result from it, provided that guidelines like those outlined below are observed. Specifically, the committee believes that the use of the adoption model is most likely to protect the children who are born to surrogate mothers from unreasonable risk of harm. Further, the liberty of adult persons to collaborate in reproduction should, in the committee's view, be respected if that liberty is exercised responsibly. Therefore, the committee concludes that surrogate parenting arrangements can be morally justifiable, in cases of medical need.

The Difficult Issue of Payment to the Surrogate Mother

Perhaps no topic related to surrogate motherhood has been more contentious than that of the surrogate mother's being paid by the commissioning couple. While payment of semen and oocyte providers (often called "donors") is routine, such payment is relatively modest, and the duration of the gamete provider's involvement in the reproductive process is usually brief. In the case of surrogate motherhood arrangements, the duration and complexity of the surrogate mother's involvement in reproduction is substantially greater, and payments have been correspondingly higher.

Several questions about payment should be distinguished. First, for what is payment made? While there is considerable confusion on this point, payment can and, in the committee's view, should be construed as payment for the surrogate mother's services of gestating and delivering an infant. These services entail the acceptance of the risks of pregnancy and childbirth and at least some loss of other employment opportunities.

Second, why is payment offered or requested? In surrogate parenthood arrangements among close friends or relatives, there will in many cases be no payment for the services of the surrogate. Rather, the surrogate will provide her services as an act of altruism, and the commissioning couple will only be asked to reimburse her for out-of-pocket expenses connected with the pregnancy. However, most women are understandably reluctant to undertake the risks of pregnancy on behalf of strangers without some kind of compensation for their time and effort. (Analogously, unless they receive financial compensation, most people are reluctant to provide child care for the children of strangers.) Thus, surrogate parenthood arrangements among strangers are likely to involve the payment of a fee.

Third, can the exploitation of poor women by rich couples be avoided in fee-for-service arrangements? Opponents of surrogate motherhood have argued that, if a fee must be paid to the surrogate mother, only well-to-do couples will be able to afford to become commissioning couples. That argument seems correct; however, it applies equally to any medical service that is not currently covered by most health insurance programs. Opponents also place proponents of surrogate parenthood on the horns of a dilemma: if the payment offered to the candidate for surrogacy is too low, it is said to exploit her by not paying her a decent wage; if the payment is too high, it said to exploit her by being irresistible and coercive. There may be procedural safeguards that help to ensure that candidate surrogates give free and informed consent. However, it may be only they themselves who can determine what is acceptable as a just wage.

In short, financial transactions clearly complicate surrogate motherhood arrangements. However, surrogacy arrangements between strangers are not likely to occur without the payment of a fee to the surrogate mother. While the committee has reservations about the introduction of financial transactions into human reproduction, it can see no overriding ethical objection to the payment of a surrogate mother for her services, provided that policy guidelines like those outlined below are carefully observed.

Toward an Ethically Acceptable Public Policy on Surrogate Parenting Arrangements

An ethically acceptable public policy on surrogate parenthood will recognize that commissioning parents and surrogate mothers have divergent interests as well as interests in common. Because of the divergent interests, one professional person or agency should not attempt to represent the interests of both major parties to surrogate parenting arrangements. As in the case of organ donation and transplantation, public policy should require separation of roles to prevent apparent or real conflicts of interest. Further, because surrogate parenthood is in many respects analogous to adoption, the same kinds of safeguards that have been established for the practice of adoption should also be instituted for surrogate parenting arrangements.

In light of these general guidelines and the discussion above, the following specific policies are proposed:

1. Surrogate motherhood arrangements should be considered only in the case of infertility or other medical need, but not for reasons of convenience alone.
2. The surrogate mother and the commissioning couple should be regarded as distinct parties agreeing to cooperate for a defined purpose. Each party should be separately represented, both medically and legally.
3. Surrogate parenting arrangements should be viewed as preconception adoption agreements in which the surrogate mother is regarded as the mother for all medical and other purposes. After the birth of the infant, the surrogate mother can decide whether or not to place the child for adoption, in accordance with applicable local adoption rules and practices. This policy includes a specified period of time after birth during which the surrogate mother is free to depart from the preconception agreement and retain custody of the child. If she decides to place the child for adoption, the members of the commissioning couple will become the parents of the child.
4. While the committee is reluctant to propose a specific regulatory framework, it recommends that, for the near future, surrogate parenting arrangements be overseen by private nonprofit agencies with credentials similar to those of adoption agencies. Such agencies should seek to ensure that the interests of all involved parties are adequately protected. The agencies should conduct confidential counseling and screening of candidate surrogates and candidate commissioning parents. Their primary goal should be to promote the welfare of the future child, as well as the welfare of any existing children of the surrogate.
5. Plans for contingencies like the following should be carefully considered in advance by the commissioning couple, the surrogate mother, and the professionals involved in this reproductive arrangement: the prenatal diagnosis of a genetic or chromosomal abnormality; the inability or unwillingness of the surrogate to carry the pregnancy to term; the death of a member of the commissioning couple or the dissolution of the couple's marriage during the pregnancy; the birth of a handicapped infant; and a decision by the surrogate mother to retain custody of an infant conceived on behalf of, and typically with the aid of gametes from, the commissioning couple.
6. The contingency plans discussed by the parties to surrogate parenting arrangements should be written down to make explicit the intentions of the parties, to facilitate later recollection of these intentions, and to help promote the interests of the future child.
7. The surrogate mother, in consultation with her physician, should be the sole source of consent for medical decisions regarding pregnancy and delivery.
8. Whatever compensation is provided to the surrogate mother should be paid solely on the basis of her service in attempting to assist an infertile or otherwise medically handicapped couple; compensation should not be based on a successful delivery or on the health status of the child.

IMPLICATIONS FOR THE PRACTICE OF OBSTETRICS–GYNECOLOGY

The physician who participates in surrogate motherhood arrangements, provides fertility services or obstetric services for a surrogate, or provides counseling services should carefully examine all relevant issues, including legal, psychological, societal, medical, and ethical aspects. Simple, clear answers cannot be anticipated.

The following recommendations are offered as guidance to physicians.

AVOIDANCE OF CONFLICT OF INTEREST

The physician should not have as patients both the commissioning couple and the surrogate mother. Conflicts of interest may arise that would not allow the physician to serve both patients properly.

INITIATION OF SURROGATE ARRANGEMENTS

1. When approached by a patient interested in surrogate motherhood, the physician should, as in all other aspects of medical care, be certain that there is a full discussion of ethical and medical risks, benefits, and alternatives, many of which have been surveyed in this statement. In particular, the physician should be sure that contingencies like

those outlined in item 5 (above) have been thoroughly considered.

2. A physician may justifiably decline to participate in initiating surrogate motherhood arrangements.

3. If a physician decides to become involved in surrogate motherhood arrangements, he or she should follow these guidelines:

- The physician should be assured that appropriate procedures are utilized to screen the commissioning couple and the surrogate. Such screening should include appropriate fertility studies and infectious-disease and genetic screening.
- The physician should receive only usual compensation for obstetric and gynecologic services. Referral fees and other arrangements for financial gain beyond usual fees for medical services are inappropriate.
- The physician should not participate in a surrogate program in which the financial arrangements are likely to exploit any of the parties.

CARE OF PREGNANT SURROGATES

1. When a woman seeks medical care for an established pregnancy, regardless of the method of conception, she should be cared for as any other obstetric patient or referred to a qualified physician who will provide that care.

2. The surrogate mother should be considered the sole source of consent with respect to clinical intervention and management of the pregnancy. Confidentiality between the physician and patient should be maintained.

NOTES

1. The most recent estimates from the National Center for Health Statistics (NCHS) are that, of all married couples in the reproductive age group in the United States, approximately 3.5 million would like to have a[nother] baby and have not been able to do so. This includes both women with what the NCHS report refers to as "impaired fecundity" and women who are surgically sterile for noncontraceptive reasons. See WD Mosher and WF Pratt, Fecundity, infertility, and reproductive health in the United States. National Center for Health Statistics, Vital and Health Statistics Series 23, no. 14. Washington, DC: Government Printing Office, 1982.
2. According to the most recent data available from the National Committee for Adoption, in 1986 there were a total of 51,157 unrelated adoptions of American children, including 24,589 infants, in the United States. In addition, there were an estimated 36,000 children who were candidates for adoption but who could not be placed for a variety of reasons, for example, because they were older or handicapped or because they could not be matched with families of the same ethnic background. However, the combined number of couples and individuals seeking to adopt exceeded the total of both adopted children and children who were candidates for adoption. The combined number of couples and individuals desiring adoption in the United States was estimated at 2 million for 1986. See Adoption Factbook (Washington, DC: National Committee for Adoption, 1989).

PROCEED WITH CARE: FINAL REPORT OF THE ROYAL COMMISSION ON NEW REPRODUCTIVE TECHNOLOGIES, 1993

INTRODUCTION. *This report, though brief in summary, was by far the most comprehensive study of the new reproductive technologies ever undertaken. Over a period of four years, the Canadian Royal Commission on New Reproductive Technologies amassed volumes of background papers and conducted scores of public hearings. Its final report comprised 1,275 printed pages in two volumes. The Royal Commission report represents a second-generation approach to the new reproductive technologies in at least two ways. First, informed by the experience of infertile couples and especially of infertile women, it questioned whether the cost, the physical and mental suffering of women patients, and the low success rates of in vitro fertilization justify the use of this technique in most cases of infertility. Second, the Royal Commission was quite prepared not only to express moral disapproval of, but also to recommend the outlawing of, paid surrogate parenting arrangements and prenatal diagnosis for gender selection. The following excerpt is the full text of the report's executive summary.*

Executive Summary

The mandate of the Royal Commission was to examine how new reproductive technologies should be handled in Canada. Having children and healthy families are important goals to most Canadians, but some people cannot reach those goals without help. If there are technologies that can be used to help, a caring society should provide these. But there are misuses and harms, as well as benefits, that may come from use of the technologies—harms to both individuals and society.

We undertook our task by consulting very widely. As well as public hearings and submitted briefs, we had toll-free telephone lines, public surveys, and other avenues for Canadians to have input. In all, more than 40,000 people were involved in our work. We carried out a canvassing and examination of the issues that was extensive in both width and depth, with research projects and analyses in many disciplines, among them the social sciences, ethics, law, and medicine. More than 300 researchers at institutions across the country conducted projects for us.

We came to our conclusions in light of this widely based input and evidence, with three considerations in mind: a set of explicit ethical principles, the values of Canadians, and a conviction that offering any medical procedure as a service must be based on evidence that it works.

In spite of the existence of standards and guidelines recommended by various professional associations, we found that a varied patchwork of practices exists. Some practices are dangerous, such as donor insemination using sperm from donors who have not been tested for HIV. Some are harmful to the interests of the children born through the use of various technologies, such as the lack of records kept on their origins. Some are not respectful of women's choices, such as the finding that a woman's chance of being referred for prenatal testing varied more than fourfold across the country, despite the fact that women's attitudes toward testing varied relatively little. We found insufficient emphasis on the prevention of infertility. We found some discriminatory practices in access to services, some clinics preparing to carry out procedures to allow surrogacy, and some commercial clinics existing to treat sperm to allow sex selection. Procedures are being offered as treatments without good evidence that they are effective, when

Canada, Royal Commission on New Reproductive Technologies, "Executive Summary," in *Proceed with Care: Final Report of the Royal Commission on New Reproductive Technologies*, Canada: Minister of Government Services, November 15, 1993.

they should be offered only in research trials. There are technologies on the horizon, such as embryo splitting and use of eggs from female fetuses for implantation. Our ethical analyses showed that some technologies and some uses of technology that are now possible or will be possible in the near future would contravene Canadian values.

It is clear that the situation with regard to the use of new reproductive technologies needs to be addressed; the issues will not go away—in fact, the field is growing, and potential uses are expanding. As this report went to press, the media were reporting the cloning of a human zygote. This vividly underscores the need to have in place a structure to deal with this evolving field in a way that takes into account the values and input of Canadians.

We conclude that government, as the guardian of the public interest, must act to put boundaries around the use of new reproductive technologies, and must put in place a system to manage them within those boundaries, not just for now, but, equally important, in an ongoing way. We therefore have two recommendations. First, we recommend legislation to prohibit, with criminal sanctions, several aspects of new reproductive technologies, such as using embryos in research related to cloning, animal/human hybrids, the fertilization of eggs from female fetuses for implantation, the sale of eggs, sperm, zygotes, or fetal tissues, and advertising for, paying for, or acting as an intermediary for preconception (surrogacy) arrangements.

Second, we recommend that the federal government establish a regulatory and licensing body—a National Reproductive Technologies Commission (NRTC)—with licensing required for the provision of new reproductive technologies to people. Only the federal government can set up such a system, and it is important that the government fulfil its responsibility to protect citizens and society by doing so.

Several requirements are common to all the technologies: the need for reliable information to guide policy and practice; the need for standards and guidelines for the organization and provision of services; the need for effective means to ensure compliance; and the need for accountability. The approach we propose builds on the best standards and practices of the medical specialties involved, which are already in use in some Canadian clinics. These standards should be expanded and should be embodied in a licensing system.

We recommend the NRTC be composed of 12 members, representing a broad range of experiences and perspectives. Consultation activities should be undertaken to further enhance public input and involvement. Women should make up a substantial proportion—normally at least half—of the Commission's membership.

To ensure wide public input into the working of the system and to deal with setting policy as new issues evolve, we recommend that membership in the proposed NRTC should include persons with a broad range of experiences and perspectives, including the perspectives of those with disabilities, those who are infertile, and those who are members of racial minorities. A range of expertise should be represented, including reproductive medicine, ethics, law, and social sciences.

We recommend the NRTC have five areas of regulatory responsibility, in which the provision of services would be subject to compulsory licensing through five sub-committees established for that purpose. These areas are:

- sperm collection, storage, and distribution, and the provision of assisted insemination services;
- assisted conception services, including egg retrieval and use;
- prenatal diagnosis;
- research involving human zygotes (embryo research); and
- the provision of human fetal tissue for research or other specified purposes.

Licence hearings should be public, and a licence would be conditional on compliance with certain standards and stipulations of license. The major functions in these five areas of regulatory authority would be to:

- license, set standards, and monitor practice;
- collect, evaluate, store, and disseminate information;
- consult, help coordinate, and facilitate intergovernmental cooperation in the field; and
- monitor future technologies and practices and set policies for them.

In addition, we recommend the establishment of a sixth subcommittee, with primary responsibility in the field of infertility prevention. Its responsibilities would include the compilation and evaluation of data pertaining to the causes of infertility, the promotion of cooperative research efforts in Canada and internationally, and regulatory, public education, or other options for preventing or reducing the incidence of infertility.

With full implementation of these recommendations, a consistent country-wide system for the regulation of reproductive technologies and the provision of related services would emerge, with the following attributes:

- Assisted insemination, *in vitro* fertilization, and related infertility treatments would be provided only by licensed facilities, with national standards of service (related to matters such as counselling, informed disclosure and consent, standardized calculation of success rates, and consistent record keeping) as conditions for obtaining and keeping licence to provide these services.
- A national sperm collection and distribution system would be in place to ensure the availability of safe sperm, quarantined until donors are tested for infectious diseases, for use in assisted insemination in a medical setting or in self-insemination. The system would in-

clude comprehensive confidential record keeping on donors and recipients, with non-identifying information on the donor available to the recipient and child, and personal identification kept secure and available only in court-ordered cases.

- Prenatal diagnostic services would be provided only by licensed facilities, with national standards established and monitored through the licensing system. Prenatal ultrasound and testing of pregnant women's blood for congenital anomalies or genetic disease in the fetus would be provided only through provincially licensed or mandated programs. The structure would assure Canadians that genetic knowledge is applied in human reproduction in an accountable way and within acceptable limits—for example, not used for purposes of sex selection.
- A mechanism would be in place to facilitate multicentre trials and other research needed to assess the safety and effectiveness of reproductive technologies. It would promote interprovincial cooperation to mount the large-scale research projects needed to provide information on which to base health care service provision and resource allocation decisions.
- Once their risks and effectiveness had been assessed, infertility treatment and prenatal diagnostic services would be provided solely through provincial health care systems. Other treatments or procedures would be provided only in the context of research, with fully informed participation by volunteer research subjects and with rigorous protections for them. To preclude the development of commercial services, licensing conditions would include a stipulation that services not be offered on a for-profit basis.
- Annual reporting to the National Commission by licensed facilities would provide data that would allow evaluation of any long-term effects of treatments on the health of women or on their children.
- Any provision of fetal tissue for research would be licensed, so that it is used only in an accountable and ethical way according to guidelines, with permission for tissue use obtained separately from and subsequent to the decision to terminate a pregnancy.
- Any embryo research would be conducted only in licensed facilities, so that such research is carried out in an accountable and ethical way and in accordance with guidelines, including limitations on the purposes for which research can be undertaken, and permitted only during the 14 days immediately following fertilization.
- A focal point for national action would be in place to support and encourage infertility prevention initiatives, to foster consultation and co-ordination of efforts among the many sectors involved, and to promote public education and research in Canada and internationally on the risk factors for and prevention of infertility.
- Canada would have a visible and continuing forum to monitor developments, promote public discussion, and develop public policy advice on the use of assisted reproductive technologies, prenatal diagnostic technologies, embryo research, research involving the use of fetal tissue, and other rapidly evolving or emerging technologies.

Getting There from Here

Commissioners are strongly of the view that the establishment of a National Reproductive Technologies Commission of the type we recommend must be an immediate federal priority. We believe that a National Commission presents the only feasible response to the clearly demonstrated need and justified public demand for coherent, effective, and appropriate national regulation of new reproductive technologies. The field is developing too rapidly, the consequences of inaction are too great, and the potential for harm to individuals and to society is too serious to allow Canada's response to be delayed, fragmented, or tentative.

A central goal of our recommendations is to enable individual Canadians to make personal decisions about their involvement with the technologies, confident in the knowledge that mechanisms are in place to assess their safety and effectiveness and to consider their ethical, legal, and social implications. Individuals have a responsibility to inform themselves as fully as possible before making such decisions, but government, on behalf of citizens, has a responsibility to ensure that inappropriate and unethical use of technology is prohibited and that the procedures and supports necessary for informed decision making are in place.

The regulatory framework we propose is essential to provide this assurance, but by itself it is not sufficient. Strong leadership and cooperation will be required among governments and professionals involved in the development and delivery of reproductive technologies, as well as among many other sectors of society. No group or institution can act effectively in isolation—partnership and cooperation among federal and provincial/territorial governments, professional organizations, patient groups, and other interested groups are critical.

Establishing such a system will take some time—although we should note that other countries have succeeded in putting their systems in place within a relatively short period after their own inquiries. Nevertheless, some time will be required to appoint members of the Commission, establish and appoint its sub-committees, and carry out detailed implementation of the licensing system. Time will be needed to hold an initial round of licensing hearings, design secure record-keeping systems, and identify specific data collection methods and reporting forms.

The need for comprehensive action at the national level does not preclude the need for provincial and professional responses. Nor do provinces or the professions need to wait for a federal response before taking action themselves.

Provinces can take immediate steps to control the provision and proliferation of reproductive technologies in the health care system through the evidence-based approach we recommend. Practitioners now offering services can respond to the concerns Canadians raised before the Royal Commission and to the issues we have identified in the report. Professional associations can ensure that all their members are aware of the existing guidelines for practice and can promote more complete adherence to these standards among their members. Technology users and groups representing them can use the report of the Royal Commission to press for government and professional action. In the meantime, individual Canadians contemplating the use of reproductive technologies can use the information we have provided, ask questions, and request information from providers about the effectiveness, consequences, and potential risks of the technology use they are considering. Indeed, an informed public is the most effective bulwark against misuse or abuse of technology.

But all of these are only stop-gap measures. Government should act as the guardian of the public interest to set limits and to regulate the use of new reproductive technologies. No other body is sufficiently broadly based or has the mandate to do this. It is important that we put in place now the structures and an open, broad process to enable Canadians to deal with these growing dilemmas, dilemmas that affect individual lives and what kind of a society we are. How we use reproductive technology is not at root a medical matter, but a social matter that reaches into lay prevention, education, commerce, science, and research policy. Matters so important to women and children, in terms not only of their health but of their legal status and how they are viewed, cannot differ from province to province. The field is growing rapidly and Canadians want the government to act. There is clearly precedent—radio and television broadcasting is regulated and monitored through a licensing agency for the Canadian public interest. The area of reproductive technology use is at least as important to us as individuals and as a society.

Conclusion

Commissioners have set out a blueprint for how Canada, with its unique institutions and social make-up, can deal with new reproductive technologies, regulate their use, and ensure that future developments or use are in the public interest. Our blueprint requires action and leadership from the federal government, but also involves the participation and commitment of provincial governments, the professions, and many sectors of society. The approach we propose is feasible and practical, and we have laid out a detailed plan for how it can be accomplished.

The reasons for such action are compelling: the potential for harm to individuals and the need to protect the vulnerable interests of individuals and society. Adopting our recommendations will enable this protection, but will also allow scientific knowledge to be used to better the lives of many Canadians. Implementing the blueprint will demonstrate that we care about each other's well-being and recognize collective values with respect to the importance people attach to having children. At the same time, it will ensure that only ethical and accountable use of technology is made, and demonstrate that Canadians have wisdom, humanity, and compassion in the way they choose to use technology.

The Commission has done its work and indicated the path it believes should be taken. The next steps belong to the government and people of Canada.

Part V

ETHICAL ISSUES IN THE CHANGING HEALTH CARE SYSTEM

THE CHANGING HEALTH CARE SCENE: INTRODUCTION

Robert Veatch

THE PERIOD FROM 1970 to the present has produced revolutionary changes in Western health care ethics. The most dramatic shifts have occurred in the ethics of human experimentation, the care of the dying, and reproductive ethics and genetics. Underlying those changes, however, are others that have also signaled dramatic revisions in medical ethics. Among the most significant of these changes in the history of medical ethics are those that affect the relationship between health care professionals and lay people.

Prior to this time, one could, without exaggeration reduce Western medical ethics to the Hippocratic dictum that the physician should always act so as to benefit the patient and protect the patient from harm. Of course, not every physician acted that way in all cases, but this dictum was, without question, the moral norm that inspired them, and the code in which lay people unthinkingly concurred.

Systematic medical research began in the nineteenth century, but really gained momentum as a major phenomenon of health care only in the mid-twentieth century. With such research, it became clear that physicians could be acting acceptably even when they were striving for other objectives—when, for example, they undertook interventions for the purpose of gaining systematic knowledge rather than simply benefiting the individual patient. Medical ethics was becoming social; the welfare of third parties was becoming an acceptable objective of medicine.

The 1960s ended with the initiation of the heart transplants era—the dramatic moment when a finite human had the hubris purposely to cut the heart from a fellow human, confident that he could replace the diseased organ with one procured from another human who had just been pronounced dead.

The removal of that heart from a newly dead human being was an example of medicine intervening in the life of a particular patient, not to benefit that patient, but to benefit another. Similar organ procurements had occurred over a decade earlier when kidneys were removed from willing relatives and transplanted into patients in end-stage renal failure. It was, however, the heart transplant that captured the public's imagination. Medical ethics had to accommodate this new-found willingness to violate the Hippocratic mandate to intervene only for the benefit of the patient.

Simultaneously, the civil rights and antiwar movements of the 1960s were generating a radical shift in the moral perspective of the United States: a movement toward social ethics. The civil rights movement resuscitated the moral language of rights, which had been so critical to the founding fathers in the United States and to the whole underlying system of eighteenth century liberal political philosophy.

The language of rights was used to put forward a claim that trumps considerations of benefit and harm, the foundation of the Hippocratic perspective. The antiwar movement built a framework for challenging the authority of elites. The melding of these two "events" resulted in a more general rights movement, first for women's rights, then students' rights, and, soon thereafter, patients' rights.

The result was a two-pronged challenge to the Hippocratic ethic: a movement away from the consequence-oriented calculation of benefits and harms in the direction of rights and duties and a movement away from the individual in the direction of social ethics. While the movement toward social ethics posed the risk of drowning the patient in a sea of social utilitarianism, the resurgence of rights and duties, offered a more deontological perspective that had the potential to hold consequentialist reasoning in check. The first result was a concern for the moral community that we see not only in the ethics of experimentation, but also in the ethics of resource allocation and the transplantation of human organs. The transplantation issue represents that development in this chapter.

The first legislative effort affecting organ transplants was the development and passage by all fifty states of the Uniform Anatomical Gift Act, the first text in this section.[1] A necessary precursor was a revised definition of death. Death pronouncements based on irreversible loss of brain function had to be acceptable before hearts could be procured, but prior to the adoption of the legislation permitting the gift of human body parts, it was not at all clear that the corpse could be used, legally and ethically, for social purposes even when consent was obtained and the welfare of another was at stake.

The passage of the Uniform Anatomical Gift Act in all states did not resolve all ethical problems. Some proposed that we abandon the gift-giving mode of organ transfer in favor of "routine salvaging," that is, treating the dead body as the property of the state to be used without additional consent or gift-giving when important social aims could be furthered. Others proposed a movement to permit money payments to increase the efficiency of organ procurement. Controversy also erupted over the transplantation of organs to foreigners, some of whom were accused of using their substantial economic and political resources to buy their way to the front of American organ transplant program lines. A system was needed to deal with these questions, and with the pragmatic logistics of moving organs and tissues rapidly throughout the nation.

In 1983 Congress held hearings[2] that eventually gave rise to legislation that created the national Task Force on Organ Transplantation—a national body charged with outlining a public policy for transplantation—and then the national Organ Procurement and Transplantation Network—the administrative and policymaking body that actually manages the national organ procurement and allocation system in the United States. Portions of the report from the Task Force on Organ Transplantation appear in this section.[3] Commissions in other countries had looked at aspects of the transplantation issue, particularly the definition of death problem,[4] but the U.S. task force report carried the analysis to a much greater depth.

The other major challenge to the Hippocratic ethic came from the shift to the deontological framework of rights and duties that potentially overrides considerations of mere benefit and harm. This ethical perspective entails the possibility that acting to benefit the patient may have to be subordinated at times to preserving the patient's rights. This viewpoint arose in demands that patients be told the truth about terminal diagnoses even if doing so would distress patients and hypothetically even lead them to make choices that were not in their best interest.

The risk is hypothetical because even though many physicians believed that such choices were being made, there is little evidence to support such a belief. The point, however, is that, if patients have rights (such as the right to consent or refuse consent to treatment based on their own values), then it may be morally wrong for the physician to withhold essential information even if doing so would make the patient better off.

This shift to a rights perspective underlies the evolution of the informed consent doctrine. Informed consent is simply the playing out of the implications of the changes involved in choosing the principle of autonomy or self-determination over the choice of always benefiting the patient. Consent has its roots in the concept of individual self-determination and began its evolution into an informed consent doctrine in the early twentieth century. A recognition of the full implications, including the duty to inform the patient of possible outcomes as well as get consent, however, really does not arrive until the Salgo case of 1957.[5] This case and the Natanson case of 1960[6] established the right of the patient to give a consent that was informed and voluntary.

Yet another potential problem remained to challenge the consent doctrine. While some people persisted in speaking of giving the patient "full" information, most began to realize that medical procedures, in fact contain countless details, many of which are utterly trivial and boring. No rational patient would want to know everything. In fact, given that the information about any procedure is virtually infinite, it is not even clear what telling "everything" could mean.

For a time the standard of disclosure appeared to be that a clinician must disclose those pieces of information about a procedure that his or her colleagues similarly situated would have disclosed. This standard often worked well, but it left a crucial problem. What if a piece of information that the patient needs to know in order to make an adequately informed judgment, is information that colleagues are not in the habit of disclosing?

Logically, if the goal is to further patient autonomy, the clinician must disclose what the patient needs to know, that is, any knowledge that is "material" to the patient's decision, whether the physician's colleagues would disclose it or not. Since it was almost impossible for the typical clinician to guess what actual patients will need to know, it was often suggested that at least the clinician was obliged to disclose what a "reasonable person" in a particular patient's situation would need to know to make an adequately informed decision to consent, or refuse consent, to treatment. This standard became known first as the *reasonable man standard* and then, as sensitivities to gender-neutral language evolved, as the *reasonable person standard*. The case of *Canterbury v. Spence* was one of the crucial cases establishing this standard.[7] The opinion in this case together with selections from the report of the President's Commission for the Study of Ethical Problems in Medicine and Biomedical and Behavioral Research on making health care decisions (the report dealing with informed consent) is reproduced here.

A final example of these recent challenges to the Hippocratic ethic illustrates both the movement to a more social ethic and the abandonment of a purely consequence-oriented ethic that has a tendency to condone paternalism. The ethical notion of confidentiality has a long history in medical ethics. It dates at least as far back as the Hippocratic Oath. While there is a confidentiality provision in the Oath, it merely proscribes disclosing "those things that ought not be spread abroad," leaving open the question of just what those things are that ought to be spread abroad.

That question was traditionally answered with Hippocratic paternalism: disclose only when it is in the patient's interest to do so. Both the British and American Medical Associations used this answer until the last half of the twentieth century. Then came the realization that disclosing when it would benefit the patient can sometimes mean disclosing when the patient does not want disclosure to be made. A direct conflict can occur between paternalistic disclosures to benefit the patient and the patient's right to insist on nondisclosure. Within a ten year period following 1970, both the British and American Medical Associations had abandoned their paternalism in favor of the more robust right of the patient to insist on confidentiality.

This development posed yet another risk: an absolute policy of nondisclosure would have to be followed even when some third party is at serious risk of major bodily harm if a disclosure is not made. Cases of confessions to psychiatrists by their patients of plans to commit homicide pose a real problem for one committed to absolute nondisclosure. Gradually, a limited justification for breaking confidence against the patient's wishes emerged, based on the rights of third parties to have information disclosed when there was a credible threat of grave bodily harm to those third parties. The legal case of a student who revealed to a university psychologist that he was planning to murder a former girl friend led to the first legal case that required health professionals to break confidence in the name of protecting the rights of third parties. Such a disclosure could never have been supported with the Hippocratic Oath, but it seems to have won great acceptance by supporters of the more socially oriented ethic of rights and duties. The case of *Tarasoff v. Regents of the University of California*[8] is presented in this section.

NOTES

1. Sadler, A. M., B. L. Sadler, and E. Blythe Stason. "The Uniform Anatomical Gift Act." *Journal of the American Medical Association* 206 (Dec. 9, 1968): 2501–06.
2. U.S. House of Representatives, Subcommittee on Investigations and Oversight of the Committee on Science and Technology. *Organ Transplants: Hearings, April 13, 14, 27, 1983*. 98th Congress. Washington, D.C.: U.S. Government Printing Office, 1983.
3. Task Force on Organ Transplantation. *Organ Transplantation: Issues and Recommendations*. Washington, D.C.: U.S. Department of Health and Human Services, 1986.
4. Ingvar, D.H., and L. Widen. "Brain Death—Summary of a Symposium." *Lakartidningen* 34 (1972): 3804–3814; Ueki, K., K. Takeuchi, and K. Katsurada. "Clinical Study of Brain Death." Presentation No. 286. Fifth International Congress of Neurological Surgery. Tokyo, Japan, 1973; Working Party. *The Removal of Cadaveric Organs for Transplantation: A Code of Practice*. Health Departments. Great Britain and Northern Ireland: H.M. Stationary Office, 1979; Law Reform Commission of Canada. *Criteria for the Determination of Death*. Ottawa, Canada: Minister of Supply and Services, 1981; Netherlands Red Cross Society. *Summary of the Report of the Ad Hoc Committee on Organ Transplantation*, 1971; German Surgical Society. "Definition of the Signs and Time of Death: Statement by the Commission on Reanimation and Organ Transplantation." *German Medical Monthly* 13 (1968): 359.
5. *Salgo v. Leland Stanford Jr. University Board of Trustees*, 317 P.2d 170 (1957).
6. *Natanson v. Kline* 186 Kan. 393, 350 P. 2d 1093 (1960).
7. *Canterbury v. Spence*, 464 F. 2d 772 (D.C. Cir. 1972); see also *Cobbs v. Grant* 502 P.2d 1 (Cal. 1972) and *Berkey v. Anderson*. 1 Cal. App. 3d 790. 82 Cal. Rptr. 67 (1969).
8. *Tarasoff v. Regents of University of California*. 17C.3d 425, 131 Cal. Rptr. 14, 551 P.2d 334.

THE UNIFORM ANATOMICAL GIFT ACT, 1968

INTRODUCTION. *In 1968 the first heart transplants in humans had just been completed and the Harvard Ad Hoc Committee on the Definition of Death was preparing a proposal to redefine death based on brain criteria. The era of transplantation was about to begin. In order to procure organs and tissues from newly dead bodies, however, a new social and legal consensus was needed. There remained concern about violating the corpse. No one was sure what was owed to the dead body. It was clear that even a corpse was in some important sense the vestige of a human life and deserved to be treated with respect, but now that important life-and-death issues were at stake for the still living, it was crucial that a clear public policy be developed.*

The main controversy was over who, if anyone, was entitled to authorize the removal of body parts. One view, finding some support in a minority of both Jewish and Christian communities concerned about mutilation of the corpse, was that the human body must be buried whole. Jewish ethics has, however, long held that one has an affirmative duty to save life when a specific, identifiable person's life is at stake. This teaching led many Jews to argue that a moral duty exists to make organs available. At the other extreme was a group perhaps reflecting ancient Platonic views, who held that, once what used to be called the soul departed from the body, the family had no further rights in it. They believed that useful parts could be salvaged by the society for a good purpose such as transplantation. Some supported a softer version permitting "opting out," by which an individual or his or her family could register a veto on the state's salvaging activities.

In between these two views was the position finally adopted. It held that a "quasi-property right" to the body of the deceased rested with the family. The family had both a right and duty to dispose of the body properly. This included consenting to organ procurement. Reflecting the liberal affirmation of the individual characteristic of modern western society, the individual's wishes had first priority, so the family had to be guided by the individual's previously expressed wishes either for or against organ procurement. The language of gift-giving reflected this notion of the priority of the individual, then the family in deciding about disposition of socially valuable body parts. The National Conference of Commissioners on Uniform State Laws formed a committee that led to a draft Uniform Anatomical Gift Act built on this model. The brothers Blair and Fred Sadler, combined with Blythe Stason, drafted the model, which eventually was adopted in all legal jurisdictions in the United States.

Prefatory Note

Human bodies and parts thereof are used in many aspects of medical science, including teaching, research, therapy and transplantation. It is a rapidly expanding branch of medical technology. Transplantation of parts may involve skin grafts, bones, blood, corneas, kidneys, livers, arteries and even hearts. It is said that 6,000 to 10,000 lives could be saved each year by renal transplants if a sufficient supply of kidneys were available.

Transplantation may be effected within narrow limits from one living person to another living person. In such case, all that is required is an appropriate "informed consent" authorizing the surgical removal on the one hand, and the implantation on the other. Tissues and organs from the dead can also be used to bring health and years of life to the living. From this source the potential supply is very great. But, if utilization of bodies and parts of bodies is to be

National Conference of Commissioners on Uniform State Laws, "The Uniform Anatomical Gift with Prefatory Note and Comments." Drafted at the 77th Annual Conference, Philadelphia, Pennsylvania, July 22-August 1, 1968; approved by the American Bar Association at its meeting in Philadelphia, Pennsylvania, August 7, 1968.

effectuated, a number of competing interests in a dead body must be harmonized, and several troublesome legal questions must be answered.

The principal competing interests are: (1) the wishes of the deceased during his lifetime concerning the disposition of his body; (2) the desires of the surviving spouse or next of kin; (3) the interest of the state in determining by autopsy, the cause of death in cases involving crime or violence; (4) the need of autopsy to determine the cause of death when private legal rights are dependent upon such cause; and (5) the need of society for bodies, tissues, and organs for medical education, research, therapy, and transplantation. These interests compete with one another to a greater or lesser extent and this creates problems.

The principal legal questions arising from these various interests are: (1) who may during his lifetime make a legally effective gift of his body or a part thereof; (2) what is the right of the next of kin, either to set aside the decedent's expressed wishes, or themselves to make the anatomical gifts from the dead body; (3) who may legally become donees of anatomical gifts; (4) for what purposes may such gifts be made; (5) how may gifts be made, can it be done by will, by writing, by a card carried on the person, or by telegraphic or recorded telephonic communication; (6) how may a gift be revoked by the donor during his life-time; (7) what are the rights of survivors in the body after removal of donated parts; (8) what protection from legal liability should be afforded to surgeons and others involved in carrying out anatomical gifts; (9) should such protection be afforded regardless of the state in which the document of gift is executed; (10) what should the effect of an anatomical gift be in case of conflict with laws concerning autopsies; (11) should the time of death be defined by law in any way; (12) should the interest in preserving life by the physician in charge of a decedent preclude him from participating in the transplant procedure by which donated tissues or organs are transferred to a new host. These are the principal legal questions that should be covered in an anatomical gift act. The Uniform Anatomical Gift Act covers them.

The laws now on the statute books do not, in general, deal with these legal questions in a complete or adequate manner. The laws are a confusing mixture of old common law dating back to the seventeenth century and state statutes that have been enacted from time to time. Some 39 states and the District of Columbia have donation statutes that deal in a variety of ways with some, but by no means all, of the above listed legal questions. Four other states have statutes providing for the gift of eyes only.

These statutes differ from each other in a variety of respects, both as to content and coverage. They differ in their enumeration of permissible donees (some require that donees be specified, others permit gifts to be made to any hospital or physician in charge at death); they vary as to acceptable purposes for anatomical gifts (some, for example, do not include licensed tissue banks); they prescribe a variety of minimum ages for the donors; others differ as to the manner of execution of gifts and the manner of revocation. Some require delivery of the instrument of gift or filing in a public office, or both, as a condition of validity; others make no such provision. Since the statutes differ in important respects, a gift adequate in one state may or may not protect the surgeon in another state who relies upon the law in effect where the transplant takes place. In short, both the common law and the present statutory picture is one of confusion, diversity, and inadequacy. This tends to discourage anatomical gifts and to create difficulties for physicians, especially for transplant surgeons.

In view of the foregoing, the need for a comprehensive act and an act applicable in all states is apparent. The Uniform Anatomical Gift Act herewith presented by the National Conference of Commissioners on Uniform State Laws carefully weighs the numerous conflicting interests and legal problems. Wherever adopted it will encourage the making of anatomical gifts, thus facilitating therapy involving such procedures. When generally adopted, even if the place of death, or the residence of the donor, or the place of use of the gift occurs in a state other than that of the execution of the gift, uncertainty as to the applicable law will be eliminated and all parties will be protected. At the same time the Act will serve the needs of the several conflicting interests in a manner consistent with prevailing customs and desires in this country respecting dignified disposition of dead bodies. It will provide a useful and uniform legal environment throughout the country for this new frontier of modern medicine.

Uniform Anatomical Gift Act

An Act authorizing the gift of all or part of a human body after death for specified purposes.

Section 1 [*Definitions.*]

(a) "Bank or storage facility" means a facility licensed, accredited, or approved under the laws of any state for storage of human bodies or parts thereof.

(b) "Decedent" means a deceased individual and includes a stillborn infant or fetus.

(c) "Donor" means an individual who makes a gift of all or part of his body.

(d) "Hospital" means a hospital licensed, accredited, or approved under the laws of any state; includes a hospital operated by the United States government, a state, or a subdivision thereof, although not required to be licensed under state laws.

(e) "Part" means organs, tissues, eyes, bones, arteries, blood, other fluids and any other portions of a human body.

(f) "Person" means an individual, corporation, government or governmental subdivision or agency, business trust, estate, trust, partnership or association, or any other legal entity.

(g) "Physician" or "surgeon" means a physician or surgeon licensed or authorized to practice under the laws of any state.

(h) "State" includes any state, district, commonwealth, territory, insular possession, and any other area subject to the legislative authority of the United States of America.

COMMENT

Subsection (f) is taken verbatim from the Uniform Statutory Construction Act, section 26 (4). In any state that has adopted the Uniform Act or its equivalent, this subsection will be unnecessary.

Subsection (h) is taken from section 26 (9) of the Uniform Statutory Construction Act.

Section 2 [*Persons Who May Execute an Anatomical Gift.*]

(a) Any individual of sound mind and 18 years of age or more may give all or any part of his body for any purpose specified in section 3, the gift to take effect upon death.

(b) Any of the following persons, in order of priority stated, when persons in prior classes are not available at the time of death, and in the absence of actual notice of contrary indications by the decedent or actual notice of opposition by a member of the same or a prior class, may give all or any part of the decedent's body for any purpose specified in section 3:

(1) the spouse,
(2) an adult son or daughter,
(3) either parent,
(4) an adult brother or sister,
(5) a guardian of the person of the decedent at the time of his death,
(6) any other person authorized or under obligation to dispose of the body.

(c) If the donee has actual notice of contrary indications by the decedent or that a gift by a member of a class is opposed by a member of the same or a prior class, the donee shall not accept the gift. The persons authorized by subsection (b) may make the gift after or immediately before death.

(d) A gift of all or part of a body authorizes any examination necessary to assure medical acceptability of the gift for the purposes intended.

(e) The rights of the donee created by the gift are paramount to the rights of others except as provided by Section 7 (d).

COMMENT

Existing state statutes differ in their respective standards establishing the donor's competence to execute an anatomical gift.

"Competence to execute a will" is used as the standard in 10 states. "Legal age" and sound mind is required in 5 states. "Twenty-one years and sound mind" is the stated standard in the statutes of 10 states. In 4 states a person who is 18 years of age or older may make the gift, and in 6 states "any person" may do so. One state requires 21 years accompanied by a certificate of a physician that the donor is "of sound mind and not under the influence of narcotic drugs."

To minimize confusion there is merit in having a uniform provision throughout the country. Also it is desirable to enlarge the class of possible donors as much as possible. Subsection (a) of Section 2, providing that any person of sound mind and 18 years or more of age may execute a gift, will afford both nationwide uniformity and a desirable enlargement of the class of donors. Persons 18 years of age or more are of sufficient maturity to make the required decisions and the Uniform Act takes advantage of this fact.

Subsection (b) spells out the right of survivors to make the gift. Taking into account the very limited time available following death for the successful removal of such critical tissues as the kidney, the liver, and the heart, it seems desirable to eliminate all possible question by specifically stating the rights of and the priorities among the survivors.

Also, Section 2 (b) provides for the effect of indicated objections by the decedent, and differences of view among the survivors. Finally it authorizes the survivors to execute the necessary documents even prior to death. In view of the fact that persons under 18 years of age are excluded from subsection (a), it is especially desirable to cover with care the status of survivors, so younger decedents may be included.

Subsection (d) is added at the suggestion of members of the medical profession who regard a post mortem examination, to the extent necessary to ascertain freedom from disease that might cause injury to the new host for transplanted parts, as essential to good medical practice.

Subsection (e) recognizes and gives legal effect to the right of the individual to dispose of his own body without subsequent veto by others.

Section 3 [*Persons Who May Become Donees; Purposes for Which Anatomical Gifts May be Made.*]

The following persons may become donees of gifts of bodies or parts thereof for the purposes stated:

(1) any hospital, surgeon, or physician, for medical or dental education, research, advancement of medical or dental science, therapy, or transplantation; or
(2) any accredited medical or dental school, college or university for education, research, advancement of medical or dental science, or therapy; or
(3) any bank or storage facility, for medical or dental education, research, advancement of medical or dental science, therapy, or transplantation; or

(4) any specified individual for therapy or transplantation needed by him.

COMMENT

Existing state statutes reveal great diversity of provisions concerning possible donees and the purposes for which anatomical gifts may be made.

As to donees, the lists include licensed hospitals, storage banks, teaching institutions, universities, colleges, medical schools, state public health and anatomy boards, and institutions approved by the state department of health. Some of the statutes are detailed and comprehensive. Others are limited, brief, and general. A few do not seek in any way to name or limit the donees. The Uniform Act attempts to achieve a maximum of clarity and precision by carefully naming the permissible donees.

The statutes in a few states specify that no donor shall ask compensation and no donee shall receive it. Several statutes provide that storage banks shall be non-profit organizations. On the other hand, most of the states have chosen not to deal with this question. The Uniform Act follows the latter course in this regard.

As to purposes, again there is great diversity among the statutes. The list of purposes includes teaching, research, advancement of medical science, therapy, transplantation, rehabilitation, and scientific uses. Again some of the statutes are detailed, and others are brief and general. A few statutes contain no limitation whatsoever—merely naming the donees, thus assuring that gifts will not be made to undesirable persons or organizations, and then they are inclusive in naming the purposes in broad terms, thus assuring flexibility. The Uniform Act follows this course.

Section 4 [*Manner of Executing Anatomical Gifts.*]

(a) A gift of all or part of the body under Section 2 (a) may be made by will. The gift becomes effective upon the death of the testator without waiting for probate. If the will is not probated, or if it is declared invalid for testamentary purposes, the gift, to the extent that it has been acted upon in good faith, is nevertheless valid and effective.

(b) A gift of all or part of the body under Section 2 (a) may also be made by document other than a will. The gift becomes effective upon the death of the donor. The document, which may be a card designed to be carried on the person, must be signed by the donor in the presence of 2 witnesses who must sign the document in his presence. If the donor cannot sign, the document may be signed for him at his direction and in his presence in the presence of 2 witnesses who must sign the document in his presence. Delivery of the document of gift during the donor's lifetime is not necessary to make the gift valid.

(c) The gift may be made to a specified donee or without specifying a donee. If the latter, the gift may be accepted by the attending physician as donee upon or following death. If the gift is made to a specified donee who is not available at the time and place of death, the attending physician upon or following death, in the absence of any expressed indication that the donor desired otherwise, may accept the gift as donee. The physician who becomes a donee under this subsection shall not participate in the procedures for removing or transplanting a part.

(d) Notwithstanding Section 7 (b), the donor may designate in his will, card, or other document of gift the surgeon or physician to carry out the appropriate procedures. In the absence of a designation or if the designee is not available, the donee or other person authorized to accept the gift may employ or authorize any surgeon or physician for the purpose.

(e) Any gift by a person designated in Section 2 (b) shall be made by a document signed by him or made by his telegraphic, recorded telephonic, or other recorded message.

COMMENT

Most existing state statutes authorizing anatomical gifts provide for doing so either by will or by other document in writing. The number of witnesses varies from state to state, but the majority require two witnesses. The Uniform Act requires two witnesses to validate a gift during the donor's lifetime, but witnesses are relatively unnecessary in the case of a gift by next of kin since they are available in person. Hence, none are required in such cases. To facilitate availability of evidence of the gift, a card may be carried on the person, a practice commonly and successfully followed in connection with gifts of eyes. This is an important provision, for we are a peripatetic people and the advantages of a card carried on the person stating the donor's intention to donate is apparent.

Also important are the provisions of subsection (c) that permit the attending physician upon or following death to be the donee when no donee is named or when the named donee is not available. The donee physician cannot participate personally in removing or transplanting a part, but he can, of course, make a further gift to another person for any authorized purpose.

Attention should also be called to subsection (e) authorizing the next of kin to make gifts by "telegraphic, recorded telephonic, or other recorded message." Frequently the next of kin are far away, and this provision, not found in any existing statute, has the advantage of expediting the procedures where time for effective action is short.

As the Uniform Act becomes widely accepted it will prove helpful if the forms by which gifts are made are similar in each of the participating states. Such forms should be as simple and understandable as possible. The following forms are suggested for the purpose:

Anatomical Gift by a Living Donor

I am of sound mind and 18 years or more of age.

I hereby make this anatomical gift to take effect upon my death. The marks in the appropriate squares and words filled into the blanks below indicate my desires.

I give: ☐ my body; ☐ any needed organs or parts; ☐ the following organs or parts ________; To the following person (or institution): ☐ the physician in attendance at my death; ☐ the hospital in which I die; ☐ the following named physician, hospital, storage bank or other medical institution ________;

☐ the following individual for treatment ________; for the following purposes:

☐ any purpose authorized by law; ☐ transplantation; ☐ therapy; ☐ research; ☐ medical education.

Dated ________ City and State ________ Signed by the Donor in the presence of the following who sign as witnesses:

____
Signature of Donor

Address of Donor

____
Witness

____
Witness

Anatomical Gift by Next of Kin or Other Authorized Person

I hereby make this anatomical gift of or from the body of ________ who died on ________ at the ________ in ________ The marks in the appropriate squares and the words filled into the blanks below indicate my relationship to the deceased and my desires respecting the gift.

I am the surviving: ☐ spouse; ☐ adult son or daughter; ☐ parent; ☐ adult brother or sister; ☐ guardian; ☐ , ________ authorized to dispose of the body;

I give ☐ the body of deceased; ☐ any needed organs or parts; ☐ the following organs or parts ________;

To the following person (or institution) ________

(insert the name of a physician, hospital, research or educational institution, storage bank, or individual), for the following purposes: ☐ any purpose authorized by law; ☐ transplantation; ☐ therapy; ☐ research; ☐ medical education.

Dated ________ City and State ________

____
Signature of Survivor

____
Address of Survivor

Section 5 [*Delivery of Document of Gift.*]

If the gift is made by the donor to a specified donee, the will, card, or other document, or an executed copy thereof, may be delivered to the donee to expedite the appropriate procedures immediately after death. Delivery is not necessary to the validity of the gift. The will, card, or other document, or an executed copy thereof, may be deposited in any hospital, bank or storage facility or registry office that accepts it for safekeeping or for facilitation of procedures after death. On request of any interested party upon or after the donor's death, the person in possession shall produce the document for examination.

COMMENT

Some of the statutes make rather formal mandatory provisions for filing of documents of gift. Thus in two states the gift must be "filed for record in the office of the judge of probate." In another the document must be filed either before death or within 60 hours after death with the State Department of Health. In another the instrument must be filed for record "in the office of the clerk of the district court of the parish wherein the person making the gift resides." In still another the instrument must be filed in the probate court. In two states it is provided that the instrument shall be delivered by the donor to the donee. On the other hand, in the great majority of the states, no provision is made for filing, recording, or delivery to the donee. The gift is by implication effective without such formality. Section 5 of the Uniform Act follows the majority permissive practice, but includes permissive filing provisions to expedite postmortem procedures.

Section 6 [*Amendment or Revocation of the Gift.*]

(a) If the will, card, or other document or executed copy thereof, has been delivered to a specified donee, the donor may amend or revoke the gift by:

(1) the execution and delivery to the donee of a signed statement, or
(2) an oral statement made in the presence of 2 persons and communicated to the donee, or
(3) a statement during a terminal illness or injury addressed to an attending physician and communicated to the donee, or
(4) a signed card or document found on his person or in his effects.

(b) Any document of gift which has not been delivered to the donee may be revoked by the donor in the manner set out in subsection (a), or by destruction, cancellation, or mutilation of the document and all executed copies thereof.

(c) Any gift made by a will may also be amended or revoked in the manner provided for amendment or revocation of wills, or as provided in subsection (a).

COMMENT

In about one half of the states no provision is made for revocation. However, in the interest of carrying out the ultimate desires of the donor, there is good reason for facilitating revocation. Accordingly, about half of the states make affirmative provisions concerning the matter. Usually it is provided that revocation may be accomplished by executing a "like instrument" filed in the manner provided for the instrument of gift and delivered to the donee. In a few states revocation is accomplished by demanding return of the document of gift. There is merit in making revocation both simple and easy to accomplish. Prospective donors are more likely to look with favor on making anatomical gifts if they realize that revocation is readily possible. The Uniform Act makes careful and complete provision for revocation under various contingencies. However, if a donor has deposited an executed copy of an undelivered document of gift as authorized by Section 5, and if the donor desires to revoke the gift, he must see to it that the executed copy which has been deposited is destroyed.

Section 7 [*Rights and Duties at Death.*]

(a) The donee may accept or reject the gift. If the donee accepts a gift of the entire body, he may, subject to the terms of the gift, authorize embalming and the use of the body in funeral services. If the gift is of a part of the body, the donee, upon the death of the donor and prior to embalming, shall cause the part to be removed without unnecessary mutilation. After removal of the part, custody of the remainder of the body vests in the surviving spouse, next of kin, or other persons under obligation to dispose of the body.

(b) The time of death shall be determined by a physician who tends the donor at his death, or, if none, the physician who certifies the death. The physician shall not participate in the procedures for removing or transplanting a part.

(c) A person who acts in good faith in accord with the terms of this Act or with the anatomical gift laws of another state [or a foreign country] is not liable for damages in any civil action or subject to prosecution in any criminal proceeding for his act.

(d) The provisions of this Act are subject to the laws of this state prescribing powers and duties with respect to autopsies.

COMMENT

Section 7 contains several important provisions. The donee may of course, reject the gift if he deems it best to do so. If he accepts the gift, all possible provision is made for taking account of the interests of the survivors in dignified memorial ceremonies. Also if the donee accepts the gift, absolute ownership vests in him. He may, if he so desires, transfer his ownership to another person, whether the gift be of the whole body or merely a part. He may "cause the part to be removed" either by himself or by another person. The only restrictions are that the part must be removed without mutilation and the remainder of the body vests in the next of kin.

Subsection (b) leaves the determination of the time of death to the attending or certifying physician. No attempt is made to define the uncertain point in time when life terminates. This point is not subject to clear cut definition and medical authorities are currently working toward a consensus on the matter. Modern methods of cardiac pacing, artificial respiration, artificial blood circulation and cardiac stimulation can continue certain bodily systems and metabolism far beyond spontaneous limits. The real question is when have irreversible changes taken place that preclude return to normal brain activity and self sustaining bodily functions. No reasonable statutory definition is possible. The answer depends upon many variables, differing from case to case. Reliance must be placed upon the judgment of the physician in attendance. The Uniform Act so provides.

However, because time is short following death for a transplant to be successful, the transplant team needs to remove the critical organ as soon as possible. Hence there is a possible conflict of interest between the attending physician and the transplant team, and accordingly subsection (b) excludes the attending physician from any part in the transplant procedures. Such a provision isolates the conflict of interest and is eminently desirable. However, the language of the provision does not prevent the donor's attending physician from communicating with the transplant team or other relevant donees. This communication is essential to permit the transfer of important knowledge concerning the donor, for example, the nature of the disease processes affecting the donor or the results of studies carried out for tissue matching and other immunological data.

Subsection (d) is necessary to preclude the frustration of the important medical examiners' duties in cases of death by suspected crime or violence. However, since such cases often can provide transplants of value to living persons, it may prove desirable in many if not most states to reexamine and amend, the medical examiner statutes to authorize and direct medical examiners to expedite their autopsy procedures in cases in which the public interest will not suffer.

The entire section 7 merits genuinely liberal interpretation to effectuate the purpose and intent of the Uniform Act, that is, to encourage and facilitate the important and ever increasing need for human tissue and organs for medical research, education and therapy, including transplantation.

Section 8 [*Uniformity of Interpretation.*]

This Act shall be so construed as to effectuate its general purpose to make uniform the law of those states which enact it.

Section 9 [*Short Title.*]

This Act may be cited as the Uniform Anatomical Gift Act.

Section 10 [*Repeal.*]

The following acts and parts of acts are repealed:

(1)
(2)
(3)

Section 11 [*Time of Taking Effect.*]

This Act shall take effect. . . .

ORGAN TRANSPLANTATION: ISSUES AND RECOMMENDATIONS, 1986

INTRODUCTION. *In the years following the passage of the Uniform Anatomical Gift Act, organ transplantation matured and became a true, life-saving procedure for thousands of patients. Moral and public policy problems began to emerge, not only with the gift of organs from the deceased, but also in other areas. In 1984, the National Organ Transport Act created the structure for a national organ transplant program. It also called for an interdisciplinary, national Task Force on Organ Transplantation to analyze public policy issues; that is, to review the appropriateness of the gift-giving mode of organ procurement and other problems related to the collection and allocation of these resources. The report of this Task Force in 1986 provided the foundation for the emergence of a national policy that wisely gave equal moral weight to the twin goals of efficiency and equity in allocation. The alternative notion, that of accepting a market in organs, which had been subjected to a moratorium in the 1984 legislation, continued to be condemned, and, despite occasional proposals to legalize such a market, remains illegal in the United States and many other jurisdictions of the world. This selection presents the recommendations of the Task Force on Organ Transplantation (i.e., the executive summary of its report) and its conclusions on organ and tissue donation (chapter 2) and patient access to and payment for organ transplants (chapter 5). Statements of exception to several recommendations in chapter 5 are also reprinted here.*

EXECUTIVE SUMMARY

In response to widespread public interest and involvement in the field of organ transplantation, the Congress enacted the National Organ Transplant Act of 1984 (PL 98-507). In addition to prohibiting the purchase of organs, the act provided for the establishment of grants to organ procurement agencies (OPAs) and a national organ-sharing system. This act also established a twenty-five member Task Force on Organ Transplantation representing medicine, law, theology, ethics, allied health, the health insurance industry, and the general public. The Office of the Surgeon General of the Public Health Service, the National Institutes of Health (NIH), the Food and Drug Administration (FDA), and the Health Care Financing Administration (HCFA) were also represented.

The mandate given to the Task Force was to conduct comprehensive examinations of the medical, legal, ethical, economic, and social issues presented by human organ procurement and transplantation and to report on these issues within one year. In addition, we were asked to assess immunosuppressive medications used to prevent rejection and to report on our findings within seven months; this report also was to include a series of recommendations, including recommending a means of assuring that individuals who need such medications can obtain them.

During the twelve months following its organizational meeting on February 11, 1985, the Task Force met in public session on eight occasions and held two public hearings. We were supported by staff from the Office of Organ Transplantation and by consultants from HCFA and other agencies and organizations. Data were obtained through surveys, literature reviews, commissioned studies, consultations, and public testimony. Five workgroups were established within the Task Force to address each of the mandated issues identified by Congress and to prepare presentations and recommendations for consideration by the full membership.

As required by the act, the Task Force completed an assessment of immunosuppressive medications and the costs of these therapies, and submitted its report and rec-

U.S. Task Force on Organ Transplantation. *Organ Transplantations: Issues and Recommendations.* Rockville, MD: U.S. Department of Health and Human Services, 1986. Endnote references, lightly edited for clarity, follow the statements of exception.

ommendations to the Secretary and the Congress on October 21, 1985. Briefly, we found that the new immunosuppressive regimens, although expensive, proved to be cost-saving due to improvement in outcome; for this reason, and in order to ensure equitable access, the Task Force recommended that the federal government establish a mechanism to provide immunosuppressive drugs to recipients otherwise unable to pay for these drugs, when Medicare paid for the transplantation procedure.

In this final report, the Task Force summarizes its arguments on the issues identified as major concerns by the Congress, and presents a series of recommendations for consideration of federal and state legislators, public health officials, the organ and tissue transplantation community, organized medicine, nursing, and the federal government.

Organ and Tissue Donation and Procurement

The serious gap between the *need* for organs and tissues and the *supply* of donors is common to all programs in organ transplantation, as well as to tissue banking and transplantation. The Task Force believes that substantial improvements in organ donation would ensue through new, innovative, and expanded programs in public and professional education and the coordination of efforts of the many organizations and agencies that engage in these activities. In particular, we support both the enactment of legislation in states that have not clarified determination of death based on irreversible cessation of brain function (the Uniform Determination of Death Act), and the enactment of legislation requiring implementation of routine hospital policies and procedures to provide the next-of-kin with the opportunity of donating organs and tissues. In addition, we found both a serious lack of uniform standards of accountability and quality assurance in organ and tissue procurement and a spectrum of effectiveness of procurement activities. Therefore, the Task Force supports the development both of minimum performance and certification standards, and of monitoring mechanisms.

RECOMMENDATIONS

1. To facilitate organ donation the Task Force recommends:

- The Uniform Determination of Death Act be enacted by the legislatures of states that have not adopted this or a similar act.
- Each state medical association develop and adopt model hospital policies and protocols for the determination of death based upon irreversible cessation of brain function that will be available to guide hospitals in developing and implementing institutional policies and protocols concerning brain death.
- States enact legislation requiring coroners and medical examiners to give permission for organ and tissue procurement when families consent unless the surgical procedure would compromise medicolegal evidence. Further, the legislation should (1) require coroners and medical examiners to develop policies that facilitate the evaluation of all nonheart-beating cadavers under their jurisdiction for organ and tissue donation, and (2) provide the next-of-kin with the opportunity to consider postmortem tissue donation. The Task Force further recommends that coroners develop agreements with local tissue banks to help implement these policies.

2. To facilitate the identification of potential donors and to provide the next-of-kin with appropriate opportunities to donate organs and tissues, the Task Force recommends that:

- All health professionals involved in caring for potential organ and tissue donors voluntarily accept the responsibility for identifying these donors and for referring such donors to appropriate organ procurement organizations.
- Hospitals adopt routine inquiry/required request policies and procedures for identifying potential organ and tissue donors and for providing next-of-kin with appropriate opportunities for donation.
- The Joint Commission on the Accreditation of Hospitals develop a standard that requires all acute care hospitals to both have an affiliation with an organ procurement agency and have formal policies and procedures for identifying potential organ and tissue donors and for providing next-of-kin with appropriate opportunities for donation.
- The Department of Defense and the Veterans Administration require their hospitals to have routine inquiry policies.
- The Health Care Financing Administration incorporate into the Medicare conditions of participation for hospitals certified under subpart U of the Code of Federal Regulations, a condition that requires hospitals to have routine inquiry policies.
- All state legislatures formulate, introduce, and enact routine inquiry legislation.
- The Commission for Uniform State Laws develop model legislation that requires acute care hospitals to develop an affiliation with an organ procurement agency and to adopt routine inquiry policies and procedures.

3. In regard to living donors and the donor pool, the Task Force recommends that:

- A study of the potential donor pool be conducted using data available through the National Hospital Discharge Survey, supplemented by regional retrospective hospital record reviews.
- Living donors be fully informed about the risks of kidney donation. Health care professionals must guarantee that the decision to donate is entirely voluntary. In the case of

all living donors, special emphasis should be placed on histocompatibility.
- A national registry of human organ donors not be established.

4. To improve public education in organ and tissue donation, the Task Force recommends that:

- Educational efforts aimed at increasing organ donation among minority populations be developed and implemented, so that the donor population will come to more closely resemble the ethnic profile of the pool of potential recipients in order to gain the advantage of improved donor and recipient immunologic matching.
- At the regional level, single consortia, composed of public, private, and voluntary groups that have an interest in education on organ and tissue donation should develop, coordinate, and implement public and professional education to supplement, but not replace, activities undertaken by local programs.
- A single organization, such as the American Council on Transplantation, composed of public, private, and voluntary groups that are national in scope and have an interest in education for organ and tissue donation, should develop and coordinate broad scale public and professional educational programs and materials on the national level. This umbrella organization would both develop and distribute model educational materials for use by national and local organizations and plan, coordinate, and develop national efforts using nationwide electronic and print media.
- A national educational program should be established, similar to the High Blood Pressure Education Program of National Institutes of Health's National Heart, Lung, and Blood Institute, aimed at increasing organ donation. This program should include development both of curricula and instructional materials for use in primary and secondary schools throughout the nation, and of programs directed to special target populations, e.g., minority groups, family units, and churches.

5. To improve professional education in organ and tissue donation the Task Force recommends that:

- Medical and nursing schools incorporate organ and tissue procurement and transplantation in the curriculum.
- The Accreditation Council of Graduate Medical Education, the body responsible for accrediting residency programs, include requirements for exposure to organ and tissue donation and transplantation in relevant programs in graduate medical education, such as emergency and critical care medicine and the neurological sciences.
- Each appropriate medical and nursing specialty require demonstration of knowledge of organ and tissue donation and transplantation for certification.
- All professional associations of physicians and nurses involved in caring for potential organ and tissue donors (especially neurosurgeons; trauma surgeons; emergency physicians; and critical care, emergency room, and trauma team nurses), establish programs to educate and encourage their members both to participate in the referral of donors and to cooperate in the organ donation process.
- Organizations of physician specialists who frequently come in contact with organ and tissue donors should establish mechanisms, such as a committee on transplantation, to facilitate communication and cooperation with physicians in the transplantation specialties.

6. The Task Force recommends that organ procurement agencies and procurement specialists be certified:

- Professional peer group organizations, e.g., the North American Transplant Coordinators Organization, should establish mechanisms for certification of non-physician organ and tissue procurement specialists and standards for evaluation of performance at regular intervals.
- The Department of Health and Human Services should certify no more than one Organ Procurement Agency in any standard metropolitan statistical area or existing organ donor referral area, whichever is larger.
- The Department of Health and Human Services should use the criteria developed by the Association of Independent Organ Procurement Agencies as a guideline to develop consistent certification standards for Independent Organ Procurement Agencies and Hospital-Based Organ Procurement Agencies.
- The Department of Health and Human Services should establish minimal performance productivity standards as part of a recertification process that could be conducted at regular intervals. Such standards should address procurement activity, organizational structure and programs, staff training and competence, and fiscal accountability.
- Appropriate peer organizations should develop standards for certifying tissue banks and for conducting performance evaluations at regular intervals. Such standards should include assessment of quality and quantity of performance, organizational structure and programs, staff training and competency, and fiscal responsibility.

7. The Task Force recommends that the Department of Health and Human Services collect uniform data on organ procurement activities of all Organ Procurement Agencies, including, at a minimum, the number of kidneys procured, kidneys transplanted, kidneys procured but not transplanted, kidneys exported abroad, and relevant cost data. (The data could be collected through the Organ Procurement and Transplantation Network or from each Organ Procurement Agency.)

- The Department of Health and Human Services require all Organ Procurement Agencies to have, as a minimum, a form of governance that would be similar to that described for the national Organ Procurement and Transplantation Network, i.e., it should include adequate representation from each of the following categories: transplant surgeons from participating transplant centers, transplant physicians from participating transplant centers, histocompatibility experts from the affiliated histocompatibility laboratories, representatives of the Organ Procurement Agencies, and members of the general public. Representatives of the general public should have no direct or indirect professional affiliation with the transplant centers or the Organ Procurement Agency. Not more than 50 percent of the Board of Directors may be surgeons or physicians directly involved in transplantation, and at least 20 percent should be members of the general public. Where the governing boards of existing Organ Procurement Agencies differ from this composition, it is desirable that those boards be modified over a maximum of two years to achieve this distribution. The Task Force believes that all Organ Procurement Agency boards should consider immediate steps to include public representatives.

8. To facilitate more effective collaboration between organ and tissue banks, the Task Force recommends that formal cooperative agreements be established among eye, skin, and bone banks.

- All Organ Procurement Agencies evaluate all potential donors for multiple organ and tissue donation.
- Organ procurement agencies and tissue banks enter into formal agreements for collaborative programs to educate the public and health professionals and to coordinate donor identifications, discussions with next-of-kin, and the procurement process.

Organ Sharing

The Task Force believes that establishment of a unified national system of organ sharing that encompasses a patient registry and coordinates organ allocation and distribution will go far in assuring equity and fairness in the allocation of organs. In addition, a national network organization, through adoption of agreed upon standards and policies, may serve as the vehicle both for improving matching of donors and recipients and for improving access of groups at special disadvantage (the sensitized and small pediatric recipients); thus, the outcome of organ transplantation in this country will surely improve. The development of a national network will permit the gathering and analysis of comprehensive data and, through the establishment of a scientific registry, will facilitate the exchange of new information vital to progress in the field. We assisted the Office of Organ Transplantation in developing specifications for a model network, and urge that the National Organ Procurement and Transplantation Network be established promptly; in addition, we urge Congress to appropriate the funds necessary to initiate the development of the scientific registry.

RECOMMENDATIONS

1. The Task Force recommends that a single national system for organ sharing be established; that its participants agree on and adopt uniform policies and standards by which all will abide; and that its governance include a broad range of viewpoints, interests, and expertise, including the public.

- The national network establish a method to systematically collect and analyze data related to both kidney and extrarenal organ procurement and transplantation. Further, to provide an ongoing evaluation of the scientific and clinical status of organ transplantation, a scientific registry of the recipients of kidney and extrarenal organ transplants should be developed and administered through the national network, and the Task Force urges the Congress to appropriate funds to initiate this activity.
- Organ sharing be mandated for perfectly matched (HLA A, B, and DR) donor-recipient pairs and for donors and recipients with zero antigen mismatches (assuming that at least one antigen has been identified at each locus for both donor and recipient).
- A system of serum sharing and/or allocation of organs based on computer-determined prediction of a negative crossmatch, be developed to increase the rate of transplantation in the highly sensitized patient group by increasing the effective size of the donor pool.
- Blood group O organs be transplanted only into blood group O recipients.
- Because of the limited local and regional donor pools available to small pediatric patients, the national organ-sharing system should be designed to provide pediatric extrarenal transplant patients access to a national pool of pediatric donors.
- The national organ-sharing network, when established, should conduct ongoing reviews of organ procurement activities, particularly organ discard rates, and develop mechanisms to assist those agencies and programs with high discard rates. In the meantime, we recommend that the Department of Health and Human Services conduct a study to identify why procured kidneys are not transplanted and why the discard rates vary widely from one organ procurement program to another.

2. The Task Force recommends regional centralization of histocompatibility testing where it is geographically fea-

sible, and standardization of key typing reagents and cross-matching techniques.

3. The Task Force recommends that the Congress appropriate funds to establish a national ESRD registry that would combine a renal transplant registry with a dialysis registry. The Task Force further recommends that the national organ-sharing network be represented on any committee responsible for management and data analysis of a national ESRD registry.

Equitable Access to Organ Transplantation

The process of selecting patients for transplantation, both in the formation of the waiting list and in the final selection for allocation of the organ, is generally fair and for the most part has succeeded in achieving equitable distribution of organs. However, the Task Force believes that these processes must be defined by each center and by the system as a whole, and that the standards for patient selection and organ allocation must be based solely on objective medical criteria that are applied fairly and are open to public examination. Moreover, as vital participants in the process, the public must be included in developing these standards and in implementing the policies. We recognized the complex conflict between need for an organ (medical urgency) and the probability of success of the transplant, and did not presume to make recommendations in this sphere; rather we believe that a thoughtful process of development of policies for organ allocation, which takes into account both medical utility and good stewardship, must take place within a broadly representative group.

The Task Force condemns commercialization of organ transplantation and the exploitation of living unrelated donors. The Task Force also addressed the difficult problem of offering organ transplantation to non-immigrant aliens. Because transplantable organs are scarce, we have recommended that no more than 10 percent of all cadaveric kidney transplants in any center be performed in non-immigrant aliens and that extrarenal transplants be offered only when no suitable recipient who is a resident of this country can be found [note omitted]. The Task Force also concluded that equitable access of patients to extrarenal organ transplantation is impeded unfairly by financial barriers, and recommends that all transplant procedures that are efficacious and cost effective be made available to patients, regardless of their ability to pay, through existing public and private health insurance or, as a last resort, through a publicly funded program for patients who are without insurance, Medicare, or Medicaid who could not otherwise afford to obtain the organ transplant.

RECOMMENDATIONS

1. The Task Force recommends that each donated organ be considered a national resource to be used for the public good; the public must participate in the decisions of how this resource can be used to best serve the public interest.

2. In order that patients and their physicians be fully informed, the Task Force recommends that:

- Health professionals provide unbiased, timely, and accurate information to all patients who could possibly benefit from organ transplantation so that they can make informed choices about whether they want to be evaluated and placed on a waiting list.
- Information be published annually for patients and physicians on the graft and patient survival data by transplant center. A clear explanation of what the data represent should preface the presentation of data. A strong recommendation should be made in the publication that each patient discuss with his or her attending physician the circumstances of medical suitability for transplantation and where that patient may best be served.

3. The Task Force recommends that selection of patients both for waiting lists and for allocation of organs be based on medical criteria that are publicly stated and fairly applied.

- The criteria for prioritization be developed by a broadly representative group that will take into account both need and probability of success. Selection of patients otherwise equally medically qualified should be based on length of time on the waiting list.
- Selection of patients for transplants not be subject to favoritism, discrimination on the basis of race or sex, or ability to pay.
- Organ-sharing programs that are designed to improve the probability of success be implemented in the interests of justice and the effective and efficient use of organs, and that the effect of mandated organ sharing be constantly assessed to identify and rectify imbalances that might reduce access of any group.

4. The Task Force recommends that non-immigrant aliens not comprise more than 10 percent of the total number of kidney transplant recipients at each transplant center, until the Organ Procurement and Transplantation Network has had an opportunity to review the issue. In addition, extrarenal organs should not be offered for transplantation to a non-immigrant alien unless it has been determined that no other suitable recipient can be found.

5. The Task Force emphatically rejects the commercialization of organ transplantation and recommends that:

- Exportation and importation of donor organs be prohibited except when distribution is arranged or coordinated by the Organ Procurement and Transplantation Network and the organs are to be sent to recognized national networks. Even then, when an organ is to be exported from the United States, documentation must be available to demonstrate that all appropriate efforts have been made to locate a recipient in the United States and/or Canada. The Task Force has every expectation that these international organ sharing programs will be reciprocal.

- The practice of soliciting or advertising for non-immigrant aliens and performing a transplant for such patients, without regard to the waiting list, cease.
- Transplanting kidneys from living unrelated donors should be prohibited when financial gain rather than altruism is the motivating factor.
- To the extent federal law does not prohibit the intrastate sale of organs, states should prohibit the sale of organs from cadavers or living donors within their boundaries.
- As a condition of membership in the Organ Procurement Transplantation Network (OPTN), each transplant center be required to report every transplant or organ procurement procedure to the OPTN. Moreover, transplantation procedures should not be reimbursed under Medicare, Medicaid, CHAMPUS, and other public payers, unless the transplant center meets payment, organ-sharing, reporting, and other guidelines to be established by the OPTN or another agency administratively responsible for the development of such guidelines. Failure to comply with these guidelines will require that the center show cause why it should not be excluded from further organ sharing through the OPTN.
- In order to insure that patients in need of an extrarenal organ transplant can obtain procedures regardless of ability to pay, the Task Force recommends that private and public health benefit programs, including Medicare and Medicaid, should cover heart and liver transplants, including outpatient immunosuppressive therapy that is an essential part of post-transplant care.
- A public program should be set up to cover the costs of people who are medically eligible for organ transplants but who are not covered by private insurance, Medicare, or Medicaid and who are unable to obtain an organ transplant due to lack of funds.

Diffusion of Organ Transplantation Technology

The number of organ transplant centers in this country is rapidly increasing. As the technical aspects of the procedures have been mastered and patient management has become better understood and standardized, it is not surprising that diffusion of this technology has taken place. The issue of designating centers for reimbursement purposes requires careful consideration of many factors, including cost, criteria for facilities, resources, staffing, and the training and experience of personnel. After lengthy debate, the majority of the Task Force agreed with the widely accepted principle within surgery that the volume of surgical procedures performed is positively associated with outcomes and inversely related to cost and believe that this principle applies to organ transplantation procedures as well. Therefore, we recommend that a minimum volume criterion be enforced, together with other criteria defining the minimal requirements for both institutional and professional support and outcome of transplantation procedures [note deleted]. In the context of scarcity of donor organs, we strongly support regulating diffusion of transplantation technology.

RECOMMENDATIONS

1. The Task Force recommends that transplant centers be designated by an explicit, formal process using well-defined, published criteria.
2. The Task Force recommends that the Department of Health and Human Services designate centers to perform kidney, heart, and liver transplants, and that the centers be evaluated against explicit criteria to ensure that only those institutions with requisite capabilities are allowed to perform the procedures.
3. The Task Force recommends that the Department of Health and Human Services adopt minimum criteria for kidney, heart, and liver transplant centers that address facility requirements, staff experience, training requirements, volume of transplants to be performed each year, and minimum patient and graft survival rates.

Research in Organ Transplantation

Organ transplantation continues to evolve and improve at a fast pace. Strong research programs in basic and applied clinical sciences have been vital to this fortunate development. As is clearly evident in the concerns of the public that resulted in the enactment of the National Organ Transplant Act, research also is needed in the social, ethical, economic, and legal aspects of organ donation and transplantation. The Task Force acknowledges the important role played by the NIH in transplantation research, and encourages the NIH to coordinate the free flow of information regarding transplant-related research through an interinstitutional council on transplantation. Moreover, we strongly urge that research on all aspects of transplantation be fostered and encouraged and that funding for this vital effort be increased. Therein lies the future of transplantation.

RECOMMENDATIONS

1. The Task Force recommends that basic research continue to receive high priority.
2. The Task Force recommends that both laboratory and clinical research of an applied nature directly related to

transplantation also be fostered, encouraged, and increasingly funded. For the immediate benefit of patients, the Task Force further recommends that research be aggressively pursued in organ preservation and optimal immunosuppression techniques. The Task Force also wishes to emphasize the importance of sponsoring prospective clinical trials, involving multiple institutions, to solve certain problems in patient management.

3. The Task Force recommends that continuing attention be devoted to collecting complete information on the status and efficacy of transplantation treatments.

4. The Task Force recognizes that the interaction and exchange of information between the agencies involved in transplantation research and its funding must be encouraged. Therefore, we recommend that the National Institutes of Health be provided with resources to establish an interagency and interinstitute Council on Transplantation that will serve as a focus for this activity.

Establishment of an Advisory Board on Organ Transplantation

At the final meeting of the Task Force, where this report was adopted, a recommendation was made to establish a National Organ Transplantation Advisory Board. The Task Force agreed in concept that a national group to advise the Secretary of Health and Human Services would continue to be needed to monitor implementation of the Task Force's findings and serve in an advisory capacity on organ procurement and transplantation issues. Therefore we adopted the following recommendation:

> The Task Force recommends that a National Organ Transplantation Advisory Board be authorized and funded to review, evaluate, and advise with regard to the implementation of the recommendations of the Task Force on Organ Transplantation, to serve in an advisory capacity to the Office of Organ Transplantation and to other transplant-related activities of the Department of Health and Human Services, and that this board be established in the Office of the Secretary.

* * *

CHAPTER 2: ORGAN AND TISSUE DONATION

The need for organs (kidneys, livers, hearts, and heart-lungs) far exceeds the current supply. The Task Force compared the number of people on waiting lists to the number of organs that were donated and determined that for every donor organ that becomes available, there are roughly three people waiting for transplantation. The consequences of the critical shortage of available organs are often fatal for those who need organ transplantation. A 1984 report underscored this fact, observing that

> eighty-four adults and 27 children died over the past two years waiting for liver transplants at the University of Pittsburgh School of Medicine. . . . At New York City's Montefiore Medical Center, 25 out of 30 patients have died over the past two years waiting for a new lung. At Stanford University Medical Center, one out of every three candidates for heart transplant dies before a suitable heart is found.[1]

Current availability of donor tissue (e.g., corneas, skin, and bone) for transplantation also is inadequate to meet the needs of thousands of people who could benefit from the therapeutic use of these resources.

The Task Force charge was to assess where the barriers to organ donation exist and to recommend ways of increasing organ donation in this country. In conducting our assessment, we examined public values, analyzed the legal framework governing organ and tissue donation, reviewed numerous opinion polls of public attitudes, analyzed literature concerning the potential organ donor pool, reviewed surveys of attitudes of health professionals regarding organ donation, assessed educational activities aimed at informing the public and health professionals about organ donation and transplantation, and assessed the feasibility of establishing a national registry of organ donors.

Ethical Framework for a Voluntary System of Organ Donation

Organ donation in this country is based on accepted societal values. These values help to define the attitudes, policies, and laws governing the current voluntary system of organ donation and procurement, and according to numerous opinion polls, receive wide support in contemporary society. These values include:

- Saving lives and improving the quality of life.
- Respecting individual autonomy.
- Promoting a sense of community through acts of generosity.
- Showing respect for the decedent.
- Showing respect for the wishes of the family.

The search for methods of increasing the supply of organs for transplantation is largely based on the first value, saving human lives and improving their quality.

In addition to being efficient and effective, the proposed methods for increasing the availability of organs must be congruent with other societal values. According to a report from the Hastings Center, even "a brief examination of the interests and values involved in cadaver organ recovery makes it clear that moral considerations other than efficiency must be acknowledged and respected even in the face of the challenge posed by life-threatening diseases and dysfunctions." The report continues by noting that it is important to develop policies that,

> not only contribute to an increase in the number of cadaver organs obtained for transplant, but also acknowledge and advance the moral values and concerns our society has regarding individual autonomy and privacy, the importance of the family, the dignity of the body, and the value of social practices that enhance and strengthen altruism and our sense of community.[2]

Any proposed policy that disregards these values can be expected to arouse vigorous and widespread opposition.

Legal Framework

Legal questions about cadaveric organ donation arose when kidney transplantation emerged as an effective medical procedure in the 1960s. The Uniform Anatomical Gift Act (UAGA), which has been enacted in every state, resolved those questions by establishing the legal right of all adult Americans to make their wishes known prior to death. In the absence of direction from the deceased, family members have the right to decide whether or not to donate organs. If no family can be located, those with legal or moral responsibility for the body may consent to organ donation. Twelve states also permit the removal of corneas in certain cases under jurisdiction of the coroner or medical examiner if the decedent has not objected and no family members object.

Donor cards, which are an explicit statement of an individual's wish to be an organ donor, play only a minor role in the current system of organ procurement. Only a relatively small percentage of the general public carry these cards. Donor cards are seldom found at the scene of fatal accidents or brought to the attention of physicians and families. Although signed donor cards constitute legally effective consent, physicians are reluctant to retrieve organs on the basis of these cards alone, and almost always require the consent of the next of kin. The UAGA requires that organs and tissues be removed only after death has been determined by a physician who is not a member of the transplant team.

Postmortem surgical recovery of organs (but not tissues) requires that death be pronounced under circumstances in which total brain function has ceased, and circulation and lung functions are temporarily mechanically maintained (i.e., a heart-beating cadaver). This condition, defined as brain death, is relatively rare. Recovering organs from heart-beating cadavers minimizes cellular injury to the organ.

Brain death has been legally recognized in forty-three states by statute or appellate court decision. The common law definition of death that prevails in the seven remaining states is not inconsistent with determination of death using brain-death criteria.[3] To provide for uniformity and to reduce all legal uncertainty, however, all states without brain death legislation should enact the Uniform Determination of Death Act. This act was jointly drafted by the President's Commission for the Study of Ethical Problems in Medicine and Biomedical and Behavioral Research and the National Conference of Commissioners on Uniform State Laws, the American Bar Association, and the American Medical Association.[3]

> The Task Force recommends that the Uniform Determination of Death Act be enacted by the legislatures of states that have not adopted this or a similar act.

Misunderstanding about brain death often occurs even where brain death statutes are in effect. This frequently is due to uncertainty about the clinical determination of brain death, regarding which the various laws are silent. Hospitals, hospital associations, and state medical associations could dispel much of this misunderstanding by adopting model criteria for determining brain death. Criteria developed by an expert group advising the President's Commission for the Study of Ethical Problems in Medicine and Biomedical and Behavioral Research could provide an excellent model for this purpose.[4]

> The Task Force recommends that each state medical association develop and adopt model hospital policies and protocols for the determination of death based upon irreversible cessation of brain function that will be available to guide hospitals in developing and implementing institutional policies and protocols concerning brain death.

Legal complications arising from organ donation have been extremely rare. Despite the recovery of organs from thousands of donors annually for more than a decade and increasing litigation throughout the health care system, lawsuits arising out of organ procurement are almost unknown. In addition, the UAGA provides legal immunity for good-faith efforts of health professionals who cooperate in organ procurement. Given this experience and the legal protection afforded by the UAGA, the Task Force finds that physicians should not avoid participating in organ procurement out of fear of legal liability.

Proposals to Change the Legal Framework

Although the annual number of potential donors cannot now be accurately pinpointed, there is good reason to believe that only a fraction of available organs and tissues are being retrieved under the current voluntary system. Several tactics that would increase the number of organs procured have been proposed, ranging from commercializing organ procurement (e.g., brokering and selling organs for profit) to greatly reducing the requirement for individual and family consent by presuming consent to donate unless a premortem objection is on record.

The National Organ Transplant Act (PL 98-507) makes buying and selling organs and tissues a federal crime. At least three states have passed similar laws. Therefore, introducing a commercial market in organs is illegal.

The enactment of laws that permit a "presumed consent" has also been proposed.[5] Unless a premortem objection has been expressed by the deceased or postmortem objections by next-of-kin, consent is presumed to have been given and organ and tissue procurement could take place at death. As mentioned earlier, twelve states have adopted variants of a presumed consent law for corneas.[2] These laws allow corneas to be taken "unless there is known objection," when the body of the deceased is under the jurisdiction of the coroner or medical examiner. These statutes are usually invoked when no family member is present from whom consent may be obtained. These laws have been effective in increasing the supply of corneal tissue, have withstood constitutional challenge, and considering the thousands of corneas retrieved every year under these laws, have generated very few objections.

Although there are recurring proposals to extend presumed consent from corneas to other tissues and vascularized organs, both consensus derived from experts in the field and public opinion polls show that there is little support for this mechanism as a way of increasing the availability of donor organs. It is clear that potential organ donors and their families want to continue to be the primary decisionmakers. Thus, the Task Force believes that present efforts should focus on enhancing the current voluntary system rather than on reducing the role of actual consent.

One modification of the legal system that would increase the number of organ and tissue donors would to be enact laws that would encourage coroners and medical examiners to give permission for organ and tissue procurement from cadavers under their jurisdiction. In some areas of the country, coroners and medical examiners refuse to allow donated organs to be removed from bodies under their jurisdiction because of their desire to preserve the integrity of medicolegal evidence. In most cases, removing organs does not interfere with the determination of the cause of death and unnecessarily reduces the number of cadaveric donors that are available each year.

> The Task Force recommends that states enact legislation requiring coroners and medical examiners to give permission for organ and tissue procurement when families consent unless the surgical procedure would compromise medicolegal evidence. The Task Force also recommends that states enact legislation that (1) requires coroners and medical examiners to develop policies that facilitate the evaluation of all nonheart-beating cadavers under their jurisdiction for organ and tissue donation, and (2) provides the next of kin with the opportunity to consider postmortem tissue donation. The Task Force further recommends that coroners develop agreements with local tissue banks to help implement these policies.

Improving the Voluntary Donation System: Routine Inquiry

The Task Force finds that a major problem with the current voluntary system of organ donation is that families often are not informed of their option to donate organs and tissues after brain death is determined. Because many families are unaware of this option, it is likely that more organs could be procured while honoring the legal commitment to voluntary consent if family members were routinely informed of the opportunity to donate organs and tissues at the time of death of a relative.

A system of routine inquiry has been recommended by many experts.[6] This would require hospitals to establish a system to ensure that the next-of-kin of all suitable donors are informed of opportunities for donating organs and tissues. This concept was supported by more than 70 percent of the respondents in a recent poll, and has been enacted into law in several states.[7] Hospitals that have adopted such policies report dramatic increases in organ donation. For example, donations in the Henry Ford Hospital in Detroit, Michigan, increased from an annual rate of six to twenty donors within nine months after this policy was enacted.[8]

Routine inquiry policies (or required request) are necessary because some health professionals are reluctant to broach the subject of organ donation with families facing the death of a loved one, and because family members fail to remember this option in their time of grief. Organ donation and tissue donation is almost always a profound source of consolation to families of patients suffering unexpected and premature death. This was eloquently illustrated at a Task Force hearing by the mother of a young child who suffered brain death following the rupture of a cerebral aneurysm. The mother told the Task Force that she had not considered organ donation until a procurement coordinator discussed it with her. She attributed her positive response both to the manner in which she was offered the opportunity to donate her daughter's organs and to the solace it provided her.

> I can honestly admit that out of my personal tragedy something beautiful has blossomed, a living memorial to my daughter. And, I truly believe that this was made possible because I was contacted by someone who epitomized my concept of what compassion is all about.[9]

Given the benefits of organ and tissue donation to both families and recipients, the Task Force believes that trained health professionals either should discuss organ donation with families of all deceased patients who are suitable candidates for organ donation or should refer the patient to a regional organ and/or tissue procurement organization, so that a procurement coordinator will have an opportunity to approach the family.

Conceived as a systems approach, routine inquiry places the responsibility for offering the family the option of organ donation on the institution, rather than on a particular staff member. These policies should be based on the premise that hospitals and health professionals have a responsibility to their communities to assist in providing organs and tissues for transplantation, and a responsibility to surviving families to help them cope with their grief through providing donation as an option.

Several features of routine inquiry should be noted. Although the concept is often called "required request," a routine inquiry policy requires neither that an unwilling person make the request, nor that families be *asked* to donate. Rather, this policy requires hospitals to adopt procedures to assure that the family is *offered* the opportunity to donate. The distinction is important because people react more positively when offered a choice. The family retains the power to decide.

Instituting required request as a hospital policy prevents health professionals from implicitly making the decision for the family by failing to provide the option. Moreover, donation discussions need not occur in cases of clinical unsuitability, nor are attending physicians or other health professionals required to initiate donation discussions themselves. Their only duty is to inform a designated hospital staff member, or representative of the regional OPA trained to approach grieving families, that there may be a potential donor.

> The Task Force recommends that all health professionals involved in caring for potential organ and tissue donors voluntarily accept the responsibility for identifying these donors and for referring such donors to appropriate organ procurement organizations.

The Task Force believes that organs and tissues, consistent with individual and family wishes, should be used for transplantation wherever possible. To this end, voluntary individual participation of health professionals should be supplemented with institutional policies designed to facilitate identification and referral of potential donors.

The Task Force recommends that hospitals adopt routine inquiry/required request policies and procedures for identifying potential organ and tissue donors and for providing next-of-kin with appropriate opportunities for donation.

This recommendation for voluntary establishment of routine inquiry policies may not be sufficient to achieve full cooperation of all hospitals. State health departments could require routine inquiry policies as part of the licensing requirement, but this process is complex and may lead to varying regulatory action. Alternatively, the Joint Commission on the Accreditation of Hospitals (JCAH) could adopt an accreditation standard that requires hospitals to adopt routine inquiry policies.

> The Task Force recommends that the Joint Commission on the Accreditation of Hospitals develop a standard that requires all acute care hospitals to have an affiliation with an organ procurement agency and formal policies and procedures for identifying potential organ and tissue donors and for providing next of kin with appropriate opportunities for donation. The Task Force further recommends that the Department of Defense and the Veterans Administration require their hospitals to have routine inquiry policies.

In addition, the Health Care Financing Administration (HCFA) certifies approximately 6,000 hospitals for Medicare reimbursement. A HCFA requirement that acute-care hospitals it certifies adopt routine inquiry policies would further encourage implementation in most of the hospitals in the United States.

> The Task Force recommends that the Health Care Financing Administration incorporate into the Medicare conditions of participation for hospitals certified under subpart U of the Code of Federal Regulations, a condition that requires hospitals to have routine inquiry policies.

State legislation that requires local hospitals to implement routine inquiry also would be effective. Such laws have already been adopted in California, New York, and Oregon, and are under consideration in at least twenty other states. . . .

These statutes differ primarily with respect to the following provisions: recording organ donation inquiry and decisions on death certificates; requiring the regional OPA to be notified; and extent of involvement of state regulatory agencies in monitoring compliance and establishing requirements for training health professionals. Of these three statutes, the Task Force believes that California law provides a desirable model for emulation by other states at the present time. The issues addressed in these statutes, and the provisions for assuring adequate monitoring for compliance and training need to be carefully considered by groups seeking enactment of routine inquiry legislation. If states develop numerous variations in routine inquiry statutes, the Commission for Uniform State Laws should become involved in developing model legislation in this area.

> The Task Force recommends that all state legislatures formulate, introduce, and enact routine inquiry legislation.

> The Task Force also recommends that the Commission for Uniform State Laws develop model legislation that requires acute care hospitals to develop an affiliation with an organ procurement agency and to adopt routine inquiry policies and procedures.

The Availability of Donors

Cadaveric Donors The potential organ donor pool is much smaller than the number of cadavers because the circumstances of brain death rule out all but a few thousand of those who die each year. Organs can be retrieved only from heart-beating cadavers. About half of the approximately two million deaths each year in the United States occur in hospitals; the number who are declared brain dead is unknown. Additionally, the number of those who can supply organs if they die under appropriate circumstances is appreciably reduced by criteria such as age, past medical history, and present quality of organ function.

The potential cadaveric donor pool has been estimated at 20,000 donors per year.[10–11] To validate this estimate, the Task Force commissioned a literature search and analysis of available data.[12] Sixteen studies that estimated the annual number of potential donors were evaluated. The estimates offered by these studies (expressed in potential donors per 100 hospital deaths) range from 0.77 to 18.0. This wide range casts doubt on the reliability of the data as a whole. In addition, most of the studies attempt to estimate the donor pool only for one organ (primarily kidneys), and not for the heart or liver. No study adequately assessed the size of the pediatric donor pool. Although the wide range of findings illustrates the crude nature of present estimates, most of the better studies do indicate that the potential donor pool for cadaveric organs probably lies between 17,000 and 26,000 donors per year.

Clarification of the potential donor pool, especially by age, organ, and geographic area, would be of enormous value. The underlying question confronting the organ procurement system is whether all potential donors are being identified. Obviously, it is difficult to assess the overall effectiveness of the organ procurement system if the size of the potential donor base is unknown. The identification of a potential pool of donors between the ages of one month and three years is a special concern.

> Therefore, the Task Force recommends that a study of the potential donor pool be conducted using data available through the National Hospital Discharge Survey, supplemented by regional retrospective hospital record reviews.

Although there is no really reliable estimate of the number of potential donors, the availability of cadaveric donors has increased slowly during recent years. No nationwide record of donors is kept, but the annual number of cadaveric donors in the United States can be approximated from the number of cadaveric kidneys transplanted, and adding an estimated 20 percent discard factor for kidneys procured but not transplanted.[13] The resulting number is divided by two to yield the estimated number of donors. In 1984, approximately 3,290 cadaveric donors were available, as shown in Table 2-1, an increase of 20 percent from 1983.

TABLE 2-1. Cadaveric Organ Donors Extrapolated from Number of Cadaveric Kidney Transplants

Year	*No. of Kidney Transplants**	*Est. No. of Donors*	*Donor Increase*
1980	3422	2138	
1981	3427	2142	<+> 1%
1982	3681	2300	<+> 8%
1983	4329	2705	<+> 10%
1984	5264	3290	<+> 20%

Source: U.S. Department of Health and Human Services, Health Care Financing Administration, End-Stage Renal Disease Medical Management Information System.

Living Donors In recent years, living donors have provided one-fourth to one-third of the kidneys that have been transplanted in the United States, a smaller proportion than in earlier years. In 1967, 46 percent of the transplanted kidneys came from living donors, while in 1984, 24 percent came from living donors. The number of living kidney donors, compared to cadaveric donors, from 1980–1984 is shown in Table 2-2.[14]

There are clear-cut benefits to recipients in the transplantation of kidneys from well-matched, genetically related living donors, but there are legitimate concerns about the minimal risks to these living donors. There are also concerns about their susceptibility to pressure and coercion. Refusing to use a kidney from a competent living donor is unduly paternalistic in cases where a donor is well informed, understands, and is willing to accept the risks of kidney donation. There is no reason to exclude all living unrelated donors, such as spouses and friends, but special care should be taken to ensure that the decision to donate is informed, voluntary, and altruistic and special emphasis should be placed on histocompatibility.

Transplant teams should make sure that living donors are competent, and understand and willingly accept the risks of donating a kidney. For example, if a non-immigrant alien provides an unrelated donor, it may be impossible to determine if the donor is donating the kidney willingly or is being coerced or paid. Where circumstances make it difficult or impossible for the transplant team to determine how informed and willing a potential donor is, the organ should not be removed.

> The Task Force recommends that living donors be fully informed about the risks of kidney donation. Health care professionals must guarantee that the decision to donate is entirely voluntary. In the case of all living donors, special emphasis should be placed on histocompatibility.

There also should be a heavy presumption against using children (especially preadolescent children) and mentally retarded persons as sources of kidneys because they are

TABLE 2-2. Number of Cadaveric and Living Donors

Year	*Total*	*Cadaver*	*Living*
1980	4697	3422 (72.8%)	1275 (27.2%)
1981	4885	3427 (70.2%)	1458 (29.8%)
1982	5358	3681 (68.7%)	1677 (31.3%)
1983	6112	4328 (70.8%)	1784 (29.2%)
1984	6968	5264 (75.5%)	1704 (24.5%)

Source: Facility Survey Tables (1980–1984), End-Stage Renal Disease Program Medical Management Information System, Health Care Financing Administration, U.S. Department of Health and Human Services.

usually unable to give valid consent. There should be an independent judicial review of any proposal to remove a kidney from an incompetent person.

Public Attitudes

To examine the attitudes of the public toward donation, the Task Force analyzed regional and national public opinion polls, consulted with experts in the field, and received testimony from knowledgeable witnesses at two public hearings. We found that Americans are well aware of the need for organs and tissues and, in fact, a large majority are supportive of organ donation and consider it praiseworthy.

Attitudes toward donation are complicated by many factors, which are reflected in public opinion polls conducted during the past 17 years.[15–19] Comparisons are difficult because of the lack of standardization in sampling methods, question formats, and polling techniques. However, these polls have consistently shown that awareness of organ transplantation is very high among the general public and that organ donation is perceived as a socially desirable action. A 1985 Gallup poll commissioned by the American Council on Transplantation reported that 93 percent of Americans surveyed knew about organ transplantation and, of these, 75 percent approved of the concept of organ donation.[16,7] Although a large majority approve of organ donation, only 27 percent indicate that they would be very likely to donate their own organs, and only 17 percent have actually completed donor cards.[16] Of those who are very likely to donate, nearly half have not told family members of their wish, even though family permission is usually requested before an organ is removed.[16]

The public is generally willing to honor a relative's wish to be a donor and to give permission if asked to donate a loved one's organs; many would not mind if their own organs were donated, even if they had never given explicit permission. A majority of the public also appears to understand the meaning of the term "brain death," but more than half do not realize that brain death is a prerequisite for organ donation. Most Americans have a very positive attitude toward organ donors whom they view as "loving, generous people who care about others."[16,7]

The public continues to have many fears and misconceptions about organ donation. The fear that doctors might do "something" to them before they are really dead or might hasten their death are the reasons people most frequently cite for not wanting to give permission to donate their organs. Religious reasons are sometimes cited as an objection to organ donation, even though no major religious group in the United States opposes organ donation as a matter of formal doctrine.[16,7] The fears and misconceptions that are barriers to organ donation are listed in Table 2-3, in descending order of importance.

TABLE 2-3. Reasons for Not Permitting Organ Donation

They might do something to me before I am really dead.
Doctors might hasten my death.
I don't like to think about dying.
I don't like someone cutting me up after I die.
Never thought about it.
Want body intact for healthy afterlife.
Family might object.
Against my religion.
Complicated to give permission.

Source: Gallup Survey, January 1985.

Individuals with more formal education and those in upper income brackets are the most likely to want to donate their organs. Nonwhites are least willing to donate their organs. Only 9 percent of nonwhite respondents to the Gallup poll said they were very likely to agree to donate their organs, as compared to 29 percent of the white respondents. Fears that doctors will do something to the potential donor before death that might hasten death appear to be the greatest barrier to organ donation by nonwhites, cited by nearly 45 percent of the nonwhite respondents to the 1985 Gallup poll. In contrast, only 20 percent of the white respondents cited this concern.[16]

The apparent reluctance of minorities, especially blacks, to become involved in organ donation is a serious concern, especially because 31 percent of all patients on kidney dialysis are black. The distribution of HLA antigens is somewhat different in the black population, and the frequency of a "blank," or unidentified, antigen is higher in black patients. For these reasons, black patients are less likely to receive a well-matched kidney from a white donor and may be at a disadvantage in organ-sharing programs if the donor pool does not contain a representative portion of black donors. . . .

A study by Howard University, which attempted to determine why blacks donate less frequently than whites, cited the following reasons: lack of knowledge, religious beliefs, fear of complications, and lack of adequate communication between the public and health providers.[20] In group discussions with the authors of the study, black respondents stressed lack of knowledge about kidney transplants and the need for improved communication and education. Physicians were viewed as being important both in making the topic of organ transplant relevant and in having a positive influence on decision making.

Public Education

Education programs regarding organ donation are conducted by transplant centers, voluntary health agencies, organ and tissue banks, state health departments, and other organizations. Lack of coordination among these programs has led to a degree of redundancy and inconsistency.

Sponsoring organizations, such as local kidney foundations or eye banks, may promote specific organs or tissues in their educational materials, thus limiting public understanding and awareness of multiple organ and/or tissue donation. Public education programs are often conventional or unimaginative, and targeted groups are frequently those already convinced of the benefits of organ donation.

To determine the current local, regional, and national scope of public education, the members of the Task Force surveyed state health departments, organ procurement agencies (OPAs), and voluntary health organizations. The surveys sought information about educational goals, activities, materials, population targeting, coordination with other educational programs, and evaluation methods.

Few of the agencies and organizations surveyed perceive education as a cumulative process aimed at both modification of values and dissemination of knowledge over a period of time. Instead, current public education activities consist of a poorly focused set of activities that are generally neither systematic in conception nor execution. With few exceptions, public education activities in organ transplantation are neither developed nor implemented by education specialists.

The surveys revealed a lack of specific, operationally defined goals and objectives. The surveys also revealed that little formal effort is made to evaluate the effectiveness of transplant education programs. Most voluntary health agencies and OPAs confine their educational activities to providing speakers for civic groups, schools, and churches. These activities are sometimes supplemented with occasional health fair exhibits, press releases, and donor information materials. The program goals that are formulated focus on distributing donor cards and related materials. Donor cards can be useful in increasing public awareness of the need for donor organs, but few Americans sign and carry them, and experience has shown that these cards are not an effective means of increasing the number of donated organs and tissues.

Special Populations Special public education efforts are needed to raise the awareness of minorities about organ transplantation and to increase their participation in donation. Black physicians, clergy, and voluntary family-oriented organizations should be involved in an effort to educate black families about organ donation. The Howard University study concluded that the message about organ donation aimed at the black community should focus on the high incidence of hypertension and kidney disease among blacks, and hence on the great need of blacks for transplantable organs, as well as the great good that organ donation does.

> The Task Force recommends that educational efforts aimed at increasing organ donation among minority populations be developed and implemented, so that the donor population will come to more closely resemble the ethnic profile of the pool of potential recipients, in order to gain the advantage of improved donor and recipient immunologic matching.

Media Campaigns Advertising campaigns by families seeking organs for relatives on waiting lists have demonstrated how effective the media can be in raising awareness. Educational programs in organ donation have not used the media to its fullest. National voluntary health agencies and some local OPAs develop public service announcements, but the quality is uneven. Use of national and local electronic media is poorly coordinated, and these announcements are seldom aired on national television. Both local OPAs and voluntary health agencies try to get media cooperation in developing news and feature stories on donation and transplantation, but this is difficult to do effectively without staff experienced in media and public relations.

State Programs At least forty-four states have programs for distributing organ donation information and donor cards in conjunction with licensing drivers.[21] Little formal *continuing* effort is made to promote distribution of donor materials by the states, however. There are a few exceptions. For example, the state program in Oregon has been supplemented by a local coalition of agencies, the Oregon Donor Program, a voluntary effort supported by the United Way, private contributions, grants, and in-kind services of member organizations. This program is sponsored by the state's five organ and tissue procurement agencies, the Department of Motor Vehicles, Red Cross, Kidney Association, police and fire departments, as well as community leaders. This group developed two audiovisual programs. One program is designed to encourage applicants for drivers licenses to complete donor cards. The other is used to train and motivate Department of Motor Vehicles employees to distribute the state's educational materials.

There is a similar program in Florida. The Florida Statewide Organ and Tissue Donor Program is a voluntary consortium formed to promote public education. Supported with state funds, this consortium is composed of representatives from the Department of Health, Department of Motor Vehicles, End-Stage Renal Disease (ESRD) Network, Florida Hospital Association, Kidney Foundation, Lions Clubs, eye banks, bone and tissue banks, Emergency Medical Services, as well as all transplant centers and individual organ procurement programs in the state. In addition to traditional educational efforts, this group has developed an educational program in support of distribution of donor materials to licensed drivers and is developing specialized education programs aimed at black and Hispanic populations. Both of these consortia coordinate statewide public and professional educational efforts with emphasis on seminars, speakers, and educational materials. These two models of public and private participation provide examples for emulation by other states.

> The Task Force recommends that at the regional level, single consortia, composed of public, private, and voluntary groups that have an interest in education on organ and tissue donation develop, coordinate, and implement public and professional education to supplement, but not replace, activities undertaken by local programs.

School Curricula The Task Force believes there is a need for curriculum models on organ and tissue donation for both primary and secondary schools. Health education curricula now available in growing numbers of school districts include a range of topics related to health issues, such as smoking, alcohol and drug abuse, and blood donation. Some of these curricula guides have been developed under the auspices of the Centers for Disease Control for national distribution. National voluntary organizations, such as the American Heart Association, the National Kidney Foundation, and the American Blood Commission, have also developed models related to particular health topics.

In one state, Virginia, a local educational consortium, The Giving for Life Council, recognized the need for instituting an educational process that is ongoing and systematic. This Richmond-based group has secured the cooperation of the State Board of Education to include organ and tissue donor education in the curriculum for health education classes throughout the state. The Virginia experience demonstrates that curriculum on organ transplantation and donation can be included in educational planning at the state level. Similar achievements in other states could make a major contribution toward improving public education for organ and tissue donation.

National Programs Programs for raising public awareness and encouraging behavioral change have emerged on a national level. One such organization, the American Council on Transplantation (ACT), evolved from two workshops convened by the Surgeon General of the Public Health Service in 1983. The workshops were attended by representatives from the transplant community who agreed that there was a need for an umbrella organization for the many national public and private groups that have an interest in increasing the availability of organs and tissues for transplantation. This organization now has more than forty national public and private groups as members. For the past two years it has helped to coordinate local, regional, and national activities during National Organ and Tissue Donor Awareness Week. If the ACT's full potential is to be realized, it will need to expand its membership to include representatives from all areas of organ and tissue procurement and transplantation.

The Task Force believes there is a need for an umbrella organization composed of representatives of private and voluntary organizations and federal agencies, to coordinate the development and distribution of public education materials. This organization would complement and coordinate local efforts and add consistency to the educational materials used by local groups.

> The Task Force recommends that a single organization, such as the American Council on Transplantation, composed of public, private, and voluntary groups that are national in scope and have an interest in education for organ and tissue donation, develop and coordinate broad scale public and professional educational programs and materials on the national level. This umbrella organization would both develop and distribute model educational materials for use by national and local organizations and plan, coordinate, and develop national efforts using nationwide electronic and print media.

Another national educational effort, the National High Blood Pressure Education Program of the National Heart, Lung, and Blood Institute has succeeded through a partnership between public and private organizations. This program was designed to develop a special education effort both to increase awareness of the benefits of hypertension control and to encourage patients and health professionals to take action. The program operates from the consensus of a multi-member coordinating committee of interested organizations and relies on the local affiliates of member and other voluntary organizations to reach out to the public and health professionals in their communities. This program operates a clearinghouse for both laymen and health professionals, and uses the mass media to reach the general public; local organizations are referenced in taglines on public service announcements and printed materials.

> The Task Force recommends establishment of a national educational program, similar to the High Blood Pressure Education Program of NIH's National Heart, Lung, and Blood Institute, aimed at increasing organ donation. This program should include development both of curricula and instructional materials for use in primary and secondary schools throughout the nation, and of programs directed to special target populations, e.g., minority groups, family units, and churches.

Materials used by regional and national programs to educate the public vary greatly in the degree of sophistication and type of information provided. We concluded that a need exists for greater uniformity in educational messages, information, and statistics, as well as for better coordination among those providing the information.

Attitudes of Health Professionals

Physicians and nurses who care for patients dying in American hospitals exercise a "gatekeeper" function in terms of identifying potential donors and raising the issue of donation with families. Physicians and nurses are in a position to facilitate organ donation but too frequently do not. This fact is the major reason for our recommendation that routine inquiry policies be adopted in American hospitals. The failure of many health professionals to participate in the organ donation process will remain a major barrier to organ donation unless measures are taken to overcome the underlying causes.

Polls consistently demonstrate that a majority of physicians understand the effectiveness of kidney transplantation and personally approve of the concept of postmortem donation. The problem then is how to account for the documented lack of enthusiasm for participation in the donation process.

The reluctance of health professionals to broach the subject of donation with families can be attributed to many factors. For some health professionals, lack of knowledge regarding the need for organ and tissue donors is a factor, as is lack of awareness of the success and cost-effectiveness of extrarenal organ transplantation. However, the problem cannot be remedied by facts alone. Organ retrieval confronts participating health professionals with the need to alter traditional professional, ethical, and attitudinal responses to death, family grief, and clinical responsibility. It forces a reorientation from preserving a patient's life, to preservation of organ function when the patient has been declared brain dead. It means that the focus of attention must change from the physician's patient to the transplant recipient, who the physician probably will never see. The care process no longer ends with death.

Many physicians and nurses are unclear about brain death and how to identify a potential organ donor. They are also concerned that families of the deceased may neither understand nor accept such a pronouncement. Legal liability as a result of declaration of brain death or participation in the donation process also is cited as a significant concern although the extreme rarity of medicolegal complications suggests that this concern is not realistic.

Physicians and nurses may be reluctant to discuss organ donation with potential donor families, fearing that this will cause the families more stress.[22,26] Those who have this attitude fail to realize that organ donation may bring consolation to grieving families.[13,27] One survey found that although 81 percent of the public believe that organ donation helps a family deal with grief, only 66 percent of neurosurgeons believe this.[22] In another survey, more than 600 neurosurgeons indicated that the emotional trauma experienced by families was the single greatest obstacle to offering organ donation.[24]

Reluctance on the part of physicians to "ask something of the family" when they were unable to "save the patient," also has been cited as a factor.[25,27] This perception that they have failed to save the patient results in an unconscious desire to distance from the next of kin. This problem could be resolved if physicians perceived these discussions with families as an opportunity to give them comfort and solace, rather than as a situation in which they are seeking to *take* organs and tissues. Physicians unwilling to enter into such discussions can refer potential donors to specialists in organ procurement.

The additional time and effort that participating in the organ donor process requires of busy health professionals also can be a problem. For this reason, many organ procurement agencies provide coordinators to assist hospital staffs with the evaluation and management of donors, as well as with securing appropriate medical consents.

The attitudes of physicians are preeminent in influencing the behavior of the other members of the health-care team. In a study of intensive care nurses, 86 percent of the respondents personally approved of organ donation in their hospitals, but only 41 percent believed that the neurologists and neurosurgeons approved. In addition, only 17 percent of the nurses believed it was their responsibility to approach donor families, while 65 percent indicated that this decision is made by physicians.[28] Another study found that only 40 percent of hospital administrators believe that physicians are strongly in favor of organ procurement; it also found that although health professionals generally are well disposed to organ procurement, they are not active in communicating this attitude to others.[22] This is the reason for our earlier recommendation that all health professionals involved in caring for potential organ and tissues donors voluntarily accept the responsibility for identifying these donors and for referring such donors to appropriate organ procurement organizations.

Professional Education

In order to assess existing professional educational efforts, the Task Force surveyed organ procurement agencies, national voluntary health organizations, and associations of health professionals, as well as health departments, hospital associations, and medical and nursing societies in all fifty states. In brief, the results indicate that aside from the efforts of local organ procurement agencies, little is being done systematically to educate health professionals about organ donation.

We believe education of health professionals is critical if the number of donor organs available for transplantation is to be increased. Educational efforts must begin in medical and nursing schools with curricula that address all aspects of the organ donation process.

> The Task Force recommends that medical and nursing schools incorporate curricula focusing on organ and tissue procurement and transplantation. The Task Force also recommends that the Accreditation Council of Graduate Medical Education, the body responsible for accrediting residency programs, include requirements for exposure to organ and tissue donation and transplantation in relevant programs in graduate medical education, such as emergency and critical care medicine and the neurological sciences.

A number of medical specialties and subspecialties have either already included questions about organ donation in their certification process or would consider doing so. The American Board of Neurological Surgery was receptive to including questions on organ donation and transplantation on its written Primary Examination. The American Board of Psychiatry and Neurology has incorporated questions regarding the psychological impact of organ transplants on the consultative/liaison portion of its examination. The American Board of Emergency Medicine also indicated it would consider including items in its certification examination concerning the role of the emergency health care professional in organ donation.

> The Task Force recommends that each appropriate medical and nursing specialty board require demonstration of knowledge of organ and tissue donation and transplantation for board certification.

A Task Force survey of national associations of health professionals revealed that although these organizations are interested in continuing education on organ donation, few provided such programs. Organizations such as the American Medical Association, the American Society of Anesthesiologists, and the American Nurses Association have passed resolutions encouraging their members to support organ procurement efforts.[29–31] The American Academy of Pediatrics has adopted a policy statement affirming that:

> Pediatricians providing care for moribund children need to know the criteria for donor suitability, how to obtain legal permission for organ donation, common problems associated with donor organ procurement, how to arrange for organ procurement, and so forth. The Academy can help educate pediatricians in these and other aspects of transplantation through programs at Academy meetings and through Pediatrics, the Pediatric Review and Education Program, and *News and Comment*.[32]

Statements of endorsement and resolutions, however, do not necessarily translate into educational programs.

We also surveyed professional associations of transplant surgeons, physicians, coordinators, and others involved in the recovery and transplantation of organs and tissues. None of the respondent organizations indicated that they formally organized activities beyond their membership, although numerous ad hoc or individual initiatives occur regularly. The goal of professional education is not only providing information but also influencing professional values and attitudes and motivating the participation of others. Physician-to-physician education and motivation should be a responsibility of every physician and surgeon engaged in transplantation activities.

> The Task Force recommends that all professional associations of physicians and nurses involved in caring for potential organ and tissue donors (especially neurosurgeons; trauma surgeons; emergency physicians; and critical care, emergency room, and trauma team nurses), establish programs to educate and encourage their members both to participate in the referral of donors and to cooperate in the organ donation process. The Task Force also recommends that organizations of physician specialists who frequently come in contact with organ and tissue donors should establish mechanisms, such as a committee on transplantation, to facilitate communication and cooperation with physicians in the transplantation specialties.

State Health Departments Responses from forty-one state health departments to the Task Force survey indicate that professional education about transplantation is a focus in only a few states where consortia have been formed. In Pennsylvania, for example, the Department of Health organized an Advisory Committee on Organ and Tissue Donation composed of representatives from the state's two Organ Procurement Agencies, the Pennsylvania Medical Society, Pennsylvania Hospital Association, Pennsylvania Nurses Association, the state Catholic Conference, the Coroners' Association, eye banks, and other interested groups. This committee worked successfully for the passage of the Uniform Determination of Death Act in the Pennsylvania legislature, the development of a model protocol by the Pennsylvania Medical Society for the determination of brain death, and the development of model hospital policies for the State Hospital Association on the determination of brain death and organ procurement. However, Pennsylvania is the exception; most state health departments reported little involvement with organ procurement groups in professional education.

State Medical Societies A Task Force survey of fifty state medical societies, to which seventeen states responded, showed that a few medical societies are involved in continuing activities related to transplantation. Several had formal relationships with state organ procurement agencies; others had standing committees or were active members of consortia to promote donation and procurement. The most comprehensive activity was reported by the Texas Medical Association, which joined forces with the Texas Hospital Association to encourage every hospital in the state to cooperate with a procurement organization and to establish organ donation policies and criteria for brain death. The emphasis placed by medical societies on legislative actions to establish hospital policies, such as routine inquiry and brain death criteria, has been particularly productive where it has occurred.

State medical societies reported providing virtually no continuing education programs on organ donation to members. Similarly, surveys of the state hospital and nursing associations also revealed, except in activities mentioned above, little or no organized educational activities and little interest in establishing organ donor education programs.

Organ Procurement Agencies Professional education surveys were sent to all OPAs. Responses were received from thirty-one of the states and the District of Columbia. This survey showed that the most intensive efforts to provide education to physicians, nurses, and ancillary health professionals are conducted by OPAs. One study found that the amount of time OPA staff devoted to educational efforts was second only to actual organ procurement activities. Each OPA is responsible for educational efforts in a selected number of hospitals within a defined catchment area. Organization and frequency of educational programs vary among OPAs, but the purpose is the same, to inform and motivate physicians and nurses to identify and refer potential donors to the OPA.

OPAs engage in other educational and technical activities, "the operational key to success at organ procurement is an effective program of medical marketing . . . a program of convincing medical professionals in ICUs to refer potential donors to the OPA."[33] A successful program requires an informative and persuasive staff and flexibility in developing and implementing strategies.

The Task Force survey confirmed statements of experts in the field that most OPA educational activity is being directed to critical care nurses and relatively little to physicians, who are often less accessible to OPA staff. Although critical care nurses are often major participants in the donation and procurement process, physicians exert the strongest influence. Because physicians generally respond best to peer education, many procurement coordinators suggest that transplant surgeons and physicians should become more active in the education of their medical colleagues. There is some evidence, however, that non-physician procurement coordinators can be effective if they have appropriate background and training.[34]

There are two primary activities employed by OPA staff to educate and motivate health professionals. The first, formal educational programs, are provided almost entirely by non-physician procurement coordinators. In some areas of the country OPAs have been successful in establishing regularly scheduled programs. The high turnover in critical care nursing positions warrants such regular programs. However, our survey revealed that only 19 percent of the responding OPAs provided fifty-one or more educational programs a year, while 35 percent provided fewer than twenty-six programs annually. The second activity employed by OPAs, frequently termed "surveillance," consists of unscheduled meetings with critical care area staff. The primary purpose of these contacts is to promote close professional relationships between key nurses and physicians and the procurement coordinator and to remind them of the need for participation in organ procurement activities.

Although professional education materials are relatively standard throughout the country, the Task Force observed some discrepancies. For example, a wide range of acceptable minimum ages for postmortem organ donors appears in literature distributed by OPAs. It is especially important that uniformity be achieved in defining the need for liver donors as young as one month. Our survey also found that almost a third of the OPAs emphasized kidney procurement rather than procurement of all organs and tissues. Many OPAs are apparently most responsive to the local need for kidneys and have not yet developed a strong orientation toward procuring extrarenal organs and tissues. In view of the urgent need to recover multiple organs and tissues from all available donors, there is a need for a more uniform educational approach emphasizing all organs and tissues and providing guidelines for acceptability for extrarenal organs.

The survey also found that relatively few OPAs coordinated their educational activities with those of other local or regional procurement programs. In many areas, eye and tissue banks mount separate educational programs rather than working in concert with OPAs. This lack of coordination impairs the effectiveness of educational efforts directed to multiple organ and tissue procurement.

Effectiveness of a National Registry of Human Organ Donors

There are individuals and groups that believe a national donor registry would help increase the supply of organs. The National Organ Transplant Act required that the Task Force include in its report "an assessment of the feasibility of establishing, and of the likely effectiveness of, a national registry of human organ donors." A registry of organ donors is a computerized list of individuals who have indicated a premortem willingness to be donors and who have agreed to be listed on a registry so that their wishes can be honored at the time of death.

As part of this assessment, the Task Force reviewed information from current and past donor registries: the Lifeline program, the Living Bank International, and a registry operated by the state of Florida. In addition, two Task Force members attended a conference on donor registries for bone marrow transplantation held in May of 1985.

Lifeline The "Lifeline" program began in 1976 as a one-year organ and tissue retrieval pilot project in a medical center at Washington University in St. Louis. During the first six months, the program concentrated on donor education as a means of encouraging medical center personnel to volunteer to register as potential donors. During the year there was a five-fold increase in the referral rate of donors, but because only three of the actual donors had been registered in the Lifeline computer it is unclear whether the increase can be attributed to the registry. However, the authors of a study on the pilot point out that the registry had some ancillary value as a data base for statistical analysis of the demographic characteristics of potential donors, a record of which tissues were to be donated to facilitate family consent, and a repository of information for postmortem examinations to expedite the identification of any medical contraindications to donation.[35] This project was ultimately taken over by the Red Cross; it no longer operates as a registry.[36]

The Living Bank International The Living Bank International is a nonprofit service organization in Houston. Since 1968 this organization has registered approximately 500,000 potential donors throughout the world, with a current list of approximately 145,000.[37] The Living Bank stresses public education and provides a donor card. It operates a 24-hour telephone referral service, and refers anatomical donations to the appropriate medical facilities closest to the place of the donor's death.

Representatives of the Living Bank emphasize that they do not keep complete statistics, but they reported that in 1984 they handled 395 deaths of which 221 were registered donors with the Living Bank. This process produced thirty kidneys, six livers, and five hearts.[37] The materials they provided contained little information about the success, effectiveness, costs, and problems of this international registry. Although it appears that the Living Bank's educational activities are effective, it is not possible to evaluate its registry and referral activities in the absence of this essential data.

Florida Florida has implemented an educational program that includes a central registry of drivers who have completed donor cards, operated by the Department of Motor Vehicle and Highway Safety. At the end of 1985 the registry listed approximately 380,000 potential donors.[38] Because the program is only about a year old, it is too early to assess its effectiveness.

Conference on Bone Marrow Registries The National Institutes of Health sponsored a conference on donor registries for bone marrow transplantation. The conference's technology assessment panel concluded "that a centralized national registry for unrelated marrow transplant donors should not be established at this time."[39] This conclusion was based on evidence about the developmental nature and the limited success of bone marrow transplantation from unrelated donors. However, the panel also concluded that "the modest success of the results obtained with matched unrelated donors . . . does warrant continuation of this form of marrow transplantation and facilitation of the efforts of local donor registries," including the development of a mechanism to enable registries to communicate more effectively with each other and with transplant centers. The panel did not believe that the data bases of individual donor programs should be merged into a single national data base because "the degree of cooperation to be anticipated from donor centers is heavily dependent on a feeling of local responsibility and community involvement,"[39] and because problems of privacy and confidentiality would be magnified in a national system.

These recommendations have only limited application to the question of whether a national registry of organ donors should be established. First, there is more debate about the efficacy of bone marrow transplantation from unrelated donors than there is about most organ transplants. Second, bone marrow is taken only from living donors, unlike most other transplant organs.

In summary, the Task Force did not find any information that clearly demonstrates that registries are effective. Registries do not appear to be necessary because there are other effective ways to increase the organ supply. Like donor cards, registries may not substantially increase the donation of organs, although possibly they may be useful as part of larger educational efforts and as a mechanism for triggering requests to the family for permission to use a decedent's organs. Furthermore, the utility of registries is questionable. The time between declaration of death and contact with the family usually is quite short. Often there is no time to query a computer; to find out if the patient is listed. Because so much emphasis is placed on next-of-kin consent, querying the registry is an unnecessary step. The costs of maintaining a registry are large and the chances are great that a name could remain in the registry long after the person is dead.

As the organ procurement system now operates, the primary focus is on securing permission from family members rather than from the actual donor. There are good reasons to think that this will continue, and that the system can be made more effective without introducing a national registry.

The Task Force recommends that a national registry of human organ donors not be established.

CHAPTER 5: PATIENT ACCESS TO AND PAYMENT FOR ORGAN TRANSPLANTATION

Equitable access is a central issue in organ transplantation. Congress recognized the importance of this issue when it directed the Task Force to make recommendations for "assuring equitable access by patients to organ transplantation and for assuring the equitable allocation of donated organs among transplant centers and among patients medically qualified for an organ transplant."

The Task Force has examined issues of equitable access and equitable allocation of donated organs as these currently arise in clinical practice. Although we find equitable access to be a continuing issue of great importance, we also find that the current system is basically fair and, to a large extent, has succeeded in distributing organs equitably. However, there are exceptions, and some emerging problems deserve attention. Continued public support for organ transplantation depends on public confidence that organs are distributed equitably to those who need them.

This chapter describes the current system of allocating organs and the meaning of equitable access and fairness in organ distribution. It also examines several ethical issues, assesses the factors that affect access (including reimbursement practices), and makes recommendations for future action.

The Nature of Patient Selection Criteria

Donor organs are scarce, and only a limited number of people can receive a transplant in a given year. Therefore, transplant recipients must be selected from a large pool of patients who need this procedure. Choices must be made about who will receive an organ transplant and live or have their quality of life improved, and who will not. Transplantation teams set the criteria for patient selection, and organ procurement agencies use these criteria to assist in the placement of organs. On the whole, they appear to make their decisions responsibly. Nevertheless, there is increasing public demand that the criteria for patient selection be public and fair. This demand stems in part from the nature of the organ procurement system, which depends on voluntary gifts to strangers. Indeed, because of the close connection between organ procurement and the policies of organ distribution, it is essential that the criteria for patient selection are fair and are perceived to be fair. Otherwise, distrust may perpetuate the scarcity of organs.

As scarce, life-saving resources, donated organs should be used in a manner that assures good patient and graft survival rates and an acceptable length and quality of life. This requires an efficient, effective, and objective method of distributing organs that is fair. The Organ Procurement and Transplantation Network (OPTN), as proposed in Chapter 4 [not reprinted in this volume], describes how such a system could function.

Central to the question of fairness is the issue of controlling the disposition of donated organs. Organs are donated on behalf of all potential recipients; this implies that the organ is to be used for the good of the community, and ultimately the community must decide what best serves the public interest. Although the gift is presently made to a person, agency, or institution, surgeons and organ procurement agencies should view themselves as stewards or trustees of this resource. The physicians who select the recipient of a donated organ are making decisions about how a scarce public resource should be used. Such a decision should be determined by criteria based on need, effectiveness, and fairness that are publicly stated and publicly defended.

> Therefore the Task Force recommends that donated organs be considered a national resource to be used for the public good; the public must participate in the decisions of how this resource can be used to best serve the public interest.

There are several questions that have been raised about the current system of allocating organs. It has a strong bias in favor of patients in the community where organs are procured, even if there is a better matched patient for the organ elsewhere. In addition, the perceived commitment of the transplant team to their patients sometimes leads to locally procured organs being used in local cases for medical urgency, retransplants, or in presensitized patients, when the organ could have been used in a better-matched patient elsewhere with more likelihood of success. There are also cases in which patients may have provided financial incentives to obtain organs ahead of others on the waiting list, though these are exceptional. Finally, where medical efficacy is roughly equal, a variety of considerations, from source of organ and time on the waiting list to social and economic factors, have influenced selection of the transplant recipient. Ability to pay also has been a major nonmedical factor in determining how a heart or liver is distributed for transplantation.

Medical Criteria and Length of Time on the Waiting List

Given the scarcity of organs and the need to select recipients for transplantation, the question is, "Which criteria for patient selection are equitable or fair?" The Task Force takes *equitable access* to mean that people are treated fairly with regard to access to waiting lists for transplantation and decisions concerning who receives a donated organ. There is evidence that blacks are neither represented on kidney transplant waiting lists, nor are transplanted in proportion to their representation in the dialysis population.[1] There is general agreement that the waiting list of transplantation candidates should be determined primarily by medical criteria. However, there is a debate about whether these medical criteria should be broad or narrow. Many believe that the fairest procedure is to use broad medical criteria to establish the waiting list and then to use narrower medical criteria to determine who actually receives an available organ.

In this connection, the Task Force heard testimony that patient access to waiting lists and ultimately to organ transplantation is affected not only by scarcity of organs or by lack of funds, but also by inadequate information about transplants generally.[2]

> The Task Force recommends that health professionals provide unbiased, timely, and accurate information to all patients who could possibly benefit from organ transplantation so that they can make informed choices about whether they want to be evaluated and placed on a waiting list. The Task Force recommends that information be published annually for patients and physicians on the graft and patient survival data by transplant center. A clear explanation of what the data represent should preface the presentation of data. A strong recommendation should be made in the publication that each patient discuss with his or her attending physician the circumstances of medical suitability for transplantation and where that patient may best be served.

Given the scarcity of organs and the cost of transplants, we believe that the most ethical means of organ distribution is to use medical criteria. Although these criteria vary depending on the type of transplant a patient receives and where the transplant is performed, the criteria are designed to use organs to maximize graft and patient survival and quality of life. The prevailing ethos and practice are to allocate organs to the recipient who will live the longest with the highest quality of life. If there is no reasonable chance that a transplant will be successful for a particular patient, it would be poor stewardship to give the organ to that patient. Probability of successful transplantation and urgency of need are the main medical criteria for patient selection; however, there is debate about how these criteria should be specified.

Judgments about the probability of success are complicated and controversial. Some contraindications are well established, such as mismatched blood group or positive donor-recipient crossmatch. . . . On the basis of current evidence, the Task Force believes that justice, effectiveness and efficiency in the use of organs indicate that a recipient with zero mismatches for HLA-A, B, and DR antigens should be offered that organ and that O blood type organs always should be offered first to suitable "O" recipients. Equally convincing is the evidence that enlarging the pool of donors will greatly increase the likelihood that a highly sensitized patient will receive an organ that is an acceptable match. Based on these findings, the Task Force developed a series of specifications for the national organ-sharing system that gives preference to well-matched recipients or presensitized patients for whom an organ is a good match. . . . These medical criteria address the probability of success, and, in the setting of organs as a scarce resource, are ethical when uniformly applied to all potential recipients.

Urgency of need may conflict with the probability of success. For example, it has been noted that

> when determining who will get a heart, it becomes a difficult ethical issue as to whether the patient with the better outcome or the individual with the greatest urgency should receive the heart. The patients themselves would opt for the patient with the greatest urgency and by and large that is the decision taken by the team. However, one is conscious of the fact that one may be affecting the overall success rate by making choices in favor of individual patient urgency rather than making them on the basis of success.[3]

The Task Force also was presented with an analysis of factors relating to outcome in a single center's experience in liver transplantation, which demonstrated an association of severity with poor outcome; the most critically ill potential recipients (comatose, requiring ICU support, and with a very brief life expectancy) had a survival rate following liver transplantation that was less than half that of patients still well enough to be at home while awaiting transplantation. The clear implication of this is that failure to provide an organ to more able patients in a timely fashion allowed their conditions to deteriorate so that their anticipated transplant outcomes worsened. Not to use an available organ in the patient with an urgent need condemns that patient to death, yet using an organ in such a patient results in an outcome far poorer than would be achieved if that organ were given to a recipient in better condition; urgency of need decreases probability of successful transplantation in this example.[4] A decision on how to apply the criterion of urgency must be developed by a thoughtful and broadly representative group, which must struggle with the concept of best use of organs in the context of compassion and humanitarianism. Because donated organs are a scarce resource, policies to resolve conflicts between equity and efficiency that arise in the distribution of organs should be determined by a broadly representative group that includes patient, community, and ethical perspectives, as well as those of the medical professionals directly involved.

Some argue that medical urgency should include not only the immediate threat of death, but also the likelihood of not receiving another organ because of presensitization, particularly because sensitized patients now constitute a hard core of the waiting lists for kidney transplants. Tension between probability of success and urgency of need also exists here. Although access to a national donor pool is essential if highly sensitized patients are to receive a compatible organ, and although the transplant teams ordinarily give priority to such patients, the success rates with transplants in highly sensitized patients are lower than those achieved when the chosen recipient is unsensitized.

If two or more patients are equally good candidates for a particular organ according to the medical criteria of need and probability of success, the principle of justice suggests that length of time on the waiting list is the fairest way to make the final selection. How often this criterion of first come, first served is used will depend on how frequently a good HLA match or compatible sensitized recipient is available to claim higher priority for the organ. Many organs will need to be allocated on criteria other than HLA match and sensitization, such as length of time on the waiting list. In many cases, this criterion of time on the waiting list would also give priority to highly sensitized patients over equivalently matched nonsensitized patients.

> The Task Force recommends that selection of patients both for waiting lists and for allocation of organs be based on medical criteria that are publicly stated and fairly applied. The Task Force also recommends that the criteria be developed by a broadly representative group that will take into account both need and probability of success. Selection of patients otherwise equally medically qualified should be based on length of time on the waiting list.

Debates about Other Criteria

Several other criteria for selecting transplant recipients have been proposed. The Task Force categorically rejects some, such as discrimination according to sex and race. However, others are controversial, and the Task Force believes it is important to examine these criteria carefully to ensure both that they reflect medical judgments rather than judgments of social worth, and that they are fair. These criteria are: age, lifestyle, access to a social support network, and previous transplants. Each is discussed briefly below.

Age is sometimes offered as a criterion. If increasing age continues to be correlated with an increased mortality and morbidity due to associated medical problems that reduce the probability of successful transplantation, age may serve as a rough rule of thumb for selecting patients. However, it is necessary to emphasize that each individual case could be different because the primary concern from a medical standpoint is physiological age rather than chronological age.[5] If length of survival after transplantation is emphasized in determining probability of success, then age could enter into the calculus. These first two reasons for assigning priority to younger candidates rest on medical utility—age as a predictor of successful outcome and a longer period of survival after transplantation. Some ethicists also argue that considerations of justice in the allocation of resources over the whole life span justify assigning priority to younger candidates over older candidates.[6] However, in view of the widespread controversy about the appropriateness of the criterion of age, we urge the utmost caution in its use in order to avoid unwarranted discrimination against older patients.

Lifestyle sometimes is used as a criterion in selecting patients for transplantation. Some have argued that it is just to assign low priority to transplant candidates whose organ failures resulted from their lifestyles. However, compassion and the uncertainty about the connection between many lifestyles and diseases militate against implementing such a policy. Furthermore, the lifestyle may not have been chosen voluntarily. However, in some cases, a behavioral pattern, such as alcoholism or drug addiction, may be medically relevant in determining the probability of successful transplantation. For example, a patient's continued heavy use of alcohol and drugs may greatly reduce the probability that a transplant will be successful.

Another controversial criterion for selecting organ transplant recipients is whether the patient has a social network of support. It can be argued that this criterion is medically relevant because such a social network may increase the probability of successful outcome, especially in rehabilitation. According to the Massachusetts Task Force on Organ Transplantation, "family support networks may be extremely important in after-hospital care," but "the absence of a family or the existence of an unconventional substitute should not serve as a reason to exclude the patient from evaluation."[7]

Yet another controversial criterion is whether a patient has already received one or more transplants. Between 1977 and 1981, 10,818 people received 11,615 kidney transplants, with 10,063 patients receiving one transplant, 713 patients receiving two and 42 patients receiving three or more.[8] Although some analysts contend that equitable access to scarce organs for transplantation should limit a patient to one transplant, others resist this conclusion, holding that to deny the patient another transplant would constitute abandonment. Judgments may differ depending on whether there are back-up or alternative treatments, such as dialysis for end-stage renal disease.

In summary, the preferential assignment of an organ to a recipient based on objective medical criteria, such as HLA matching, a compatible presensitized recipient, or length of time on the waiting list, is well recognized and widely accepted. Other criteria such as urgency of need, age, lifestyle, the presence of social support, or the need for retransplantation, must be individualized and carefully applied so that medical judgments are reflected rather than judgments of social worth.

> The Task Force recommends that selection of patients for transplants not be subject to favoritism, discrimination on the basis of race or sex, or ability to pay.

Technical, Practical, and Ethical Limitations on Sharing Organs

The principle that donated cadaveric organs are a national resource implies that

> in principle, and to the extent technically and practically achievable, any citizen or resident of the United States in need of a transplant should be considered as a potential recipient of each retrieved organ on a basis equal to that of a patient who lives in the area where the organs or tissues are retrieved. Organs and tissues ought to be distributed on the basis of objective priority criteria, and not on the basis of accidents of geography.[9]

Practical and technical limitations exist, however, which must be accommodated when organ distribution policies are developed. The ideal, as portrayed above, may not always be achievable, and efforts to achieve it may result in inequities.

Some organ-sharing issues are pertinent only to kidney transplantation. The success rates of kidney transplantation, especially in unsensitized patients, are so high that the additional benefits of mandated organ sharing on the basis of HLA matching may be overshadowed by the costs and risks of transportation and the decline of interest by the surgical team. Another potential disadvantage of transporting kidneys over long distances is that the resulting delays may increase the risk of delayed function due to the known effects of cyclosporine toxicity on kidneys subject to prolonged *ex vivo* preservation. Yet, the Task Force is convinced that the advantages of achieving a good match or of giving a highly sensitized patient a unique opportunity to receive a kidney outweigh this potential disadvantage. The OPTN, when organized and established, should be able to minimize logistic delays.

It has been estimated that 15 to 20 percent of kidneys obtained from cadaveric donors will meet the criteria for mandated organ sharing . . . (six HLA antigen match, zero antigen mismatch, or negative crossmatch for a highly sensitized recipient). It is important to safeguard against the risk of reducing access of certain segments of the population to renal transplantation by implementing mandated organ-sharing programs. In a system that shares organs on the basis of histocompatibility testing, patients are at a disadvantage whose HLA types either are not currently well defined or are different from the donor population. The frequencies of certain HLA phenotypes are different in black, Hispanic, and white populations. The identification of HLA phenotypes is somewhat less complete in black and Hispanic individuals (the best available data suggests that the relative risk of having a "blank," or unidentified, antigen is 1.3 in blacks compared to whites).[10] An additional factor is the higher frequency of end-stage renal disease (ESRD) in black populations (estimated to be four to five times the rate of ESRD in whites).[11]

In cities or regions with large black and Hispanic populations, a disproportionate number of the potential transplant recipients are black or Hispanic, while most of the donors are white.[12] Under those circumstances, a system of sharing based on histocompatibility may result in more of the kidneys procured in such a city or region being assigned to white recipients elsewhere than can be matched to local nonwhite patients. These same local patients also will be at a disadvantage on a national list because their HLA phenotypes will differ from the national donor profile, and fewer organs will be sent to them from elsewhere. Thus, transplant centers with a majority of black patients may have a decreased incentive for organ procurement because their patients will not benefit; minority patients may have to wait longer for an organ than white patients.

Because the majority of kidneys will remain under the jurisdiction of regional organizations whose rules for allocating organs will rely on objective medical criteria, the patients who are "left out" of obtaining a good match probably will have adequate access to cadaveric renal transplantation based on other criteria, such as length of time on the waiting list or urgent medical need. However, it is necessary to be certain that this occurs, and that the system does not deprive them of a timely opportunity for transplantation.

The Task Force recommends that organ-sharing programs that are designed to improve the probability of success be implemented in the interests of the effective and efficient use of organs and justice, and the effect of mandated organ sharing be constantly assessed to identify and rectify imbalances that might reduce access of any group.

Non-Immigrant Aliens

The issue of transplanting non-immigrant aliens with organs obtained in the United States is ethically complex. A number of reasons have been cited for such a practice. One is compassion for families who have come to this country in the hopes of saving the life of a loved one, often pauperizing themselves to do so. Another is that political pressure is often brought to bear on transplant teams by our government, which for political motives has encouraged patients to come to the United States for transplants. Although giving non-immigrant aliens priority based on their willingness to pay higher prices is ethically unacceptable, the issue raises the question of whether residents of this country should be given priority for organs retrieved in the United States and whether any non-immigrant aliens should have an opportunity to receive an organ in this country. The Task Force considered the following policy options in addressing this issue:

1. Allowing non-immigrant aliens on the waiting list and giving them priority.
2. Excluding them from the waiting list altogether.
3. Accepting non-immigrant aliens on the waiting list without assigning any numerical restrictions or giving any priority to American citizens.
4. Including some on the waiting list after informing them that they would not receive an organ unless it was clear that no American citizen could benefit from it.
5. Accepting a quota (perhaps 5 to 10 percent) of foreign nationals on the waiting list and treating them equally with American citizens (perhaps excluding them altogether from some categories of extreme scarcity, or those with long waiting lists, such as patients with blood group O).

There is some evidence that giving non-immigrant aliens priority on a waiting list has sometimes been the actual (though not the stated) policy of some centers. There is no justification for this policy. It threatens to undermine the voluntary, cooperative system of organ procurement in the United States. If money is the real reason for assigning priority to non-immigrant aliens, then some transplant institutions are selling organs that have been donated to them without charge. The Task Force rejects the commercialization of organ transplantation, whether the sales are by individuals and families or by physicians and institutions. Other bases of favoritism also are unjustified.

The second option, excluding non-immigrant aliens altogether, has been opposed as unfeeling and unfair, particularly because suitable recipients cannot always be found in this country for all organs. In past years, up to 10 to 15 percent of the retrieved kidneys could not be used; several hundred viable kidneys have been exported when no recipient could be found. However, it is possible that the number of Americans on the waiting list for renal transplantation will increase; currently only 8,000 to 10,000 of the 75,000 dialysis patients are on the waiting list.[8] Also, implementation of a national computerized recipient list will facilitate placement of organs with recipients in this country. The supply of donors will be a serious limiting factor under these circumstances. The policy of totally excluding non-immigrant aliens has also been criticized for neglecting the international goodwill that American transplant programs can generate, especially if these centers combine transplantation of some foreign nationals with efforts to develop transplant programs in those countries.

The main argument for transplanting some non-immigrant aliens is that medical humanitarianism does not recognize criteria for sex, race, nationality, etc. In addition, there might be an obligation to share organs with foreign nationals whose countries participate in a *reciprocal* arrangement with the United States, as Canada does. It is not clear, however, that there is an obligation to accept nonresident, non-immigrant aliens from countries that do not participate at all in systems of giving and receiving organs, even though it may be generous to do so.

The third policy, accepting non-immigrant aliens without assigning any numerical restrictions or giving them priority over American citizens, is difficult to defend in view of the shortage of organs for American residents whose tax dollars support a system of kidney retrieval and who participate in a voluntary, cooperative system of donation.

The major debate centers on the fourth and fifth policy options. The fourth option is to give Americans priority for organs but put some non-immigrant aliens at the bottom of the waiting list or on a separate waiting list. This list would be checked only if the organ did not match anyone on the list of potential American recipients. The major objection to this policy is that such patients are then treated as second-class patients. Many believe this is unethical because it leads non-immigrant aliens to come to the United States in the false hope of a realistic opportunity to obtain an organ.

Many favor the fifth policy, accepting a limited number of non-immigrant aliens, because it avoids these inequities. Whether charity to neighbors is a duty or an ideal, some limits are reasonable, both morally and politically. The figure of 10 percent is often used in religious and moral traditions that recognize a principle of tithing. This policy probably would be politically feasible, because public protest has been directed against the favoritism and injustice of the first policy, not against sharing with non-immigrant aliens per se. However, critics contend that any figure is arbitrary, and that this policy is still unfair to American residents, who should have priority over non-immigrant aliens in the competition for scarce organs.

It is possible to develop one policy for renal organs and another for extrarenal organs. For example, it could be argued that the policy of assigning a quota is acceptable for kidneys because these are not as scarce as other organs and because dialysis is usually available as an alternative treatment, while at the same time the policy of putting non-immigrant aliens at the bottom of the waiting list is acceptable for extrarenal organs because no practical means of life support is available for patients on these waiting lists and many will die before an organ is assigned. A similar compromise was reached by the Task Force, with anticipation of further review by the OPTN when it is established. After considerable debate, the Task Force adopted the following recommendation regarding this issue. Eight Task Force members took exception to this recommendation. Their statement appears at the end of this report [not reprinted in this volume].

> The Task Force recommends that non-immigrant aliens not comprise more than 10 percent of the total number of kidney transplant recipients at each transplant center, until the Organ Procurement and Transplantation Network has had an opportunity to review the issue. In addition, extrarenal organs should not be offered for transplantation to a non-immigrant alien unless it has been determined that no other suitable recipient can be found.

> The Task Force also recommends that as a condition of membership in the Organ Procurement Transplantation Network, each transplant center be required to report every transplant or organ procurement procedure to the OPTN. Moreover, transplantation procedures should not be reimbursed under Medicare, Medicaid, CHAMPUS, and other public payers, unless the transplant center meets payment, organ sharing, reporting, and other guidelines to be established by the OPTN or another agency administratively responsible for the development of such guidelines. Failure to comply with these guidelines will require that the center show cause why it should not be excluded from further organ sharing through the OPTN.

Commercialization of Organ Transplantation

One major reason for rejecting commercialization of organ procurement is that society's moral values militate against regarding the body as a commodity.

> The view that the body is intimately tied to our conceptions of personal identity, dignity, and self-worth is reflected in the unique status accorded to the body within our legal tradition as something which cannot and should not be bought or sold. Religious and secular attitudes make it plain just how widespread is the ethical stance maintaining that the body ought to have special moral standing. The powerful desire to accord respect to the dignity, sanctity, and identity of the body, as well as the moral attitudes concerning the desirability of policies and practices which encourage altruism and sharing among the members of society produced an emphatic rejection of the attempt to commercialize organ [donation and] recovery and make a commodity of the body.[13]

Although transfer of an organ for valuable consideration is a felony under federal law, punishable by up to five years imprisonment and a $50,000 fine, the Task Force became aware of reports of serious abuses in the procurement, distribution, and use of human organs for transplantation. These abuses generally involved the use of kidneys and were reported in the press, in testimony delivered at public hearings held by the Task Force, and in an article that appeared in *The Lancet* in 1985.[14] The reported abuses fell into four categories:

- Exporting and selling cadaveric kidneys abroad.
- Advertising for, or soliciting, non-immigrant aliens to receive transplants in the United States without regard to established waiting lists and medical criteria.
- Brokering kidneys from living unrelated donors.
- Selling organs within the United States and within states.

These activities are discussed below.

Exporting and Selling Cadaveric Kidneys Abroad

The Task Force became aware of several reports that donor organs have been shipped abroad under circumstances suggesting sale or inappropriate remuneration. Although many of those organs could not be used in the United States and there is justification for international sharing of kidneys, instances in which large payments are made for organs suggest that the organs are being sold or transferred for "valuable consideration." Even if an institution rather than an individual profits from the transaction, the practice of accepting a payment for an organ that is more than the reasonable cost of procuring and shipping that organ could amount to an organ sale that violates Federal law. Such practices can lead to American patients being denied access to transplants, while others reap a profit from shipping organs abroad.

The Task Force adopted the following position with regard to the sale of cadaveric kidneys abroad:

> Human organs are a scarce resource that should be allocated fairly and on the basis of medical criteria. Although there may be certain legitimate reasons for sending kidneys abroad, we are alarmed at the large numbers of cadaveric kidneys that have been exported from this country when there are so many patients in America who are currently on waiting lists. The Task Force is concerned that export of cadaveric kidneys is being influenced by the potential for monetary gain or other non-medical reasons. In the interest of assuring equitable allocation of organs among transplant centers and patients, as well as improving access to organ transplantation generally, the Task Force recommends that exportation and importation of donor organs be prohibited except when distribution is arranged or coordinated by the Organ Procurement and Transplantation Network and the organs are to be sent to recognized national networks. Even then, when an organ is to be exported from the United States, documentation must be available to demonstrate that all appropriate efforts have been made to locate a recipient in the United States and/or Canada. The Task Force has every expectation that these international organ sharing programs will be reciprocal.

The Task Force urges that the Health Resources and Services Administration proceed expeditiously with implementation of the OPTN required by law.

Soliciting Non-immigrant Aliens to Receive Transplants in the United States The Task Force received reports that some American centers were providing transplants to a large number of non-immigrant aliens, and in some cases advertised abroad for transplant candidates, offering transplants within several days or weeks of arrival. The suspicion is that financial incentives have played a role in the favoritism shown some non-immigrant alien transplant recipients.

> The Task Force recommends that the practice of soliciting or advertising for non-immigrant aliens and performing a transplant for such patients, without regard to the waiting list, cease.

Brokering Kidneys from Living Unrelated Donors

In the United States, 30 percent of kidney donations come from living donors. In nearly all cases, the living donor is related to the recipient, and the practice is widely accepted. The use of unrelated living donors is more controversial, and occurs to a much more limited extent. In many cases, the unrelated donor is a foreign national who has been brought to the United States for the transplant by a foreign national recipient. In Great Britain, evidence that foreign national donors were paid for their donation has greatly reduced the use of living unrelated donors.

Payment to a living donor is payment for the organ. The donor has sold his organ to the patient, who then hires the doctor and transplant program to complete the transaction. Because the broad consensus that organs should not be sold includes direct sales to patients as well as sales brokered through middlemen, all such transactions are unethical and illegal and should be treated as such. Although the main problem is exploitation of the poor and denigration of the dignity of the donor, payments to living unrelated donors also violate equitable access, because it gives a recipient who can afford to buy an organ a chance to have a transplant that is denied to someone who cannot pay. The Task Force adopted the following position on this issue:

> We are alarmed that even with a statute prohibiting the sale of human organs, certain transplant centers are reportedly brokering kidneys from living unrelated donors. We find this practice to be unethical and to raise serious questions about the exploitation and coercion of people, especially the poor. The Task Force recommends that transplanting kidneys from living unrelated donors should be prohibited when financial gain rather than altruism is the motivating factor. Furthermore, because transplantation involving living related donors is difficult to monitor, particularly as it relates to non-immigrant aliens, for such patients to receive transplants in the United States there must be objective evidence of consanguinity. An independent donor advocate must be assigned to represent the donor.

Selling Organs within the United States and within States The arguments relating to the use of unrelated living donors also apply here. Several members of the Task Force received copies of an offer from a white male to sell his kidney for $2 million, non-negotiable; the document has since been referred to the Inspector General for investigation. There is a question of the applicability of the federal law when the sale does not represent "interstate commerce." Therefore, the Task Force adopted the following position on this issue:

> Title III of PL 98-508, prohibits the transfer of any human organ for "valuable consideration that affects interstate commerce." The Task Force urges the appropriate federal officials to strictly enforce this provision. To the extent that federal law does not prohibit the intrastate sale of organs, the Task Force recommends that states prohibit the sale of organs from cadavers or living donors within their boundaries. The Task Force also opposes insurance policies that guarantee policy holders priority in receiving human organs for transplantation.

Payment for Organ Transplantation

Costs The cost of heart and liver transplantation procedures is a major factor in the decision whether or not to seek this treatment. The average cost of a heart transplantation procedure is $95,000 (range: $57,000–$110,000); the average cost of a liver transplantation procedure is $130,000 (range: $68,000–$238,000). Meeting these high costs is a major source of financial and emotional strain for many patients and their families. Unless they are covered by adequate health insurance or by public programs, only the wealthy or those who can raise sufficient funds through public appeals can receive a heart or liver transplant.

Existing Payment Mechanisms Virtually all kidney transplantation procedures are paid for by Medicare, Medicaid, or private insurance. Medicare also pays for corneal and bone marrow transplants, as well as liver transplants for Medicare eligible children younger than eighteen with biliary atresia or other forms of end-stage liver disease. Medicare does not pay for drugs that are self-administered or given on an outpatient basis, such as the immunosuppressant medications that prevent organ rejection. The Task Force addressed this issue in its October 1985 *Report to the Secretary and the Congress on Immunosuppressive Therapies*, and recommended coverage of immuno-suppressive therapy. Although HCFA commissioned a major technology assessment of heart transplantation and received the report in May 1985, no decision on Medicare coverage of heart transplantation had been made at the time this report was prepared.

Although state Medicaid programs traditionally have followed Medicare policies in determining what procedures to pay for, this has not necessarily been the practice with organ transplantation. Many states pay for transplantation procedures that Medicare does not cover, usually on a case-by-case, or exception, basis. Thus, while a state may "cover" a transplantation procedure, in the absence of a formal policy with stated criteria specifying conditions under which such coverage will be provided, there is no assurance that an agreement to reimburse will be either consistently or fairly applied. States without formal policies regarding payment for heart and liver transplants have been reluctant to develop any in the absence of more definitive information regarding long-term costs. In those instances where transplants are paid for, the federal government provides matching funds. Medicaid pays for liver transplants in thirty-three states, heart transplants in twenty-four states, heart-lung transplants in thirteen states, and pancreas transplants in three states. . . .

CHAMPUS provides health care benefits for active military personnel, their dependents, and retired military personnel, and pays for kidney, liver, and bone marrow transplants. The medical programs of each of the uniform services either pay for or provide kidney, heart, and bone marrow transplants.

As heart and liver transplantation have become accepted treatments, private insurance programs have begun to offer coverage for these procedures. In general, coverage for extrarenal organ transplantation by private insurers exceeds that provided by the public sector. Private sector coverage is summarized in Table 5-1.

However, this coverage is not universal and many people do not have policies that pay for organ transplantation procedures. Also, coverage varies considerably among payers. This uneven coverage is the result of a number of influences affecting reimbursement for almost all evolving health care technologies, including the need for the procedure, the supply and distribution of resources, precedents set by other payers, and public demand. Because these are complicated factors to evaluate, it is difficult for all third-party payers to reach timely or uniform decisions.

The need for a particular transplant procedure is determined by the incidence of disease leading to organ failure and by the effectiveness of the treatment procedure. With improvements in the outcome of the transplant, the indications for the procedure broaden and the number of contraindications are reduced. For example, as transplantation

TABLE 5-1. Summary of Surveys: Percentage of Respondents Providing Coverage by Transplant Procedures, 1985

	Heart	*Heart-Lung*	*Liver**	*Pancreas*
BC/BS	80	72	84	53
HIAA	85	69	80	57
GHAA (HMOs)	30	23	74	18

*Data on liver transplant coverage include some members who provide coverage only for children younger than eighteen with biliary atresia.

Source: Spring, 1985, membership surveys on organ transplantation issues: the Blue Cross and Blue Shield Association (BC/BS); Health Insurance Association of America (HIAA); and the Group Health Association of America (GHAA).

becomes safer, older patients may become eligible to receive an organ, thus greatly increasing the potential pool of recipients. Given that the determinants of need are so dynamic, it is not possible to accurately project the reimbursement risks of third-party payers.

However, transplantation is unique among advanced medical technologies because, in addition to the institutional resources, it also requires a supply of organs. It is the supply of donor organs, rather than institutional or professional resources, that limits the number of transplant procedures that can be performed. Consequently, the costs and reimbursement requirements associated with transplantation are also limited. As long as this limitation exists, third-party payers can have some confidence that, as a whole, reimbursement risks will remain manageable, or at least predictable. Indeed, private insurers have noted that, because of the small volume of transplant procedures performed relative to the number of insured beneficiaries, the incremental increases in insurance premiums due to including transplant coverage have been small, especially when the carrier's risk has been shared through reinsurance. If the supply of organs significantly increases, the effect on reimbursement costs and coverage by third-party payers could be substantial.

Most payers have cited the experimental status of the procedure as the justification for not covering certain transplant procedures. Whether a particular procedure is experimental or is an accepted medical treatment is a professional judgment regarding safety, efficacy, and the long-term outcome of the procedure and is usually determined by peer review. Peer review may be informal and unstructured, such as the gradual accumulation of evidence in the medical literature leading to "conventional wisdom" about the status of a procedure, or it may be a part of a formal, explicit technology evaluation, conducted by an agency such as the National Center of Health Services Research and Health Care Technology Assessment. The major third-party payers each have a process for evaluating health care technology and medical procedures. These processes differ in detail, but all incorporate peer review by medical professionals. These different processes contribute to the lack of uniform coverage for evolving health care technologies, such as transplantation.

For the most part, cost-effectiveness considerations have not been an important factor. The most important factor in determining whether a procedure is covered by either public or private payers is whether it is medically necessary or "reasonable and necessary." An individual policyholder or employee preference or interest could also determine whether a procedure is covered. Once a procedure is determined to be an accepted or necessary medical treatment, it becomes difficult to deny that treatment to beneficiaries on the grounds of cost.

Many medical procedures become eligible for reimbursement by third-party payers as a result of gradual accumulation of *ad hoc*, unrelated decisions by individual insurers rather than through a formal, directed process. Precedents set by other payers, especially competitors in the private sector, may play an important role in determining whether a procedure is covered. As the largest single payer, Medicare has often been regarded as the most important precedent setter for major coverage decisions. This has not been true for extrarenal transplants however. Private insurers and state Medicaid programs have opted to pay for transplants that Medicare will not cover.

The high public visibility of organ transplantation has exerted considerable pressure on both third-party payers and public officials to find ways of paying for these procedures, particularly when patients have inadequate insurance coverage or no coverage at all. The public perception of transplantation as an acceptable, last-resort treatment for certain end-stage diseases has been a considerable force in increasing reimbursement coverage for these procedures.

Access and Ability to Pay

Since the passage of the Social Security Amendments of 1972 (PL 92-603), which established the End-Stage Renal Disease Program, patient wealth has not been a major factor in determining who obtains a kidney transplant, except to the extent that immunosuppressant therapy has not been available. However, some patients who meet medical eligibility criteria but lack third-party payer coverage are denied access to heart or liver transplantation because of inability to pay. The Task Force believes that the federal government should ensure that all patients have access to all efficacious organ transplantation procedures, regardless of ability to pay. There are two arguments that support this position. . . .

The Commitment of Society to Meet Basic Health Needs The question of providing extrarenal transplants to those who are unable to pay for them, like questions of funding other health needs, concerns the obligation of society to meet the basic health care needs of its citizens. There is a widespread recognition that the government should ensure access to a decent minimum or adequate level of health care. The President's Commission for the Study of Ethical Problems in Medicine and Biomedical and Behavioral Research held that a standard of "equitable access to health care requires that all citizens be able to secure an adequate level of health care without excessive burdens."[15] Although opinions may differ over what constitutes an "adequate level of care" and "excessive burdens," life-saving procedures that are comparable in cost and efficacy to other procedures that are routinely funded would seem to qualify.

The Task Force believes that heart and liver transplants belong in this category. These procedures are neither experimental nor unproven, but produce outcomes in terms of longevity and quality of life that are equivalent to treatments that are covered by public and private insurance (e.g., treatment of patients with AIDS, certain malignancies, or serious burns). The National Heart Transplant Study found that 80 percent of heart recipients survive one year, and 50 percent are alive at the end of five years, with a good quality of life applying both objective and subjective criteria.[16] Comparable results have also been achieved for liver transplants in several centers.[17]

Given the nonexperimental, established status of heart and liver transplantation, denying coverage under existing private and public health insurance programs has the effect of denying one group of patients the support of society while granting it to others. At a time when treatment for other life-threatening health conditions is paid for without question, it would be anomalous to deny funding for heart or liver transplantation when it is comparable in cost and efficacy.

The recognition that society is obligated to meet the basic health needs of those unable to pay for themselves has been the linchpin of federal policy for the past twenty years. Medicare and Medicaid programs are the result of the federal commitment to eliminate wealth disparity in access to health care. These programs are committed to funding those services that are "reasonable and necessary for the diagnosis or treatment of illness or injury or to improve the function of a malformed body member."[18]

The question of wealth discrimination in heart and liver transplantation thus arises in the context of a system that is already strongly committed to meeting basic health care needs, regardless of ability to pay. A strong precedent exists in the 1972 decision to end wealth discrimination in kidney transplantation by funding it through the ESRD program. At that time, the outcome of kidney transplantation was considerably poorer than the outcome of heart or liver transplantation is today. Given this context, and the fact that transplantation of the heart or liver is a "necessary" treatment for certain end-stage diseases in certain patients, it would seem clear that these procedures should be paid for by public and private insurance.

The Task Force is cognizant of the need to conserve health funds and recognizes that it may no longer be possible for public funds to be used to meet the health needs of everyone who qualifies. But the Task Force believes that the burden of conserving public health funds should be spread equally, not borne by one disease group alone. The lack of consistent public and private health insurance coverage for heart and liver transplantation may cause some people with end-stage heart and liver disease to bear the burden of the need to economize in health care costs. A person who has end-stage renal disease would receive treatment, while a person who contracts end-stage liver or heart disease would not. The latter patient therefore is denied equitable access to a life-saving procedure.

The Task Force wishes to emphasize that the recommendation to end wealth discrimination in heart and liver transplantation is not based on a belief that society is obligated to fund every health or medical procedure that might benefit someone. Rather, this recommendation is based on the fact that our society is already committed to funding a wide variety of basic health care needs. Given this commitment, it is arbitrary to exclude one life-saving procedure while funding others of equal life-saving potential and cost. If a transplant or other procedure is not shown to be "reasonable and necessary . . . for the treatment of illness," there is no obligation to fund it. Once a therapy is determined to be medically effective, there would be compelling reasons to fund it under existing public and private insurance programs, providing its cost effectiveness is equivalent to other comparable therapies that are funded. However, it is recognized that private insurers must also consider market forces and demand, including selective offerings and customer willingness to pay for such costly services.

The Special Nature of Organ Transplantation: Organs as a Public Resource A separate argument for eliminating wealth discrimination in extrarenal transplantation derives from the special nature of organ transplantation—organs are donated by individuals for the good of the public as a whole. Whether or not there is an obligation to provide equal access to health care, it seems unfair and even exploitative for society to ask people to donate organs if those organs will then be distributed on the basis of ability to pay. This argument connects organ procurement with organ distribution and focuses attention on the nature of the gift of a donated organ. Organs are a public resource and all members of the public who need a transplant should have equal access to an organ. This argument offers an independent justification for the societal funding of organ transplants, without building on a general right to health care or on what the society already funds.

When the President's Commission held that there is a "societal obligation" to provide equitable access to health care, it referred to "society in the broadest sense—the collective American community," which consists of "individuals, who are in turn members of many other, overlapping groups, both public and private; local, state, regional, and national units; professional and workplace organizations; religious, educational, and charitable organizations; and family, kinship, and ethnic groups." Within this pluralistic approach, the President's Commission cited the federal government as the institution of last resort; it held that the "ultimate responsibility" rests with the federal government "for seeing that health care is available to all when the market, private charity, and government efforts at the state and local level are insufficient in achieving equity."[15]

The Task Force concludes that equitable access to extrarenal transplantation means access regardless of wealth. Because of the social commitment to meet basic health needs and the special status of donated organs as a community resource, the Task Force believes that donated organs should be distributed to medically eligible recipients regardless of their ability to pay for the transplant.

Accordingly, the Task Force makes the following recommendations:

> Private and public health benefit programs, including Medicare and Medicaid, should cover heart and liver transplants, including outpatient immunosuppressive therapy that is an essential part of post-transplant care. . . .

> A public program should be set up to cover the costs of people who are medically eligible for organ transplants but who are not covered by private insurance, Medicare, or Medicaid and who are unable to obtain an organ transplant due to lack of funds.

* * *

STATEMENTS OF EXCEPTION

Accepting a Limited Number of Non-immigrant aliens for Transplantation

We the undersigned dissent from the recommendation in chapter 5 that "non-immigrant aliens should not comprise more than 10 percent of the total number of kidney transplant recipients at each transplant center until such time as the organ procurement and transplantation network has had an opportunity to review the issue."

We prefer to substitute the following for that recommendation:

A kidney should not be offered for transplantation to a non-immigrant alien unless it has been determined that no other suitable recipient can be found.

- This recommendation is identical to the one adopted by the Task Force regarding the distribution of extrarenal organs and rests on essentially similar reasoning.
- There is a significant shortage of donated organs. Although the number of organs donated has increased during the past few years, the number of patients on waiting lists has increased at a greater rate during that same time. In effect, this leads to competition for this scarce resource. Inevitably, some individuals who are medically eligible for and wish to receive a transplant are denied this opportunity.
- United States citizens and residents make organ transplantation possible by the voluntary and altruistic donation of organs. All transplantable organs come from this community.
- In the case of kidney transplantation, tax payers in the United States also support the entire cost of organ procurement programs and the cost of dialysis treatments for those awaiting a renal transplant.
- Under these circumstances, the national community that donates the organs and operates the organ procurement and transplantation system can reasonable expect to be offered the opportunity to receive a donated organ whenever a suitable one is available.
- Specifically, we believe that members of this community should not be denied an organ transplant because an organ is given to others. We believe this applies to donated kidneys as well as to donated livers and hearts. We further believe that when no American citizen or resident can benefit from an available donor organ, that organ should be offered overseas or to a non-immigrant alien.

It is a sad fact that as long as a shortage of organs continues, some individuals in need must be denied a transplant. Under these circumstances members of the giving community (both American citizens and aliens living in the United States) have a right to expect that their medical needs will be met and that patient selection decisions will not be made to their detriment.

[Eight members of the Task Force signed this exception.]

VOLUME OF ANNUAL KIDNEY TRANSPLANTS FOR DESIGNATED TRANSPLANT CENTERS

The undersigned disagree with the requirement of a minimum of twenty-five kidney transplants per center per year.

- The Task Force was presented with a study conducted by Dr. Philip J. Held (of the Urban Institute) which clearly showed no adverse graft or patient survival in kidney transplants performing 16–20, 21–25, 26–30, and 31 and over kidney transplants per year.
- Some Task Force members criticized Dr. Held's study on the grounds that the analysis did not control for case-mix. This simply is not true as Table 3 of the analysis states: covariates considered in both periods (1979–1981, 1982–1984) were: age, sex, race, known presence of diabetes, numbers of HLA matches, lymphocyte culture results, number of transplants per patient. An additional covariate for 1979–1981 was proportion of kidneys obtained from outside the transplant center. Additional covariates for 1982–1984 were: use or nonuse of Cyclosporine A, splenectomy, kidney preservation time, pre-transplant blood transfusions.
- If the majority of the Task Force believes these case-mix variables are inadequate such that the conclusions of Dr. Held's analysis are not valid, the Task Force must remember that Dr. Held's study and Dr. Krakauer's HCFA

study of the effectiveness and costs of Cyclosporine A *not only used the same HCFA data, but used identical covariates to control for case-mix.*

- One can only conclude that the majority of the Task Force in accepting Dr. Krakauer's study but not Dr. Held's, did so not because of methodological criticism. We know of no good reason for criticizing the results of the analysis and therefore cannot support the Task Force's recommended minimum of twenty-five annual kidney transplants per center.
- There are no data showing a negative correlation between kidney transplant outcome and low volume centers in the range of 15–30 transplants per year.
- Currently unenforced Medicare regulations require a minimum of fifteen kidney transplants per year per center for unconditional certification for Medicare reimbursement.
- The ESRD program data for 1984 (see chapter 6 . . . of the . . . Report [not reprinted here]) indicates 42 percent (71 of 169) of kidney transplant centers performed fewer than twenty-five transplants in 1984. The Task Force's recommendation would put these centers at risk of closure.

Based on these facts, we made the following recommendation in place of the majority position recommending a minimum volume of 25 annual kidney transplants per center:

> [that] A minimum volume of fifteen annual kidney transplants per center be required. [And that] Over a two-year period additional analysis of the relationship of volume to renal graft and patient survival be undertaken. Continuance and/or revision of this standard should be made based upon the results of the study.

[Signed by five Task Force members]

NOTES TO ORGAN TRANSPLANTATION: ISSUES AND RECOMMENDATIONS

Notes to Chapter 2

1. Emergency Care Research Institute (ECRI). Issues in Health Care Technology. Organ Transplants: Policy Issues and Donor Organ Procurement, 1984; section 9.12: 1.
2. The Hastings Center. Ethical, Legal and Policy Issues Pertaining to Solid Organ Procurement: A Report of the Project on Organ Transplantation, 1985 (October) 2.
3. President's Commission for the Study of Ethical Problems in Medicine and Biomedical and Behavioral Research. *Defining Death: Medical, Legal, and Ethical Issues in the Determination of Death*, 1981; 61, Washington, D.C.: U.S. Government Printing Office.
4. Ibid., p. 159.
5. Caplan A. "Organ Transplantation: The Costs of Success." *The Hastings Center Report* 1983; 13: (December) 28.
6. Caplan A. "Organ Procurement: It's Not in the Cards." *The Hastings Center Report* 1984; 14: (October) 6.
7. Prottas, J.M., and H.L. Batten. Attitudes and Incentives in Organ Procurement. Part II: Attitudes of the American Public. Report to the Health Care Financing Administration, 1986.
8. Oh, H.K., and M.H. Uniewski. "Enhancing Organ Recovery by Initiation of Required Request within a Major Medical Center." *Transplant Proc* (in press).
9. Heck, E. Texas Eye Bank. Testimony before the Task Force on Organ Transplantation, Dallas, Texas, September 30, 1985.
10. Council on Scientific Affairs. "Organ Donor Recruitment." *JAMA* 1981, 246: 2157.
11. Mertz, B. "The Organ Procurement Problem: Many Causes, No Easy Solution." *JAMA* 1985, 254: 3258.
12. Maximus, Inc. Phase I Report: Assessment of the Potential Organ Donor Pool: Literature Review and Data Source Assessment. McLean, Virginia, 1985.
13. Stuart, F.P. "Need, Supply and Legal Issues Related to Organ Transplantation in the United States." *Transplant Proc* 1984; 16: 88.
14. Department of Health and Human Services, Health Care Financing Administration. End-Stage Renal Disease Facility Survey, 1980–1984.
15. "Most in the U.S. Found Willing to Donate Organs." *New York Times*. January 17, 1968.
16. Gallup Organization, Inc. The U.S. Public's Attitudes toward Organ Transplant/Organ Donation. Gallup Survey, 1985.
17. Gallup Organization, Inc. Attitudes and Opinions of the American Public toward Kidney Donation. Gallup Survey, 1983.
18. Kidney Foundation of Eastern Missouri and Metro-East. Assessment of Public and Professional Attitudes Regarding Organ Donation, 1975.
19. Transplantation Council of Southern California. Public Opinions and Attitudes about Medical Transplantation among Los Angeles Residents. 1975.
20. Callender, C.O., J.A. Bayton, C. Yeager, and J.E. Clark. "Attitudes among Blacks toward Donating Kidneys for Transplantation: A Pilot Project." *J. Natl. Assoc.* 1984, 74: 808.
21. Overcast, T.D., R.W. Evans, L.E. Bowen, M.M. Hoe, and C.L. Livak. "Problems in the identification of Potential Organ Donors." *J. Natl. Assoc.* 1984, 251: 1560.
22. Prottas, J.M., and H.L. Batten. Attitudes and Incentives in Organ Procurement. Part I: Professional Attitudes toward Organ Procurement. Report to the Health Care Financing Administration, 1986.
23. Hall, G. Testimony before the Subcommittee on Investigations and Oversight of the Committee on Science and Technology, U.S. House of Representatives, April 13, 1983.
24. Organ Recovery, Inc. Factors Affecting Organ Donation from the Perspective of the Neurological Surgeon. Cleveland, Ohio, 1985.
25. Kaufman, H.H., J.D. Huchton, M.M. McBride, C.A. Beardsley, and B.D.Kahan. "Kidney Donation: Needs and Possibilities." *Neurosurgery* 1979; 5: 237.
26. Minister's Task Force on Kidney Donation. Organ Donation in the Eighties. The Ontario Ministry of Health, 1985.

27. Simmons, R.G., and R.L. Simmons. *Gift of Life*. New York: John Wiley and Sons, 1977: 338.
28. Sophie, L.R., J.C. Salloway, G. Sorock, P. Volek, and F.K. Merkel. "Intensive Care Nurses' Perceptions of Cadaver Organ Procurement." *Heart and Lung* 1983; 12: 263.
29. American Medical Association. Board of Trustees Report. 1985.
30. American Society of Anesthesiologists. House of Delegates Resolution No. 12, 1984.
31. American Nurses Association. House of Delegates Resolution No. 4, 1985.
32. American Academy of Pediatrics. Policy Statement: Organ Transplantation, 1984.
33. Prottas, J.M. "Structure and Effectiveness of the United States Organ Procurement System." *Inquiry* 1985; 22: 365.
34. Denny, D.W. "The Non-Physician Coordinator's Contribution to the Development of an Organ Procurement Program." *Transplant Proc* 1985 ; 17: 6.
35. Anderson, C.B., E.E. Etheredge, G.A. Sicard, P.E. Lacy, M.W. May and W.F. Ballinger. "A Pilot Program of Multiple Organ Cadaver Organ and Tissue Retrieval." *Surgery* 1979; 95: 291.
36. Anderson, C.B., Department of Surgery, School of Medicine, Washington University, St. Louis, Missouri. Personal communication, April 6, 1986.
37. Rasco, J.E., Written personal communication. Living Bank International, October 29, 1985.
38. Mousatsos, S. Executive Director, Florida Tissue and Organ Donor Consortium. Personal communication. March 31, 1986.
39. National Institutes of Health, Technology Assessment Meeting Statement. Donor Registries for Bone Marrow Transplantation. May 13–15, 1986.

Notes to Chapter 5

1. The End-Stage Renal Disease Network of the Greater Capital Area. Outcomes of Renal Transplantation in the Washington, D.C. Area 1983–1984, Chevy Chase, Maryland.
2. Task Force on Organ Transplantation Public Hearings, Chicago, Illinois, May 22, 1985.
3. Stiller, C.R., F.N. McKenzie, and W.J. Jostuk. "Cardiac Transplantation: Ethical and Economic Issues." *Transplantation Today*, 1985; (February) 2: 24.
4. Peters, T.G. Public Hearings, Task Force on Organ Transplantation, Dallas, Texas, September 30, 1985.
5. Young, J. Testimony. Secretary's Conference on Families. National Institutes of Health, December 4, 1985.
6. Veatch, R. Public statement. Task force on Organ Transplantation, Rosslyn, Virginia, January 9, 1986.
7. Department of Public Health, Commonwealth of Massachusetts. Report of the Massachusetts Task Force on Organ Transplantation, Boston University School of Public Health, Boston, October 1984.
8. Department of Health and Human Services. Office of Organ Transplantation, Organ Transplantation Background Information, February 1985.
9. Hunsicker, L.G. Public hearings. Task Force on Organ Transplantation, Chicago, Illinois, May 22, 1985.
10. Mickey, M.R., and Terasaki, P.I. Personal communication. Task Force on Organ Transplantation [no date].
11. Baur, M.P., et al. "Population Analysis on the Basis of Deduced Haplotypes from Random Families," *Histocompatibility Testing 1984*, Springer-Verlag, Berlin, Germany, p. 333.
12. Ibid.
13. The Hastings Center. Ethical, Legal and Policy Issues Pertaining to Solid Organ Procurement: A Report of the Project on Organ Transplantation, October, 1985.
14. The Council of the Transplantation Society. "Commercialization in Transplantation: The Problems and Some Guidelines for Practice." *Lancet* 1985; ii: 715.
15. President's Commission for the Study of Ethical Problems in Medicine and Biomedical and Behavioral Research. *Securing Access to Health Care: The Ethical Implications of Differences in the Availability of Health Services*, 1983; Washington, D.C.: U.S. Government Printing Office.
16. Evans, R.W., et al. The National Heart Transplantation Study: Final Report, vols. 1–5. Battelle Human Affairs Research Centers, Seattle, 1984.
17. Najarian, J.S., and N.L. Ascher. "Liver Transplantation," *New England Journal of Medicine* 1984; 311: 1179.
18. The Social Security Act, Section 1862(a)(1)(A).

CANTERBURY V. SPENCE, 464 F. 2D 772 (1972)

INTRODUCTION. *The doctrine of informed consent was one of the defining characteristics of the movement of biomedical ethics away from the paternalistic Hippocratic tradition toward an ethic more focused on the rights of patients. Informed consent is a notion that does not appear at all in the Hippocratic Oath or in any other medical ethical writings until the twentieth century. The concept of patients consenting to medical treatment was introduced first without much attention being paid to whether patients were adequately informed. As the doctrine of consent developed, however, more emphasis was placed on assuring that the consent was both informed and voluntary. Both criteria would seem to be implied in the philosophical commitment to autonomy or self-determination on which the consent doctrine rests.*

When the courts and proponents of medical ethics began insisting on patients being informed, the question arose of how much information had to be disclosed. The first answer was "as much as that which medical colleagues similarly situated would have disclosed." This focus became known as the professional standard. The problem with that standard, however, was that sometimes physicians could show that they had disclosed all that their colleagues would have, although they had still not disclosed a piece of information that may have helped their patients make informed decisions for or against a proposed treatment. A reasonable person standard then emerged as the plausible basis for deciding how much to disclose. Under this standard, a physician must tell the patient what a reasonable person (called the "reasonable man" in the early cases) would find relative to making a choice. The case of Jerry Canterbury was one of the key cases establishing the reasonable person standard.

THIS APPEAL is from a judgment entered in the District Court on verdicts directed for the two appellees at the conclusion of plaintiff-appellant Canterbury's case in chief. His action sought damages for personal injuries allegedly sustained as a result of an operation negligently performed by appellee Spence, a negligent failure by Dr. Spence to disclose a risk of serious disability inherent in the operation, and negligent post-operative care by appellee Washington Hospital Center. On close examination of the record, we find evidence which required submission of these issues to the jury. We accordingly reverse the judgment as to each appellee and remand the case to the District Court for a new trial.

U.S. Court of Appeals, District of Columbia Circuit. *Jerry W. Canterbury, Appellant, v. William Thornton Spence and the Washington Hospital Center.* Cited as Canterbury v. Spence 464 F.2d. 772 (1972).

I

The record we review tells a depressing tale. A youth troubled only by back pain submitted to an operation without being informed of a risk of paralysis incidental thereto. A day after the operation he fell from his hospital bed after having been left without assistance while voiding. A few hours after the fall, the lower half of his body was paralyzed, and he had to be operated on again. Despite extensive medical care, he has never been what he was before. Instead of the back pain, even years later, he hobbled about on crutches, a victim of paralysis of the bowels and urinary incontinence. In a very real sense this lawsuit is an understandable search for reasons.

At the time of the events which gave rise to this litigation, appellant was nineteen years of age, a clerk-typist employed by the Federal Bureau of Investigation. In December, 1958, he began to experience severe pain between his shoulder blades.[1] He consulted two general practitioners, but the medications they prescribed failed to eliminate the pain. Thereafter, appellant secured an appointment with Dr. Spence, who is a neurosurgeon.

Dr. Spence examined appellant in his office at some length but found nothing amiss. On Dr. Spence's advice appellant was x-rayed, but the films did not identify any abnormality. Dr. Spence then recommended that appellant undergo a myelogram—a procedure in which dye is injected into the spinal column and traced to find evidence of disease or other disorder—at the Washington Hospital Center.

Appellant entered the hospital on February 4, 1959.[2] The myelogram revealed a "filling defect" in the region of the fourth thoracic vertebra. Since a myelogram often does no more than pinpoint the location of an aberration, surgery may be necessary to discover the cause. Dr. Spence told appellant that he would have to undergo a laminectomy—the excision of the posterior arch of the vertebra—to correct what he suspected was a ruptured disc. Appellant did not raise any objection to the proposed operation nor did he probe into its exact nature.

Appellant explained to Dr. Spence that his mother was a widow of slender financial means living in Cyclone, West Virginia, and that she could be reached through a neighbor's telephone. Appellant called his mother the day after the myelogram was performed and, failing to contact her, left Dr. Spence's telephone number with the neighbor. When Mrs. Canterbury returned the call, Dr. Spence told her that the surgery was occasioned by a suspected ruptured disc. Mrs. Canterbury then asked if the recommended operation was serious and Dr. Spence replied "not anymore than any other operation." He added that he knew Mrs. Canterbury was not well off and that her presence in Washington would not be necessary. The testimony is contradictory as to whether during the course of the conversation Mrs. Canterbury expressed her consent to the operation. Appellant himself apparently did not converse again with Dr. Spence prior to the operation.

Dr. Spence performed the laminectomy on February 11[3] at the Washington Hospital Center. Mrs. Canterbury traveled to Washington, arriving on that date but after the operation was over, and signed a consent form at the hospital. The laminectomy revealed several anomalies: a spinal cord that was swollen and unable to pulsate, an accumulation of large tortuous and dilated veins, and a complete absence of epidural fat which normally surrounds the spine. A thin hypodermic needle was inserted into the spinal cord to aspirate any cysts which might have been present, but no fluid emerged. In suturing the wound, Dr. Spence attempted to relieve the pressure on the spinal cord by enlarging the dura—the outer protective wall of the spinal cord—at the area of swelling.

For approximately the first day after the operation appellant recuperated normally, but then suffered a fall and an almost immediate setback. Since there is some conflict as to precisely when or why appellant fell,[4] we reconstruct the events from the evidence most favorable to him.[5] Dr. Spence left orders that appellant was to remain in bed during the process of voiding. These orders were changed to direct that voiding be done out of bed, and the jury could find that the change was made by hospital personnel. Just prior to the fall, appellant summoned a nurse and was given a receptacle for use in voiding, but was then left unattended. Appellant testified that during the course of the endeavor he slipped off the side of the bed, and that there was no one to assist him, or side rail to prevent the fall.

Several hours later, appellant began to complain that he could not move his legs and that he was having trouble breathing; paralysis seems to have been virtually total from the waist down. Dr. Spence was notified on the night of February 12, and he rushed to the hospital. Mrs. Canterbury signed another consent form and appellant was again taken into the operating room. The surgical wound was reopened and Dr. Spence created a gusset to allow the spinal cord greater room in which to pulsate.

Appellant's control over his muscles improved somewhat after the second operation but he was unable to void properly. As a result of this condition, he came under the care of a urologist while still in the hospital. In April, following a cystoscopic examination, appellant was operated on for removal of bladder stones, and in May was released from the hospital. He reentered the hospital the following August for a 10-day period, apparently because of his urologic problems. For several years after his discharge he was under the care of several specialists, and at all times was under the care of a urologist. At the time of the trial in April, 1968, appellant required crutches to walk, still suffered from urinal incontinence and paralysis of the bowels, and wore a penile clamp.

In November, 1959 on Dr. Spence's recommendation, appellant was transferred by the F.B.I. to Miami where he could get more swimming and exercise. Appellant worked three years for the F.B.I. in Miami, Los Angeles and Houston, resigning finally in June, 1962. From then until the time of the trial, he held a number of jobs, but had constant trouble finding work because he needed to remain seated and close to a bathroom. The damages appellant claims include extensive pain and suffering, medical expenses, and loss of earnings.

II

Appellant filed suit in the District Court on March 7, 1963, four years after the laminectomy and approximately two years after he attained his majority. The complaint stated several causes of action against each defendant. Against Dr. Spence it alleged, among other things, negligence in the performance of the laminectomy and failure to inform him beforehand of the risk involved. Against the hospital the complaint charged negligent post-operative care in permitting appellant to remain unattended after the laminectomy, in failing to provide a nurse or orderly to assist him at the time of his fall, and in failing to maintain a side rail on his bed. The answers denied the allegations of negligence and defended on the ground that the suit was barred by the statute of limitations.

Pretrial discovery—including depositions by appellant, his mother and Dr. Spence—continuances and other delays consumed five years. At trial, disposition of the threshold question whether the statute of limitations had run was held in abeyance until the relevant facts developed. Appellant introduced no evidence to show medical and hospital practices, if any, customarily pursued in regard to the critical aspects of the case, and only Dr. Spence, called as an adverse witness, testified on the issue of causality. Dr. Spence described the surgical procedures he utilized in the two operations and expressed his opinion that appellant's disabilities stemmed from his pre-operative condition as symptomized by the swollen, non-pulsating spinal cord. He stated, however, that neither he nor any of the other physicians with whom he consulted was certain as to what that condition was, and he admitted that trauma can be a cause of paralysis. Dr. Spence further testified that even without trauma paralysis can be anticipated "somewhere in the nature of one percent" of the laminectomies performed, a risk he termed "a very slight possibility." He felt that communication of that risk to the patient is not good medical practice because it might deter patients from undergoing needed surgery and might produce adverse psychological reactions which could preclude the success of the operation.

At the close of appellant's case in chief, each defendant moved for a directed verdict and the trial judge granted both motions. The basis of the ruling, he explained, was that appellant had failed to produce any medical evidence indicating negligence on Dr. Spence's part in diagnosing appellant's malady or in performing the laminectomy; that there was no proof that Dr. Spence's treatment was responsible for appellant's disabilities; and that notwithstanding some evidence to show negligent post-operative care, an absence of medical testimony to show causality precluded submission of the case against the hospital to the jury. The judge did not allude specifically to the alleged breach of duty by Dr. Spence to divulge the possible consequences of the laminectomy.

We reverse. The testimony of appellant and his mother that Dr. Spence did not reveal the risk of paralysis from the laminectomy made out a prima facie case of violation of the physician's duty to disclose which Dr. Spence's explanation did not negate as a matter of law. There was also testimony from which the jury could have found that the laminectomy was negligently performed by Dr. Spence, and that appellant's fall was the consequence of negligence on the part of the hospital. The record, moreover, contains evidence of sufficient quantity and quality to tender jury issues as to whether and to what extent any such negligence was causally related to appellant's post-laminectomy condition. These considerations entitled appellant to a new trial.

Elucidation of our reasoning necessitates elaboration on a number of points. In Parts III and IV we explore the origins and rationale of the physician's duty to reasonably inform an ailing patient as to the treatment alternatives available and the risks incidental to them. In Part V we investigate the scope of the disclosure requirement and in Part VI the physician's privileges not to disclose. In Part VII we examine the role of causality, and in Part VIII the need for expert testimony in non-disclosure litigation. In Part IX we deal with appellees' statute of limitations defense and in Part X we apply the principles discussed to the case at bar.

III

Suits charging failure by a physician[6] adequately to disclose the risks and alternatives of proposed treatment are not innovations in American law. They date back a good half-century,[7] and in the last decade they have multiplied rapidly.[8] There is, nonetheless, disagreement among the courts and the commentators[9] on many major questions, and there is no precedent of our own directly in point.[10] For the tools enabling resolution of the issues on this appeal, we are forced to begin at first principles.[11]

The root premise is the concept, fundamental in American jurisprudence, that "[e]very human being of adult years and sound mind has a right to determine what shall be done with his own body. . . ."[12] True consent to what happens to one's self is the informed exercise of a choice, and that entails an opportunity to evaluate knowledgeably the options available and the risks attendant upon each.[13] The average patient has little or no understanding of the medical arts, and ordinarily has only his physician to whom he can look for enlightenment with which to reach an intelligent decision.[14] From these almost axiomatic considerations springs the need, and in turn the requirement, of a reasonable divulgence by physician to patient to make such a decision possible.[15]

A physician is under a duty to treat his patient skillfully[16] but proficiency in diagnosis and therapy is not the full measure of his responsibility. The cases demonstrate that the physician is under an obligation to communicate specific information to the patient when the exigencies of reasonable care call for it.[17] Due care may require a physician perceiving symptoms of bodily abnormality to alert the patient to the condition.[18] It may call upon the physician confronting an ailment which does not respond to his ministrations to inform the patient thereof.[19] It may command the physician to instruct the patient as to any limitations to be presently observed for his own welfare,[20] and as to any precautionary therapy he should seek in the future.[21] It may oblige the physician to advise the patient of the need for or desirability of any alternative treatment promising greater benefit than that being pursued.[22] Just as plainly, due care normally demands that the physician warn the patient of any risks to his well-being which contemplated therapy may involve.[23]

The context in which the duty of risk-disclosure arises is invariably the occasion for decision as to whether a particular treatment procedure is to be undertaken. To the physician, whose training enables a self-satisfying evaluation, the answer may seem clear, but it is the prerogative of the patient, not the physician, to determine for himself the direction in which his interests seem to lie.[24] To enable the patient to chart his course understandably, some familiarity with the therapeutic alternatives and their hazards becomes essential.[25]

A reasonable revelation in these respects is not only a necessity but, as we see it, is as much a matter of the physician's duty. It is a duty to warn of the dangers lurking in the proposed treatment, and that is surely a facet of due care.[26] It is, too, a duty to impart information which the patient has every right to expect.[27] The patient's reliance upon the physician is a trust of the kind which traditionally has exacted obligations beyond those associated with arms-length transactions.[28] His dependence upon the physician for information affecting his well-being, in terms of contemplated treatment, is well-nigh abject. As earlier noted, long before the instant litigation arose, courts had recognized that the physician had the responsibility of satisfying the vital informational needs of the patient.[29] More recently, we ourselves have found "in the fiducial qualities of [the physician-patient] relationship the physician's duty to reveal to the patient that which in his best interests it is important that he should know."[30] We now find, as a part of the physician's overall obligation to the patient, a similar duty of reasonable disclosure of the choices with respect to proposed therapy and the dangers inherently and potentially involved.[31]

This disclosure requirement, on analysis, reflects much more of a change in doctrinal emphasis than a substantive addition to malpractice law. It is well established that the physician must seek and secure his patient's consent before commencing an operation or other course of treatment.[32] It is also clear that the consent, to be efficacious, must be free from imposition upon the patient.[33] It is the settled rule that therapy not authorized by the patient may amount to a tort—a common law battery—by the physician.[34] And it is evident that it is normally impossible to obtain a consent worthy of the name unless the physician first elucidates the options and the perils for the patient's edification.[35] Thus the physician has long borne a duty, on pain of liability for unauthorized treatment, to make adequate disclosure to the patient.[36] The evolution of the obligation to communicate for the patient's benefit as well as the physician's protection has hardly involved an extraordinary restructuring of the law.

IV

Duty to disclose has gained recognition in a large number of American jurisdictions,[37] but more largely on a different rationale. The majority of courts dealing with the problem have made the duty depend on whether it was the custom of physicians practicing in the community to make the particular disclosure to the patient.[38] If so, the physician may be held liable for an unreasonable and injurious failure to divulge, but there can be no recovery unless the omission forsakes a practice prevalent in the profession.[39] We agree that the physician's noncompliance with a professional custom to reveal, like any other departure from prevailing medical practice,[40] may give rise to liability to the patient. We do not agree that the patient's cause of action is dependent upon the existence and nonperformance of a relevant professional tradition.

There are, in our view, formidable obstacles to acceptance of the notion that the physician's obligation to disclose is either germinated or limited by medical practice. To begin with, the reality of any discernible custom reflecting a professional consensus on communication of option and risk information to patients is open to serious doubt.[41] We sense the danger that what in fact is no custom at all may be taken as an affirmative custom to maintain silence, and that physician-witnesses to the so-called custom may state merely their personal opinions as to what they or others would do under given conditions.[42] We cannot gloss over the inconsistency between reliance on a general practice respecting divulgence and on the other hand, realization that the myriad of variables among patients[43] makes each case so different that its omission can rationally be justified only by the effect of its individual circumstances.[44] Nor can we ignore the fact that to bind the disclosure obligation to medical usage is to arrogate the decision on revelation to the physician alone.[45] Respect for the patient's right of self-determination on particular therapy[46] demands a standard set by law for physicians rather than one which physicians may or may not impose upon themselves.[47]

More fundamentally, the majority rule overlooks the graduation of reasonable-care demands in Anglo-American jurisprudence and the position of professional custom in the hierarchy. The caliber of the performance exacted by the reasonable-care standard varies between the professional and non-professional worlds, and so also the role of professional custom. "With but few exceptions," we recently declared, "society demands that everyone under a duty to use care observe minimally a general standard."[48] "Familiarly expressed judicially," we added, "the yardstick is that degree of care which a reasonably prudent person would have exercised under the same or similar circumstances."[49] "Beyond this," however, we emphasized, "the law requires those engaging in activities requiring unique knowledge and ability to give a performance commensurate with the undertaking."[50] Thus physicians treating the sick must perform at higher levels than non-physicians in order to meet the reasonable care standard in its special application to physicians[51]—"that degree of care and skill ordinarily exercised by the profession in [the physician's] own or similar localities."[52] And practices adopted by the profession have indispensable value as evidence tending to establish just what that degree of care and skill is.[53]

We have admonished, however, that "[t]he special medical standards[54] are but adaptions of the general standard to a group who are required to act as reasonable men possessing their medical talents presumably would."[55] There is, by the same token, no basis for operation of the special medical standard where the physician's activity does not bring his medical knowledge and skills peculiarly into play.[56] And where the challenge to the physician's conduct is not to be gauged by the special standard, it follows that medical custom cannot furnish the test of its propriety, whatever its relevance under the proper test may be.[57] The decision to unveil the patient's condition and the chances as to remediation, as we shall see, is ofttimes a non-medical judgment[58] and, if so, is a decision outside the ambit of the special standard. Where that is the situation, professional custom hardly furnishes the legal criterion for measuring the physician's responsibility to reasonably inform his patient of the options and the hazards as to treatment.

The majority rule, moreover, is at war with our prior holdings that a showing of medical practice, however probative, does not fix the standard governing recovery for medical malpractice.[59] Prevailing medical practice, we have maintained, has evidentiary value in determinations as to what the specific criteria measuring challenged professional conduct are and whether they have been met,[60] but does not itself define the standard.[61] That has been our position in treatment cases, where the physician's performance is ordinarily to be adjudicated by the special medical standard of due care.[62] We see no logic in a different rule for nondisclosure cases, where the governing standard is much more largely divorced from professional considerations.[63] And surely in nondisclosure cases the factfinder is not invariably functioning in an area of such technical complexity that it must be bound to medical custom as an inexorable application of the community standard of reasonable care.[64]

Thus we distinguished, for purposes of duty to disclose, the special and general-standard aspects of the physician-patient relationship. When medical judgment enters the picture and for that reason the special standard controls, prevailing medical practice must be given its just due. In all other instances, however, the general standard exacting ordinary care applies, and that standard is set by law. In sum, the physician's duty to disclose is governed by the same legal principles applicable to others in comparable situations, with modifications only to the extent that medical judgment enters the picture.[65] We hold that the standard measuring performance of that duty by physicians, as by others, is conduct which is reasonable under the circumstances.[66]

V

Once the circumstances give rise to a duty on the physician's part to inform his patient, the next inquiry is the scope of the disclosure the physician is legally obliged to make. The courts have frequently confronted this problem but no uniform standard defining the adequacy of the divulgence emerges from the decisions. Some have said "full" disclosure,[67] a norm we are unwilling to adopt literally. It seems obviously prohibitive and unrealistic to expect physicians to discuss with their patients every risk of proposed treatment—no matter how small or remote[68] —and generally unnecessary from the patient's viewpoint as well. Indeed, the cases speaking in terms of "full" disclosure appear to envision something less than total disclosure,[69] leaving unanswered the question of just how much.

The larger number of courts, as might be expected, have applied tests framed with reference to prevailing fashion within the medical profession.[70] Some have measured the disclosure by "good medical practice,"[71] others by what a reasonable practitioner would have bared under the circumstances,[72] and still others by what medical custom in the community would demand.[73] We have explored this rather considerable body of law but are unprepared to follow it. The duty to disclose, we have reasoned, arises from phenomena apart from medical custom and practice.[74] The latter, we think, should no more establish the scope of the duty than its existence. Any definition of scope in terms purely of a professional standard is at odds with the patient's prerogative to decide on projected therapy himself.[75] That prerogative, we have said, is at the very foundation of the duty to disclose,[76] and both the patient's right to know and the physician's correlative obligation to tell him are diluted to the extent that its compass is dictated by the medical profession.[77]

In our view, the patient's right of self-decision shapes the boundaries of the duty to reveal. That right can be effectively exercised only if the patient possesses enough information to enable an intelligent choice. The scope of the physician's communications to the patient, then, must be measured by the patient's need,[78] and that need is the information material to the decision. Thus the test for determining whether a particular peril must be divulged is its materiality to the patient's decision: all risks potentially affecting the decision must be unmasked.[79] And to safeguard the patient's interest in achieving his own determination on treatment, the law must itself set the standard for adequate disclosure.[80]

Optimally for the patient, exposure of a risk would be mandatory whenever the patient would deem it significant to his decision, either singly or in combination with other risks. Such a requirement, however, would summon the physician to second-guess the patient, whose ideas on materiality could hardly be known to the physician. That would make an undue demand upon medical practitioners, whose conduct, like that of others, is to be measured in terms of reasonableness. Consonantly with orthodox negligence doctrine, the physician's liability for nondisclosure is to be determined on the basis of foresight, not hindsight; no less than any other aspect of negligence, the issue on nondisclosure must be approached from the viewpoint of the reasonableness of the physician's divulgence in terms of what he knows or should know to be the patient's informational needs. If, but only if, the fact-finder can say that the physician's communication was unreasonably inadequate is an imposition of liability legally or morally justified.[81]

Of necessity, the content of the disclosure rests in the first instance with the physician. Ordinarily it is only he who is in position to identify particular dangers; always he must make a judgment, in terms of materiality, as to whether and to what extent revelation to the patient is called for. He cannot know with complete exactitude what the patient would consider important to his decision, but on the basis of his medical training and experience he can sense how the average, reasonable patient expectably would react.[82] Indeed, with knowledge of, or ability to learn, his patient's background and current condition, he is in a position superior to that of most others—attorneys, for example—who are called upon to make judgments on pain of liability in damages for unreasonable miscalculation.[83]

From these considerations we derive the breadth of the disclosure of risks legally to be required. The scope of the standard is not subjective as to either the physician or the patient; it remains objective with due regard for the patient's informational needs and with suitable leeway for the physician's situation. In broad outline, we agree that "[a] risk is thus material when a reasonable person, in what the physician knows or should know to be the patient's position, would be likely to attach significance to the risk or cluster of risks in deciding whether or not to forego the proposed therapy."[84]

The topics importantly demanding a communication of information are the inherent and potential hazards of the proposed treatment, the alternatives to that treatment, if any, and the results likely if the patient remains untreated. The factors contributing significance to the dangerousness of a medical technique are, of course, the incidence of injury and the degree of the harm threatened.[85] A very small chance of death or serious disablement may well be significant; a potential disability which dramatically outweighs the potential benefit of the therapy or the detriments of the existing malady may summon discussion with the patient.[86]

There is no bright line separating the significant from the insignificant; the answer in any case must abide a rule of reason. Some dangers—infection, for example—are inherent in any operation; there is no obligation to communicate those of which persons of average sophistication are aware.[87] Even more clearly, the physician bears no responsibility for discussion of hazards the patient has already discovered,[88] or those having no apparent materiality to patients' decision on therapy.[89] The disclosure doctrine, like others marking lines between permissible and impermissible behavior in medical practice, is in essence a requirement of conduct prudent under the circumstances. Whenever nondisclosure of particular risk information is open to debate by reasonable-minded men, the issue is for the finder of the facts.[90]

VI

Two exceptions to the general rule of disclosure have been noted by the courts. Each is in the nature of a physician's privilege not to disclose, and the reasoning underlying them is appealing. Each, indeed, is but a recognition that, as important as is the patient's right to know, it is greatly outweighed by the magnitudinous circumstances giving rise to the privilege. The first comes into play when the patient is unconscious or otherwise incapable of consenting, and harm from a failure to treat is imminent and outweighs any harm threatened by the proposed treatment. When a genuine emergency of that sort arises, it is settled that the impracticality of conferring with the patient dispenses with need for it.[91] Even in situations of that character the physician should, as current law requires, attempt to secure a relative's consent if possible.[92] But if time is too short to accommodate discussion, obviously the physician should proceed with the treatment.[93]

The second exception obtains when risk-disclosure poses such a threat of detriment to the patient as to become unfeasible or contraindicated from a medical point of view. It is recognized that patients occasionally become so ill or emotionally distraught on disclosure as to foreclose a rational decision, or complicate or hinder the treatment, or perhaps even pose psychological damage to the patient.[94] Where that is so, the cases have generally held that the physician is armed with a privilege to keep the information from the patient,[95] and we think it clear that portents of that type may justify the physician in action he deems medically warranted. The critical inquiry is whether the physician responded to a sound medical judgment that communication of the risk information would present a threat to the patient's well-being.

The physician's privilege to withhold information for therapeutic reasons must be carefully circumscribed, however, for otherwise it might devour the disclosure rule itself. The privilege does not accept the paternalistic notion that the physician may remain silent simply because divulgence might prompt the patient to forego therapy the physician feels the patient really needs.[96] That attitude presumes instability or perversity for even the normal patient, and runs counter to the foundation principle that the patient should and ordinarily can make the choice for himself.[97] Nor does the privilege contemplate operation save where the patient's reaction to risk information, as reasonable foreseen by the physician, is menacing.[98] And even in a situation of that kind, disclosure to a close relative with a view to securing consent to the proposed treatment may be the only alternative open to the physician.[99]

VII

No more than breach of any other legal duty does nonfulfillment of the physician's obligation to disclose alone establish liability to the patient. An unrevealed risk that should have been made known must materialize, for otherwise the omission, however unpardonable, is legally without consequence. Occurrence of the risk must be harmful to the patient, for negligence unrelated to injury is nonactionable.[100] And, as in malpractice actions generally,[101] there must be a causal relationship between the physician's failure to adequately divulge and damage to the patient.[102]

A causal connection exists when, but only when, disclosure of significant risks incidental to treatment would have resulted in a decision against it.[103] The patient obviously has no complaint if he would have submitted to the therapy notwithstanding awareness that the risk was one of its perils. On the other hand, the very purpose of the disclosure rule is to protect the patient against consequences which, if known, he would have avoided by foregoing the treatment.[104] The more difficult question is whether the factual issue on causality calls for an objective or a subjective determination.

It has been assumed that the issue is to be resolved according to whether the factfinder believes the patient's testimony that he would not have agreed to the treatment if he had known of the danger which later ripened into injury.[105] We think a technique which ties the factual conclusion on causation simply to the assessment of the patient's credibility is unsatisfactory. To be sure, the objective of risk-disclosure is preservation of the patient's interest in intelligent self-choice on proposed treatment, a matter the patient is free to decide for any reason that appeals to him.[106] When, prior to commencement of therapy, the patient is sufficiently informed on risks and he exercises his choice, it may truly be said that he did exactly what he wanted to do. But when causality is explored at a post-injury trial with a professedly uninformed patient, the question whether he actually would have turned the treatment down if he had known the risks is purely hypothetical: "Viewed from the point at which he had to decide, would the patient have decided differently had he known something he did not know?"[107] And the answer which the patient supplies hardly represents more than a guess, perhaps tinged by the circumstance that the uncommunicated hazard has in fact materialized.[108]

In our view, this method of dealing with the issue on causation comes in second-best. It places the physician in jeopardy of the patient's hindsight and bitterness. It places the factfinder in the position of deciding whether a speculative answer to a hypothetical question is to be credited. It calls for a subjective determination solely on testimony of a patient-witness shadowed by the occurrence of the undisclosed risk.[109]

Better it is, we believe, to resolve the causality issue on an objective basis: in terms of what a prudent person in the patient's position would have decided if suitably informed of all perils bearing significance.[110] If adequate disclosure could reasonably be expected to have caused that person to decline the treatment because of the revelation of the kind of risk or danger that resulted in harm, causation is shown, but otherwise not.[111] The patient's testimony is relevant on that score of course but it would not threaten to dominate the findings. And since that testimony would probably be appraised congruently with the factfinder's belief in its reasonableness, the case for a wholly objective standard for passing on causation is strengthened. Such a standard would in any event ease the fact-finding process and better assure the truth as its product.

VIII

In the context of trial of a suit claiming inadequate disclosure of risk information by a physician, the patient has the burden of going forward with evidence tending to establish prima facie the essential elements of the cause of action, and ultimately the burden of proof—the risk of nonpersuasion[112]—on those elements.[113] These are normal impositions upon moving litigants, and no reason why they should not attach in nondisclosure cases is apparent. The burden of going forward with evidence pertaining to a privilege not to disclose,[114] however, rests properly upon the physician. This is not only because the patient has made out a prima facie case before an issue on privilege is reached, but also because any evidence bearing on the privilege is usually in the hands of the physician alone. Requiring him to open the proof on privilege is consistent with judicial policy laying such a burden on the party who seeks shelter from an exception to a general rule and who is more likely to have possession of the facts.[115]

As in much malpractice litigation,[116] recovery in nondisclosure lawsuits has hinged upon the patient's ability to prove through expert testimony that the physician's performance departed from medical custom. This is not surprising since, as we have pointed out, the majority of American jurisdictions have limited the patient's right to know to whatever boon can be found in medical practice.[117] We have already discussed our disagreement with the majority rationale.[118] We now delineate our view on the need for expert testimony in nondisclosure cases.

There are obviously important roles for medical testimony in such cases, and some roles which only medical evidence can fill. Experts are ordinarily indispensable to identify and elucidate for the factfinder the risks of therapy and the consequences of leaving existing maladies untreated. They are normally needed on issues as to the cause of any injury or disability suffered by the patient and, where privileges are asserted, as to the existence of any emergency claimed and the nature and seriousness of any impact upon the patient from risk-disclosure. Save for relative infrequent instances where questions of this type are resolvable wholly within the realm of ordinary human knowledge and experience, the need for the expert is clear.[119]

The guiding consideration our decisions distill, however, is that medical facts are for medical experts[120] and other facts are for any witnesses—expert or not—having sufficient knowledge and capacity to testify to them.[121] It is evident that many of the issues typically involved in nondisclosure cases do not reside peculiarly within the medical domain. Lay witness testimony can competently establish a physician's failure to disclose particular risk information, the patient's lack of knowledge of the risk, and the adverse consequences following the treatment.[122] Experts are unnecessary to a showing of the materiality of a risk to a patient's decision on treatment, or to the reasonably, expectable effect of risk disclosure on the decision.[123] These conspicuous examples of permissible uses of nonexpert testimony illustrate the relative freedom of broad areas of the legal problem of risk nondisclosure from the demands for expert testimony that shackle plaintiffs' other types of medical malpractice litigation.[124]

IX

We now confront the question whether appellant's suit was barred, wholly or partly, by the statute of limitations. The statutory periods relevant to this inquiry are one year for battery actions[125] and three years for those charging negligence.[126] For one a minor when his cause of action accrues, they do not begin to run until he has attained his majority.[127] Appellant was nineteen years old when the laminectomy and related events occurred, and he filed his complaint roughly two years after he reached twenty-one. Consequently, any claim in suit subject to the one-year limitation came too late.

Appellant's causes of action for the allegedly faulty laminectomy by Dr. Spence and allegedly careless post-operative care by the hospital present no problem. Quite obviously, each was grounded in negligence and so was governed by the three-year provision.[128] The duty-to-disclose claim appellant asserted against Dr. Spence, however, draws another consideration into the picture. We have previously observed that an unauthorized operation constitutes a battery, and that an uninformed consent to an operation does not confer the necessary authority.[129] If, therefore, appellant had at stake no more than a recovery of damages on account of a laminectomy intentionally done without intelligent permission, the statute would have interposed a bar.

It is evident, however, that appellant had much more at stake.[130] His interest in bodily integrity commanded protection, not only against an intentional invasion by an unauthorized operation[131] but also against a negligent invasion by his physician's dereliction of duty to adequately disclose.[132] Appellant has asserted and litigated a violation of that duty throughout the case.[133] That claim, like the others, was governed by the three-year period of limitation applicable to negligence actions[134] and was unaffected by the fact that its alternative was barred by the one-year period pertaining to batteries.[135]

X

This brings us to the remaining question, common to all three causes of action: whether appellant's evidence was of such caliber as to require a submission to the jury. On the first, the evidence was clearly sufficient to raise an issue as to whether Dr. Spence's obligation to disclose information on risks was reasonably met or was excused by the surrounding circumstances. Appellant testified that Dr. Spence revealed to him nothing suggesting a hazard associated with the laminectomy. His mother testified that, in response to her specific inquiry, Dr. Spence informed her that the laminectomy was no more serious than any other operation. When, at trial, it developed from Dr. Spence's testimony that paralysis can be expected in one percent of laminectomies, it became the jury's responsibility to decide whether that peril was of sufficient magnitude to bring the disclosure duty into play.[136] There was no emergency to frustrate an opportunity to disclose,[137] and Dr. Spence's expressed opinion that disclosure would have been unwise did not foreclose a contrary conclusion by the jury. There was no evidence that appellant's emotional makeup was such that concealment of the risk of paralysis was medically sound.[138] Even if disclosure to appellant himself might have bred ill consequences, no reason appears for the omission to communicate the information to his mother, particularly in view of his minority.[139] The jury, not Dr. Spence, was the final arbiter of whether nondisclosure was reasonable under the circumstances.[140]

Proceeding to the next cause of action, we find evidence generating issues as to whether Dr. Spence performed the laminectomy negligently and, if so, whether that negligence contributed causally to appellant's subsequent disabilities. A report Dr. Spence prepared after the second operation indicated that at the time he felt that too-tight sutures at the laminectomy site might have caused the paralysis. While at trial Dr. Spence voiced the opinion that the sutures were not responsible, there were circumstances lending support to his original view. Prior to the laminectomy, appellant had none of the disabilities of which he now complains. The disabilities appeared almost immediately after the laminectomy. The gusset Dr. Spence made on the second operation left greater room for the spinal cord to pulsate, and this alleviated appellant's condition somewhat. That Dr. Spence's in-trial opinion was hardly the last word is manifest from the fact that the team of specialists consulting on appellant was unable to settle on the origin of the paralysis.

We are advertent to Dr. Spence's attribution of appellant's disabilities to his condition preexisting the laminectomy, but that was a matter for the jury. And even if the jury had found that theory acceptable, there would have remained the question whether Dr. Spence aggravated the preexisting condition. A tortfeasor takes his victim as he finds him, and negligence intensifying an old condition creates liability just as surely as negligence precipitating a new one.[141] It was for the jury to say, on the whole evidence, just what contributions appellant's preexisting condition and Dr. Spence's medical treatment respectively made to the disabilities.

In sum, judged by legal standards, the proof militated against a directed verdict in Dr. Spence's favor. True it is that the evidence did not furnish ready answers on the dispositive factual issues, but the important consideration is that appellant showed enough to call for resolution of those issues by the jury. As in Sentilles v. Inter-Carribbean Shipping Corporation,[142] a case resembling this one, the Supreme Court stated,

> The jury's power to draw the inference that the aggravation of petitioner's tubercular condition, evident so shortly after the accident, was in fact caused by that accident, was not impaired by the failure of any medical witness to testify that it was in fact the cause. Neither can it be impaired by the lack of medical unanimity as to the respective likelihood of the potential causes of the aggravation, or by the fact that other potential causes of aggravation existed and were not conclusively negated by the proofs. The matter does not turn on the use of a particular form of words by the physicians in giving their testimony. The members of the jury, not the medical witnesses, were sworn to make a legal determination of the question of causation. They were entitled to take all the circumstances, including the medical testimony into consideration.[143]

We conclude, lastly, that the case against the hospital should also have gone to the jury. The circumstances surrounding appellant's fall—the change in Dr. Spence's order that appellant be kept in bed,[144] the failure to maintain a side rail on appellant's bed, and the absence of any attendant while appellant was attempting to relieve himself—could certainly suggest to jurors a dereliction of the hospital's duty to exercise reasonable care for the safety and well-being of the patient.[145] On the issue of causality, the evidence was uncontradicted that appellant progressed after the operation until the fall but, a few hours thereafter, his condition had deteriorated, and there were complaints of paralysis and respiratory difficulty. That falls tend to cause or aggravate injuries is, of course, common knowledge, which in our view the jury was at liberty to utilize.[146] To this may be added Dr. Spence's testimony that paralysis can be brought on by trauma or shock. All told, the jury had available a store of information enabling an intelligent resolution of the issues respecting the hospital.[147]

We realize that, when appellant rested his case in chief, the evidence scarcely served to put the blame for appellant's disabilities squarely on one appellee or the other. But this does not mean that either could escape liability at the hand of the jury simply because appellant was unable to do more. As ever so recently we ruled, "a showing of negligence by each of two (or more) defendants with uncertainty as to which caused the harm does not defeat recovery but passes the burden to the tortfeasors for each to prove, if he can, that he did not cause the harm."[148] In the case before us, appellant's evidentiary presentation on negligence survived the claims of legal insufficiency, and appellees should have been put to their proof.[149]

Reversed and remanded for a new trial.

NOTES

1. Two months earlier, appellant was hospitalized for diagnostic tests following complaints of weight loss and lassitude. He was discharged with a final diagnosis of neurosis and thereafter given supportive therapy by his then attending physician.
2. The dates stated herein are taken from the hospital records. At trial, appellant and his mother contended that the records were inaccurate, but the one-day difference over which they argued is without significance.
3. The operation was postponed five days because appellant was suffering from an abdominal infection.
4. The one fact clearly emerging from the otherwise murky portrayal by the record, however, is that appellant did fall while attempting to void and while completely unattended.
5. See Aylor v. Intercounty Constr. Corp., 127 U.S.App.D.C. 151, 153, 381 F.2d 930, 932 (1967), and cases cited in n. 2 thereof.
6. Since there was neither allegation nor proof that the appellee hospital failed in any duty to disclose, we have no occasion to inquire as to whether or under what circumstances such a duty might arise.

7. See, *e. g.*, Theodore v. Ellis, 141 La. 709, 75 So. 655, 660 (1917); Wojciechowski v. Coryell, 217 S.W. 638, 644 (Mo.App. 1920); Hunter v. Burroughs, 123 Va. 113, 96 S.E. 360, 366–368 (1918).
8. See the collections in Annot., 79 A.L.R. 2d 1028 (1961); Comment, Informed Consent in Medical Malpractice, 55 Calif.L.Rev. 1396, 1397 n. 5 (1967).
9. For references to a considerable body of commentary, see Waltz & Scheuneman, Informed Consent to Therapy, 64 Nw.U.L.Rev. 628 n. 1 (1970).
10. In Stivers v. George Washington Univ., 116 U.S.App.D.C. 29, 320 F.2d 751 (1963), a charge was asserted against a physician and a hospital that a patient's written consent to a bi-lateral arteriogram was based on inadequate information, but our decision did not touch the legal aspects of that claim. The jury to which the case was tried found for the physician, and the trial judge awarded judgment for the hospital notwithstanding a jury verdict against it. The patient confined the appeal to this court to the judgment entered for the hospital, and in no way implicated the verdict for the physician. We concluded "that the verdict constitutes a jury finding that [the physician] was not guilty of withholding relevant information from [the patient] or in the alternative that he violated no duty owed her in telling her what he did tell her or in withholding what he did not tell her. . . ." 116 U.S.App.D.C. at 31, 320 F.2d at 753. The fact that no review of the verdict as to the physician was sought thus became critical. The hospital could not be held derivatively liable on the theory of a master-servant relationship with the physician since the physician himself had been exonerated. And since there was no evidence upon which the verdict against the hospital could properly have been predicated independently, we affirmed the trial judge's action in setting it aside. 116 U.S.App.D.C. at 31–32, 320 F.2d at 753–754. In these circumstances, our opinion in *Stivers* cannot be taken as either approving or disapproving the handling of the risk-nondisclosure issue between the patient and the physician in the trial court.
11. We undertake only a general outline of legal doctrine on the subject and, of course, a discussion and application of the principles which in our view should govern this appeal. The rest we leave for future litigation.
12. Schloendorff v. Society of New York Hospital, 211 N.Y. 125, 105 N.E. 92, 93 (1914). See also Natanson v. Kline, 186 Kan. 393, 350 P.2d 1093, 1104 (1960), clarified, 187 Kan. 186, 354 P.2d 670 (1960); W. Prosser, Torts § 18 at 102 (3d ed. 1964); Restatement of Torts § 49 (1934).
13. See Dunham v. Wright, 423 F.2d 940, 943–946 (3d Cir. 1970) (applying Pennsylvania law); Campbell v. Oliva, 424 F.2d 1244, 1250–1251 (6th Cir. 1970) (applying Tennessee law); Bowers v. Talmage, 159 So.2d 888 (Fla.App.1963); Woods v. Brumlop, 71 N.M. 221, 377 P.2d 520, 524–525 (1962); Mason v. Ellsworth, 3 Wash.App. 298, 474 P.2d 909, 915, 918–919 (1970).
14. Patients ordinarily are persons unlearned in the medical sciences. Some few, of course, are schooled in branches of the medical profession or in related fields. But even within the latter group variations in degree of medical knowledge specifically referable to particular therapy may be broad, as for example, between a specialist and a general practitioner, or between a physician and a nurse. It may well be, then, that it is only in the unusual case that a court could safely assume that the patient's insights were on a parity with those of the treating physician.
15. The doctrine that a consent effective as authority to form therapy can arise only from the patient's understanding of alternatives to and risks of the therapy is commonly denominated "informed consent." See, *e.g.*, Waltz & Scheuneman, Informed Consent to Therapy, 64 Nw.U.L. Rev. 628, 629 (1970). The same appellation is frequently assigned to the doctrine requiring physicians, as a matter of duty to patients, to communicate information as to such alternatives and risks. See, *e.g.*, Comment, Informed Consent in Medical Malpractice, 55 Calif.L.Rev. 1396 (1967). While we recognize the general utility of shorthand phrases in literary expositions, we caution that uncritical use of the "informed consent" label can be misleading. See, *e.g.*, Plante, An Analysis of "Informed Consent." 36 Ford.L. Rev. 639, 671–72 (1968).

    In duty-to-disclose cases, the focus of attention is more properly upon the nature and content of the physician's divulgence than the patient's understanding or consent. Adequate disclosure and informed consent are, of course, two sides of the same coin—the former a *sine qua non* of the latter. But the vital inquiry on duty to disclose relates to the physician's performance of an obligation, while one of the difficulties with analysis in terms of "informed consent" is its tendency to imply that what is decisive is the degree of the patient's comprehension. As we later emphasize, the physician discharges the duty when he makes a reasonable effort to convey sufficient information although the patient, without fault of the physician, may not fully grasp it. See text *infra* at notes 82–89. Even though the factfinder may have occasion to draw an inference on the state of the patient's enlightenment, the factfinding process on performance of the duty ultimately reaches back to what the physician actually said or failed to say. And while the factual conclusion on adequacy of the revelation will vary as between patients—as, for example, between a lay patient and a physician-patient—the fluctuations are attributable to the kind of divulgence which may be reasonable under the circumstances.
16. Brown v. Keaveny, 117 U.S.App.D.C. 117, 118, 326 F.2d 660, 661 (1963); Quick v. Thurston, 110 U.S.App.D.C. 169, 171, 290 F.2d 360, 362, 88 A.L.R.2d 299 (en banc 1961); Rodgers v. Lawson, 83 U.S.App.D.C. 281, 282, 170 F.2d 157, 158 (1948).
17. See discussion in McCoid, The Care Required of Medical Practitioners, 12 Vand.L.Rev. 549, 586–97 (1959).
18. See Union Carbide & Carbon Corp. v. Stapleton, 237 F.2d 229, 232 (6th Cir. 1956); Maertins v. Kaiser Foundation Hosp., 162 Cal.App.2d 661, 328 P.2d 494, 497 (1958); Doty v. Lutheran Hosp. Ass'n, 110 Neb. 467, 194 N.W. 444, 445, 447 (1923); Tvedt v. Haugen, 70 N.D. 338, 294 N.W. 183, 187 (1940). See also Dietze v. King, 184 F.Supp. 944, 948, 949 (E.D.Va.1960); Dowling v. Mutual Life Ins. Co., 168 So.2d 107, 116 (La.App.1964), writ refused, 247 La. 248, 170 So.2d 508 (1965).
19. See Rahn v. United States, 222 F.Supp. 775, 780–781 (S.D.Ga.1963) (applying Georgia law); Baldor v. Rogers, 81

So.2d 658, 662, 55 A.L.R.2d 453 (Fla.1955); Manion v. Tweedy, 257 Minn. 59, 100 N.W.2d 124, 128, 129 (1959); Tvedt v. Haugen, *supra* note 18, 294 N.W. at 187; Ison v. McFall, 55 Tenn.App. 326, 400 S.W.2d 243, 258 (1964); Kelly v. Carroll, 36 Wash.2d 482, 219 P.2d 79, 88, 19 A.L.R.2d 1174, cert. denied, 340 U.S. 892, 71 S.Ct. 208, 95 L.Ed. 646 (1950).

20. Newman v. Anderson, 195 Wis. 200, 217 N.W. 306 (1928). See also Whitfield v. Daniel Constr. Co., 226 S.C. 37, 83 S.E. 2d 460, 463 (1954).
21. Beck v. German Klinik. 78 Iowa 096, 43 N.W. 617, 618 (1889); Pike v. Honsinger, 155 N.Y. 201, 49 N.E. 760, 762 (1898); Doan v. Griffith, 402. S.W.2d 855, 856 (Ky.1966).
22. The typical situation is where a general practitioner discovers that the patient's malady calls for specialized treatment, whereupon the duty generally arises to advise the patient to consult a specialist. See the cases collected in Annot., 35 A.L.R.3d 349 (1971). See also Baldor v. Rogers, *supra* note 19, 81 So.2d at 662; Garafola v. Maimonides Hosp., 22 A.D.2d 85, 253 N.Y.S.2d 856, 858, 28 A.L.R.3d 1357 91964); aff'd, 19 N.Y.2d 765, 279 N.Y.S.2d 523, 226 N.E.2d 311, 28 A.L.R. 3d 1362 (1967); McCoid, The Care Required of Medical Practitioners, 12 Vand.L.Rev. 549, 597–98 (1959).
23. See, *e.g.*, Wall v. Brim, 138 F.2d 478. 480–481 (5th Cir. 1943), consent issue tried on remand and verdict for plaintiff aff'd., 145 F.2d 492 (5th Cir. 1944), cert. denied, 324 U.S. 857, 65 S.Ct. 858, 89 L. Ed. 1415 (1945); Belcher v. Carter, 13 Ohio App.2d 113, 234 N.E.2d 311, 312 (1967); Hunter v. Burroughs, *supra* note 7, 96 S.E. at 366; Plante, An Analysis of "Informed Consent," 36 Ford.L.Rev. 639, 653 (1968).
24. See text *supra* at notes 12–13.
25. See cases cited *supra* notes 14–15.
26. See text *supra* at notes 17–23.
27. Some doubt has been expressed as to ability of physicians to suitably communicate their evaluations of risks and the advantages of optional treatment, and as to the lay patient's ability to understand what the physician tells him. Karchmer, Informed Consent: A Plaintiff's Medical Malpractice "Wonder Drug," 31 Mo.L.Rev. 29, 41 (1966). We do not share these apprehensions. The discussion need not be a disquisition, and surely the physician is not compelled to give his patient a short medical education; the disclosure rule summons the physician only to a reasonable explanation. See Part V, *infra*. That means generally informing the patient in nontechnical terms as to what is at stake: the therapy alternatives open to him, the goals expectably to be achieved, and the risks that may ensue from particular treatment and no treatment. See Stinnett v. Price, 446 S.W.2d 893, 894, 895 (Tex.Civ.App.1969). So informing the patient hardly taxes the physician, and it must be the exceptional patient who cannot comprehend such an explanation at least in a rough way.
28. That element comes to the fore in litigation involving contractual and property dealings between physician and patient. See, *e.g.*, Campbell v. Oliva, supra note 13, 424 F.2d at 1250; In re Bourquin's Estate, 161 Cal.App.2d 289, 326 P.2d 604, 610 (1958); Butler v. O'Brien, 8 Ill.2d 203, 133 N.E.2d 274, 277 (1956); Woodbury v. Woodbury, 141 Mass. 329, 5 N.E. 275, 278, 279 (1886); Clinton v. Miller, 77 Okl. 173, 186 P. 932, 933 (1919); Hodge v. Shea, 252 S.C. 601, 168 S.E.2d 82, 84, 87 (1969).
29. See, *e.g.*, Sheets v. Burman, 322 F.2d 277, 279–280 (5th Cir. 1963); Hudson v. Moore, 239 Ala. 130, 194 So. 147, 149 (1940); Guy v. Schuldt, 236 Ind. 101, 138 N.E.2d 891, 895 (1956); Perrin v. Rodriguez, 153 So. 555, 556–557 (La.App. 1934); Schmucking v. Mayo, 183 Minn. 37, 235 N.W. 633 (1931); Thompson v. Barnard, 142 S.W.2d 238, 241 (Tex.Civ. App.1940), aff'd, 138 Tex. 277, 158 S.W. 2d 486 (1942).
30. Emmett v. Eastern Dispensary & Cas. Hosp., 130 U.S.App.D.C. 50, 54, 396 F.2d 931, 935 (1967). See also, Swan, The California Law of Malpractice of Physicians, Surgeons, and Dentists, 33 Calif.L.Rev. 248, 251 (1945).
31. See cases cited *supra* note 16–28; Berkey v. Anderson, 1 Cal.App.3d 790, 82 Cal.Rptr. 67, 78 (1970); Smith, Antecedent Grounds of Liability in the Practice of Surgery. 14 Rocky Mt.L.Rev. 233, 249–50 (1942); Swan, The California Law of Malpractice of Physicians, Surgeons, and Dentists, 33 Calif.L.Rev. 248, 251 (1945); Note, 40 Minn.L.Rev. 876, 879–80 (1956).
32. See cases collected in Annot., 56 A.L.R. 2d 695 (1967). Where the patient is incapable of consenting, the physician may have to obtain consent from someone else. See, *e.g.*, Bonner v. Moran. 75 U.S.App. D.C. 156, 157–158, 126 F.2d 121, 122–123, 139 A.L.R. 1366 (1941).
33. See Restatement (Second) of Torts §§ 55–58 (1965).
34. See, *e.g.*, Bonner v. Moran, *supra* note 32, 75 U.S.App.D.C. at 157, 126 F.2d at 122, and cases collected in Annot., 56 A.L.R.2d 695, 697–99 (1957). See also Part IX, *infra*.
35. See cases cited *supra* note 13. See also McCoid, The Care Required of Medical Practitioners, 12 Vand.L.Rev. 549, 587–91 (1959).
36. We discard the thought that the patient should ask for information before the physician is required to disclose. Caveat emptor is not the norm for the consumer of medical services. Duty to disclose is more than a call to speak merely on the patient's request, or merely to answer the patient's questions; it is a duty to volunteer, if necessary, the information the patient needs for intelligent decision. The patient may be ignorant, confused, overawed by the physician or frightened by the hospital, or even ashamed to inquire. See generally Note, Restructuring Informed Consent: Legal Therapy for the Doctor-Patient Relationship, 79 Yale L.J. 1533, 1545–51 (1970). Perhaps relatively few patients could in any event identify the relevant questions in the absence of prior explanation by the physician. Physicians and hospitals have patients of widely divergent socio-economic backgrounds, and a rule which presumes a degree of sophistication which many members of society lack is likely to breed gross inequities. See Note, Informed Consent as a Theory of Medical Liability, 1970 Wis.L.Rev. 879, 891–97.
37. The number is reported at 22 by 1967. Comment, Informed Consent in Medical Malpractice, 55 Calif.L.Rev. 1396, 1397, and cases cited in n. 5 (1967).
38. See, *e.g.*, DiFilippo v. Preston, 3 Storey 539, 53 Del. 539, 173 A.2d 333, 339 (1961); Haggerty v. McCarthy, 344 Mass. 136, 181 N.E.2d 562, 565, 566 (1962); Roberts v. Young, 369 Mich. 133, 119 N.W.2d 627, 630 (1963); Aiken v. Clary, 396 S.W.2d 668, 675, 676 (Mo. 1965). As these

cases indicate, majority-rule courts hold that expert testimony is necessary to establish the custom.

39. See cases cited *supra* note 38.
40. See, *e.g.*, W. Prosser, Torts § 33 at 171 (3d ed. 1964).
41. See, *e.g.*, Comment, Informed Consent in Medical Malpractice, 55 Calif.L.Rev. 1396, 1404–05 (1967); Comment, Valid Consent to Medical Treatment: Need the Patient Know?, 4 Duquesne L.Rev. 450, 458–59 (1966); Note, 75 Harv.L.Rev. 1445, 1447 (1962).
42. Comment, Informed Consent in Medical Malpractice, 55 Calif.L.Rev. 1396, 1404 (1967); Note, 75 Harv.L.Rev. 1445, 1447 (1962).
43. For example, the variables which may or may not give rise to the physician's privilege to withhold risk information for therapeutic reasons. See text Part VI, *infra*.
44. Note, 75 Harv.L.Rev. 1445, 1447 (1962).
45. *E.g.*, W. Prosser, Torts § 32 at 168 (3d ed. 1964); Comment, Informed Consent in Medical Malpractice, 55 Calif.L. Rev. 1396, 1409 (1967).
46. See text *supra* at notes 12–13.
47. See Berkey v. Anderson, *supra* note 31, 82 Cal.Rptr. at 78; Comment, Informed Consent in Medical Malpractice, 55 Calif. L.Rev. 1396, 1409–10 (1967). Medical custom bared in the cases indicates the frequency with which the profession has not engaged in self-imposition. See, *e.g.*, cases cited *supra* note 23.
48. Washington Hosp. Center v. Butler, 127 U.S.App.D.C. 379, 383, 384 F.2d 331, 335 (1967).
49. *Id.*
50. *Id.*
51. *Id.*
52. Rodgers v. Lawson, *supra* note 16, 83 U.S.App.D.C. at 282, 170 F.2d at 158. See also Brown v. Keaveny, *supra* note 16, 117 U.S.App.D.C. at 118, 326 F.2d at 661; Quick v. Thurston, *supra* note 16, 110 U.S.App.D.C. at 171, 290 F.2d at 362.
53. *E.g.*, Washington Hosp. Center v. Butler, *supra* note 48, 127 U.S.App.D.C. at 383, 384 F.2d at 335. See also cases cited *infra* note 119.
54. *Id.* at 383 ns. 10–12, 384 F.2d at 335 ns. 10–12.
55. *Id.* at 384 n. 15, 384 F.2d at 336 n. 15.
56. *E.g.*, Lucy Webb Hayes Nat. Training School v. Perotti, 136 U.S.App.D.C. 122, 127–129, 419 F.2d 704, 710–711 (1969); Monk v. Doctors Hosp., 131 U.S.App.D.C. 174, 177, 403 F.2d 580, 583 (1968); Washington Hosp. Center v. Butler, *supra* note 48.
57. Washington Hosp. Center v. Butler, *supra* note 48, 127 U.S.App.D.C. at 387–388, 384 F.2d at 336–337. See also cases cited *infra* note 59.
58. See Part V, *infra*.
59. Washington Hosp. Center v. Butler, *supra* note 48, 127 U.S.App.D.C. at 387–388, 884 F.2d at 336–337; Garfield Memorial Hosp. v. Marshall, 92 U.S.App. D.C. 234, 240, 204 F.2d 721, 726–727, 37 A.L.R.2d 1270 (1953); Byrom v. Eastern Dispensary & Cas. Hosp., 78 U.S. App.D.C. 42, 43, 136 F.2d 278, 279 (1943).
60. *E.g.*, Washington Hosp. Center v. Butler, *supra* note. 48, 127 U.S.App.D.C. at 383, 384 F.2d at 335. See also cases cited *infra* note 119.
61. See cases cited *supra* note 59.
62. See cases cited *supra* note 59.
63. See Part V. *infra*.
64. Comment, Informed Consent in Medical Malpractice, 55 Calif.L.Rev. 1396, 1405 (1967).
65. See Part VI, *infra*.
66. See Note, 75 Harv.L.Rev. 1445, 1447 (1962). See also authorities cited *supra* notes 17–23.
67. *E.g.*, Salgo v. Leland Stanford Jr. Univ. Bd. of Trustees, 154 Cal.App.2d 560, 317 P.2d 170, 181 (1957); Woods v. Brumlop, *supra* note 13, 377 P.2d at 524–525.
68. See Stottlemire v. Cawood, 213 F.Supp. 897, 898 (D.D.C.), new trial denied, 215 F.Supp. 266 (1963); Yeates v. Harms, 193 Kan. 320, 393 P.2d 982, 991 (1964), on rehearing, 194 Kan. 675, 401 P.2d 659 (1965); Bell v. Umstattd, 401 S.W.2d 306, 313 (Tex.Civ.App.1966); Waltz & Scheuneman, Informed Consent to Therapy, 64 Nw.U.L.Rev. 628, 635–38 (1970).
69. See, Comment, Informed Consent in Medical Malpractice, 55 Calif.L.Rev. 1396, 1402–03 (1967).
70. *E.g.*, Shetter v. Rochelle, 2 Ariz.App. 358, 409 P.2d 74, 86 (1965), modified, 2 Ariz.App. 607, 411 P.2d 45 (1966); Ditlow v. Kaplan, 181 So.2d 226, 228 (Fla.App.1965); Williams v. Menehan, 191 Kan. 6, 379 P.2d 292, 294 (1963); Kaplan v. Haines, 96 N.J.Super. 242, 232 A.2d 840, 845 (1967) aff'd, 51 N.J. 404, 241 A.2d 235 (1968); Govin v. Hunter, 374 P.2d 421, 424 (Wyo.1962). This is not surprising since, as indicated, the majority of American jurisdictions find the source, as well as the scope, of duty to disclose in medical custom. See text *supra* at note 38.
71. Shetter v. Rochelle, *supra* note 70, 409 P.2d at 86.
72. *E.g.*, Ditlow v. Kaplan, *supra* note 70, 181 So.2d at 228; Kaplan v. Haines, *supra* note 70, 232 A.2d at 845.
73. *E.g.*, Williams v. Menehan, *supra* note 70, 379 P.2d at 294; Govin v. Hunter, *supra* note 70, 374 P.2d at 424.
74. See Part III, *supra*.
75. See text *supra* at notes 12–13.
76. See Part III, *supra*.
77. For similar reasons, we reject the suggestion that disclosure should be discretionary with the physician. See Note, 109 U.Pa.L.Rev. 768, 772–73 (1961).
78. See text *supra* at notes 12–15.
79. See Waltz & Scheuneman, Informed Consent to Therapy, 64 N.W.U.L.Rev. 628, 639–41 (1970).
80. See Comment, Informed Consent in Medical Malpractice, 55 Calif.L.Rev. 1396, 1407–10 (1967).
81. See Waltz & Scheuneman, Informed Consent to Therapy, 64 N.W.U.L.Rev. 628, 639–40 (1970).
82. *Id.*
83. *Id.*
84. *Id.* at 640. The category of risks which the physician should communicate is, of course, no broader than the complement he could communicate. See Block v. McVay, 80 S.D. 469, 126 N.W.2d 808, 812 (1964). The duty to divulge may extend to any risk he actually knows, but he obviously cannot divulge any of which he may be unaware. Nondisclosure of an unknown risk does not, strictly speaking, present a problem in terms of the duty to disclose although it very well might pose problems in terms of the physician's duties to have known of it and to have acted accordingly. See Waltz & Scheuneman, Informed Consent to Therapy, 64 N.W.U.L. Rev. 628, 630–35 (1970). We have no occasion to explore problems of the latter type on this appeal.

85. See Comment, Informed Consent in Medical Malpractice, 55 Calif.L.Rev. 1396, 1407 n. 68 (1967).

86. See Bowers v. Talmage, *supra* note 13 (3% chance of death, paralysis or other injury, disclosure required); Scott v. Wilson, 396 S.W.2d 532 (Tex.Civ.App. 1965), aff'd, 412 S.W.2d 299 (Tex.1967) (1% chance of loss of hearing, disclosure required). Compare, where the physician was held not liable. Stottlemire v. Cawood, *supra* note 68, (1/800,000 chance of aplastic anemia); Yeates v. Harms, supra note 68 (1.5% chance of loss of eye); Starnes v. Taylor, 272 N.C. 386, 158 S.E.2d 339, 344 (1968) (1/250 to 1/500 chance of perforation of esophagus).

87. Roberts v. Young, *supra* note 38, 119 N.W.2d at 629–630; Starnes v. Taylor, *supra* note 86, 158 S.E.2d at 344; Comment, Informed Consent in Medical Malpractice, 55 Calif.L.Rev. 1396, 1407 n. 69 (1967); Note, 75 Harv.L.Rev. 1445, 1448 (1962).

88. Yeates v. Harms, *supra* note 68, 393 P. 2d at 991; Fleishman v. Richardson-Merrell, Inc., 94 N.J.Super. 90, 226 A.2d 843, 845–840 (1967). See also Natanson v. Kline, *supra* note 12, 350 P.2d at 1106.

89. See text *supra* at note 84. And compare to the contrary, Oppenheim, Informed Consent to Medical Treatment, 11 Clev.-Mar. L.Rev. 249, 264–65 (1962); Comment, Valid Consent to Medical Treatment: Need the Patient Know?, 4 Duquesne L.Rev. 450, 457–58 (1966), a position we deem unrealistic. On the other hand, we do not subscribe to the view that only risks which would cause the patient to forego the treatment must be divulged, see Johnson, Medical Malpractice—Doctrines of Res Ipsa Loquitur and Informed Consent, 37 U.Colo.L.Rev. 182, 185–91 (1965); Comment, Informed Consent in Medical Malpractice, 55 Calif.L.Rev. 1396, 1407 n. 68 (1967); Note, 75 Harv.L.Rev. 1445, 1446–47 (1962), for such a principle ignores the possibility that while a single risk might not have that *effect*, two or more might do so. Accord, Waltz & Scheuneman, Informed Consent to Therapy. 64 Nw.U.L. Rev. 628, 635–41 (1970).

90. *E.g.*, Bowers v. Talmage, *supra* note 13. 159 So.2d at 889; Aiken v. Clary, *supra* note 38, 396 S.W.2d at 676; Hastings v. Hughes, 59 Tenn.App. 98, 438 S.W.2d 349, 352 (1968).

91. *E.g.*, Dunham v. Wright, *supra* note 13, 423 F.2d at 941–942 (applying Pennsylvania law); Koury v. Follo, 272 N.C. 366, 158 S.E.2d 548, 555 (1968); Woods v. Brumlop, *supra* note 13, 377 P.2d at 525; Gravis v. Physicians & Surgeons Hosp., 415 S.W.2d 674, 677, 678 (Tex.Civ.App.1967).

92. Where the complaint in suit is unauthorized treatment of a patient legally or factually incapable of giving consent, the established rule is that, absent an emergency, the physician must obtain the necessary authority from a relative. See, *e.g.*, Bonner v. Moran, *supra* note 32, 75 U.S.App.D.C. at 157–158, 126 F.2d at 122–123 (15-year old child). See also Koury v. Follo, *supra* note 91 (patient a baby).

93. Compare, *e.g.*, Application of President & Directors of Georgetown College, 118 U.S.App.D.C. 80, 331 F.2d 1000, rehearing en banc denied, 118 U.S.App.D.C. 90, 331 F.2d 1010, cert. denied, Jones v. President and Directors of Georgetown College, Inc., 377 U.S. 978, 84 S.Ct. 1883, 12 L.Ed.2d 746 (1964).

94. See, *e.g.*, Salgo v. Leland Stanford Jr. Univ. Bd. of Trustees, *supra* note 67, 317 P.2d at 181 (1957); Waltz & Scheuneman, Informed Consent to Therapy, 64 Nw.U.L.Rev. 628, 641–43 (1970).

95. *E.g.*, Roberts v. Wood, 206 F.Supp. 579, 583 (S.D.Ala.1962); Nishi v. Hartwell, 52 Haw. 188, 473 P.2d 116, 119 (1970); Woods v. Brumlop, *supra* note 13, 377 P.2d at 525; Ball v. Mallinkrodt Chem. Works, 53 Tenn.App. 218, 381 S.W.2d 563, 567–568 (1964).

96. *E.g.*, Scott v. Wilson, *supra* note 86, 396 S.W.2d at 534–535; Comment, Informed Consent in Medical Malpractice, 55 Calif.L.Rev. 1396, 1409–10 (1967); Note, 75 Harv.L.Rev. 1445, 1448 (1962).

97. See text *supra* at notes 12–13.

98. Note, 75 Harv.L.Rev. 1445, 1448 (1962).

99. See Fiorentino v. Wenger, 26 A.D.2d 693, 272 N.Y.S.2d 557, 559 (1966), appeal dismissed, 18 N.Y.2d 908, 276 N.Y.S. 2d 639, 223 N.E.2d 46 (1966), reversed on other grounds, 19 N.Y.2d 407, 280 N.Y.S.2d 373, 227 N.E.2d 296 (1967). See also note 92, *supra*.

100. Becker v. Colonial Parking, Inc., 133 U.S.App.D.C. 213, 219–220, 409 F.2d 1130, 1136–1137 (1969); Richardson v. Gregory, 108 U.S.App.D.C. 263, 266–267, 281 F.2d 626, 629–630 (1960); Arthur v. Standard Eng'r. Co., 89 U.S.App.D.C. 399, 401, 193 F.2d 903, 905, 32 A.L.R.2d 408 (1951), cert. denied, 343 U.S. 964, 72 S.Ct. 1057, 96 L.Ed. 1361 (1952); Industrial Savs. Bank v. People's Funeral Serv. Corp., 54 App.D.C. 259, 260, 296 F. 1006, 1007 (1924).

101. See Morse v. Moretti, 131 U.S.App.D.C. 158, 403 F.2d 564 (1968); Kosberg v. Washington Hosp. Center, Inc., 129 U.S. App.D.C. 322, 324, 394 F.2d 947, 949 (1968); Levy v. Vaughan, 42 U.S.App.D.C. 146, 153, 157 (1914).

102. Shetter v. Rochelle, *supra* note 70, 409 P.2d at 82–85; Waltz & Scheuneman, Informed Consent to Therapy, 64 Nw.U.L. Rev. 628, 646 (1970).

103. Shetter v. Rochelle, *supra* note 70, 409 P.2d at 83–84. See also Natanson v. Kline, *supra* note 12, 350 P.2d at 1106–1107; Hunter v. Burroughs, *supra* note 7, 96 S.E. at 369.

104. See text *supra* at notes 23–35, 74–79.

105. Plante, An Analysis of "Informed Consent," 36 Fordham L.Rev. 639, 666–67 (1968); Waltz & Scheuneman, Informed Consent to Therapy, 64 Nw.U.L.Rev. 628, 646–48 (1970); Comment, Informed Consent in Medical Malpractice, 55 Calif.L. Rev. 1396, 1411–14 (1967).

106. See text *supra* at notes 12–13.

107. Waltz & Scheuneman, Informed Consent to Therapy, 64 Nw.U.L.Rev. 628, 647 (1970).

108. *Id.* at 647.

109. *Id.* at 646.

110. *Id.* at 648.

111. See cases cited *supra* note 103.

112. See 9 J. Wigmore, Evidence § 2485 (3d ed. 1940).

113. *See, e.g.*, Morse v. Moretti, *supra* note 101, 131 U.S.App.D.C. at 158, 403 F.2d at 564; Kosberg v. Washington Hosp. Center, Inc., *supra* note 101, 129 U.S. App.D.C. at 324, 394 F.2d at 949; Smith v. Reitman, 128 U.S.App.D.C. 352, 353, 389 F.2d 303, 304 (1967).

114. See Part VI, *supra.*
115. See 9 J. Wigmore, Evidence § 2486, 2488, 2489 (3d ed. 1940). See also Raza v. Sullivan, 139 U.S.App.D.C. 184, 186–188, 432 F.2d 617, 619–621 (1970), cert. denied, 400 U.S. 992, 91 S.Ct. 458, 27 L.Ed.2d 440 (1971).
116. See cases cited *infra* note 119.
117. See text *supra* at notes 37–39.
118. See Part IV, *supra.*
119. Lucy Webb Hayes Nat. Training School v. Perotti, *supra* note 56, 136 U.S. App.D.C. at 126–127, 419 F.2d at 708–709 (hospital's failure to install safety glass in psychiatric ward); Alden v. Providence Hosp., 127 U.S.App.D.C. 214, 217, 382 F.2d 163, 166 (1967) (caliber of medical diagnosis); Brown v. Keaveny, *supra* note 16, 117 U.S.App.D.C. at 118, 326 F.2d at 661 (caliber of medical treatment); Quick v. Thurston, *supra* note 16, 110 U.S.App.D.C. at 171–173, 290 F.2d at 362–364 (sufficiency of medical attendance and caliber of medical treatment); Rodgers v. Lawson, *supra* note 16, 83 U.S.App.D.C. at 285–286, 170 F.2d at 161–162 (sufficiency of medical attendance, and caliber of medical diagnosis and treatment); Byrom v. Eastern Dispensary & Cas. Hosp., *supra* note 59, 78 U.S.App.D.C. at 43, 136 F.2d at 279 (caliber of medical treatment), Christie v. Callahan, 75 U.S.App.D.C. 133, 136, 124 F.2d 825, 828 (1941) (caliber of medical treatment); Carson v. Jackson, 52 App.D.C. 51, 55, 281 F. 411, 415 (1922) (caliber of medical treatment).
120. See cases cited *supra* note 119.
121. Lucy Webb Hayes Nat. Training School v. Perotti, *supra* note 56, 136 U.S. App.D.C. at 127–129, 419 F.2d at 709–711 (permitting patient to wander from closed to open section of psychiatric ward); Monk v. Doctors Hosp., *supra* note 56, 131 U.S.App.D.C. at 177, 403 F.2d at 583 (operation of electro-surgical machine); Washington Hosp. Center v. Butler, *supra* note 48 (fall by unattended x-ray patient); Young v. Fishback, 104 U.S.App.D.C. 372, 373, 262 F.2d 469, 470 (1958) (bit of gauze left at operative site); Garfield Memorial Hosp. v. Marshall, supra note 59, 92 U.S.App. D.C. at 240, 204 F.2d at 726 (newborn baby's head striking operating table); Goodwin v. Hertzberg, 91 U.S.App.D.C. 385, 386, 201 F.2d 204, 205 (1952) (perforation of urethra); Byrom v. Eastern Dispensary & Cas. Hosp., *supra* note 59, 78 U.S.App.D.C. at 43, 136 F.2d at 279 (failure to further diagnose and treat after unsuccessful therapy); Grubb v. Groover, 62 App.D.C. 305, 306, 67 F.2d 511, 512 (1933), cert. denied, 291 U.S. 660, 54 S.Ct. 377, 78 L.Ed. 1052 (1934) (burn while unattended during x-ray treatment). See also Furr v. Herzmark, 92 U.S.App.D.C. 350, 353–354, 206 F.2d 468, 470–471 (1953); Christie v. Callahan, *supra* note 119, 75 U.S.App.D.C. at 136, 124 F.2d at 828; Sweeney v. Erving, 35 App.D.C. 57, 62, 43 L.R.A.,N.S. 734 (1910), aff'd, 228 U.S. 233, 33 S.Ct. 416, 57 L.Ed. 815 (1913).
122. See Waltz & Scheuneman, Informed Consent to Therapy, 64 Nw.U.L.Rev. 628, 645, 647 (1970); Comment, Informed Consent in Medical Malpractice, 55 Calif.L.Rev. 1396, 1410–11 (1967).
123. See Waltz & Scheuneman, Informed Consent to Therapy, 64 Nw.U.L.Rev. 628. 639–40 (1970); Comment, Informed Consent in Medical Malpractice, 55 Calif.L. Rev. 1396, 1411 (1967).
124. One of the chief obstacles facing plaintiffs in malpractice cases has been the difficulty, and all too frequently the apparent impossibility, of securing testimony from the medical profession. See, *e.g.,* Washington Hosp. Center v. Butler, *supra* note 48, 127 U.S.App.D.C. at 386 n. 27, 384 F.2d at 338 n. 27; Brown v. Keaveny, *supra* note 16, 117 U.S.App. D.C. at 118, 326 F.2d at 661 (dissenting opinion); Huffman v. Lindquist, 37 Cal.2d 465, 234 P.2d 34, 46 (1951) (dissenting opinion); Comment, Informed Consent in Medical Malpractice, 55 Calif. L.Rev. 1396, 1405–06 (1967); Note, 75 Harv.L.Rev. 1445, 1447 (1962).
125. D.C.Code § 12-301(4) (1967).
126. D.C.Code § 12-301(8), specifying a three-year limitation for all actions not otherwise provided for. Suits seeking damages for negligent personal injury or property damage are in this category. Finegan v. Lumbermens Mut. Cas. Co., 117 U.S.App.D.C. 276, 329 F.2d 231 (1963); Keleket X-Ray Corp. v. United States, 107 U.S.App.D.C. 138, 275 F.2d 167 (1960); Hanna v. Fletcher, 97 U.S. App.D.C. 310, 313, 231 F.2d 469, 472, 58 A.L.R.2d 847, cert. denied, Gichner Iron Works, Inc. v. Hanna, 351 U.S. 989, 76 S.Ct. 1051, 100 L.Ed. 1501 (1956).
127. D.C.Code § 12-302(a) (1) (1967). See also Carson v. Jackson, *supra* note 119, 52 App.D.C. at 53, 281 F. at 413.
128. See cases cited *supra* note 126.
129. See text *supra* at notes 32–36.
130. For discussions of the differences between battery and negligence actions, see, McCoid, A Reappraisal of Liability for Unauthorized Medical Treatment, 41 Minn.L.Rev. 381, 423–25 (1957); Comment, Informed Consent in Medical Malpractice, 55 Calif.L.Rev. 1396, 1399–1400 n. 18 (1967); Note 75 Harv.L.Rev. 1445, 1446 (1962).
131. See Natanson v. Kline, *supra* note 12, 350 P.2d at 1100; Restatement (Second) of Torts §§ 13, 15 (1965).
132. The obligation to disclose, as we have said, is but a part of the physician's general duty to exercise reasonable care for the benefit of his patient. See Part III, *supra.*
133. Thus we may distinguish Morfessis v. Baum, 108 U.S.App.D.C. 303, 305, 281 F. 2d 938, 940 (1960), where an action labeled one for abuse of process was, on analysis, found to be really one for malicious prosecution.
134. See Maercklein v. Smith, 129 Colo. 72, 266 P.2d 1095, 1097–1098 (*en banc* 1954); Hershey v. Peake, 115 Kan. 562, 223 P. 1113 (1924); Mayor v. Dowsett, 240 Or. 196, 400 P.2d 234, 250–251 (*en banc* 1965); McCoid, A Reappraisal of Liability for Unauthorized Medical Treatment, 41 Minn.L.Rev. 381, 424–25, 434 (1957); McCoid, The Care Required of Medical Practitioners, 12 Vand.L.Rev. 586–87 (1959); Plante, An Analysis of "Informed Consent," 36 Fordham L.Rev. 639, 669–71 (1968); Comment, Informed Consent in Medical Malpractice, 55 Calif. L.Rev. 1396, 1399–4100 n. 18 (1967); Note, 75 Harv.L.Rev. 1445, 1446 (1962).
135. See Mellon v. Seymoure, 56 App.D.C. 301, 303, 12 F.2d 836, 837 (1926); Pedesky v. Bleiberg, 251 Cal.App.2d 119, 59 Cal.Rptr. 294 (1967).
136. See text *supra* at notes 81–90.
137. See text *supra* at notes 91–92.

138. See Part VI, *supra*. With appellant's prima facie case of violation of duty to disclose, the burden of introducing evidence showing a privilege was on Dr. Spence. See text *supra* at notes 114115. Dr. Spence's opinion—that disclosure is medically unwise—was expressed as to patients generally, and not with reference to traits possessed by appellant. His explanation was:

> I think that I always explain to patients the operations are serious, and I feel that any operation is serious. I think that I would not tell patients that they might be paralyzed because of the small percentage, one per cent, that exists. There would be a tremendous percentage of people that would not have surgery and would not therefore be benefited by it, the tremendous percentage that get along very well, 99 per cent.

139. See Part VI, *supra*. Since appellant's evidence was that neither he nor his mother was informed by Dr. Spence of the risk of paralysis from the laminectomy, we need not decide whether a parent's consent to an operation on a nineteen-year-old is ordinarily required. Compare Bonner v. Moran, *supra* note 32, 75 U.S.App.D.C. at 157–158, 126 F.2d at 122–123.
140. See Part V, *supra*.
141. Bourne v. Washburn, 142 U.S.App.D.C. 332, 336, 441 F.2d 1022, 1026 (1971); Clark v. Associated Retail Credit Men, 70 App.D.C. 183, 187, 105 F.2d 62, 66 (1939); Baltimore & O. R. R. v. Morgan, 35 App.D.C. 195, 200–201 (1910); Washington A. & M. V. Ry. v. Lukens, 32 App. D.C. 442, 453–454 (1909).
142. 361 U.S. 107, 80 S.Ct. 173, 4 L.Ed.2d 142 (1959).
143. *Id.* at 109–110, 80 S.Ct. at (footnote omitted).
144. Even if Dr. Spence himself made the change, the result would not vary as to the hospital. It was or should have been known by hospital personnel that appellant had just undergone a serious operation. A jury might fairly conclude that at the time of the fall he was in no condition to be left to fend for himself. Compare Washington Hosp. Center v. Butler, *supra* note 48, 127 U.S.App.D.C. at 385, 384 F. 2d at 337.
145. Compare *id.* See also cases cited *supra* note 121.
146. See *id.* at 383–385, 384 F.2d at 335–337.
147. See *id.*
148. Bowman v. Redding & Co., 145 U.S. App.D.C. 294, 305, 449 F.2d 956, 967 (1971).
149. Appellant's remaining points on appeal require no elaboration: He contends that his counsel, not the trial judge, should have conducted the voir dire examination of prospective jurors, but that matter lay within the discretion of the judge, Fed.R. Civ.P. 47(a). He argues that Mrs. Canterbury, a rebuttal witness, should not have been excluded from the courtroom during other stages of the trial. That also was within the trial judge's discretion and, in any event, no prejudice from the exclusion appears. He complains of the trial judge's refusal to admit into evidence bylaws of the hospital pertaining to written consent for surgery, and the judge's refusal to permit two physicians to testify as to medical custom and practice on the same general subject. What we have already said makes it unnecessary for us to deal further with those complaints.

MAKING HEALTH CARE DECISIONS: THE ETHICAL AND LEGAL IMPLICATIONS OF INFORMED CONSENT IN THE PATIENT-PRACTITIONER RELATIONSHIP

INTRODUCTION. *The President's Commission realized that the evolution of the informed consent doctrine was redefining medical ethics. The Commission reviewed the debate that had occurred in the decade since the Canterbury decision and formulated a strong position endorsing informed consent as a process of shared decisionmaking based on mutual respect and participation. It recognized informed consent as necessary to promote self-determination and patient well-being. While affirming informed consent as the notion that adults are entitled to accept or reject health care interventions on the basis of their own personal values, it also recognized that patient choice is not absolute. Such choice is dependent on patients having what the Commission calls "decisionmaking capacity," a concept the Commission is careful to distinguish from the legal status of "competency." The Commission's report sets out the contemporary understanding of the consent doctrine. Parts of the introduction and chapter one, and all of chapters two, three, seven and nine are reprinted in this volume.*

INTRODUCTION

What is informed consent to health care, and why has it assumed such an important place in legal and ethical discussions? Is it merely a rhetorical construct, imposed half-heartedly upon medicine by the law? Or is it perhaps a token of larger changes in the relationship between patients and health care professionals, especially physicians? And why does the concept have such importance in the United States today—because of a particular cultural attachment to independence and autonomy? The growing importance of biomedicine in people's lives? Skepticism over "expertise" in many spheres? Or perhaps some combination of these and other factors?

These were among the basic issues before the President's Commission during its Congressionally mandated study of "the ethical and legal implications of the requirements for informed consent to . . . undergo medical procedures."[1] Rather than embroider the doctrine of informed consent within the confines of the case and statutory law that was its source, the Commission decided early in its study to examine the subject within the broader context of relations and communications between patients and health care professionals. It wished to see whether means could be found to promote a fuller understanding by patients and professionals of their common enterprise, so that patients can participate, on an informed basis and to the extent they care to do so, in making decisions about their health care.

Summary of Conclusions and Recommendations

Before the Commission could consider means of improvement, it had to address the underlying theoretical issues. The ethical foundation of informed consent can be traced to the promotion of two values: personal well-being and

President's Commission for the Study of Ethical Problems in Medicine and Biomedical and Behavioral Research, *Making Health Care Decisions: The Ethical and legal Implications of Informed Consent in the Patient-Practitioner Relationship*, 3 vols. Washington, D.C.: U.S. Government Printing Office, 1982.

self-determination. To ensure that these values are respected and enhanced, the Commission finds that patients who have the capacity to make decisions about their care must be permitted to do so voluntarily and must have all relevant information regarding their condition and alternative treatments, including possible benefits, risks, costs, other consequences, and significant uncertainties surrounding any of this information. This conclusion has several specific implications:

(1) Although the informed consent doctrine has substantial foundations in law, it is essentially an ethical imperative.

(2) Ethically valid consent is a process of shared decisionmaking based upon mutual respect and participation, not a ritual to be equated with reciting the contents of a form that details the risks of particular treatments.

(3) Much of the scholarly literature and legal commentary about informed consent portrays it as a highly rational means of decisionmaking about health care matters, thereby suggesting that it may only be suitable for and applicable to well-educated, articulate, self-aware individuals. Whether this is what the legal doctrine was intended to be or what it has inadvertently become, it is a view the Commission unequivocally rejects. Although subcultures within American society differ in their views about autonomy and individual choice and about the etiology of illness and the roles of healers and patients,[2] a survey conducted for the Commission found a universal desire for information, choice, and respectful communication about decisions.[3] Informed consent must remain flexible, yet the process, as the Commission envisions it throughout this Report, is ethically required of health care practitioners in their relationships with all patients, not a luxury for a few.

(4) Informed consent is rooted in the fundamental recognition—reflected in the legal presumption of competency—that adults are entitled to accept or reject health care interventions on the basis of their own personal values and in furtherance of their own personal goals. Nonetheless, patient choice is not absolute.

- Patients are not entitled to insist that health care practitioners furnish them services when to do so would violate either the bounds of acceptable practice or a professional's own deeply held moral beliefs or would draw on a limited resource on which the patient has no binding claim.
- The fundamental values that informed consent is intended to promote—self-determination and patient well-being—both demand that alternative arrangements for health care decisionmaking be made for individuals who lack substantial capacity to make their own decisions. Respect for self-determination requires, however, that in the first instance individuals be deemed to have decisional capacity, which should not be treated as a hurdle to be surmounted in the vast majority of cases, and that incapacity be treated as a disqualifying factor in the small minority of cases.
- Decisionmaking capacity is specific to each particular decision. Although some people lack this capacity for all decisions, many are incapacitated in more limited ways and are capable of making some decisions but not others. The concept of capacity is best understood and applied in a functional manner. That is, the presence or absence of capacity does not depend on a person's status or on the decision reached, but on that individual's actual functioning in situations in which a decision about health care is to be made.
- Decisionmaking incapacity should be found to exist only when people lack the ability to make decisions that promote their well-being in conformity with their own previously expressed values and preferences.
- To the extent feasible people with no decisionmaking capacity should still be consulted about their own preferences out of respect for them as individuals.

(5) Health care providers should not ordinarily withhold unpleasant information simply because it is unpleasant. The ethical foundations of informed consent allow the withholding of information from patients only when they request that it be withheld or when its disclosure per se would cause substantial detriment to their well-being. Furthermore, the Commission found that most members of the public do not wish to have "bad news" withheld from them.

(6) Achieving the Commission's vision of shared decisionmaking based on mutual respect is ultimately the responsibility of individual health care professionals. However, health care institutions such as hospitals and professional schools have important roles to play in assisting health care professionals in this obligation. The manner in which health care is provided in institutional settings often results in a fragmentation of responsibility that may neglect the human side of health care. To assist in guarding against this, institutional health care providers should ensure that ultimately there is one readily identifiable practitioner responsible for providing information to a particular patient. Although pieces of information may be provided by various people, there should be one individual officially charged with responsibility for ensuring that all the necessary information is communicated and that the patient's wishes are known to the treatment team.

(7) Patients should have access to the information they need to help them understand their conditions and make treatment decisions. To this end the Commission recommends that health care professionals and institutions not only provide information but also assist patients who request additional information to obtain it from relevant sources, including hospital and public libraries.

(8) As cases arise and new legislation is contemplated, courts and legislatures should reflect this view of ethically valid consent. Nevertheless, the Commission does not look to legal reforms as the primary means of bringing about changes in the relationship between health care professionals and patients.

(9) The Commission finds that a number of relatively simple changes in practice could facilitate patient participation in health care decisionmaking. Several specific techniques—such as having patients express, orally or in writing, their understanding of the treatment consented to—deserve further study. Furthermore, additional societal resources need to be committed to improving the human side of health care, which has apparently deteriorated at the same time there have been substantial gains in health care technology. The Department of Health and Human Services, and especially the National Institutes of Health, is an appropriate agency for the development of initiatives and the evaluation of their efficacy in this area.

(10) Because health care professionals are responsible for ensuring that patients can participate effectively in decisionmaking regarding their care, educators have a responsibility to prepare physicians and nurses to carry out this obligation. The Commission therefore concludes that:

- Curricular innovations aimed at preparing health professionals for a process of mutual decisionmaking with patients should be continued and strengthened, with careful attention being paid to the development of methods for evaluating the effectiveness of such innovations.
- Examinations and evaluations at the professional school and national levels should reflect the importance of these issues.
- Serious attention should be paid to preparing health professionals for team practice in order to enhance patient participation and well-being.

(11) Family members are often of great assistance to patients in helping to understand information about their condition and in making decisions about treatment. The Commission recommends that health care institutions and professionals recognize this and judiciously attempt to involve family members in decisionmaking for patients, with due regard for the privacy of patients and for the possibilities for coercion that such a practice may entail.

(12) The Commission recognizes that its vision of health care decisionmaking may involve greater commitments of time on the part of health professionals. Because of the importance of shared decisionmaking based on mutual trust, not only for the promotion of patient well-being and self-determination but also for the therapeutic gains that can be realized, the Commission recommends that all medical and surgical interventions be thought of as including appropriate discussion with patients. Reimbursement to the professional should therefore take account of time spent in discussion rather than regarding it as a separate item for which additional payment is made.

(13) To protect the interests of patients who lack decisionmaking capacity and to ensure their well-being and self-determination, the Commission concludes that:

- Decisions made by others on patients' behalf should, when possible, attempt to replicate the ones patients would make if they were capable of doing so. When this is not feasible, decisions by surrogates on behalf of patients must protect the patients' best interests. Because such decisions are not instances of personal self-choice, limits may be placed on the range of acceptable decisions that surrogates make beyond those that apply when a person makes his or her own decisions.
- Health care institutions should adopt clear and explicit policies regarding how and by whom decisions are to be made for patients who cannot decide.
- Families, health care institutions, and professionals should work together to make health care decisions for patients who lack decisionmaking capacity. Recourse to courts should be reserved for the occasions when concerned parties are unable to resolve their disagreements over matters of substantial import, or when adjudication is clearly required by state law. Courts and legislatures should be cautious about requiring judicial review of routine health care decisions for patients who lack capacity.
- Health care institutions should explore and evaluate various informal administrative arrangements, such as "ethics committees," for review and consultation in nonroutine matters involving health care decisionmaking for those who cannot decide.
- As a means of preserving some self-determination for patients who no longer possess decisionmaking capacity, state courts and legislatures should consider making provision for advance directives through which people designate others to make health care decisions on their behalf and/or give instructions about their care.

The Commission acknowledges that the conclusions contained in this Report will not be simple to achieve. Even when patients and practitioners alike are sensitive to the goal of shared decisionmaking based on mutual respect, substantial barriers will still exist.[4] Some of these obstacles, such as longstanding professional attitudes or difficulties in conveying medical information in ordinary language, are formidable but can be overcome if there is a will to do so. Others, such as the dependent condition of very sick patients or the ever-growing complexity and subspecialization of medicine, will have to be accommodated because they probably cannot be eliminated. Nonetheless, the Commission's vision of informed consent still has value as a measuring stick against which actual performance may be judged and as a goal toward which all participants in health care decisionmaking can strive. . . .

CHAPTER 1

* * *

The Context of Consent

The Commission believes that an analysis of "the ethical and legal implications of requirements for informed consent to . . . undergo medical procedures"[1] is best undertaken in the context of a broader examination of relationships between patients and health care professionals in American society. At issue is the definition of the patient-professional relationship, as well as the appropriate role of formal and informal modes of social regulation in shaping it. Clearly, the resolution of these issues requires more than a simple review of the existing law of informed consent. Thus, the remainder of this Report considers patterns of communication between patients and health care professionals and how decisions are made. These inquiries are framed by the Commission's ultimate question about this aspect of its work: how can a fuller, shared understanding by patient and professional of their common enterprise be promoted, so that patients can participate, on an informed basis and to the extent they care to do so, in making decisions about their health care?

Historical Development While the law has proclaimed, if not always given effect to, such propositions as "Anglo-American law starts with the premise of thorough-going self-determination"[2] and "each man is considered to be his own master,"[3] recent scholarship has suggested that such sentiments have played little role in traditional health care and are indeed antithetical to the proclaimed norms of the medical profession.[4] Medical skepticism of patients' capacities for self-determination can be traced to the time of Hippocrates:

> Perform [these duties] calmly and adroitly, concealing most things from the patient while you are attending to him. Give necessary orders with cheerfulness and sincerity, turning his attention away from what is being done to him; sometimes reprove sharply and emphatically, and sometimes comfort with solicitude and attention, revealing nothing of the patient's future or present condition.[5]

These attitudes continued to be reflected both in professional codes of ethics and in influential scholarly writings on medical ethics throughout the nineteenth and early twentieth centuries, and indeed survive to this day.[6] Studies of the records of daily medical practice (rather than normative statements of professional ethics) have found distinct "indigenous medical traditions" of truth-telling and consent-seeking, grounded on the theory that such knowledge "had demonstrably beneficial effects on most patients' health."[7] But little evidence exists that such traditions combined in anything like the modern doctrine of informed consent. Nor did they derive from or imply any commitment by the medical profession to patient autonomy. Indeed, when patients' wishes regarding treatment were respected it was largely because providers recognized their limited therapeutic capabilities and the substantial risks accompanying medical interventions (for example, surgery without antiseptic) as well as the impracticability of forcing treatments on resisting patients.[8]

Contemporary Trends Recent changes in health care practices, as well as broader societal changes in contemporary American life, have led to an intense reexamination of relationships between patients and health care practitioners. Gradually, a new understanding of the proper levels and limits of health care is emerging; from this flow changes in the relative rights and obligations of patients and professionals concerning matters such as disclosure and consent for medical interventions.

Perhaps the most significant single factor in this process is the emergence of the scientific, technological approach to medical care over the course of the past century. The rapidly evolving technical prowess of medicine has, of course, brought with it improved health, greater quality and length of life, and new sources of hope for the ill. This revolution in the capacities of medicine has also had profound effects on the structure of the health care delivery system and on the nature of the patient-professional relationship.

Several of these changes are particularly relevant to informed consent. First, health care is now provided in a vast array of settings, ranging from home visits by traditional family doctors to clinics, health maintenance organizations, and multispecialty group practices, to nursing homes and other long-term or chronic care facilities, to high-technology tertiary care centers. Care is frequently provided by teams of highly specialized professionals whose individual responsibilities may be defined less by the overall needs of the patient than by particular diseases or organ systems. When this occurs there may be no single professional in effective command of the entire care of the patient, no one who knows the patient well and to whom the patient may turn for information, advice, and comfort. In such instances the health care system's increased capacity and determination to overcome a disease or defect may be accompanied by a diminished capacity and inclination to care for the patient in more human terms.[9]

Such situations pose a far more serious threat to patient well-being and autonomy than any formal disclosure of remote risks on informed consent forms could possibly remedy. Indeed, the Commission believes that serious efforts by health care institutions to ensure that patients have one identifiable and reliable source of information concerning their care would do far more to remedy the current ills of the health care system than would legal prescriptions with which compliance can be neither assumed nor enforced.[10]

The expanded potential of medicine has also widened the range of choices about health care. Increasingly, the question is not simply whether to accept a single intervention that is available for a particular condition, but which intervention to choose. Often the alternatives vary markedly in their prospects for success, their intrusiveness, their potential side effects, and their other implications for patients' ability to conduct their lives as they see fit. A determination of what is "indicated" is thus inextricably intertwined with the needs and values of the particular patient.

These changes in medicine have been accompanied by broader trends in American society and culture that have reinforced their impact. Since the early 1960s there has been an extraordinary emphasis on the rights of citizens to direct the course of their lives, from voting rights to consumer rights. This stress on the individual has been coupled with a skepticism toward claims of specialized expertise and a suspicion of powerful institutions and the "establishment." Health care has not escaped its share of criticism in the process.

Some commentators have seen in these trends the basis for a new view of the role of medicine and the nature of the patient-provider relationship:

> The traditional paternal model of medicine was premised on trust in the physician's technical competence and moral sensitivity and was characterized by patient dependency and physician control. This model is being replaced gradually by one in which patients are increasingly involved in decisionmaking concerning their own medical care. The rise of consumerism and the associated emergence of "rights" language in medicine has encouraged some individuals to view medicine as a "serving" profession and to regard themselves not as patients but as "medical consumers." Such "medical consumers" sometimes wish to invert the traditional model of medicine and to make the physician a passive agent, a hired technician who practices under the direction and control of his "client." However, despite these changes which affect some patients and some physicians, many patients and physicians continue to interact in a fairly traditional, paternalistic physician-patient relationship.[11]

The survey done for the Commission lends support to the conclusion that changes are occurring in the relationship between physicians and patients. Compared with previous studies, the current results demonstrate a clear sense of physicians' responsibilities for making disclosures and reaching mutual decisions.[12] Although the results from the separate surveys of the public and of physicians indicate substantial agreement on these expectations, some lack of congruence remains. Moreover, the observational studies done for the Commission make it apparent that in actual relationships even more divergence occurs between laypeople's and professionals' expectations.

The role of the health care professional thus appears to be in a "phase of incomplete redefinition," as one Commission witness noted.[13] During this time "judgments of conscientious persons have become divergent and perplexed" and societal consensus does not exist.[14] No longer are the proper ends and limits of health care commonly understood and broadly accepted; a new concept of health care, characterized by changing expectations and uncertain understanding between patient and practitioner, is evolving. The need to find an appropriate balance of the rights and responsibilities of patients and health care professionals in this time of change has been called "the critical challenge facing medicine in the coming decades."[15]

The Commission's View

Two models of the patient-professional relationship have dominated the debate surrounding this challenge. For the sake of simplicity, while recognizing the caricatures involved, these may be referred to as "medical paternalism" and "patient sovereignty." Medical paternalism is based on a traditional view of health professionals—typically physicians—as the dominant, authoritarian figure in the relationship, with both the right and the responsibility to make decisions in the medical best interests of the patient. In reaction to this view, some have sought to take over the physician's dominant position. Proponents of maximal patient sovereignty assign patients full responsibility for and control over all decisions about their own care. According to this view, practitioners should act as servants of their patients, transmitting medical information and using their technical skills as the patient directs, without seeking to influence the patient's decisions, much less actually make them.

Both positions attempt to vest exclusive moral agency, ethical wisdom, and decisionmaking authority on one side of the relationship, while assigning the other side a dependent role. In the view of the Commission, neither extreme adequately reflects the current nature and needs of health care. The debate has increasingly become an arid exercise, which the Commission believes should be replaced by a view that reflects the tremendous diversity of health care situations and relationships today. In this Report, the Commission attempts to shift the terms of the discussion toward how to foster a relationship between patients and professionals characterized by mutual participation and respect and by shared decisionmaking. The Commission believes such a shift in focus will do better justice to the realities of health care and to the ethical values underlying the informed consent doctrine.

Although described in a single phrase, the Commission's view is intended to encompass a multitude of different realities, each one shaped by the particular medical encounter and each one subject to change as the participants move toward accommodation through the process of shared decisionmaking:

> The nature of the patient involved—his personality, character, attitude, and values—and the factors which led him to seek a

medical encounter with this particular physician are central components of the process. Similarly, the personality, character, attitude, values, and technical skills of the physician affect the accommodation. Further, the quality of the interaction between patient and physician—the chemistry of the interaction—modify the process. Of course, the nature of the medical problem, including its type, acuteness, gravity, and its potential for remediation, will be a major determinant of whether a physician-patient accommodation is achieved. For example, the entire process will be modified profoundly and telescoped if the patient is acutely or critically ill and alternative medical resources are unavailable. Finally, other considerations which may affect the achievement of a physician-patient accommodation include the clinical setting, *e.g.*, a hospital, doctor's office, or the patient's home; the organization of the medical service, Health Maintenance Organization, or fee-for-service; and also, occasionally, the claims of relevant third party interests such as those of family, insurers, or the state.[16]

At each point, the patient and physician will arrive at a joint decision in which the physician agrees to care for the patient and the patient agrees to be treated by the physician. The particular resolution of rights and responsibilities reached at a given point of the relationship may change with time and circumstances. The resiliency of the relationship will depend importantly on the extent of trust and confidence exchanged between patient and professional.[17]

Whether society should accept whatever accommodation the parties agree to regarding the communication process and the allocation of decisionmaking authority is a complex issue. It raises the question of whether patient-professional relationships are best seen as purely contractual ones, subject to modification solely on the basis of agreement by the parties, or are instead invested with a certain public interest that justifies the imposition by society of limits on the acceptable range of consensual arrangements. The contractual view has strong roots in American traditions of voluntarism and individual responsibility. Yet for reasons of history, tradition, expectations, and disparities in educational, class, and health status, patients and professionals often start out on substantially unequal footing, raising serious questions about the ability of many patients to have an effective role in shaping the relationship.

Through law, American society has regulated relationships between patients and health care practitioners for almost a century. The control of advertising by doctors (to prevent the deception of unknowing patients) and the licensing of practitioners (to prohibit quackery and establish minimum standards of expertise) are some of the earliest examples. Medical malpractice law and criminal law also establish some limits on the freedom of practitioners in the interests of patients. Informed consent is merely one of the newer ways that society places some limits on the range of relationships between patients and practitioners.

The Commission concludes that considerable flexibility should be accorded to patients and professionals to define the terms of their own relationships. The resolution favored by the Commission is a presumption that certain fundamental types of information should be made available to patients and that all patients competent to do so have a right to accept or reject medical interventions affecting them. Similarly, a professional who has been as flexible about possible avenues of treatment as his or her beliefs and standards allow is not generally obligated to accede to the patient in a way that violates the bounds of acceptable medical practice or the provider's own deeply held moral beliefs.

Nevertheless, in light of the disparities between the positions of the parties, the interaction should, at a minimum, provide the patient with a basis for effective participation in sound decisionmaking regardless of the particular form of the accommodation. It will usually consist of discussions between professional and patient that bring the knowledge, concerns, and perspective of each to the process of seeking agreement on a course of treatment.[18] Simply put, this means that the physician or other health professional invites the patient to participate in a dialogue in which the professional seeks to help the patient understand the medical situation and available courses of action, and the patient conveys his or her concerns and wishes.[19] This does not involve a mechanical recitation of abstruse medical information, but should include disclosures that give the patient an understanding of his or her condition and an appreciation of its consequences.

The Commission encourages, to perhaps a greater degree than is explicitly recognized by current law, the ability of patients and health care professionals to vary the style and extent of discussion from that mandated by this general presumption. Such variations might take any of several directions: in one relationship, the patient might prefer not to be burdened by detailed discussion of risks unlikely to arise or to affect the decision; in another relationship, a patient might request unusually detailed information on unconventional alternative therapies; in a third, a patient with a longstanding and close relationship of trust with a particular physician might ask that physician to proceed as he or she thinks best, choosing the course of therapy and revealing any information that the physician thinks would best serve the interests of the patient. Inherent in allowing such variations is the difficulty of ensuring they are genuinely agreeable to both parties and do not themselves arise out of an imbalance in status or bargaining power.

The health professional's expert knowledge, focused through the particular diagnosis and prognosis for the patient, usually confers on that person the natural role of leader and initiator in building this shared understanding. The patient, on the other hand, is especially well placed to assess the overall effects of the medical condition and possible treatments, in light of his or her own particular goals and values. Thus each party brings to the relationship special knowledge and perspectives that can help to clarify for both parties what is actually at issue in any decision to be reached.

The Commission is aware that its description of mutual participation and shared decisionmaking sets a high ideal. Both professional and patient in this dialogue are liable to misunderstandings and confusions, false hope or despair, unvoiced fears, anxiety, and questions. Even when each is sensitive to the presence of these barriers to full understanding and seeks to surmount them in the interest of agreeing on their common venture—that is, treating the patient successfully—difficulties will persist. Yet it remains a goal worth striving toward. In this Report the Commission not only fills out the contours of the concept sketched here but also explores its roots in basic values and in contemporary opinion and its implications for the education of health professionals, the delivery of care, the attitudes of patients and providers, and the rules of society as expressed through the law.

CHAPTER 2: THE VALUES UNDERLYING INFORMED CONSENT

What are the values that ought to guide decisionmaking in the provider-patient relationship or by which the success of a particular interaction can be judged? The Commission finds two to be central: promotion of a patient's well-being and respect for a patient's self-determination.[1] Before turning to the components of informed consent (Part Two of this Report) or the means for promoting its achievement (Part Three), these central values will be explored. They are in many ways compatible, but their potential for conflict in actual practice must be recognized.[2]

Serving the Patient's Well-Being

Therapeutic interventions are intended first and foremost to improve a patient's health. In most circumstances, people agree in a general way on what "improved health" means. Restoration of normal functioning (such as the repair of a fractured limb) and avoidance of untimely death (such as might occur without the use of antibiotics to control life-threatening infections in otherwise healthy persons) are obvious examples. Health care is, in turn, usually a means of promoting patients' well-being. The connection between a particular health care decision and an individual's well-being is not perfect, however. First, the definition of health can be quite controversial: does wrinkled skin or uncommonly short stature constitute impaired health, such that surgical repair or growth hormone is appropriate? Even more substantial variation can be found in ranking the importance of health with other goals in an individual's life. For some, health is a paramount value; for others—citizens who volunteer in time of war, nurses who care for patients with contagious diseases, hang-glider enthusiasts who risk life and limb—a different goal sometimes has primacy.

Absence of Objective Medical Criteria Even the most mundane case—in which there is little if any disagreement that some intervention will promote health—may well have no objective medical criteria that specify a single best way to achieve the goal. A fractured limb can be repaired in a number of ways; a life-threatening infection can be treated with a variety of antibiotics; mild diabetes is subject to control by diet, by injectable natural insulin, or by oral synthetic insulin substitutes. Health care professionals often reflect their own value preferences when they favor one alternative over another; many are matters of choice, dictated neither by biomedical principles or data nor by a single, agreed-upon professional standard.

In the Commission's survey it was clear that professionals recognize this fact: physicians maintained that decisional authority between them and their patients should depend on the nature of the decision at hand. Thus, for example, whether a pregnant woman over 35 should have amniocentesis was viewed as largely a patient's decision, whereas the decision of which antibiotic to use for strep throat was seen as primarily up to the doctor. Furthermore, on the question of whether to continue aggressive treatment for a cancer patient with metastases in whom such treatment had already failed, two-thirds of the physicians felt it was not a scientific, medical decision, but one that turned principally on personal values. And the same proportion felt the decision should be made jointly (which 64% of the doctors claimed it usually was).

Patient's Reasonable Subjective Preferences Determining what constitutes health and how it is best promoted also requires knowledge of patients' subjective preferences. In pursuit of the other goals and interests besides health that society deems legitimate, patients may prefer one type of medical intervention to another, may opt for no treatment at all, or may even request some treatment when a practitioner would prefer to follow a more conservative course that involved, at least for the moment, no medical intervention. For example, a slipped disc may be treated surgically or with medications and bed rest. Which treatment is better can be unclear, even to a physician. A patient may prefer surgery because, despite its greater risks, in the past that individual has spent considerable time in bed and become demoralized and depressed. A person with an injured knee, when told that surgery has about a 30% chance of reducing pain but almost no chance of eliminating it entirely, may prefer to leave the condition untreated. And a baseball pitcher with persistent inflammation of the elbow may prefer to take cortisone on a continuing basis even though the doctor suggests that a new position on the team would eliminate the inflammation permanently. In each case the goals and interests of particular patients incline them in different directions not only as to how, but even as to whether, treatment should proceed.

Given these two considerations—the frequent absence of objective medical criteria and the legitimate subjective preferences of patients—ascertaining whether a health care intervention will, if successful, promote a patient's well-being is a matter of individual judgment. Societies that respect personal freedom usually reach such decisions by leaving the judgment to the person involved.

The Boundaries of Health Care This does not mean, however, that well-being and self-determination are really just two terms for the same value. For example, when an individual (such as a newborn baby) is unable to express a choice, the value that guides health care decisionmaking is the promotion of well-being—not necessarily an easy task but also certainly not merely a disguised form of self-determination.

Moreover, the promotion of well-being is an important value even in decisions about patients who can speak for themselves because the boundaries of the interventions that health professionals present for consideration are set by the concept of well-being. Through societal expectations and the traditions of the professions, health care providers are committed to helping patients and to avoiding harm. Thus, the well-being principle circumscribes the range of alternatives offered to patients: informed consent does not mean that patients can insist upon anything they might want. Rather, it is a choice among medically accepted and available options, all of which are believed to have some possibility of promoting the patient's welfare, including always the option of no further medical interventions, even when that would not be viewed as preferable by the health care providers.

In sum, promotion of patient well-being provides the primary warrant for health care. But, as indicated, well-being is not a concrete concept that has a single definition or that is solely within the competency of health care providers to define. Shared decisionmaking requires that a practitioner seek not only to understand each patient's needs and develop reasonable alternatives to meet those needs but also to present the alternatives in a way that enables patients to choose one they prefer. To participate in this process, patients must engage in a dialogue with the practitioner and make their views on well-being clear. The majority of physicians (56%) and the public (64%) surveyed by the Commission felt that increasing the patient's role in medical decisionmaking would improve the quality of health care.[3]

Since well-being can be defined only within each individual's experience, it is in most circumstances congruent to self-determination, to which the Report now turns.

Respecting Self-Determination

Self-determination (sometimes termed "autonomy") is an individual's exercise of the capacity to form, revise, and pursue personal plans for life.[4] Although it clearly has a much broader application, the relevance of self-determination in health care decisions seems undeniable. A basic reason to honor an individual's choices about health care has already emerged in this Report: under most circumstances the outcome that will best promote the person's well-being rests on a subjective judgment about the individual. This can be termed the instrumental value of self-determination.

More is involved in respect for self-determination than just the belief that each person knows what's best for him or herself, however. Even if it could be shown that an expert (or a computer) could do the job better, the worth of the individual, as acknowledged in Western ethical traditions and especially in Anglo-American law, provides an independent—and more important—ground for recognizing self-determination as a basic principle in human relations, particularly when matters as important as those raised by health care are at stake. This noninstrumental aspect can be termed the intrinsic value of self-determination.

Intrinsic Value of Self-Determination The value of self-determination readily emerges if one considers what is lost in its absence. If a physician selects a treatment alternative that satisfies a patient's individual values and goals rather than allowing the patient to choose, the absence of self-determination has not interfered with the promotion of the patient's well-being. But unless the patient has requested this course of conduct, the individual will not have been shown proper respect as a person nor provided with adequate protection against arbitrary, albeit often well-meaning, domination by others. Self-determination can thus be seen as both a shield and a sword.

Freedom from interference. Self-determination as a shield is valued for the freedom from outside control it is intended to provide. It manifests the wish to be an instrument of one's own and "not of other men's acts of will."[5] In the context of health care, self-determination overrides practitioner-determination even if providers were able to demonstrate that they could (generally or in a specific instance) accurately assess the treatment an informed patient would choose. To permit action on the basis of a professional's assessment rather than on a patient's choice would deprive the patient of the freedom not to be forced to do something—whether or not that person would agree with the choice. Moreover, denying self-determination in this way risks generating the frustration people feel when their desires are ignored or countermanded.

The potential for dissatisfaction in this regard is great. In the Commission's survey, 72% of the public said that they would prefer to make decisions jointly with their physicians after treatment alternatives have been explained. In contrast, 88% of the physicians believe that patients want doctors to choose for them the best alternative. Despite these differences in perception, only 7% of the public reports dissatisfaction with their doctors' respect for their treatment preferences.[6]

Creative self-agency. As a sword, self-determination manifests the value that Western culture places on each person having the freedom to be a creator—"a subject, not an object."[7] Within the broad framework of personal characteristics fixed during the years of development, individuals define their own particular values.[8] In these ways, individuals are capable of creating their own character and of taking responsibility for the kind of person they are. Respect for self-determination thus promotes personal integration within a chosen life-style.

This is an especially important goal to be nourished regarding health care. If it is not fostered regarding such personal matters, it may not arise generally regarding public matters. The sense of personal responsibility for decisionmaking is one of the wellsprings of a democracy. Similarly, when people feel little real power over their lives—in the economy, in political affairs, or even in their daily interactions with other people and institutions—it is not surprising that they are passive in encounters with health care professionals.

If people have been able to form their own values and goals, are free from manipulation, and are aware of information relevant to the decision at hand, the final aspect of self-determination is simply the awareness that the choice is their own to make. Although the reasons for a choice cannot always be defined, decisions are still autonomous if they reflect someone's own purposes rather than external causes unrelated to the person's "self." Consequently, the Commission's concept of health care decisionmaking includes informing patients of alternative courses of treatment and of the reasoning behind all recommendations. Self-determination involves more than choice; it also requires knowledge.

The importance of information to self-determination emerged in the Commission's study of treatment refusals in hospitals. There it was found that, regarding routine treatments, information was frequently so lacking that patient self-determination was compromised.

> Often patients were not told what treatment or procedure had been ordered for them, much less asked to decide whether or not to accept it. The purpose of the procedure was frequently obscure and the risks commonly went unmentioned. Presentation of alternatives was extraordinarily rare. The main concern of the patients we interviewed was not to select the best treatment from those available, but to find out what was being selected for them and why.[9]

Implications of Self-Determination Despite the importance of self-determination, its exercise is sometimes impermissible and at other times impossible. That is, society sometimes must impose restrictions on the range of acceptable patient choices; at other times, patients either cannot, or at least do not, exercise self-determination.

External limitations. Two restrictions are recognized on the range of patient decisions that should be respected. First, some objectives are so contrary to the public interest or the interests of others that society bars the use of medical interventions toward these ends. For example, physicians may not assist patients in criminal activity (such as defacing fingertips so they will not leave identifiable fingerprints). The professional norms or moral integrity of health care professionals (individually, or collectively in health care institutions) may also conflict with the desires of a patient. When this occurs, the practitioner must first reexamine his or her own beliefs and preconceptions. If the proposed intervention would actually compromise the provider's integrity or standards, the patient will either have to accept the limitation on available interventions or seek another health care provider. Finally, a particular treatment preferred by a patient occasionally calls on very scarce resources that society (or some legitimate resource-controlling segment of the health care system) has decided to allocate to another use. Even as a "sword," self-determination does not invest a patient with rights to demand use of resources that have legitimately been allocated to others—as in the case, for example, of a patient who cannot have elective surgery on a desired date because all beds in a hospital are being used by disaster victims.

A second limitation on self-determination arises when a person's decisionmaking is so defective or mistaken that the decision fails to promote the person's own values or goals. This can happen in many ways: someone could fail to understand relevant information, such as the risks of a particular treatment, or unconsciously distort unpleasant information, such as the frightening diagnosis of cancer, and so forth. For example, a man in the prime of a full and rewarding life who has great plans for the future suddenly suffers a myocardial infarction in the middle of a poker game in which he has already won handsomely. Yet he refuses to permit himself to be transported to a hospital because he wants to play out his hand. The quality of his decisionmaking capacity is certainly in doubt. If his expressed wishes are respected nonetheless, the results in terms of self-determination would be mixed. Self-determination would be promoted in the sense that he has made the decision for himself, as opposed to having someone else make it, but self-determination would be contravened in that the decision is not the one that would best advance the man's apparent wish to live a long, full life.

Self-determination is valuable in both its roles—in letting an individual be his or her own decisionmaker and in securing each person's own goals. In situations where there is a choice of respecting the individual's decision or overriding it—that is, of favoring one aspect of self-determination at the expense of the other—overriding an individual decision is usually justified on the ground of promotion of well-being rather than of respect for self-choice.[10]

The absence of contemporaneous choice. Sometimes people anticipate that they will be unable to participate in future decisions about their own health care. A patient, for example, may be under anesthesia during surgery at a time when diagnostic tests force a decision about a further operation. Similarly, patients with an early diagnosis of senile dementia of the Alzheimer's type can expect that their physical functioning might continue long after they are mentally incapable of deciding about care. Through an "advance directive" such people can specify the types of care they want (or do not want) to receive or the person they want to make such decisions if they are unable to do so.[11] Honoring such a directive shows respect for self-determination in that it fulfills two of its three underlying values.

First, following a directive, particularly one that gives specific instructions about types of acceptable and unacceptable interventions, fulfills the instrumental role of self-determination by providing reassurance that a course of conduct promotes the patient's subjective, individual evaluation of well-being. Second, honoring the directive shows respect for the patient as a person. To disregard it would be nearly as great an insult as to disregard the wishes of a patient who expresses them at that time.

An advance directive does not, however, provide self-determination in the sense of active moral agency by the patient on his or her own behalf.[12] Although any discussion between patient and health care professional leading up to a directive would involve active participation and shared decisionmaking, that would have been in the past by the time the decision actually needs to be made about the patient's health care. At that point, there is no "self," in the active, mental sense, to determine what should be done.

Consequently, self-determination is involved when a patient establishes a way to project his or her wishes into a time of anticipated incapacity. Yet it is a sense of self-determination lacking in one important attribute: active, contemporaneous personal choice. Hence a decision not to follow an advance directive may sometimes be justified even when it would not be ethical to disregard a competent patient's contemporaneous choice.[13]

Active participation. Because patient noninvolvement in treatment decisions occurs frequently in medical care,[14] it is important to understand whether it is compatible with patient self-determination. First and foremost, patients must be aware that they are entitled to make a decision about treatment rather than merely acquiescing in a professional's recommendation. Some patients feel, for example, that making a particular treatment decision will cause them great distress, or that the complexity and uncertainty of certain decisions make them poor decisionmakers and that trusted physicians or family members would be more likely to choose the treatment most in accord with the patients' own goals and values. Alternatively, some patients simply wish others to decide so that they can spend their time and energy on other matters. This, too, could constitute a transfer of the right to decide.

In contrast, some patients defer to physicians because they believe they have no business interfering in the exercise of medical judgment. Such patients do not think they are transferring their "right to decide" to a physician because they do not in the first place believe they have any right to decide about medical treatment. This is not an exercise of self-determination. Rather, self-determination occurs when patients understand decisions are theirs to make—and also to countermand if they are dissatisfied.[15] In other words, self-determination requires that patients either make a choice or actually give the decisionmaking authority to another, not merely fail to act out of fear or ignorance of their rights.[16]

In recognizing that a self-determining person may waive active involvement in each decision, the Commission does not intend to belittle the moral ideal of the free, self-governing person who attempts to make decisions responsibly by applying his or her own values to relevant facts during deliberations about alternative actions. The ideal certainly justifies encouraging patients to play an active part in treatment decisions and argues for structuring medical practices and institutions in ways that facilitate and encourage effective patient participation. Nevertheless, it remains a moral *ideal*—people may strive to meet it but will often fall short of it. The principle of self-determination, the bedrock on which the Commission's concept of shared decisionmaking in health care rests, is best understood as respecting people's right to define and pursue their own view of what is good, which is compatible with people freely giving to others the authority to make particular health care decisions for them.

CHAPTER 3: DECISIONMAKING CAPACITY AND VOLUNTARINESS

Effective patient participation in health care decisionmaking rests on three foundations that correspond to the traditionally accepted elements of legally effective informed consent: decisionmaking capacity and voluntariness, which are treated in this Chapter, and information, which is discussed in Chapter Four. Throughout, the goals articulated by the Commission are compared with the realities of present practice, as evidenced by the Commission's studies and other empirical reports.

Capacity to Make Particular Decisions

For patients to participate effectively in making decisions about their health care, they must possess the mental, emotional, and legal capacity to do so. In the Commission's view, decisionmaking capacity is specific to a particular decision and depends not on a person's status (such as age) or on the decision reached, but on the person's actual functioning in situations in which a decision about health care is to be made. Some patients clearly possess such a capacity; others just as clearly lack it. In obvious instances of decisionmaking incapacity—for example, with infants and young children, the comatose, the severely mentally handicapped, and the severely mentally ill[1]—the responsibility of the health care professional is to recognize the incapacity and to find another way to reach a decision that will advance the patient's goals and interests. Such alternative means of decisionmaking are discussed in Part Four of this Report.

In other instances, a patient's capacity to decide on a course of treatment will be less clear-cut. Professionals may initially be uncertain of a particular patient's decisionmaking capacity. In such cases, the situation should be evaluated over time, as care providers assess the patient's understanding of information and reasoning about possible treatment. Efforts can also be made to enhance the patient's capacity by counseling, providing more information, minimizing untoward effects of psychoactive drugs, and giving other forms of support. Ultimately, however, someone must decide whether the patient is capable of making a particular decision that should then have binding force.

Questions of capacity to make health care decisions may be raised from several perspectives. The law treats the issue under the heading of "competence" and generally presumes that adults can make decisions for themselves unless they have been formally judged to be incompetent.[2] Consent granted by a competent adult normally authorizes a practitioner to provide health care, whereas consent granted by an incompetent individual is usually not legally sufficient to authorize professionals to proceed. Similarly, a competent individual's refusal of treatment as a rule has legal effect and must be respected,[3] but the refusal of a treatment by an incompetent patient lacks such legal effect (although it may be taken into account in deciding how to proceed).

The legal tests and standards governing determinations of incompetence are discussed elsewhere in this Report,[4] and are not the primary concern here. Rather, the objective is to explain why the patient's capacity to make health care decisions is important to a sound decision, and to investigate the foundations of that decisionmaking capacity.[5]

Importance of Capacity The doctrine of informed consent is founded on the premise that self-determination ought not be blind. That is, patients' interests and well-being are best served when patients understand their medical situation and participate in deciding on treatment or care. This premise is to some degree an empirical proposition and to some degree a statement of faith. Insofar as the premise is an empirical one, there are clearly patients to whom it does not apply. That is to say, some patients (for a variety of reasons) are simply unable to make decisions that will advance their own interests. Following the directives of such patients can be seriously injurious to their well-being and may fail to respect their own long-term values and objectives.

By not applying informed consent norms to patients who are incapable of joining with professionals to decide on their health care, society seeks to enhance their well-being by protecting them from substantial harms (or loss of benefits) that could result from serious defects in their decisionmaking abilities. The Commission believes that most people would desire such protection if they lost their capacity to participate effectively in medical decisionmaking, and concludes that such societal protection of the well-being of its members is, in principle, appropriate.

Society's protection does, however, impose certain costs—costs that become particularly clear when the action results in the countermanding or disregard of the expressed preferences of a patient deemed to lack capacity to make a particular decision. At least to some degree, such protection infringes on the patient's ability to determine his or her own fate. Thus, a conclusion about a patient's decisionmaking capacity necessarily reflects a balancing of two important, sometimes competing objectives: to enhance the patient's well-being and to respect the person as a self-determining individual. Commentators have sometimes failed to recognize this balancing element, viewing "capacity" or "competence" as having intrinsic meaning apart from consideration of particular circumstances or situations. Although this view may be appropriate in some instances (with, for example, the comatose or infants and small children), the Commission believes it is inadequate in more ambiguous or troublesome instances. The Commission concludes, therefore, that determinations of incapacity to participate in medical decisionmaking should reflect the balance of possibly competing interests.

Elements of Capacity In the view of the Commission, any determination of the capacity to decide on a course of treatment must relate to the individual abilities of a patient, the requirements of the task at hand, and the consequences likely to flow from the decision. Decisionmaking capacity requires, to greater or lesser degree: (1) possession of a set of values and goals[6]; (2) the ability to communicate and to understand information; and (3) the ability to reason and to deliberate about one's choices.

The first, a framework for comparing options, is needed if the person is to evaluate possible outcomes as good or bad. The framework, and the values that it embodies, must be reasonably stable; that is, the patient must be able to make reasonably consistent choices. Reliance on a patient's decision would be difficult or impossible if the patient's values were so unstable that the patient could not reach or adhere to a choice at least long enough for a course of therapy to be initiated with some prospect of being completed.

The second element includes the ability to give and receive information, as well as the possession of various linguistic and conceptual skills needed for at least a basic understanding of the relevant information. These abilities can be evaluated only as they relate to the task at hand and are not solely cognitive, as they ordinarily include emotive elements.[7] To use them, a person also needs sufficient life experience to appreciate the meaning of potential alternatives: what it would probably be like to undergo various medical procedures, for example, or to live in a new way required by a medical condition or intervention.[8]

Some critics of the doctrine of informed consent have argued that patients simply lack the ability to understand medical information relevant to decisions about their care.[9] Indeed, some empirical studies purport to have demonstrated this by showing that the lay public often does not know the meaning of common medical terms,[10] or by showing that, following an encounter with a physician, patients are unable to report what the physician said about their illness and treatment.[11] Neither type of study establishes the fact that patients cannot understand. The first merely finds that they do not currently know the right definitions of some terms; the second, which usually fails to discover what the physician actually did say, rests its conclusions on an assumption that information was provided that was subsequently not understood. In the Commission's own survey, physicians were asked: "What percentage of your patients would you say are able to understand most aspects of their treatment and condition if reasonable time and effort are devoted to explanation?" Overall, 48% of physicians reported that 90–100% of their patients could understand and an additional 34% said that 70–89% could understand.[12]

The third element of decisionmaking capacity—reasoning and deliberation—includes the ability to compare the impact of alternative outcomes on personal goals and life plans. Some ability to employ probabilistic reasoning about uncertain outcomes is usually necessary, as well as the ability to give appropriate weight in a present decision to various future outcomes.

Standards for Assessing Capacity The actual measurement of these various abilities is by no means simple. Virtually all conscious adults can perform some tasks but not others.[13] In the context of informed consent, what is critical is a patient's capacity to make a specific medical decision. An assessment of an individual's capacity must consider the nature of the particular decisionmaking process in light of the these developments: Does the patient possess the ability to understand the relevant facts and alternatives? Is the patient weighing the decision within a framework of values and goals? Is the patient able to reason and deliberate about this information? Can the patient give reasons for the decision, in light of the facts, the alternatives, and the impact of the decision on the patient's own goals and values?

To be sure, a patient may possess these abilities but fail to exercise them well; that is, the decision may be the result of a mistaken understanding of the facts or a defective reasoning process. In such instances, the obligation of the professional is not to declare, on the basis of a "wrong" decision, that the patient lacks decisionmaking capacity, but rather to work with the patient toward a fuller and more accurate understanding of the facts and a sound reasoning process.

How deficient must a decisionmaking process be to justify the assessment that a patient lacks the capacity to make a particular decision? Since the assessment must balance possibly competing considerations of well-being and self-determination, the prudent course is to take into account the potential consequences of the patient's decision. When the consequences for well-being are substantial, there is a greater need to be certain that the patient possesses the necessary level of capacity. When little turns on the decision, the level of decisionmaking capacity required may be appropriately reduced (even though the constituent elements remain the same) and less scrutiny may be required about whether the patient possesses even the reduced level of capacity. Thus a particular patient may be capable of deciding about a relatively inconsequential medication, but not about the amputation of a gangrenous limb.

This formulation has significant implications. First, it denies that simply by expressing a preference about a treatment decision an individual demonstrates the capacity to make that decision. The "expressed preference" standard does nothing to preclude the presence of a serious defect or mistake in a patient's reasoning process. Consequently, it cannot ensure that the patient's expressed preference accords with the patient's conception of future well-being. Although it gives what appears to be great deference to self-determination, the expressed preference standard may actually fail to promote the values underlying self-determination, which include the achievement of personal values and goals. For these reasons, the Commission rejects the expressed preference standard for decisions that might compromise the patient's well-being.[14]

The Commission also rejects as the standard of capacity any test that looks solely to the content of the patient's decision. Any standard based on "objectively correct" decisions would allow a health professional (or other third party) to declare that a patient lacks decisionmaking capacity whenever a decision appears "wrong," "irrational," or otherwise incompatible with the evaluator's view of what is best for the patient. Use of such a standard is in sharp conflict with most of the values that support self-determination: it would take the decision away from the patient and place it with another, and it would inadequately reflect the subjective nature of each individual's conception of what's good. Further, its imprecision opens the door to manipulation of health care decisionmaking through selective application.

Logically, just as a patient's disagreement with a health care professional's recommendation does not prove a lack of decisionmaking capacity, concurrence with the recommendation would not establish the patient's capacity. Yet, as testimony before the Commission made clear, coherent adults are seldom said to lack capacity (except, perhaps, in the mental health context) when they acquiesce in the course of treatment recommended by their physicians. (Challenges to patients' capacity are rarer still when family members expressly concur in the decision.) This divergence between theory and reality is less significant than it might appear, however, since neither the self-determination nor the well-being of a patient would usually be advanced by insisting upon an inquiry into the patient's decisionmaking capacity (or lack thereof) when patient, physician, and family all agree on a course of treatment. Even if the course being adopted might not, in fact, best match the patient's long-term view of his or her own welfare, a declaration of lack of capacity will lead to a substitute making a decision for the patient (which means full self-determination will not occur), yet will rarely result in a different health care decision being made (which means no change in well-being). Substitution of a third party for an acquiescent patient will lead to a different outcome only if the new decisionmaker has a strong commitment to promoting previously expressed values of the patient that differ significantly from those that guided the physician. If, as would usually be the case, the substitute would be a family member or other individual who would defer to the physician's recommendation, there would be little reason to initiate an inquiry into capacity. The existing practice thus seems generally satisfactory.[15]

Questions of patient capacity in decisionmaking typically arise only when a patient chooses a course—often a refusal of treatment—other than the one the health professional finds most reasonable.[16] A practitioner's belief that a decision is not "reasonable" is the beginning—not the end—of an inquiry into the patient's capacity to decide. If every patient decision that a health professional disagreed with were grounds for a declaration of lack of capacity, self-determination would have little meaning. Even when disagreement occurs, an assessment of the patient's decisionmaking capacity begins with a presumption of such capacity. Nonetheless, a serious disagreement about a decision with substantial consequences for the patient's welfare may appropriately trigger a more careful evaluation. When that process indicates that the patient understands the situation and is capable of reasoning soundly about it, the patient's choice should be accepted. When it does not, further evaluation may be required, and in some instances a determination of lack of capacity will be appropriate.[17]

Voluntariness in Decisionmaking

A second requirement for informed consent is that the patient's participation in the decisionmaking process and ultimate decision regarding care must be voluntary. A choice that has been coerced, or that resulted from serious manipulation of a person's ability to make an intelligent and informed decision, is not the person's own free choice. This has long been recognized in law: a consent forced by threats or induced by fraud or misrepresentation is legally viewed as no consent at all.[18] From the perspective of ethics, a consent that is substantially involuntary does not provide moral authorization for treatment because it does not respect the patient's dignity and may not reflect the aims of the patient.

Of course, the facts of disease and the limited capabilities of medicine often constrict the choices available to patient and physician alike. In that sense, the condition of illness itself is sometimes spoken of as "coercive" or involuntary. But the fact that no available alternative may be desirable in itself, and that the preferred course is, at best, only the least bad among a bad lot, does not render a choice coerced in the sense employed here. No change in human behavior or institutional structure could remove this limitation. Such constraints are merely facts of life that should not be regarded as making a patient's choice involuntary.

Voluntariness is best regarded as a matter of degree, rather than as a quality that is wholly present or absent in particular cases. Forced treatment—the embodiment of coercive, involuntary action—appears to be rare in the American health care system.[19] Health care professionals do, however, make limited intrusions on voluntary choice through subtle, or even overt, manipulations of patients' wills when they believe that patients would otherwise make incorrect decisions.

Forced Treatment The most overt forms of involuntariness in health care settings involve interventions forced on patients without their consent (and sometimes over their express objection) and those based on coerced consent. Although rare in mainstream American health care, such situations do arise in certain special settings, and therefore require brief discussion. Society currently legitimates certain forced medical interventions to serve important social goals such as promoting the public health (with, for example, compulsory vaccination laws), enforcing the criminal law (removing bullets needed as evidence for criminal prosecutions), or otherwise promoting the well-being of others (sedating uncontrollable inmates of mental institutions on an emergency basis, for example, to protect other inmates or staff).[20]

Although it is typically not viewed as forced treatment, a good deal of routine care in hospitals, nursing homes, and other health care settings is provided (usually by health professionals such as nurses) without explicit and voluntary consent by patients. The expectation on the part of professionals is that patients, once in such a setting, will simply go along with such routine care. However, the Commission's study of treatment refusals found that in a hospital setting it was the routine tests that were most likely to be refused. At least some patients expected that participation was voluntary and refused tests and medications ordered without their knowledge until adequate information was provided about the nature, purpose, and risks of these undertakings. Lack of information in such cases may not only preclude voluntary participation but also raise questions about a patient's rationality, and hence competence.

When a situation offers the patient an opportunity to refuse care, then patient compliance or acquiescence may be viewed as implicit consent. But when the tacit communication accompanying such care is that there is no choice for the patient to make, and compliance is expected and enforced (at least in the absence of vigorous objections), the treatment can be properly termed "forced." The following conversation between a nurse and a patient regarding postoperative care, obtained in one of the Commission's observational studies, illustrates forced treatment that follows routinely from another decision (surgery) that was made voluntarily.

NURSE: Did they mention anything about a tube through your nose?

PATIENT: Yes, I'm gonna have a tube in my nose.

NURSE: You're going to have the tube down for a couple of days or longer. It depends. So you're going to be NPO, nothing by mouth, and also you're going to have IV fluid.

PATIENT: I know. For three or four days they told me that already. I don't like it, though.

NURSE: You don't have any choice.

PATIENT: Yes, I don't have any choice, I know.

NURSE: Like it or not, you don't have any choice. (laughter) After you come back, we'll ask you to do a lot of coughing and deep breathing to exercise your lungs.

PATIENT: Oh, we'll see how I feel.

NURSE: (Emphasis) No matter how you feel, you have to do that![21]

The interview ended a few minutes later with the patient still disputing whether he was going to cooperate with the postoperative care.

Coerced Treatment Unlike forced treatment, for which no consent is given, coerced treatment proceeds on the basis of a consent that was not freely given. As used in this sense, a patient's decision is coerced when the person is credibly threatened by another individual, either explicitly or by implication, with unwanted and avoidable consequences unless the patient accedes to the specified course of action.[22] Concern about coercion is accordingly greatest when a disproportion in power or other significant inequality between a patient and another individual lends credibility to the threat of harm and when the perceived interests of the individuals diverge.[23]

The disparity in power between patient and health care professional may be slight or substantial, depending on the nature of the patient's illness, the institutional setting, the personalities of the individuals involved, and several other factors. In nonemergency settings, a patient typically can change practitioners or simply forego treatment, thus avoiding the potential for coercion. Further, although health care professionals do have interests distinct from and sometimes in conflict with those of their patients, strong social and professional norms usually ensure that priority is accorded to patients' welfare. To be sure, coercion can be exercised with benevolent motives if practitioner and patient differ in their assessments of how the patient's welfare is best served. Nonetheless, there is little reason to believe that blatant forms of coercion are a problem in mainstream American health care. When isolated instances of abuse do arise, the law provides suitable remedies.

A patient's family and other concerned persons may often play a useful role in the decisionmaking process. Sometimes, however, they may try to coerce a particular decision, either because of what they perceive to be in the patient's best interests or because of a desire to advance their own interests. In such instances, since the health care professional's first loyalty is to the patient, he or she should attempt to enhance the patient's ability to make a voluntary, uncoerced decision and to overcome any coercive pressures.[24]

Manipulation Blatant coercion may be of so little concern in professional-patient relationships because, as physicians so often proclaim, it is so easy for health professionals to elicit a desired decision through more subtle means. Indeed, some physicians are critical of the legal requirement for informed consent on the grounds that it must be mere window dressing since "patients will, if they trust their doctor, accede to almost any request he cares to make."[25] On some occasions, to be sure, this result can be achieved by rational persuasion, since the professional presumably has good reasons for preferring a recommended course of action. But the tone of such critics suggests they have something else in mind: an ability to package and present the facts in a way that leaves the patient with no real choice. Such conduct, capitalizing on disparities in knowledge, position, and influence, is manipulative in character and impairs the voluntariness of the patient's choice.[26]

Manipulation has more and less extreme forms. At one end of the spectrum is behavior amounting to misrepresentation or fraud. Of particular concern in health care contexts is the withholding or distortion of information in order to affect the patient's beliefs and decisions. The patient might not be told about alternatives to the recommended course of action, for example, or the risks or other negative characteristics of the recommended treatment might be minimized. Such behavior is justly criticized on two grounds: first, that it interferes with the patient's voluntary choice (and thus negates consent) and, second, that it interferes with the patient's ability to make an informed decision. At the other end of the spectrum are far more subtle instances: a professional's careful choice of words or nuances of tone and emphasis might present the situation in a manner calculated to heighten the appeal of a particular course of action.

It is well known that the way information is presented can powerfully affect the recipient's response to it. The tone of voice and other aspects of the practitioner's manner of presentation can indicate whether a risk of a particular kind with a particular incidence should be considered serious. Information can be emphasized or played down without altering the content. And it can be framed in a way that affects the listener—for example, "this procedure succeeds most of the time" versus "this procedure has a 40 percent failure rate." Health professionals who are aware of the effects of such minor variations can choose their language with care; if, during discussions with a patient, they sense any unintended or confused impressions being created, they can adjust their presentation of information accordingly.

Because many patients are often fearful and unequal to their physicians in status, knowledge, and power, they may be particularly susceptible to manipulations of this type. Health care professionals should, therefore, present information in a form that fosters understanding. Patients should be helped to understand the prognosis for their situation and the implications of different courses of treatment. The difficult distinction, both in theory and in practice, is between acceptable forms of informing, discussion, and rational persuasion on the one hand, and objectionable forms of influence or manipulation on the other.

Since voluntariness is one of the foundation stones of informed consent, professionals have a high ethical obligation to avoid coercion and manipulation of their patients. The law penalizes those who ignore the requirements of consent or who directly coerce it. But it can do little about subtle manipulations without incurring severe disruptions of private relationships by intrusive policing, and so the duty is best thought of primarily in ethical terms.

* * *

CHAPTER 7: LEGAL REFORMS AND THEIR IMPLICATIONS

The Law as a Means of Improvement

The law has an important function as a moral teacher, both for the professions and for the general public. Even though they do not always give full effect to the value of self-determination, legal rules and court decisions remind society of its commitment to this value.[1] Beyond this symbolic function, law establishes minimum, enforceable standards for disclosure that enable injured patients to receive compensation for injuries caused by health professionals' failure to meet these standards. Although the existence of this potential liability has generated anxiety among practitioners, it has also spurred valuable reassessment of ethical norms and professional practices and has made practitioners more sensitive to patients' needs and expectations.[2] The Commission firmly believes that the law can and should continue to perform these essential functions.

The Commission appreciates the practical difficulties of adopting its approach to patient-professional relationships as the normative legal expectation for informed consent. Transcending these practical difficulties is a more fundamental issue: the Commission is not convinced that its vision of the patient-professional relationship can be achieved primarily through reliance on the law.[3] Having analyzed the relationship in a way that recognizes the complexities and variations of individual cases, the Commission is aware that the informed consent process may not be susceptible to detailed regulation by so blunt an instrument as the law of battery or of medical negligence. Indeed, the Commission is concerned that efforts to draw the law further into regulating the subtler aspects of relationships between patients and health care professionals may prove ineffective, burdensome, and ultimately counterproductive.[4]

Nevertheless, in this Report the Commission has set forth a vision of informed consent that could, if incorporated into state law as cases arise, bring the law closer to its ethical roots as well as to the realities and potentialities of day-to-day health care. Although the Commission does not regard changes in the law as the major way its conclusions about informed consent will be translated into practice, it does believe that it would be appropriate—even desirable—for the law on the subject to adjust its minimum expectations in the direction pointed to in this Report.

Most fundamentally, the law could emphasize the process of continuing communication and decisionmaking, rather than the pro forma disclosure of particular risks that now strikes many practitioners as a hollow charade.[5] Such a shift in focus would make clear that a professional's obligation is not satisfied—and the professional is not insulated from legal liability—simply by obtaining the patient's signature on a consent form.[6] Instead, courts could engage in a more qualitative evaluation of the entire process that would account for the professional's overall effort to elicit matters of particular concern to the patient and to respond to the patient's worries, insofar as reasonably possible, through disclosure and discussion. Instead of focusing, as is now the case, on whether the practitioner warned the patient of risks, courts would inquire into whether or not the practitioner took sufficient steps to involve the patient in the decisionmaking process. The questions before the court could include, for example, whether the practitioner made reasonable efforts to impart information, to determine whether the patient understood it, to elicit the patient's values and preferences, to create a noncoercive atmosphere for the decision, and to encourage the patient to decide on the basis of the available information and the patient's own values.[7]

Efforts to translate the Commission's recommendations of ethical norms for the communication process directly into detailed legal rules may create evidentiary difficulties. To the extent that the issues to be examined in a lawsuit would be more subtle and subjective than they currently are if the Commission's recommendations were to form the ethical basis of law, proof of what occurred would be complicated. Of course, the direct testimony of both professional and patient could provide accounts of the decisionmaking process. Yet as discussed in Chapter One, the tendency of such testimony to be selective and self-serving is familiar and difficult to overcome.[8] Documentary evidence could be introduced as well, but the production of a full documentary record reflecting not merely a formal written consent but the entire process of communication and decisionmaking over an extended time would impose substantial burdens. Of particular concern would be the time needed to generate and ensure the accuracy of such records from the viewpoints of all parties.

The implication to be drawn from these difficulties is not, however, that professionals should comply with the limited requirements of the law, and then go about their business as they see fit. The Commission rejects the attitude that divides obligations into two categories: those that are legally established and must be obeyed under pain of penalty, and those that are not so established and hence can be ignored. Throughout this Report the Commission has employed the terminology of "professional-patient relationships" rather than the language of the marketplace, which treats patients as "consumers," to underline the importance of recapturing a sense of professional norms and obligations. Such norms are more than gratuitous advice; they are to be taken seriously, both by individual professionals and by their organizations.[9]

In distinguishing between a strictly legal obligation to secure consent and a professional's broader obligation to provide patients with a basis for effective participation in decisionmaking, the Commission hopes to remind health care professionals that their obligations transcend legal requirements and incorporate objectives that the law cannot readily enforce. The roots of the broader obligation are ethical and reside with the mutual trust and expectations that are appropriate for parties to the relationship. The Commission believes that recognition and fulfillment of these professional obligations by health care practitioners will go a long way toward alleviating the sometimes adversary character that has encroached upon patient-professional relationships in recent years and will reinforce the mutual trust on which successful relationships are ultimately founded.

Enhancing Self-Determination of the Formerly Competent

In addition to any judicial modification in the law of consent to bring it into line with the Commission's conclusions, states should direct legislative attention to giving patients the means to have at least some say about treatment decisions in the event they become incapable of participating in decisions directly.[10] More than one-third of the public in the Commission's survey have given instructions (though only one-quarter of those are in writing) to someone about how they would like to be treated if they become too sick to make decisions themselves. While this issue has gained prominence largely because of the attention recently accorded to so-called living wills for dying patients, people can and do set forth instructions to guide a wide variety of health care decisions.

As discussed in Chapter Two, such means would permit two of the goals of self-determination to be fulfilled: individualizing the meaning of well-being and showing respect for personal dignity. The third goal—that a patient be an active agent in decisions about his or her own care—would be impossible to achieve at all in the case of an unconscious patient and impossible to achieve fully with patients who are less seriously incapacitated. Although this Report focuses on patients' direct decisions about their own care, no discussion of legal reforms would be complete without some attention to how a person's informed consent might carry forward to a time when he or she is no longer able to participate directly through the use of written directions (known as "advance directives") prepared in anticipation of some future incapacitating illness.

Without changes in the law, the problem facing a person who wants to direct the care he or she will receive if incompetent is that the authorization provided to a family member or physician ceases to be legally effective at just the time when it is needed, namely when the person becomes incompetent, because of the legal rule (which is quite sensible in other contexts) that an agent's authority is terminated by incompetence of the person who appointed that agent.[11] Thus, special provision must be made if a person's directions about medical care, set down while he or she is competent, are to be effective in determining, or even officially guiding, the decisions actually made if the person becomes incompetent.

Instruction Directives Two types of advance directives have already been recognized by some states: instruction directives and proxy decisionmaking directives. The best known examples of the first type are the "natural death" statutes that have been enacted in 14 states since the first was adopted in 1976 in California.[12] These specify certain circumstances under which a directive to a treating physician (the wording of which is usually set forth in the statute) will be effective in limiting the extent of life-sustaining treatment administered to a patient whose condition has been diagnosed as imminently fatal. Instruction directives are, in theory, limited neither to terminal illness nor to orders to desist from treatment. They could be employed by patients who have been told that they may soon become incapable of making decisions (for example, because of a brain tumor) or by those who simply wish to have "standing orders" about some aspect of their care (such as no blood transfusions). Instructions could authorize the use of certain types of treatments, as in the case of people diagnosed as having progressive senile dementia of the Alzheimer's type who, before they become incompetent, give their permission for research procedures of more than minimal risk. And rather than specifying that under particular circumstances an individual does or does not authorize a particular type of medical intervention, instructions could describe a person's attitude toward a particular state of affairs.[13]

Whether the instructions are quite precise or very general, for several reasons an advance directive of this type is of limited use in providing effective self-determination. First, it would be extremely difficult to draft a directive that did not leave considerable range for interpretation; both the existence of the circumstances making the directive effective and the steps to be taken under it will often require discretion by health care professionals and family. Second, if the terms of the document were made more precise in order to leave the choices more with the patient and less with the treating professionals, the range of circumstances to which the document would apply would have to be narrowed or its length and complexity would have to be increased.

Third, and perhaps most important in light of the analysis of informed consent contained in this Report, instruction directives are likely to address only a limited range of medical situations that occur frequently enough to be of general concern to people. Beyond these, a directive would itself be an example of knowing and voluntary self-determination only if it emerged from a patient-professional relationship in which the patient had been counseled about the future risk of a particular disability and about the courses of treatment that would probably then be available. Even then, decisionmaking under an instruction has a truncated quality since the patient will have dictated specific decisions before all the particulars of the situation were clear and before the process of mutual participation and shared decisionmaking had fully ripened. Consequently, such directives are likely to be more useful in excluding certain procedures that are totally unacceptable to a patient than in fine-tuning decisionmaking about a full range of possible health care choices.

Proxy Directives[14] An alternative type of directive, which would avoid the difficulties both of anticipating all possible treatment choices and of leaving full discretion to health care professionals, would designate a person as authorized to make treatment decisions on a patient's behalf under specified circumstances.[15] Both the range of circumstances in which the proxy may act and the range of choices he or she is authorized to make could be broad or narrow. For example, a person who wanted vigorous treatment could authorize a proxy to make all necessary decisions, subject only to the requirement that all therapies be aggressively pursued if they offered any possibility of benefit.

Although a proxy's decisions are not directly acts of the patient, proxy directives meet the objective of allowing patients to limit what happens to them if they appoint proxies with whom they have discussed their views and who are willing to insist on treatment decisions that are consistent with those views. The proxy can participate in the process of shared decisionmaking in the patient's stead, so that that process is not artificially truncated. The degree to which this proxy process actually substitutes for a patient's direct participation depends upon how extensively the patient had previously talked over the relevant issues with health professionals.

By combining a proxy directive with specific instructions, an individual could control both the content and the process of decisionmaking about care in case of incapacity. The use of instructions would help overcome the open-ended nature of designating a proxy by increasing the likelihood that in the process of deciding on instructions a person would have discussed relevant considerations with both the potential proxy and the health care professionals—in other words, that the person would go through a process of prospective informed consent.

The possibility of appointing a proxy for health care decisionmaking already exists in the laws of 37 states that have adopted statutes authorizing what is usually termed a durable power of attorney.[16] Although these were fashioned over the past 30 years primarily to provide a less expensive means than court-ordered guardianship or conservatorship for dealing with small property interests, there is nothing in the acts that would explicitly preclude the use of durable powers of attorney to designate or instruct a proxy to make health care decisions. Commentators have suggested such use and there is anecdotal evidence that it has occurred, but this use has not been the subject of any reported judicial decisions.[17]

Statutory Developments In addition to the existing statutes that provide a means for patients to create one type of advance directive or another, several model statutes have been proposed specifically to allow such directives in health care.[18] In evaluating existing or proposed means or in devising new ones, several factors need to be taken into account. Four groupings of such considerations are presented here to suggest the range of issues the Commission believes should be addressed in evaluating statutory alternatives.

Requisites for a valid directive. Special attention needs to be given to the basic requisites for a valid directive, particularly since some of the statutes that might be employed—such as the durable power of attorney acts—were not designed specifically for the appointment of proxy health care decisionmakers.

Decisionmaking capacity of principal: There should be some way to establish that a person filling out a directive (the principal) was legally competent to do so at the time. The emphasis of this Report (as discussed in Chapters Three and Eight) is on patients possessing decisional capacity rather than on legal competence. Should a statute insist that when a directive is executed the person has the capacity to understand the choice embodied in the directive? To certify a signatory's capacity, statutes often require one or two witnesses to a document. It would seem advisable for a statute to be clear on whether the witnesses must attest to the principal's capacity or merely serve as safeguards against fraudulent signatures. Since such witnesses are likely to be laypeople, the standard of decisionmaking capacity they apply will rest on common sense, not psychological expertise.

Due regard for the step being taken: The related concern that everyone involved in the execution of a directive, particularly the principal and the prospective proxy, recognize the seriousness of the step is something that would be more difficult to guarantee by statute. It is, however, a consideration that arises in evaluating the wisdom of using existing durable power statutes, which were intended to address only property matters. One way to increase the likelihood that due regard is given to the subject matter would be to provide that before a directive is executed, the principal (and proxy, where one is involved) must have had a discussion with a health care professional of the patient's objectives and of the directive's potential consequences. This would also help ensure that any instructions reflect a process of active self-determination on the part of the patient-to-be.

Legal effect of directives. Several questions arise about the effects that a directive should have in the law and about how these effects might be achieved.

Registration: Certain documents are officially registered, so that they will not be ignored and so there can be no doubt that all concerned parties are aware of their existence. The process of registration also provides an opportunity to ensure that all the basic documentary requisites have been met; for example, an official who is charged with registering directives could be trained to determine the competence of signers. On the other hand, the additional formality of required registration might seriously discourage the use of directives, and it is doubtful whether in this context—unlike in a commercial or real estate setting—there is really much need for a directive to be on file in a governmental office in order for it to have its desired effect at the time it would be needed.

Legal immunity: A statute should make clear that people acting pursuant to a directive are not subject to civil or criminal liability for any action they take that they would not be liable for were they acting on the direct consent of a competent patient. Yet since directives—particularly those including instructions—may contain unavoidable ambiguities, some leeway must be offered if this legal immunization is to provide adequate reassurance for health care professionals. Some of the existing statutes speak of protection for actions taken in "good faith."[19] Language of this sort provides sensible protection for subsidiary health personnel who follow the orders of the physician in charge of the patient, provided they believe the physician's orders are in line with the directive or have been authorized by a proxy. Some standard of reasonable interpretation of the directive may need to be imposed, however, on an attending physician's reading of the document, lest "good faith" offer too wide a scope for discretion. Such a standard might best be developed in case law and scholarly commentary rather than in the statute itself.

Penalties for noncompliance: In order to make directives legally binding, several states have included penalties in their statutes (fines, for example, or suspension or revocation of professional licenses) for failing to follow an advance directive.[20] The wisdom or necessity of such penalty clauses depends upon the problem a statute is attempting to remedy. If health care providers are unwilling to share responsibility with patients and, in particular, tend to overtreat patients whose physical or mental condition leaves them unable to resist, then—unless they are made legally binding—advance directives are unlikely to protect effectively patients who want to limit their treatment. On the other hand, if health care professionals are simply unsure of what patients want, or if they are anxious to share decisionmaking responsibility but are apprehensive about their legal liability if they follow the instructions of a person whose decisionmaking capacity is in doubt, then the threat of penalties would be unnecessary. Indeed, it could even be counterproductive if it fostered an adversarial relationship between patient and provider.

Proxy's characteristics and authority. Several special questions arise in the context of health care concerning who may act as a proxy and what the proxy may do.

Competency of the proxy: The basic consideration about a proxy is that he or she should have the capacity to make a particular health care decision when needed. The means for assuring this capacity are not so simply stated, however. Basically, they would seem to be the same ones that are applied to patients themselves, as discussed in Chapter Eight.[21]

Disqualifications: Another issue, which could also be treated as a prerequisite for appointing a proxy, concerns whether limitations should be placed on who may serve. The main consideration is to avoid the appointment of anyone with interests that are adverse to a patient's. In some "natural death" statutes, this has led to explicit exclusion of anyone financially involved (as debtor, creditor, or heir) with the patient.[22] Special concern may also be warranted for patients in nursing homes.[23] Unfortunately, in the absence of a special group of people who serve as proxies for patients there, the people most readily available—the nursing staff and institutional officers—are typically not disinterested.

Redelegation: In certain circumstances a proxy may be temporarily or permanently unable or unwilling to serve as a substitute decisionmaker. When that occurs, should alternate proxies be limited to people who were named by the principal in an original or amended directive, or, in the absence of such alternates, should a proxy be allowed to delegate his or her authority to another person of the proxy's choosing?[24] This issue might be affected by whether either the original or a substitute proxy was a close relative of the patient, as opposed to a stranger.

Access to information: Since the proxy stands in the shoes of the patient and is expected to engage in a comparable decisionmaking process, logically the proxy should have access to the patient's medical record. Yet it may be advisable to limit the proxy's access only to that information needed for the health care decision at hand, in order to respect the patient's interest in privacy.

Bases of decision: In the case of a proxy directive, a proxy would be expected to decide about health care in a way calculated to serve the patient's best interests. Although that concept is an elastic one, the law of each state gives it some meaning, and it has received extensive attention in legal and philosophical commentary.[25] Ought the concept of best interests be uniform, or should it vary, within certain outer limits, if the surrogate is the next-of-kin rather than a stranger? An instruction directive, whether by itself or joined with a proxy directive, creates the potential for decisions based upon the particular (and perhaps idiosyncratic) wishes of the patient. The interpretation of such a directive would seem to lie with the surrogate decisionmaker, particularly in the case of a proxy designated by the patient, at least in the first instance. Provision may have to be made, of course, for an administrative mechanism to decide situations in which a health care professional challenges the decision of a proxy on the ground that it is not based on the patient's best interests or on a reasonable interpretation of the patient's instructions.

Administrative aspects. Several procedural concerns probably need to be addressed in any statute for advanced health care directives.

Triggering event: A statute needs to specify how a directive becomes effective. Two sets of concerns are involved. The first, already mentioned, relates to the necessary guarantee that the directive reflects the wishes of the patient. Some of the "natural death" acts, for example, require that a directive must be executed after the patient has been informed of a diagnosis, so that the patient's instructions are arrived at in the context of the actual, not hypothetical, choices to be made.[26] Statutes also typically provide that the designation of a surrogate or the content of specific instructions be renewed every few years so that the signatory can reconsider the instructions or designation in light of changed circumstances or opinions.[27] Once it is determined that a directive is valid, a separate issue needs to be addressed: what makes it operative? A statute may leave that question to the document itself, to be specified by the person executing the directive. Or it may provide that a particular event or condition brings the document into play. In either case, the triggering event will require both a standard for action and a specification of who will make the determination. For example, a directive may become operative when a physician makes a particular prognosis ("terminal illness") or determines that a patient lacks decisional capacity regarding a particular health care choice.

Revocation: Provision must be made for the process and standard by which a document can be revoked. The theory of self-determination suggests that as long as the principal remains competent, he or she should unquestionably have the power to revoke a directive. But what about an incompetent (incapacitated) person? The "natural death" acts have uniformly provided that *any* revocation by a principal negates a directive.[28] In the context of termination of life-sustaining treatment, that result may be sensible, since it would generally seem wrong to cease such treatment based upon a proxy's orders when a patient, no matter how confused, asks that treatment be continued. In other circumstances, however, allowing revocations by an incompetent patient could wreak havoc on a course of treatment authorized by the proxy. Perhaps when a proxy does not believe he or she should be guided by a principal's contemporaneous instructions, on the grounds that the principal is incompetent and is contradicting earlier competent instructions and/or acting against the principal's own best interests, the question of whether to follow the proxy or the principal ought to be subject to independent review.

Review and safeguards: When disputes arise, either about the choice made by a proxy or about an attempted revocation by an apparently incapacitated principal, some means of review will be necessary to safeguard the patient's interests. In some circumstances the review mechanism need only judge the process by which a decision has been reached. In other circumstances it may seem advisable to review the health care decision itself, which in turn may involve either a subjective or an objective approach to the patient's well-being. In the absence of a special provision in the statute, questions of this sort would lead to review by institutional bodies and, eventually, to judicial proceedings.

In sum, serious issues need to be addressed, either in the applicability to health care of existing statutes created to resolve other problems, such as the durable power of attorney acts, or in the drafting or revision of statutes specifically to permit advance directives for health care. Many people are concerned that, as they become old or ill or especially if they are hospitalized, decisions about their health care will pass out of their hands and into those of health care professionals, who may be strangers to them. This widespread concern justifies continued attempts to find a simple way to extend at least basic self-determination into a period of decisional incapacity. Although the issue has received particular public attention in the context of terminal illness,[29] it is not limited to that setting, and there are good reasons to treat the entire subject of advance directives within a single statute. Without endorsing any particular statute, the Commission does endorse the development of advance directives and encourages patients and professionals to use them as appropriate whether or not there is a specific statute that regulates and enforces their use.

* * *

CHAPTER 9: SUBSTANTIVE AND PROCEDURAL PRINCIPLES OF DECISIONMAKING FOR INCAPACITATED PATIENTS

Substantive Principles

As described in Chapter Two, there are two values that guide decisionmaking for competent patients: promoting patient welfare and respecting patient self-determination. They should also guide decisionmaking for incapacitated patients, though of necessity their implementation must differ. They are reflected, roughly speaking, in the two different standards that have traditionally guided decisionmaking for the incapacitated: "substituted judgment" and "best interests." Although these standards are now used in health care situations, they have their origins in a different context—namely, the resolution of family disputes and decisions about the control of the property of legal incompetents. When people become seriously disabled and unable to manage their property, they may be judged incompetent and a guardian appointed to make financial and property decisions. These doctrines were developed to instruct guardians about the boundaries of their powers without issuing detailed and specific guidelines and to provide a standard for guidance of courts that must review decisions proposed by a guardian.[1]

Simply stated, under the substituted judgment standard, the decisions made for an incapacitated person should attempt to arrive at the same choice the person would make if competent to do so (but within boundaries of "reasonableness" intended to protect the incompetent).[2] Under the best interests standard, decisions are acceptable if they would promote the welfare of the hypothetical "average person" in the position of the incompetent, which may not be the same choice the individual would make (but which may still have some aspects of subjectivity to it).[3]

Despite the long legal history of both these standards, they provide only hazy guidance for decisionmaking even in their original contexts, not to mention in the often far more complex, urgent, and personal setting of health care. Although a number of recent cases involving decisions about health care for incapacitated patients have given courts the opportunity to clarify these often vague guidelines, increased confusion may have accompanied some of the attempts to add precision to these doctrines.

Substituted Judgment The substituted judgment standard requires that the surrogate attempt to replicate faithfully the decision that the incapacitated person would make if he or she were able to make a choice. In so doing, the patient's interest in achieving well-being as he or she defines it in accordance with personal values and goals, as well as the individual's interest in self-determination, are both honored to the maximum extent possible, given the fundamental reality that the patient literally cannot make a contemporaneous choice. The surrogate's decision is limited, however, by two general external constraints. First, the surrogate is circumscribed by the same limitations that society legitimately imposes on patients who are capable of deciding for themselves,[4] such as not compromising public health (*e.g.*, by refusing a mandatory vaccination) or not taking steps contrary to the criminal law (*e.g.*, intentional maiming). Second, there are certain decisions that a patient might be permitted to make but that are outside the discretion of substitute decisionmaking and must therefore be decided by the standards of "reasonableness." This is especially true for cases in which the decision risks imposing substantial harm on patients or depriving them of substantial benefit; people may volunteer for risky research with no direct therapeutic benefits to themselves but guardians may not enroll people in such research merely because it is known that, when they were competent, they believed that such research was very important. Thus even the essentially subjective substituted judgment standard is constrained by external limitations—that is, limitations not arising from the patient's own views.

For the substituted judgment standard to be employed there must be evidence of the patient's views, which could be derived from various sources. The surrogate may be guided in decisionmaking by prior directives expressly made by that patient governing the precise matter at issue. A person might, for instance, have clearly stated that he or she wished to avoid a potentially beneficial treatment that poses a risk of crippled mental faculties if there were another treatment available that, although promising more limited benefits, also poses substantially smaller risks of damaging the mind.

The substituted judgment standard is markedly simpler to use—and contains greater assurance of being faithfully implemented—when a competent individual has given clear directives regarding medical care in the event of incapacity, although such a directive does not necessarily resolve all problems.[5] When directives are written rather than oral, it is more likely that the surrogate (or a third party who may report the incapacitated patient's putative directions to the surrogate) will not forget or misunderstand the patient's advance directives.

In the absence of advance directives, surrogates may be guided by the known values, goals, and desires of an incapacitated patient. It can reasonably be presumed, for example, that a person who is known to have had a particular aversion to painful medical interventions would wish to continue avoiding them if possible.

Best Interests Decisionmaking guided by the best interests standard requires a surrogate to do what, from an objective standpoint, appears to promote a patient's good without reference to the patient's actual or supposed preferences. This does not mean the surrogate must choose the means the practitioner thinks is "best" for promoting the patient's well-being, but only a means reasonably likely to achieve that goal. Where, for example, there is more than one therapy available, a decision in favor of any one of those considered appropriate by health care professionals will be acceptable under the best interests standard. However, the best interests standard would preclude the surrogate from choosing a therapy that is totally unacceptable by professional standards, even if the surrogate might choose that treatment for him or herself. Fundamentally, the standard of "reasonableness" is inherently cautious.

In assessing whether a procedure or course of treatment would be in a patient's best interests, the surrogate must take into account such factors as the relief of suffering, the preservation or restoration of functioning, and the quality as well as the extent of life sustained.[6] An accurate assessment will encompass consideration of the satisfaction of present desires, the opportunities for future satisfactions, and the possibility of developing or regaining the capacity for self-determination.

The impact of a decision on an incapacitated patient's loved ones may be taken into account in determining someone's best interests, for most people do have an important interest in the well-being of their families or close associates. To avoid abuse, however, especially stringent standards of evidence should be required to support a claim that reasonable people would disregard their exclusively self-regarding interests (for example, in prolonging or avoiding suffering) in favor of their interest in avoiding psychological or financial burdens on the people to whom they were attached.

The Standard for Surrogate Decisionmaking The Commission believes that decisionmaking for incapacitated patients ought, when possible, to be guided by the principle of substituted judgment, since it promotes the underlying values of self-determination and well-being better than the best interests standard does. However, the principle of substituted judgment cannot be employed universally; what some patients would want if competent cannot always be ascertained because of insufficient evidence about a patient's values and preferences or because the patient's cognitive abilities have always been so limited that he or she was never capable of developing or expressing preferences about the decision in question.[7] When a patient's likely decision is not known, the best interests standard presumes that the individual would prefer what most reasonable people would want in similar circumstances. On certain points, of course, no consensus may exist about what "most reasonable people" would prefer. Furthermore, whenever a range of choices exists, even a best interests determination will display an element of subjectivity on the part of the surrogate in defining and weighing the patient's interests.

To the extent feasible, efforts should be made with patients who are incapacitated though able to engage in communication to take into account their expressions of their own values and goals.[8] Doing so will both promote their welfare as they understand and conceive of it and honor self-determination, though of an attenuated kind. When recovery of the capacity to make decisions is a reasonable possibility, enhancing its prospect should be another goal.

Procedures for Surrogate Decisionmaking

Regardless of the substantive principle used to guide decisionmaking for patients lacking decisional capacity, policies and procedures are needed for the selection and guidance of surrogate decisionmakers. Furthermore, there is a need to specify the circumstances under which review of the surrogate's decision should be permitted or required and who should undertake such a review. The Commission recommends that however these problems are actually to be resolved, health care institutions should have clear policies about who has the authority and responsibility to determine incapacity, to speak for the patient, and to review determinations and decisions.

The Selection of a Surrogate A sound policy for decisionmaking for incapacitated patients should take into account the urgency of the need to make a decision and the existence of suitable substitutes such as interested family members or a legal guardian.

Emergencies. When a decision must be made immediately, in order to avoid seriously jeopardizing a patient's life or well-being, health care professionals are the proper decisionmakers.[9] Since such emergency care is so often provided in institutional settings involving many practitioners, one aspect of a sound policy is having the means to assign decisionmaking authority to a particular member of the treatment team. This person should usually be the available professional who is most qualified to make the decision, according to the provider's estimate of the patient's best interests.

The line between emergency and nonemergency decisions will sometimes be hard to draw and will depend in part upon the type of facility and the ready availability of additional personnel for quick consultation. Institutional policy should minimize any tendency to overextend the exceptionally broad decisionmaking authority that genuine emergencies confer on practitioners. As soon as possible, without compromising the patient's well-being, other surrogates (such as family members) should be located, informed about the choices to be made, and involved in the decisionmaking.[10]

Nonemergency situations. In nonemergency situations, the proper presumption is that the family, defined to include closest relatives and intimate friends,[11] should make health care decisions for an incapacitated patient. There are several grounds for this stance:

(1) The family is generally most concerned about the good of the patient.
(2) The family will also usually be most knowledgeable about the patient's goals, preferences, and values.
(3) The family deserves recognition as an important social unit that ought to be treated, within limits, as a single decisionmaker in matters that intimately affect its members.

Especially in a society in which many other traditional forms of community have been eroded, participation in a family is often an important dimension of personal fulfillment. Since a protected sphere of privacy and autonomy is required for the flourishing of this interpersonal union, institutions and the state should be reluctant to intrude, particularly regarding matters that are personal and on which there is a wide range of opinion in society.

The presumption that the family is the principal decisionmaker may be challenged for any of a number of reasons: decisional incapacity of family members, unresolvable disagreement among competent adult members of the family about the correct decision, evidence of physical or psychological abuse or neglect of the patient by the family, evidence of bias against the patient's interest due to conflicting interests, or evidence that the family intends to disregard the patient's advance directive or the patient's undistorted, stable values and preferences.[12] Even if, for one or more of these reasons, the family is disqualified from being the principal decisionmaker, it will often be appropriate to include family members in the decisionmaking process.

Nonemergency situations in which an incapacitated patient has no family but does have a court-appointed guardian raise special issues that are sometimes overlooked. The considerations that support a strong presumption in favor of the family's being the principal decisionmaker are weaker in the case of a court-appointed guardian, unless the guardian had been nominated by the patient prior to his or her incapacitation (in which case the guardian would be included in the definition of family used here).[13] In the absence of disqualifying reasons, a guardian should act as health care decisionmaker since the person was already making the patient's other, nonhealth-related decisions. Through involvement in past decisionmaking, the guardian may have acquired a knowledge of the patient's beliefs, concerns, and values. Finally, in addition to the ethical grounds there are legal ones: the guardian has the sanction of court authority, which should reduce the concerns of practitioners that following this particular surrogate's decisions will expose them to civil liability.

If no family or legal guardian is initially available, a suitable surrogate decisionmaker should be designated to ensure a clear assignment of authority for decisionmaking and of responsibility for the exercise of this authority. Unless a suitable surrogate decisionmaker is identified, treatment decisions may lack continuity or may rest on an unclear foundation, making it difficult if not impossible to ensure that the process by which decisions are made is ethically and legally sound.

Review Procedures Many people have "natural guardians" whose authority is either recognized as a matter of law (for example, parents deciding for children) or as a matter of custom (for example, one spouse deciding for the other).[14] The decisions made by such surrogates are not routinely subjected to formal review. Such review is more likely to occur when very significant medical interventions are being contemplated, when disagreement arises between health professionals and surrogate decisionmakers, or when decisions are made by a guardian appointed by the court.

Formal review appears to be occurring with greater frequency; at the least, it is being more widely reported in the press. Review may be more frequent because of practitioners' growing sensitivity to the need to protect the interests of patients or because of their increased fear of legal liability, from which an advance ruling by a court could insulate them.[15]

Although state law may require judicial review of certain decisions by a surrogate, well-conceived and carefully executed institutional guidelines may eliminate recourse to the courts that is unnecessary for adequate protection of patients' interests. Certainly, formal court proceedings on each and every health care determination would be unduly intrusive, slow, and costly and would frame treatment decisions in misleadingly adversarial terms.[16]

Judicial review. The most important kind of formal review at the moment is judicial. The justifications for turning to the courts are: (1) the state has a proper role, as *parens patriae*, in protecting the helpless, such as patients lacking health care decisionmaking capacity; (2) the authority of the state is legitimately exercised by courts in life-and-death matters, as in other important situations requiring individual decision; and (3) courts can reach appropriate judgments because of their expertise and disinterested stance in the resolution of disputes.[17]

Greater reliance on advance judicial review has raised a number of concerns about the relative costs and benefits of relying on courts to pass on the decisions of surrogates for incapacitated patients. Judicial review in such cases is costly in terms of time and expense; it can disrupt the process of providing care for a patient, since medical decisionmaking is evolutionary rather than static; it can create unnecessary strains in the relationship between the surrogate decisionmaker and others, such as the health care providers, who may be forced into the role of formal adversaries in the litigation; and it exposes delicate matters that are usually regarded as private to the scrutiny of the courtroom and sometimes even to the glare of the communications media.[18]

These costs may be justifiable if wiser decisions are made and if patients are provided with additional protection from harm. Frequently, however, it appears that the process of judicial review is merely a formality. Judges may not feel that they are able to add very much to the decisions already reached by those most intimately involved, particularly in cases that are brought simply to obtain judicial sanction for an agreed course of conduct.[19] Rather than being an issue the courts are accustomed to addressing, such as whether the surrogates are appropriate decisionmakers or should be disqualified because they are incompetent or have a conflict of interest, the question typically addressed is whether the treatment chosen is the right one.[20] Since this judgment requires substantial understanding of the patient's medical condition and options, the court may simply defer to the recommendation of the treating physicians. The courts' vaunted disinterest may be closer, in practical effect, to lack of interest.

Institutional review. To provide an alternative that is more responsive to the needs of all parties, "institutional ethics committees"[21] are increasingly being used.[22] Because they are closer to the treatment setting, because their deliberations are informal and typically private (and are usually regarded by the participants as falling within the general rules of medical confidentiality), and because they can reconvene easily or can delegate decisions to a separate subgroup of members, ethics committees may have some marked advantages over judicial review when it comes to decisionmaking that is rapid and sensitive to the issues at hand. Furthermore, testimony presented to the Commission indicated that these committees have had a valuable educational role for professionals.[23]

Very little is known, however, about the actual effectiveness of institutional ethics committees, especially in comparison with private, informal mechanisms or with judicial decisionmaking for patients who lack decisionmaking capacity. The composition and functions of existing ethics committees vary substantially from one institution to another. Not enough experience has accumulated to date to know the appropriate and most effective functions and hence the suitable composition of such committees. If their role is to serve primarily as "prognosis committees" to pass on the accuracy of an attending physician's judgment, then committees composed largely of physicians would seem appropriate.[24] If the ethics committees are supposed to reach decisions that best reflect the individually defined well-being of patients or the ethicality of decisions, however, it seems doubtful that an exclusively medical group would be suitable. And if the appropriate role of such review bodies should be to determine whether a surrogate decisionmaker is qualified to make medical decisions on a patient's behalf (and to set only outer boundaries on the nature of the decision reached rather than second-guessing the choice), membership should be diverse.

Alternative institutional and private arrangements, formal and informal, deserve careful examination and evaluation. Furthermore, important details, such as means of case referral, range of functions, committee composition, protection of privacy, and legal status, have not been debated, much less resolved. From what little is already known, it seems that ethics committees may be able to take a leading role in formulating and disseminating policy on decisionmaking for incapacitated patients, assisting in the resolution of difficult situations, and protecting the interests of incapacitated patients. Although committees can be reasonably prompt, efficient, sensitive, and private, having many of the decisions about health care for the incapacitated made in an informal manner between surrogate and provider is plainly a desirable objective as well, just as routine decisions for competent patients should be made by patient and provider without any outside intervention. Furthermore, just as judicial review may sometimes be an unnecessarily onerous means of reviewing medical decisions, review by an ethics committee may also sometimes be inappropriate.

The Commission believes there should be various kinds of review mechanisms available. Thus, the Commission recommends that health care institutions not only develop appropriate mechanisms but also encourage and cooperate in comparative evaluations of such approaches.[25] The results of these studies will have particular importance for society because one presumed advantage of institutional mechanisms is that they avoid the undesirable aspects of having to turn to more formal means of review. Assurance that any new mechanisms have been well thought out and are appropriate to the task is needed before widespread official sanctions can be expected.

NOTES TO MAKING HEALTH CARE DECISIONS

Introduction

1. 42 U.S.C. § 300v-1(a)(1)(A) (1981) also instructs the Commission to study the implications of "informed consent to participation in research projects." The Commission treats issues of human research generally in its biennial reports, Protecting Human Subjects. Furthermore, although they developed initially along independent lines, *see* note 19, Chapter One *infra,* the legal rules for informed consent to treatment and to participation in research spring from common legal and philosophical ground, have had parallel courses of development, and are now basically congruent, so that a separate discussion is not required in this Report.
2. Robert A. Hahn, *Culture and Informed Consent: An Anthropological Perspective* (1982), Appendix F, in Volume Three of this Report.
3. The Commission's survey of the public broke down these responses on the basis of variables such as age, gender, race, education, and income.

Notes to Chapter 1

1. Courts may not, in any event, be inclined to enforce truly shared decisionmaking, even if they were able to do so. Law has often been reluctant to intrude on the autonomy of the medical profession, out of deference to medical expertise, respect for the values of life and health served by the medical profession, and perhaps an unspoken recognition that rules created for health professionals may someday be applied to the legal profession as well. The very history of informed consent litigation, as well as other areas of medical malpractice, provides ample (although not unmixed) evidence for these views.
2. 42 U.S.C. § 300v-1 (a)(1)(A) (1981) the statutory mandate adopted in 1978, under which the Commission examines this issue.
3. Natanson v. Kline, 186 Kan. 393, 350 P.2d 1093 (1960).
4. Scott v. Bradford, 606 P.2d 554, 556 (Okla. 1980).
5. *See* Jay Katz, "Disclosure and Consent in Psychiatric Practice: Mission Impossible?" in Charles K. Hofling, ed., *Law and Ethics in the Practice of Psychiatry*, Brunner/Mazel, Inc., New York (1980) at 91.
6. Hippocrates, "Decorum," in *Hippocrâtes*, Harvard University Press, Cambridge, Mass. (W.H.S. Jones trans. 2d ed. 1967). . . .
7. *See* Katz, *supra* note 5, at 91, 97–100.
8. Martin S. Pernick, "The Patient's Role in Medical Decisionmaking: A Social History of Informed Consent in Medical Therapy" (1981), appendix E, in vol. 3. . . .
9. *Id.*
10. Dissatisfaction by both patients and some professionals with these depersonalizing tendencies of modern medicine is suggested by the renaissance of interest in holistic medicine and the rise of the self-care movement.
11. The problems of not having one person coordinating care are illustrated in this quote from a patient with leukemia:

> I kept fighting through all the fevers and transfusions. I felt I could only survive it by insisting on control. And there would be plenty of chances to test my resolve. The personnel assigned to monitor various functions never coordinated their blood sample requirements on a given day, so they'd come two or three times to leech my tender, collapsing veins. I finally put my foot down.
>
> "You're not going to take more blood," I shouted. "You take it once a day. Get together and find out how much you want and for what purpose, and, goddam it, in the absence of an emergency, don't you touch my veins. Also, no one's going to draw blood except the intravenous nurse team," I said, "because that's all they do, and they know how to do it."
>
> I got my way in both instances, thereby saving myself considerable pain.

Morris B. Abram, *The Day Is Short*, Harcourt Brace Jovanovich, New York (1982) at 209.

12. Mark Siegler, "Searching for Moral Certainty in Medicine: A Proposal for a New Model of the Doctor-Patient Encounter," 57 *Bull. N.Y. Acad. Med.* 56, 60 (1981).
13. The legal doctrine of informed consent has been severely criticized by medical professionals for going too far in its requirements for disclosure. *See* note 5 in Chapter Seven *infra*. Such criticism has diminished substantially in recent years. Furthermore, there is considerable evidence that physicians today actually do disclose a great deal more information to patients than they did 10–20 years ago. *See* Chapter Four [not reprinted in this volume].
14. Siegler, *supra* note 12, at 61.
15. *Id.*
16. *Id.*
17. *Id.* at 62.
18. *Id.* at 63.
19. The Commission's focus in this discussion on the process of reaching agreement is quite deliberate. For perhaps understandable reasons, much of the scholarly legal and philosophical literature concentrates on the "hard case," the case in which no agreement can be reached: when it comes to the crunch, who ultimately has the power to decide? Although such questions cannot be ignored, the Commission's effort in this Report is to readjust the balance toward fuller consideration of those less dramatic issues that arise routinely in the day-to-day practice of responsible medicine and nursing but that have received less attention and emphasis.
20. This image of reaching out to a patient is captured well in the following: "The skillful doctor, metaphorically speaking, throws out a rope to the patient drowning in illness and by encouraging the patient to hold on furthers the healing process." Abram, *supra* note 10, at 116.

Notes to Chapter 2

1. Although these principles have been discussed in judicial decisions and legal commentary on informed consent, the concern of the Commission with patient-provider communication and with decisionmaking in health care in general causes it to consider the issue in a way that is broader and more complex than the legal doctrine. The implications of this discussion for law are noted at appropriate points, however, and conclusions about those implications are given in Part Three.
2. Pursuit of these two values is constrained in various ways, most notably by society's overall interest in equity, justice, and maximum social welfare. These issues are the central concerns of the Commission's forthcoming report *Securing Access to Health Care*. Because these goals need not be central to the decisionmaking process of patients and providers, this report does not take up the complications arising from conflicts between legitimate societal goals and individual patient goals. The Commission's forthcoming report on decisions about life-sustaining therapy explores the relationship between societal and individual concerns in the context of a particular set of health care decisions.
3. Many physicians and patients said they believed an increased patient role would give the patient a better understanding of the medical condition and treatment, would improve physician performance in terms of the honesty and scope of discussion, and would generally improve the doctor-patient relationship. However, a number of physicians claimed that greater patient involvement would improve the quality of care because it would improve compliance and would make patients more cooperative and willing to accept the doctor's judgment.
4. Gerald Dworkin, "Autonomy and Informed Consent" (1982), appendix G, in vol. 3 . . . at section 5.
5. Isaiah Berlin, "Two Concepts of Liberty," in *Four Essays on Liberty*, Clarendon Press, Oxford (1969) at 118–38.
6. This finding should be viewed cautiously since it is well known that surveys overstate the extent of actual satisfaction, as measured during on-site interviews immediately following doctor-patient encounters.
7. Berlin, *supra* note 5.
8. This is not to deny, of course, people's interdependence nor the ways in which each person's values are influenced by others. But people either incorporate or reject such influences into their own conception of what is good. In this view, self-determination lies in the relation between people's values and their actual desires and actions. An individual is self-determined or autonomous when that person is the kind of person he or she wants to be. Self-determination does not imply free will in the sense of a will free of causal determination.
9. Paul S. Appelbaum and Loren H. Roth, "Treatment Refusal In Medical Hospitals" (1982), appendix D, in vol 2 of this Report. Although this lack of information and resulting patient noninvolvement in decisionmaking seems to have been a cause of treatment refusal they also occurred in many cases in which patients did not refuse treatment. Nonprovision of relevant information was also observed in the other on-site study.

   One caveat must be noted, however. The Appelbaum-Roth team observed house-staff/patient interactions extensively but generally did not have a chance to observe interactions between attending physicians and patients. One would expect that discussions of major treatments and procedures, especially major surgical procedures, which were more often left to the attendings, might correspond more closely to the doctrine of informed consent. However, the investigators' conclusions are probably valid for the discussions about diagnostic procedures, medications, and adjunctive therapies as discussed in the other observational study conducted for the Commission. *See* Charles W. Lidz and Alan Meisel, "Informed Consent and the Structure of Medical Care" (1982), appendix C, in vol. 2 of this Report.
10. Likewise, self-determination is not an adequate guiding principle regarding decisions for persons who suffer permanent or chronic mental impairment, such as those who are severely mentally retarded or demented, who are incapable of forming a set of values or of applying them in particular decisions. The decisions for these patients rest instead on an assessment of what would promote their "best interests" (*i.e.*, well-being); *see* [chapter 9]. . . .

    For an interesting example of some of the difficulties that may exist in determining whether an individual's choice reflects his or her long-term goals and values, *see* Albert R. Jonsen, Mark Siegler, and William J. Winslade, *Clinical Ethics*, Macmillan Publishing Co., New York (1982) at 78–81.
11. In the Commission's survey, 36% of the public reported that they have given instructions to someone about how they would like to be treated if they become too sick to make decisions, although only 23% of those instructions are in writing.
12. *See generally* Paul Ramsey, *The Patient as Person*, Yale University Press, New Haven (1970).
13. In some states, advance directives made pursuant to a statute may achieve "binding" legal effect (subject, usually, to considerable room for interpretation). *See* [chapter 7 of this report]. . . . In such a case, whatever the moral justifications, one may not be legally justified in disregarding the directions.
14. One of the observational studies conducted for the Commission concludes that "on balance the normative patient role in [health care decisionmaking] is one of passive acquiescence." Lidz and Meisel, *supra* note 9, at section 6.
15. A possible exception to this requirement would be an irrevocable grant of decisionmaking power to another, as when Odysseus, wishing both to hear and to resist the lure of the Sirens' call, had himself tied to the mast of his ship and instructed his crew not to release him however much he might entreat them to do so.
16. The critical element is the patient's attitude toward "involvement" in the decision, not the mere existence of some "delegation," for all decisions about matters as complex as medical care require a large measure of delegation. Self-determination is not lacking simply because a patient does not insist that the physician review the reasoning and empirical evidence that led up to the physician's recommendation (and its alternatives, if any), including each standardized laboratory test, each anatomical or metabolic

finding, and so forth. Rather, patients' decisions are always the end points of a long series of earlier choices made by physicians and others (where many of the steps in action and reasoning are so ingrained that those involved do not even recognize them for the choices they are). What is at issue, then, is merely the *degree* of delegation of decisionmaking authority by the patient to the professional, not the *fact* of delegation. While some patients want to explore every hypothesis, others want to know only the final recommendation; both may be exercising appropriate self-determination.

Notes to Chapter 3

1. This Report does not address the distinctive issues posed by consent to mental health care or consent to health care by the mentally ill, whether or not institutionalized.
2. *See, e.g.*, Lotman v. Security Mutual Life Ins. Co., 478 F.2d 868 (3d Cir. 1973).
3. *See, e.g.*, *In re* Brooks' Estate, 32 Ill. 2d 361, 205 N.E.2d 435 (1965).
4. *See* [chapter 8; omitted in this edition].
5. The terms "decisionmaking capacity" and "incapacity" are being used in this discussion to avoid the sometimes confounding legal overtones associated with the terms competence and incompetence.
6. At certain outer limits, an individual's goals may be so idiosyncratic that they give rise to questions about the person's capacity for decisionmaking. Assessment of incapacity is further explored in Chapter Eight . . . [omitted in this edition].
7. *See* Paul S. Appelbaum and Loren H. Roth, "Clinical Issues in the Assessment of Competency," 138 *Am. J. Psychiatry* 1462 (1981).
8. Albert R. Jonsen, Mark Siegler, and William J. Winslade, *Clinical Ethics*, Macmillan Publishing Co., New York (1982) at 56–57.
9. "[I]nformed consent may create delay, apprehension, and restrictions on the use of new techniques that will impair the progress of medicine. It is questionable whether the 'average prudent man' will understand and comprehend. . . ." Milton Oppenheim, "Informed Consent to Medical Treatment," 11 *Clev.-Mar. L. Rev.* 249, 261 (1962). *See also* George Robinson and Avraham Merav, "Informed Consent: Recall by Patients Tested Postoperatively," 22 *Annals Thoracic Surgery* 209, 212 (1976); Amelia L. Schultz, Geraldine P. Pardee, and John W. Ensinck, "Are Research Subjects Really Informed?," 123 *W. J. Med.* 76, 78 (1975). Some claim that patients can never truly comprehend what a procedure entails until they have experienced it. *See, e.g.*, Franz J. Ingelfinger, "Informed (But Uneducated) Consent," 287 *New Eng. J. Med.* 465, 465 (1972).
10. For example, in one of the observational studies conducted for the Commission, one patient asked whether his spleen had anything to do with having children. For a discussion of patient misunderstanding of medical terms, see, e.g., B.M. Korsch and V.F. Negrette, "Doctor-Patient Communication," 227 *Scientific American* 66 (1972); F.C. Tring and M.C. Hayes-Allen, "Understanding and Misunderstanding of Some Medical Terms," 7 *Brit. J. Med. Educ.* 53 (1973); and Samuel Gorovitz, *Doctors' Dilemmas: Moral Conflict and Medical Care*, Macmillan Publishing Co., New York (1982) at 19–20.
11. *See, e.g.*, Robinson and Merav, *supra* note 9, at 210–212; Gorovitz, *supra* note 10, at 40.
12. Obstetricians were most likely (57%) and subspecialists least likely (38%) to report that more than 90% could understand. Office-based physicians were more likely than hospital-based doctors to think that their patients could understand. Older doctors were more likely than younger doctors (53% versus 38%) to feel that 90–100% of patients could understand, and physicians who treated few patients with serious illness were more likely than physicians who treated more patients with serious illness to report that patients could understand (55% versus 36%).
13. Bernard Gert and Charles Culver, "What Would It Mean to Be Competent Enough to Consent to or Refuse Participation in Research?—Philosophical Overview," in Natalie Reating, ed., *Competency and Informed Consent: Papers and Other Materials Developed for the Workshop "Empirical Research on Informed Consent with Subjects of Uncertain Competence,"* National Institutes of Mental Health (Jan. 12–13, 1981).
14. Of course, extreme care must be exercised lest pronouncements of "what the patient really wants" become a cover for "what I think is best for the patient." Properly circumscribed, however, a choice made on behalf of a patient who lacks capacity may be a truer example of one fundamental interest undergirding self-determination than following the patient's preference would be.
15. Plainly, this conclusion rests on practical and prudential, rather than theoretical, considerations. A system could be instituted in which all patients facing significant decisions receive a thorough evaluation of their decisionmaking capacity. Those showing psychiatric morbidity that might undermine their decisionmaking capacity could then be channeled through an alternative process designed to protect their interests and well-being. Though this would undoubtedly result in "better" decisions for some patients, it would impose substantial additional costs and burdens on the health care system.
16. Loren H. Roth, Alan Meisel, and Charles W. Lidz, "Tests of Competency to Consent to Treatment," 134 *Am. J. Psychiatry* 279 (1977).
17. The procedural and substantive standards that apply in this assessment are discussed in Chapter Nine *infra*. The factors that prompt an inquiry about a patient's capacity are related, but not necessarily equivalent, to those that govern the resolution of the inquiry.
18. *See generally*, *Restatement (Second) of Torts*, American Law Institute Publishers, St. Paul, Minn. (1979) at § 892B; *see also* Robert E. Powell, "Consent to Operative Procedures," 21 *Md. L. Rev* 181, 203 (1961). Indeed, many of the eighteenth, nineteenth, and early twentieth century legal cases often cited as precursors of the modern doctrine of informed consent imposed liability for unauthorized medical procedures on precisely these grounds. . . .
19. Charles W. Lidz and Alan Meisel, "Informed Consent and the Structure of Medical Care" (1982), appendix C, in vol. 2 of this Report, at section 4.

20. Of course, not all forced interventions that employ medical procedures in such institutions are necessarily intended to promote the well-being of others. Drawing the line between the protection of others and the abuse of inmates is a difficult task. *See, e.g.,* Rogers v. Okin, 778 F. Supp. 1342 (D.Mass. 1979).
21. Lidz and Meisel, *supra* note 19.
22. In this respect, threats should be distinguished from warnings of unpleasant occurrences that may be the natural consequences of certain decisions. A physician's discussion of the natural history of a disease does not constitute threats, while a statement that a physician will discharge the patient from the hospital if the patient requests a second opinion (or asks too many questions, or complains excessively about hospital food) probably does. In many cases, the distinction depends on whether the professional can bring about the unwanted consequences, but this is not always true. For example, a surgeon who tells a breast cancer patient of an inability to continue in charge of her care if she rejects surgery in favor of chemotherapy or radiation is probably not issuing a threat, although in some circumstances the suggestion that a health professional would abandon a highly dependent patient if medical advice were not followed might constitute an improper and coercive threat.
23. These concerns are particularly acute in certain settings, such as so-called total institutions, where whole populations are placed in a special condition of inequality and dependency on powerful others, even for ordinary care and sustenance. Choices made in such settings are particularly subject to coercive influences, and careful scrutiny of their voluntariness is often warranted.
24. The role of the family is discussed in more detail in Chapter Five . . . [not included in this edition].
25. Henry K. Beecher, "Some Guiding Principles for Clinical Investigation," 195 *J.A.M.A.* 1135, 1135 (1966). *See also* Norman Fost, "A Surrogate System for Informed Consent," 233 *J.A.M.A.* 800 (1975); Ingelfinger, *supra* note 9, at 466.
26. "In spite of . . . federal requirements that clients participating as 'subjects' in research give 'informed consent,' and in spite of the legal releases required for such procedures as surgery, it is my impression that clients are more often bullied than informed into consent, their resistance weakened in part by their desire for the general service if not the specific procedure, in part by the oppressive setting they find themselves in, and in part by the calculated intimidation, restriction of information, and covert threats of rejection by the professional staff itself." Eliot Freidson, *The Profession of Medicine*, Dodd, Mead & Co., New York (1970) at 376. *See also* Jon R. Waltz and Thomas W. Scheuneman, "Informed Consent to Therapy," 64 *Nw. U.L. Rev.* 628, 64546 (1970).

Notes to Chapter 7

1. *See* Jay Katz, "Informed Consent—A Fairy Tale?: Law's Vision," 39 *U. Pitt. L. Rev.* 137 (1977); Joseph Goldstein, "For Harold Lasswell: Some Reflections on Human Dignity, Entrapment, Informed Consent, and the Plea Bargain," 84 *Yale L.J.* 693 (1975).
2. From the Commission's survey it is apparent that several aspects of the legal doctrine of informed consent and its implementation (*i.e.*, increased disclosure, increased patient involvement in decisionmaking, and consent forms) have made physicians more sensitive to patients' needs and expectations. As discussed in Chapter Four [omitted in this edition], these aspects are generally viewed as beneficial to the doctor-patient relationship because they tend to provoke discussion, enhance understanding on the part of both doctor and patient, lead to better decisions, and aid compliance.
3. One obstacle to the implementation of the Commission's vision through law is the difficulty of formulating an appropriate means of enforcement. When a health care professional does not engage in ethically proper discussion with a patient, and the failure to do so causes no bodily harm to the patient, the amount of damages to which the patient would be entitled are nominal, and thus few if any patients (and lawyers) would be willing to bring suit under such circumstances. Instead of relying on traditional litigation to implement the Commission's vision,

   > [t]his could be achieved by establishing a system of noninsurable tort-fines for violation of the duty to disclose and a compensation fund. The fines would be paid into the fund, which would be used to compensate those persons the legislature defines as injured by nondisclosure. Under this arrangement doctors are provided with guidance and are subject to specific deterrence. All physicians who violate a duty to disclose would be liable for fines that could be set in accordance with their deterrence objective. Only those patients suffering injury, as defined by the legislature, would be compensated.

   Leonard L. Riskin, "Informed Consent: Looking for the Action, 1975 *U. Ill. L. F.* 580, 606–07.
4. One unfortunate by-product of the legal regulation, through malpractice suits, of the doctor-patient relationship in an attempt to establish a minimum level of quality in the provision of medical services is practice of what is referred to as "defensive" medicine, which "consist[s] of medically unjustified care provided by the physician for the purpose of reducing the possibility of a malpractice suit. . . ." Project, "The Medical Malpractice Threat: A Study of Defensive Medicine," 1971 *Duke L.J.* 939, 942. This study concludes that "[t]he threat of a malpractice suit does induce physicians to overutilize diagnostic tests and procedures in particular cases, but . . . the practice is not extensive and probably not a contributing factor to the rising costs of medical care." *Id.* at 964. *But see* Elliot Sagall, "Medical Malpractice: Are the Doctors Right?," 10 *Trial* (July/Aug 1974) at 59, 60, suggesting that reports on the extent of the practice of defensive medicine are exaggerated.

   In Texas, informed consent is legally governed by a set of detailed regulations describing what doctors are supposed to disclose for particular procedures. *See* 3 Tex. Reg. 4293–96, §§ 319.01.03.001.003 (Dec. 12, 1978), issued pursuant to Tex. Rev. Civ. Stat. Ann. art. 4590i, § 6.03 (Vernon

Cum. Supp. 1980). The limitations of law in regulation of the relationship between doctors and patients is well developed by Fox and Swazey in their discussion of the famous heart transplant case of Karp v. Cooley, 493 F.2d 408 (5th Cir. 1974). *See* Renee C. Fox and Judith P. Swazey, *The Courage to Fail: A Social View of Organ Transplants and Dialysis*, Univ. of Chicago Press, Chicago (1974) at 201 *et seq*.

5. The requirement of informed consent has frequently been described by physicians as a myth or a fiction. *See, e.g.*, Henry K. Beecher, "Consent in Clinical Experimentation—Myth and Reality," 195 *J.A.M.A.* 34–35 (1966); Preston J. Burnham, "Medical Experimentation on Humans," 152 *Science* 448 (1966); William P. Irvin, "Now, Mrs. Blare, About the Complications. . . ." 40 *Med. Econ.* 102 (1963); Eugene G. Laforet, "The Fiction of Informed Consent," 235 *J.A.M.A.* 1579 (1976); Edmund B. Middleton, "Informed Consent," 233 *J.A.M.A.* 1049 (1975); Mark Ravitch, "Informed Consent—Descent to Absurdity," 101 *Med. Times* No. 9, 164 (1973). The articles critical of informed consent appear to have diminished in frequency in the last few years.
6. . . . If informed consent is viewed as a process—as this Report envisions—rather than as an event, proposals to embody "informed consent" in a written or "electronic" document are ultimately unavailing. *See, e.g.*, Note, 44 *Brooklyn L. Rev.* 241, 27381 (1978).
7. Several current dilemmas in informed consent law would remain problematic in this view. For example, what causal relationship needs to be established between the professional's failure to provide a basis for effective participation and the physical injury associated with treatment? When the professional's failure to provide such a basis did not result in physical injury to the patient, there would be no readily ascertainable monetary damages to serve as a basis for redress (or to encourage an attorney to take the case on a contingent-fee basis). A standard for money damages to redress dignitary injuries may be needed, or the governmental and voluntary organizations that regulate licensure and certification may need to investigate allegations of systematic violation of patients' rights, as a ground for professional discipline.
8. *See* pp. 25–26 supra [omitted in this edition].
9. Indeed, although the broad generalities of battery and malpractice law, which aim largely at redressing past misconduct, may not be helpful here, the rules spelled out by hospital boards, medical societies, and licensing bodies could provide more detailed prospective guidance and encouragement.
10. Standards and procedures for assessing which patients are incapable of participating in a health care decision are discussed in Chapter Eight *infra*.
11. *See* American Law Institute, *Restatement (Second) of Agency*, American Law Institute Publishers, St. Paul, Minn. (1957) at § 122.
12. *See* Ala. Code §§ 22-8A-1 to 22-8A-10 (Supp. 1981); Ark. Stat. Ann. §§ 82-3801–.3804 (Supp. 1981); Cal. Health and Safety Code §§ 7185–7195 (Deering Supp. 1982); D.C. Code §§ 6-2421 to 2430 (Supp. 1982); Del. Code Ann. tit. 16, §§ 2501–2509 (1982); Idaho Code §§ 39-4501 to 4508 (Supp. 1982); Kan. Stat. Ann. §§ 65-28,101 to 65-28,109 (Supp. 1981); Nev. Rev. Stat. §§ 449.540–.690 (1979); N.M. Stat. Ann. §§ 24-7-1 to 24-711 (1981); N.C. Gen. Stat. §§ 90-320 to 90-322 (1981); Or. Rev. Stat. §§ 97.050–.090 (1981); Tex. Rev. Civ. Stat. Ann. art. 4590h §§ 1–11 (Vernon 1982); 18 Vt. Stat. Ann. §§ 5251–5262 (1982); Wash. Rev. Code Ann. 70.122.010–70.122.905 (West 1982).
13. An example of such a directive would be one stating: "I feel that I would rather not live than remain in an unconscious state from which I have no likelihood of recovering." This might provide a clearer sense of a person's feelings and wishes than a directive that merely specifies the treatment a person does or does not want under certain circumstances.
14. The term "surrogate" is used in this report (*see* Chapter Eight . . . [omitted in this edition]) to designate an agent authorized to make a health care decision on behalf of a patient who lacks the capacity to do so personally. Within this category, a "proxy" is a surrogate appointed by a patient.
15. In the context of the present discussion, the triggering event under a directive designating a proxy would be (at the least) that the signer had become incapable of participating in decisions about his or her own care. Directives could, in theory, designate a proxy to step into the decisionmaking shoes of a person who remained capable of making his or her own choices but who chose not to.
16. *See* Alaska Stat. §§ 13.26.325, .330 (1979); Ariz. Rev. Stat. §§ 14-5501 to 5502 (1975); Ark. Stat. Ann. §§ 58-501 to 511 (1971); Colo. Rev. Stat. §§ 15-14-501 to 502 (Supp. 1979); Conn. Gen. Stat. § 45-690 (1979); Del. Code tit. 25, §§ 175–180 (Supp. 1978); Fla. Stat. Ann. § 709.08 (West 1980); Ga. Code Ann. § 4-214.1 (1975); Haw. Rev. Stat. §§ 560:5-501 to 502 (Supp. 1979); Idaho Code §§ 15-5-501 to 502 (1979); Ind. Code Ann. §§ 30-2-1.5-1 to 2 (Burns Supp. 1979–1981); Iowa Code Ann. §§ 633.705.706 (West Supp. 1980–1981); Ky. Rev. Stat. § 386.093 (Supp. 1978); Me. Rev. Stat. tit. 18-A, §§ 5-501 to 502 (1979); Md. Est. & Trusts Code Ann. §§ 13-601 to 602 (1974); Mass. Ann. Laws, ch. 201, § 50 (Michie Supp. 1980); Mich. Comp. Laws Ann. §§ 700.495–.499 (Supp. 1980–1981); Minn. Stat. Ann §§ 524.5-501 to 502 (West 1975); Miss. Code Ann. § 87-3-15 (1973); Mont. Code Ann. §§ 72-5-501 to 502 (1979); Neb. Rev. Stat. §§ 302662 to 2663 (1975); N.J. Stat. Ann. §§ 46:2B-8 to 9 (West Supp. 1979–1980); N.M. Stat. Ann. §§ 45-5-501 to 502 (1978); N.Y. Gen. Oblig. Law § 5-1601 (McKinney 1978); N.C. Gen. Stat. § 47-115.1 (1976 & Supp. 1979); N.D. Cent. Code §§ 30.1-30-01 to 02 (1976); Ohio Rev. Code Ann. §§ 1337.09-.091 (Page 1979); Okla. Stat. Ann. tit. 58, §§ 1051–1062 (West Supp. 1979–1980); Or. Rev. Stat. §§ 126.407, .413 (1979); Pa. Stat. Ann. tit. 20, §§ 5601–5602 (Purdon 1975); S.C. Code § 32-13-10 (Supp. 1979); Tex. Prob. Code Ann. tit. 17A, § 36A (Vernon Supp. 1980); Utah Code Ann. §§ 75-5-501 to 502 (1978); Vt. Stat. Ann. tit. 14, §§ 3-51-3052 (Supp. 1979); Va. Code §§ 11-9.1 to .2 (1978); Wash. Rev. Code Ann. §§ 11.94.010–.020 (Supp. 1980–1981); Wyo. Stat. §§ 34-9-101 to 110 (1977). *See also* Uniform Durable Power of Attorney Act, 8 U.L.A. 74–80 (1981).
17. "Legal Problems of the Aged and Infirm—The Durable Power of Attorney—Planned Protective Services and the

Living Will," 13 *Real Property, Probate and Trust Journal* 1, 2–4, 35–36, 41 (Spring 1978).

18. Yale Law School Legislative Services Project, Medical Treatment Decision Act, Society for the Right to Die, New York (1981) at § 3; Uniform Health Care Consent Act, National Conference of Commissioners on Uniform State Laws, New York (1982) at § 6; Uniform Right to Refuse Treatment Act, Concern for Dying, Chicago (Draft, May 1982) at §§ 3–5.
19. *See* Ala. Code § 22-8A-7 (Supp. 1981); Del. Code Ann. tit. 16 § 2505 (1982); Kan. Stat. Ann. § 65-28,106 (Supp. 1981); N.M. Stat. Ann. § 24-7-7 (1981); Or. Rev. Stat. § 97.065 (1981); Wash. Rev. Code Ann. § 70.122.050 (West 1982). *See also* Medical Treatment Decision Act, *supra* note 18, at § 9; Uniform Right to Refuse Treatment Act, *supra* note 18, at § 12.
20. Cal. Health and Safety Code § 7191(b) (Deering Supp. 1982); Kan. Stat. Ann. § 65-28, 107(a) (Supp. 1981); Tex. Rev. Civ. Stat. Ann. art. 4590h § 7(b) (Vernon 1982). *See also* Medical Treatment Act, *supra* note 18, at § 12.
21. *See* pp. 172–73 . . . [omitted in this edition].
22. *See* Ala. Code § 22-8A-4 (Supp. 1981); Cal. Health and Safety Code § 7188 (Deering Supp. 1982); Del. Code Ann. tit. 16, § 2503(b) (1982); Idaho Code § 39-4505 (Supp. 1982); Kan. Stat. Ann. § 65-28,103(a) (Supp. 1981); Nev. Rev. Stat. § 449.600 (1979); N.C. Gen. Stat. § 90321(c) (1981); Or. Rev. Stat. § 97.055 (1981); Tex. Rev. Civ. Stat. Ann. art. 4590h § 3 (Vernon 1982); 18 Vt. Stat. Ann. § 5254 (1982); Wash. Rev. Code Ann. § 70.122.030 (West 1982).
23. *See, e.g.*, Cal. Health and Safety Code § 7188.5 (Deering Supp. 1982): "A directive shall have no force or effect if the declarant is a patient in a skilled nursing facility . . . at the time the directive is executed unless one of the two witnesses to the directive is a patient advocate or ombudsman as may be designated by the State Department of Aging for this purpose . . . ." The explanation given by the legislature for enacting this provision is "that some patients in skilled nursing facilities may be so insulated from a voluntary decisionmaking role, by virtue of the custodial nature of their care, as to require special assurance that they are capable of willfully and voluntarily executing a directive."
24. The Uniform Health Care Consent Act addresses this issue in several sections. Section 5 provides for a limited delegation of power by some individuals authorized to consent to health care for another under § 4(a)(2), (b)(2), and (b)(3). According to § 5, the only individuals authorized to consent for another who may delegate their decisional authority are *family members*. Nonfamily health care representatives, who may be appointed according to the terms of § 6, are not authorized to delegate their decisional authority. All delegations must be in writing, and unless the writing so specifies, no further delegation of decisional authority is permitted. Any delegated authority terminates six months after the effective date of the writing.
25. *See* Joel Feinberg, *Rights, Justice, and the Bounds of Liberty*, Princeton Univ. Press, Princeton, N.J. (1980); Ruth Macklin, "Return to the Best Interests of the Child," in Willard Gaylin and Ruth Macklin, eds., *Who Speaks for the Child*, Plenum Press, New York (1982); A. M. Capron, "The Authority of Others to Decide about Biomedical Intervention with Incompetents," in Gaylin and Macklin, *id.*; Joseph Goldstein, Anna Freud, and Albert J. Solnit, *Beyond the Best Interests of the Child*, Free Press, New York (1979).
26. *See* Cal. Health and Safety Code § 7188 (Deering Supp. 1982); Idaho Code § 39-4504 (Supp. 1982); Or. Rev. Stat. § 97.055 (1981); Tex. Rev. Civ. Stat. Ann. art. 4590h § 3 (Vernon 1982).
27. See Cal. Health and Safety Code § 7188 (Deering Supp. 1982); Del. Code Ann. tit. 16, § 2506(c) (1982); Idaho Code § 39-4504 (Supp. 1982); Or. Rev. Stat. § 97.055 (1981).
28. See Ala. Code § 22-8A-5 (Supp. 1981); Cal. Health and Safety Code § 7189 (Deering Supp. 1982); Del. Code Ann. tit. 16, § 2504 (1982); Idaho Code § 39-4505 (Supp. 1982); Kan. Stat. Ann. § 65-28,104 (Supp. 1981); Nev. Rev. Stat. § 449.620 (1979); N.M. Stat. Ann. § 24-7-6 (1981); N.C. Gen. Stat. § 90-321(e) (1981); Or. Rev. Stat. § 97.055 (1981); Tex. Rev. Civ. Stat. Ann. art. 4590h § 4(a) (Vernon 1982); Wash. Rev. Code Ann. § 70.122.040 (West 1982).
29. Indeed, the subject receives further attention from the Commission in its forthcoming report on deciding about life-sustaining therapy.

Notes to Chapter 9

1. *See generally* Lawrence A. Frolik, "Plenary Guardianship: An Analysis, a Critique, and a Proposal for Reform," 23 *Ariz. L. Rev.* 599 (1981).
2. For example, the substituted judgment doctrine permits a surrogate to make a gift of some of an incompetent's assets to a relative to whom the incompetent person had previously made gifts. The court will approve such a gift to the extent that it does not endanger funds needed for the incompetent's support—even if the incompetent person would have been willing to be more generous.
3. The best interests doctrine has received most attention in law in cases involving questions of the custody and care of children, *see generally* 2 C.J.S. *Adoption of Persons* §§ 90–91 (1972), and in cases involving the expenditure of trust funds, *see generally* 76 *Am. Jur.* 2d, "Trusts" § 288 (1975), neither of which are entirely accurate guides to understanding how the standard ought to operate in instances of surrogate health care decisionmaking for adults who lack decisionmaking capacity.
4. *See* Chapter Two *supra.*
5. *See* Chapter 7's Enhancing Self-Determination of the Formerly Competent, *supra.*
6. The phrase "quality of life" has been used in differing ways; sometimes it refers to the value that the continuation of life has for the patient, and other times to the value that others find in the continuation of the patient's life, perhaps in terms of their estimates of the patient's actual or potential productivity or social contribution. In applying the best interest principle, the Commission is concerned with the value of the patient's life for the patient.
7. Allen E. Buchanan, "The Limits of Proxy Decision Making for Incompetents," 29 *UCLA L. Rev.* 393 (1981); John A. Robertson, "Legal Criteria for Orders Not to Resuscitate: A Response to Justice Liacos," in A. Edward Doudera and J. Douglas Peters, eds., Legal and Ethical Aspects of Treating

Critically and Terminally Ill Patients, AUPHA Press, Washington, D.C. (1982) at 159–63.

8. The only necessary implication of a determination of incapacity to decide about health care is that the patient's decision, if any, may be overruled. Even if patients' decisionmaking capacities are sufficiently impaired that it would be inappropriate to take their preferences as binding, patients may still be able to appreciate many aspects of the decision and may feel they have been treated more respectfully if those vested with the power to make decisions about them recognize the extent to which they are sentient beings with values and preferences of their own. Encouraging participation in the decisionmaking process may in fact facilitate recovery of capacity under some circumstances. These patients would be well served if their surrogates were to let them make such decisions for themselves, although the surrogate's permission may also be required.
9. Allen Buchanan, "Medical Paternalism or Legal Imperialism: Not the Only Alternatives for Handling Saikewicz-type Cases," 5 *Law & Med.* 97, 105–06 (1979); Alan Meisel, "The 'Exceptions' to the Informed Consent Doctrine: Striking a Balance Between Competing Values in Medical Decisionmaking," 1979 *Wis. L. Rev.* 413, 476.
10. Meisel, *supra* note 9, at 476.
11. The Commission's broad use of the term "family" reflects a recognition of the fact that many of those with most knowledge and concern for the patient may not be his or her actual relatives. The fact that more than one person may fall within this category points to the need to designate one person as the principal decisionmaker for the incapacitated patient. One possibility is to define a presumptive priority, *e.g.*, that a person living with his or her spouse will speak for that spouse, that adult children will speak for elderly widowed parents, etc. In some cases such presumptions may be helpful. Nevertheless, the Commission believes that it is the responsibility of the practitioner to determine who acts as the patient's "surrogate." No neat formulas or serial orderings will suffice to capture the complexities involved in determining who among the individuals presenting themselves as friends and relatives of the patient knows the patient best and has his or her best interests in view. The responsibility is therefore on the practitioner either to determine who this spokesperson is or to go to court to have a guardian appointed.
12. Buchanan, *supra* note 9, at 111.
13. If an incapacitated patient has both a competent family and a legal guardian, they should function together as principal decisionmakers to the extent permitted by local law.
14. *See* note 10, Chapter Eight . . . [omitted in this edition].
15. *See generally* Robert A. Burt, *Taking Care of Strangers*, The Free Press, New York (1979).
16. Nevertheless, arrangements should be made to ensure that the appropriate cases do come before a formal tribunal, as when, for example, the patient expresses a desire for judicial review, or the patient's health needs will require continual decisionmaking on a broad range of issues. Further, it is incumbent upon health care providers to seek review when they believe that a surrogate's decision about treatment fails to reflect the patient's values and goals (to the extent that they are ascertainable) or the patient's best interests.
17. The argument for judicial review is well stated by Professor Baron. *See* Charles H. Baron, "Assuring 'Detached But Passionate Investigation and Decision': The Role of Guardians Ad Litem in Saikewicz-Type Cases, 4 *Am. J. Law & Med.* 111 (1978); Charles H. Baron, "Medical Paternalism and the Rule of Law: A Reply to Dr. Relman," 4 *Am. J. Law & Med.* 337 (1979). *See also, In re* Roe, 421, N.E.2d 40, 51–56 (Mass. 1981); Superintendent of Belchertown State School v. Saikewicz, 370 N.E.2d 417, 432–35 (1977). The view that judicial review is inappropriate is well stated by Dr. Relman, the editor of the *New England Journal of Medicine. See* Arnold S. Relman, "The Saikewicz Decision: A Response to Allen Buchanan's Views on Decision Making for Terminally Ill Incompetents," 5 *Am. J. Law & Med.* 119 (1979).
18. Buchanan, *supra* note 9, at 105–06.
19. *See, e.g., In re* Nemser, 51 Misc.2d 616, 273 N.Y.S.2d 624, 629 (S.Ct. 1966), in which a trial court judge to whom a petition for the appointment of a guardian to consent to surgery on an elderly, somewhat incapacitated, but objecting woman, chided the woman's family, the hospital, and the doctors for seeking his imprimatur:

> [I]t is apparent that this proceeding was necessitated only because of the current practice of members of the medical profession and their associated hospitals of shifting the burden of their responsibilities to the courts, to determine, in effect, whether doctors should proceed with certain medical procedures definitively found necessary or deemed advisable for the health, welfare, and perhaps even the life of a patient who is either unwilling or unable to consent thereto. . . . [ellipsis in original].
>
> It seems incongruous in light of the physicians' oath that they even seek legal immunity prior to action necessary to sustain life. [H]ow legalistic minded our society has become, and what an ultra-legalistic maze we have created to the extent that society and the individual have become enmeshed and paralyzed by its unrealistic entanglements!

See also William J. Curran, "A Problem of Consent, Kidney Transplantation in Minors," 34 *N.Y.U.L. Rev.* 891 (1959)

20. *See, e.g., In re* Quinlan, 70 N.J. 10, 355 A.2d 647, 664, *cert. denied*, 429 U.S. 922 (1976):

> If a putative decision by Karen to permit this non-cognitive, vegetative existence to terminate by natural forces is regarded as a valuable incident of her right of privacy, as we believe it to be, then it should not be discarded solely on the basis that her condition prevents her conscious exercise of the choice. The only practical way to prevent destruction of the right is to permit the guardian and family of Karen to render their best judgment subject to the qualification hereinafter stated, as to whether she would exercise it in these circumstances. If their conclusion is in the affirmative this decision should be accepted by a society the overwhelming majority of whose members would, we think, in similar circumstances exercise such a choice in the same way for themselves or for those closest to them.

21. The Commission uses the term "institutional ethics committee" rather than "hospital ethics committee" because

such committees could well function in other health care institutions such as nursing homes.

22. In the past decade, 5% of large hospitals (that is, those with more than 200 beds) have established such committees. Stuart Youngner, "Hospital Ethics Committees" (1982), Appendix to Commission's forthcoming Report on decisions about life-sustaining treatment.
23. Testimony of Ronald Cranford, M.D., transcript of 21st meeting of the President's Commission (June 10, 1982) at 18, 39.
24. Carole Levine, "Hospital Ethics Committees: A Guarded Prognosis," 7(3) *Hastings Ctr. Rep.* 25, 27 (1977); Robert Veatch, "Hospital Ethics Committees: Is There a Role?," 7(3) *Hastings Ctr. Rep.* 22, 24 (1977).
25. To assist in this endeavor, the Commission's forthcoming report on decisions about life-sustaining treatment will provide a more detailed examination of the potentials, liabilities, and reported experience with institutional ethics committees and other mechanisms for ensuring that decisionmaking of high quality occurs.

TARASOFF V. REGENTS OF UNIVERSITY OF CALIFORNIA, SUPREME COURT OF CALIFORNIA, 1974

INTRODUCTION. *A distinguishing mark of medical ethics is the rule that generally requires that information received by the health care professional from patients be kept confidential. The confidentiality rule has always had potential exceptions, however. Two general classes of exceptions exist: one for cases in which the welfare of the patient would be served by breaking a confidence; the other for cases in which the welfare of third parties would be served. The more paternalistic ethical traditions such as those of the Hippocratic Oath would accept breach of confidentiality in order to benefit the patient (even if the patient did not concur). The pre-1980 American Medical Association Code permitted such breaches. The ethical traditions more committed to the rights of patients insist that confidences can be broken to benefit patients only with the patient's permission.*

While the newer codes are less likely to permit breaking confidence to benefit the patient, they have opened the door to certain disclosures for the welfare of others. Though a professional ethic committed only to the welfare of the patient would not permit such disclosures, most recent codes, including that of the American Medical Association since 1980, recognize that in some cases the clinician has a duty to warn others of serious threats of bodily harm. The case of Tatiana Tarasoff, whose former boy friend disclosed to a psychologist a credible threat against her, illustrates the issue.

ON OCTOBER 27, 1969, Prosenjit Poddar killed Tatiana Tarasoff.[1] Plaintiffs, Tatiana's parents, allege that two months earlier Poddar confided his intention to kill Tatiana to Dr. Lawrence Moore, a psychologist employed by the Cowell Memorial Hospital at the University of California at Berkeley. They allege that on Moore's request, the campus police briefly detained Poddar, but released him when he appeared rational. They further claim that Dr. Harvey Powelson, Moore's superior, then directed that no further action be taken to detain Poddar. No one warned Tatiana of her peril. Concluding that these facts neither set forth causes of action against the therapists and policemen involved, nor against the Regents of the University of California as their employer, the superior court sustained defendants' demurrers to plaintiffs' second amended complaints without leave to amend.[2] This appeal ensued.

Plaintiffs' complaints predicate liability on two grounds: defendants' failure to warn plaintiffs of the impending danger and their failure to use reasonable care to bring about Poddar's confinement pursuant to the Lanterman-Petris-Short Act (Welf. & Inst.Code, § 5000ff.) Defendants, in turn, assert that they owed no duty of reasonable care to Tatiana and that they are immune from suit under the California Tort Claims Act of 1963 (Gov.Code, § 810 ff.).

We shall explain that defendant therapists, merely because Tatiana herself was not their patient, cannot escape liability for failing to exercise due care to warn the endangered Tatiana or those who reasonably could have been expected to notify her of her peril. When a doctor or a psychotherapist, in the exercise of his professional skill and knowledge, determines, or should determine, that a warning is essential to avert danger arising from the medical or psychological condition of his patient, he incurs a legal obligation to give that warning. Primarily, the relationship between defendant therapists and Poddar as their patient imposes the described duty to warn. We shall point out that a second basis for liability lies in the fact that

Tarasoff v. The Regents of the University of California 1974. Cite as Sup. 118 Cal.Rptr. 129.

defendants' bungled attempt to confine Poddar may have deterred him from seeking further therapy and aggravated the danger to Tatiana; having thus contributed to and partially created the danger, defendants incur the ensuing obligation to give the warning.

We reject defendants' asserted defense of governmental immunity; no specific statutory provision shields them from liability for failure to warn, and Government Code section 820.2 does not protect defendants' conduct as an exercise of discretion. We conclude that plaintiffs' complaints state, or can be amended to state, a cause of action against defendants for negligent failure to warn.

Defendants, however, may properly claim immunity from liability for their failure to *confine* Poddar. Government Code section 856 bars imposition of liability upon defendant therapists for their determination to refrain from detaining Poddar and Welfare and Institutions Code section 5154 protects defendant police officers from civil liability for releasing Poddar after his brief confinement. We therefore conclude that plaintiffs cannot state a cause of action for defendants' failure to detain Poddar. Since plaintiffs base their claim to punitive damages against defendant Powelson solely upon Powelson's failure to bring about such detention, not upon Powelson's failure to give the above described warnings, that claim likewise fails to state a cause of action.

1. Plaintiffs' complaints. Plaintiffs, Tatiana's mother and father, filed separate but virtually identical second amended complaints. The issue before us on this appeal is whether those complaints now state, or can be amended to state, causes of action against defendants. We therefore begin by setting forth the pertinent allegations of the complaints.[3]

Plaintiffs' first cause of action, entitled "Failure to Detain a Dangerous Patient," alleges that on August 20, 1969, Poddar was a voluntary outpatient receiving therapy at Cowell Memorial Hospital. Poddar informed Moore, his therapist, that he was going to kill an unnamed girl, readily identifiable as Tatiana, when she returned home from spending the summer in Brazil. Moore, with the concurrence of Dr. Gold, who had initially examined Poddar, and Dr. Yandell, assistant to the director of the department of psychiatry, decided that Poddar should be committed for observation in a mental hospital. Moore orally notified Officers Atkinson and Teel of the campus police that he would request commitment. He then sent a letter to Police Chief William Beall requesting the assistance of the police department in securing Poddar's confinement.

Officers Atkinson, Brownrigg, and Halleran took Poddar into custody, but, satisfied that Poddar was rational, released him on his promise to stay away from Tatiana. Powelson, director of the department of psychiatry at Cowell Memorial Hospital, then asked the police to return Moore's letter, directed that all copies of the letter and notes that Moore had taken as therapist be destroyed, and "ordered no action to place Prosenjit Poddar in 72-hour treatment and evaluation facility."

Plaintiffs' second cause of action, entitled "Failure to Warn On a Dangerous Patient," incorporates the allegations of the first cause of action, but adds the assertion that defendants negligently permitted Poddar to be released from police custody without "notifying the parents of Tatiana Tarasoff that their daughter was in grave danger from Posenjit Poddar." Poddar persuaded Tatiana's brother to share an apartment with him near Tatiana's residence; shortly after her return from Brazil, Poddar went to her residence and killed her.

Plaintiffs' third cause of action, entitled "Abandonment of a Dangerous Patient," seeks $10,000 punitive damages against defendant Powelson. Incorporating the crucial allegations of the first cause of action, plaintiffs charge that Powelson "did the things herein alleged with intent to abandon a dangerous patient, and said acts were done maliciously and oppressively."

Plaintiff's fourth cause of action, for "Breach of Primary Duty to Patient and the Public" states essentially the same allegations as the first cause of action, but seeks to characterize defendants' conduct as a breach of duty to safeguard their patient and the public. Since such conclusory labels add nothing to the factual allegations of the complaint, the first and fourth causes of action are legally indistinguishable.

2. Plaintiffs can state a cause of action for negligent failure to warn. The second cause of action in plaintiffs' complaints alleges that Tatiana's death proximately resulted from defendants' negligent failure to warn plaintiffs of Poddar's intention to kill Tatiana and claims general and special damages. Ordinarily such allegations of negligence, proximate causation, and damages would establish a cause of action. (See Dillon v. Legg (1968) 68 Cal.2d 728, 733–734, 69 Cal.Rptr. 72, 441 P.2d 912.) Defendants, however, contend that in the circumstances of the present case they owed no duty of care to Tatiana or her parents and that, in the absence of such duty, they were free to act in careless disregard of Tatiana's life and safety.

In analyzing this contention, we bear in mind that legal duties are not discoverable facts of nature, but merely conclusory expressions that, in cases of a particular type, liability should be imposed for damage done. As stated in Dillon v. Legg, *supra*, at page 734, 69 Cal.Rptr. at page 76, 441 P.2d at page 916. "The assertion that liability must . . . be denied because defendant bears no 'duty' to plaintiff 'begs the essential question—whether the plaintiff's interests are entitled to legal protection against the defendant's conduct. . . . [Duty] is not sacrosanct in itself, but only an expression of the sum total of those considerations of policy which lead the law to say that the particular plaintiff is entitled to protection.' (Prosser, Law of Torts [3d ed. 1964] at pp. 332–333.)" Rowland v. Christian (1968) 69 Cal.2d 108, 113, 70 Cal.Rptr. 97, 100, 443 P.2d 561, 564, listed the principal considerations: "the foreseeability of harm to the plaintiff, the degree of certainty that the plaintiff suffered injury, the closeness of the connection between the defendant's conduct and the injury suffered, the moral blame attached to the defendant's conduct, the policy of preventing future harm, the extent of the burden to the defendant and consequences to the community of imposing a duty to exercise care with resulting liability for breach, and the availability, cost, and prevalence of insurance for the risk involved."[4]

Although under the common law, as a general rule, one person owed no duty to control the conduct of another[5] (Richards v. Stanley (1954) 43 Cal.2d 60, 65, 271 P.2d 23; Wright v. Arcade School Dist. (1964) 230 Cal.App.2d 272, 277, 40 Cal.Rptr. 812; Rest.2d Torts (1965) 315), nor to warn those endangered by such conduct (Rest.2d Torts, supra, § 314, com. c; Prosser, Law of Torts (4th ed. 1971) § 56, p. 341), the courts have noted exceptions to this rule. In two classes of cases the courts have imposed a duty of care: (1) cases in which the defendant stands in some special relationship to either the person whose conduct needs to be controlled or in a relationship to the foreseeable victim of that conduct (see Rest.2d Torts, *supra*, §§ 315–320); and (2) cases in which the defendant has engaged, or undertaken to engage, in affirmative action to control the anticipated dangerous conduct or protect the prospective victim. (See Rest.2d Torts, *supra*, §§ 321–324a.)[6] Both exceptions apply to the facts of this case.

Turning, first, to the special relationships present in this case, we note that a relationship of defendant therapists to either Tatiana or to Poddar will suffice to establish a duty of care; as explained in section 315 of the Restatement Second of Torts, a duty of care may arise from either "(a) a special relation . . . between the actor and the third person which imposes a duty upon the actor to control the third person's conduct, or (b) a special relation . . . between the actor and the other which gives to the other a right to protection."

Although plaintiffs' pleadings assert no special relation between Tatiana and defendant therapists, they establish as between Poddar and defendant therapists the special relation that arises between a patient and his doctor or psychotherapist.[7] Such a relationship may support affirmative duties for the benefit of third persons. (See Fleming & Maximov, The Patient or His Victim: The Therapist's Dilemma (1974) 62 Cal.L.Rev. 1025, 1027–1031.) Thus, for example, a hospital must exercise reasonable care to control the behavior of a patient which may endanger other persons.[8] A doctor must also warn a patient if the patient's condition or medication renders certain conduct, such as driving a car, dangerous to others.[9]

Although the California decisions that recognize this duty have involved cases in which the defendant stood in a special relationship *both* to the victim and to the person whose conduct created the danger,[10] we do not think that the duty should logically be constricted to such situations. Decisions of other jurisdictions hold that the single relationship of a doctor to his patient is sufficient to support the duty to use reasonable care to warn of dangers emanating from the patient's illness. The courts hold that a doctor is liable to persons infected by his patient if he negligently fails to diagnose a contagious disease (Hofmann v. Blackmon (Fla.App.1970) 241 So. 2d 752), or, having diagnosed the illness, fails to warn members of the patient's family (Wojcik v. Aluminum Co. of America (1959) 18 Misc.2d 740, 183 N.Y.S. 2d 351, 357–358; Davis v. Rodman (1921) 147 Ark. 385, 227 S.W. 612; Skillings v. Allen (1919) 143 Minn. 323, 173 N.W. 663; see also Jones v. Stanko (1928) 118 Ohio St. 147, 160 N.E. 456.)

More closely on point, since it involved a dangerous mental patient, is the decision in Merchants Nat. Bank & Trust Co. of Fargo v. United States (D.N.D.1967) 272 F.Supp. 409. The Veterans Administration arranged for the patient to work on a local farm, but did not warn the farmer of the man's background. The farmer consequently permitted the patient to come and go freely during nonworking hours; the patient borrowed a car, drove to his wife's residence and killed her. Notwithstanding the lack of any "special relationship" between the Veterans Administration and the wife, the court found the Veterans Administration liable for the wrongful death of the wife.

As the present case illustrates, a patient with severe mental illness and dangerous proclivities may, in a given case, present a danger as serious and as foreseeable as does the carrier of a contagious disease or the driver whose condition or medication affects his ability to drive safely. We conclude that a doctor or a psychotherapist treating a mentally ill patient, just as a doctor treating physical illness, bears a duty to use reasonable care to give threatened persons such warnings as are essential to avert foreseeable danger arising from his patient's condition or treatment.

As we stated previously, a duty to warn may also arise from a voluntary act or undertaking by a defendant. Once the defendant has commenced to render service, he must employ reasonable care; if reasonable care requires the giving of warnings, he must do so. Numerous cases hold that if a defendant's prior conduct has created or contributed to a danger, even if that conduct itself is non-negligent or protected by governmental immunity, the defendant bears a duty to warn affected persons of such impending danger. (See Johnson v. State of California (1968) 69 Cal.2d 782, 796–797, 73 Cal.Rptr. 240, 447 P.2d 352, and cases there cited; Rest.2d Torts, supra, § 321 and illus. to com. (a), § 323 and com. (c).)

The record in People v. Poddar (1974) 10 Cal.3d 750, 111 Cal.Rptr. 910, 518 P.2d 342 indicates, and plaintiffs' complaints could be amended to assert, that following Poddar's encounter with the police, Poddar broke off all contact with the hospital staff and discontinued psychotherapy. From those facts one could reasonably infer that defendants' actions led Poddar to halt treatment which, if carried through, might have led him to abandon his plan to kill Tatiana, and thus that defendants, having contributed to the danger, bear a duty to give warning.

Defendant therapists advance two policy considerations which, they suggest, justify a refusal to impose a duty upon a psychotherapist to warn third parties of danger arising from the violent intentions of his patient. We explain why, in our view, such considerations do not preclude imposition of the duty in question.

First, defendants point out that although therapy patients often express thoughts of violence, they rarely carry out these ideas. Indeed the open and confidential character of psychotherapeutic dialogue encourages patients to voice such thoughts, not as a device to reveal hidden danger, but as part of the process of therapy. Certainly a therapist should not be encouraged routinely to reveal such threats to acquaintances of the patient; such disclosures could seriously disrupt the patient's relationship with his therapist and with the persons threatened. In singling out those few patients whose threats of violence present a serious danger and in weighing against this danger the harm to the patient that might result from revelation, the psychotherapist renders a decision involving a high order of expertise and judgment.

The judgment of the therapist, however, is no more delicate or demanding than the judgment which doctors and professionals must regularly render under accepted rules of responsibility. A professional person is required only to exercise "that reasonable degree of skill, knowledge, and care ordinarily possessed and exercised by members of [his] profession under similar circumstances." (Bardessono v. Michels. (1970) 3 Cal.3d 780, 788, 91 Cal. Rptr. 760, 764, 478 P.2d 480, 484.) As a specialist, the psychotherapist, whether doctor or psychologist, would also be "held to that standard of learning and skill normally possessed by such specialist in the same or similar locality under the same or similar circumstances." (Quintal v. Laurel Grove Hospital (1964) 62 Cal.2d 154, 159160, 41 Cal.Rptr. 577, 580, 397 P.2d 161, 164.) But within that broad range in which professional opinion and judgment may differ respecting the proper course of action, the psychotherapist is free to exercise his own best judgment free from liability; proof, aided by hindsight, that he judged wrongly is insufficient to establish liability.

In other words, the fact that a decision calls for considerable expert skill and judgment means, in effect, that it be tested by a standard of care which takes account of those circumstances; the standard used in measuring professional malpractice does so. But whatever difficulties the courts may encounter in evaluating the expert judgments of other professions, those difficulties cannot justify total exoneration from liability.

Second, defendants argue that free and open communication is essential to psychotherapy (see In re Lifschutz (1970) 2 Cal. 3d 415, 431–432, 85 Cal.Rptr. 829, 467 P.2d 557); that "Unless a patient . . . is assured that . . . information [revealed by him] can and will be held in utmost confidence, he will be reluctant to make the full disclosure upon which diagnosis and treatment . . . depends." (Sen. Committee on the Judiciary, comments on Evid.Code, § 1014.) The giving of a warning, defendants contend, constitutes a breach of trust which entails the revelation of confidential communications.

We recognize the public interest in supporting effective treatment of mental illness and in protecting the rights of patients to privacy (see In re Lifschutz, *supra*, 2 Cal.3d at p. 432, 85 Cal.Rptr. 829, 467 P.2d 557), and the consequent public importance of safeguarding the confidential character of psychotherapeutic communication. Against this interest, however, we must weigh the public interest in safety from violent assault. The Legislature has undertaken the difficult task of balancing the countervailing concerns. In Evidence Code section 1014, it established a broad rule of privilege to protect confidential communications between patient and psychotherapist. In Evidence Code section 1024, however, the Legislature created a specific and limited exception to the psychotherapist-patient privilege: "There is no privilege . . . if the psychotherapist has reasonable cause to believe that the patient is in such mental or emotional condition as to be dangerous to himself or to the person or property of another and that disclosure of the communication is necessary to prevent the threatened danger."[11]

The revelation of a communication under the above circumstances is not a breach of trust or a violation of professional ethics; as stated in the Principles of Medical Ethics of the American Medical Association (1957) section 9: "A physician may not reveal the confidences entrusted to him in the course of medical attendance . . . *unless he is required to do so by law or unless it becomes necessary in order to protect the welfare of the individual or of the community.*" (Emphasis added.) We conclude that the public policy favoring protection of the confidential character of patient-psychotherapist communications must yield in instances in which disclosure is essential to avert danger to others. The protective privilege ends where the public peril begins.

Our current crowded and computerized society compels the interdependence of its members. In this risk-infested society we can hardly tolerate the further exposure to danger that would result from a concealed knowledge of the therapist that his patient was lethal. If in the exercise of reasonable care the therapist can warn the endangered party or those who can reasonably be expected to notify him, we see no sufficient societal interest that would protect and justify concealment. The containment of such risks lies in the public interest.

For the foregoing reasons, we find that plaintiffs' complaints can be amended to state a cause of action against defendants Moore, Powelson, Gold, and Yandell and against the Regents as their employer, for breach of a duty to warn Tatiana arising from the relationship of these defendants to Poddar.[12] The complaints can also be amended to assert causes of action against the police defendants for failure to warn on the theory that the officers' conduct increased the risk of violence. The judgment of the superior court, sustaining defendants' demurrers without leave to amend must therefore be reversed.

3. Defendants are not immune from liability for failure to warn. We turn to the issue of whether defendants are protected by governmental immunity for having failed to warn Tatiana or those who reasonably could have been expected to notify her of her peril. We focus our analysis on section 820.2 of the Government Code.[13] That provision declares, with exceptions not applicable here, that "a public employee is not liable for an injury resulting from his act or omission where the act or omission was the result of the exercise of the discretion vested in him, whether or not such discretion [was] abused."[14]

Noting that virtually every public act admits of some element of discretion, we drew the line in Johnson v. State of California (1968) 69 Cal.2d 782, 73 Cal.Rptr. 240, 447 P.2d 352, between discretionary policy decisions which enjoy statutory immunity and ministerial administrative acts which do not. We concluded that section 820.2 affords immunity only for "*basic* policy decisions." (Emphasis added.) (See also Elton v. County of Orange (1970) 3 Cal.App.3d 1053, 1057–1058, 84 Cal.Rptr. 27; 4 Cal.Law Revision Com.Rep. (1963) p. 810; Van Alstyne, Supplement to Cal. Government Tort Liability (Cont.Ed.Bar 1969) § 5.54, pp. 16–17; Comment, California Tort Claims Act: Discretionary Immunity (1966) 39 So.Cal.L.Rev. 470, 471; cf. James, Tort Liability of Governmental Units and their Officers (1955) 22 U.Chi. L.Rev. 610, 637–638, 640, 642, 651.)

We also observed that if courts did not respect this statutory immunity, they would find themselves "in the unseemly position of determining the propriety of decisions expressly entrusted to a coordinate branch of government." (Johnson v. State of California, *supra*, 69 Cal.2d at p. 793, 73 Cal.Rptr. at p. 248, 447 P.2d. at p. 360.) It therefore is necessary, we concluded, to "isolate those areas of quasi-legislative policy-making which are sufficiently sensitive to justify a blanket rule that courts will not entertain a tort action alleging that careless conduct contributed to the governmental decision." (Johnson v. State of California, *supra*, at p. 794, 73 Cal.Rptr. at p. 248, 447 P.2d at p. 360.) After careful analysis we rejected, in *Johnson*, other rationales commonly advanced to support governmental immunity,[15] and concluded that the immunity's scope should be no greater than is required to give legislative and executive policymakers sufficient breathing space in which to perform their vital policymaking functions.

Relying on *Johnson*, we conclude that defendants in the present case are not immune from liability for their failure to warn of Tatiana's peril. *Johnson* held that a parole officer's determination whether to warn an adult couple that their prospective foster child had a background of violence "present[ed] no . . . reasons for immunity" (Johnson v. State of California, *supra*, at p. 795, 73 Cal.Rptr. 240, 447 P.2d 352), was "at the lowest, ministerial rung of official action" (*id.* at p. 796, 78 Cal.Rptr. at p. 250, 447 P.2d at p. 362), and indeed constituted "a classic case for the imposition of tort liability." *Id.*, p. 797, 73 Cal.Rptr. at p. 251, 447 P.2d at p. 363; cf. Morgan v. County of Yuba (1964) 230 Cal.App.2d 938, 942943, 41 Cal.Rptr. 508.) Although defendants in *Johnson* argued that the decision whether to inform the foster parents of the child's background required the exercise of considerable judgmental skills, we concluded that the state was not immune from liability for the parole officer's failure to warn because such a decision did not rise to the level of a "basic policy decision."

We also noted in *Johnson* that federal courts have consistently categorized failures to warn of latent dangers as falling outside the scope of discretionary omissions immunized by the Federal Tort Claims Act.[16] (See United Air Lines, Inc. v. Weiner (9th Cir. 1964) 335 F.2d 379, 397398, cert. den. sub nom. United Air Lines, Inc. v. United States, 379 U.S. 951, 85 S. Ct. 452, 13 L.Ed.2d 549 (decision to conduct military training flights was discretionary but failure to warn commercial airline was not); United States v. Washington (9th Cir. 1965) 351 F.2d 913, 916 (decision where to place transmission lines spanning canyon was assumed to be discretionary but failure to warn pilot was not); United States v. White (9th Cir. 1954) 211 F.2d 79, 82 (decision not to "dedud" army firing range assumed to be discretionary but failure to warn person about to go onto range of unsafe condition was not); Bulloch v. United States (D. Utah 1955) 133 F.Supp. 885, 888 (decision how and when to conduct nuclear test deemed discretionary but failure to afford proper notice was not); Hernandez v. United States (D.Hawaii 1953) 112 F.Supp. 369, 371 (decision to erect road block characterized as discretionary but failure to warn of resultant hazard was not).

We conclude, therefore, that the defendants' failure to warn Tatiana or those who reasonably could have been expected to notify her of her peril does not fall within the absolute protection afforded by section 820.2 of the Government Code. We emphasize that our conclusion does not raise the specter of therapists employed by government indiscriminately held liable for damages despite their exercise of sound professional judgment. We require of publicly employed therapists only that quantum of care which the common law requires of private therapists, that they use that reasonable degree of skill, knowledge, and conscientiousness ordinarily exercised by members of their profession. The imposition of liability in those rare cases in which a public employee falls short of this standard does not contravene the language or purpose of Government Code section 820.2.

4. Defendant therapists are immune from liability for failing to confine Poddar. We sustain defendant therapists' contention that Government Code section 856 insulates them from liability for failing to confine Poddar. Section 856 affords public entities and their employees absolute protection from liability for "any injury resulting from determining in accordance with any applicable enactment . . . whether to confine a person for mental illness."[17] The section includes an exception to the general rule of immunity, however, "for injury proximately caused by . . . negligent or wrongful act[s] or omission[s] in carrying out or failing to carry out . . . a determination to confine or not to confine a person for mental illness. . . ."

Turning first to Dr. Powelson's status with respect to section 856, we observe that the actions attributed to him by plaintiffs' complaints fall squarely within the protections furnished by that provision. Plaintiffs allege Powelson ordered that no detention action be taken. This conduct definitionally reflected Powelson's "determining . . . [not] to confine [Poddar]." Powelson therefore is immune from liability for any injuries stemming from his decision. (See Hernandez v. State of California (1970) 11 Cal.App.3d 895, 90 Cal. Rptr. 205.)

Section 856 also insulates Dr. Moore for his conduct respecting confinement, although the analysis in his case is a bit more subtle. Clearly, Moore's decision that Poddar *be* confined was not a proximate cause of Tatiana's death, for indeed if Moore's efforts to bring about Poddar's confinement had been successful, Tatiana might still be alive today. Rather, any confinement claim against Moore must rest upon Moore's failure to overcome Powelson's decision and actions opposing confinement.

Such a claim, based as it necessarily would be upon a subordinate's failure to prevail over his superior, obviously would derive from a rather onerous duty. Whether to impose such a duty we need not decide, however, since we can confine our analysis to the question whether Moore's failure to overcome Powelson's decision realistically falls within the protections afforded by section 856. Based upon the allegations before us, we conclude that Moore's conduct is protected.

Plaintiffs' complaints imply that Moore acquiesced in Powelson's countermand of Moore's confinement recommendation. Such acquiescence is functionally equivalent to "determining . . . [not] to confine" and thus merits protection under section 856. At this stage we are unaware, of course, precisely how Moore responded to Powelson's actions; he may have debated the confinement issue with Powelson, for example, or taken no initiative whatsoever, perhaps because he respected Powelson's judgment, feared for his future at the hospital, or simply recognized that the proverbial handwriting was on the wall. None of these possibilities constitutes, however, the type of careless or wrongful behavior subsequent to a decision respecting confinement which is stripped of protection by the exceptionary language in section 856. Rather, each is in the nature of a decision not to continue to press for Poddar's confinement. No language in plaintiffs' original or amended complaints suggests that Moore determined to fight Powelson but failed successfully to do so due to negligent or otherwise wrongful acts or omissions. Under the circumstances, we conclude that plaintiffs' second amended complaints allege facts which trigger immunity for Dr. Moore under section 856.[18]

5. Defendant police officers are immune from liability for failing to continue Poddar in their custody. Confronting, finally, the question whether the defendant police officers are immune from liability for releasing Poddar after his brief confinement, we conclude that they are. The source of their immunity is section 5154 of the Welfare and Institutions Code, which declares that "[t]he professional person in charge of the facility providing 72-hour treatment and evaluation, his designee, *and the peace officer responsible for the detainment of the person* shall not be held civilly or criminally liable for any action by a person released at or before the end of 72 hours. . . ." (Emphasis added.)

Although defendant police officers technically were not "peace officers" as contemplated by the Welfare and Institutions Code,[19] plaintiffs' assertion that the officers incurred liability by failing to continue Poddar's confinement clearly contemplates that the officers were "responsible for the detainment of [Poddar]." We could not impose a duty upon the officers to keep Poddar confined yet deny them the protection furnished by a statute immunizing those "responsible for . . . [confinement]." Because plaintiffs would have us treat defendant officers as persons who were capable of performing the functions of the "peace officers" contemplated by the Welfare and Institutions Code, we must accord defendant officers the protections which that code prescribes for such "peace officers."

6. Plaintiffs' complaints state no cause of action for exemplary damages. Plaintiffs' third cause of action seeks punitive damages against defendant Powelson. Incorporating by reference the factual allegations of the first cause of action, plaintiffs assert that Powelson "did the things herein alleged with intent to abandon a dangerous patient, and said acts were done maliciously and oppressively."[20] The incorporated allegations speak only of Powelson's failure to bring about Poddar's commitment; they do not refer to his failure to warn Tatiana or her parents. Since we have concluded that Powelson is protected by governmental immunity from liability for his decision not to commit Poddar, plaintiffs' complaints state no basis for recovery of exemplary damages against Powelson.

7. Conclusion For the reasons stated, we conclude that plaintiffs can assert the elements essential to a cause of action for breach of a duty to warn. The judgment of the superior court dismissing plaintiffs' action is reversed, and the cause remanded for further proceedings consistent with the views expressed herein.

[Chief Justice Wright, Justices Mosk and Sullivan, and retired Associate Justice Burke (sitting under assignment by the Chairman of the Judicial Council) concurred. There follows the dissenting opinion of Justice Clark.]

JUSTICE CLARK'S DISSENT

The majority's opinion correctly holds that when a psychiatrist, in terminating treatment to a patient, increases the risk of his violence, the psychiatrist must warn the potential victim. However, I do not agree with the majority's conclusion that the psychiatrist must also disclose threats of violence based solely on his prior psychiatrist-patient relationship. Further, I do not agree with the majority's holding that police officers shall become subject to the same duty.

Duty to Disclose Based on Psychiatrist-Patient Relationship

Generally, one person owes no duty to control the conduct of another. (Richards v. Stanley (1954) 43 Cal.2d 60, 65, 271 P.2d 23; Wright v. Arcade School Dist. (1964) 230 Cal.App.2d 272, 277, 40 Cal.Rptr. 812; Rest.2d Torts (1965) § 315.) Exceptions arise only in limited situations where (1) a special relationship exists between the defendant and the injured party giving the latter a right to protection, or (2) a special relationship exists between the defendant and the active wrongdoer imposing a duty on the defendant to control the wrongdoer's conduct. The majority does not contend the first exception is applicable to this case.

Overriding considerations of policy compel the conclusion that the duty to warn a potential victim may not be founded on the mere existence of a psychiatrist-patient relationship.

The imposition of a duty-depends on policy considerations. (Dillon v. Legg (1968) 68 Cal.2d 728, 734, 69 Cal.Rptr. 72, 441 P.2d 912.) The principal considerations include the burden on the defendant, the consequence to the community, the prevention of future violence, and the foreseeability of harm to the plaintiff. (Rowland v. Christian (1968) 69 Cal.2d 108, 113, 70 Cal.Rptr. 97, 443 P.2d 561.)

Although the majority fleetingly acknowledges these considerations, it neglects applying them to our case. More specifically, the majority opinion fails to realistically evaluate the devastating impact their new duty will have on the field of mental health—and the repercussions resulting to society.

The importance of psychiatric treatment is well-recognized in California, reflected in this court's recent statement, "We recognize the growing importance of the psychiatric profession in our modern, ultracomplex society. The swiftness of change—economic, cultural, and moral—produces accelerated tensions in our society, and the potential for relief of such emotional disturbances offered by psychological therapy undoubtedly establishes it as a profession essential to the preservation of societal health and well-being." (In re Lifschutz (1970) 2 Cal.3d 415, 421–422, 85 Cal.Rptr. 829, 832, 467 P.2d 557, 560.)

Successful psychotherapy demands confidentiality. (In re Lifschutz, *supra*, 2 Cal. 3d 415, 422, 85 Cal.Rptr. 829, 467 P.2d 557.) "It is clearly recognized that the very practice of psychiatry vitally depends upon the reputation in the community that the psychiatrist will not tell." (Slovenko, Psychiatry and a Second Look at the Medical Privilege (1960) 6 Wayne L.Rev. 175, 188.)

Assurance of confidentiality is important in three ways.

First, without a substantial guarantee of confidentiality, people requiring treatment will be deterred from seeking assistance. (See Senate Judiciary Committee's comment accompanying section 1014 of the Evid.Code; Slovenko, *supra*, 6 Wayne L. Rev. 175, 187–188; Goldstein and Katz, Psychiatrist-Patient Privilege. The GAP Proposal and the Connecticut Statute (1962) 36 Conn.Bar J. 175, 178.) It remains an unfortunate fact in our society that a stigma attaches to people seeking psychiatric guidance (apparently increased by the propensity of people considering treatment to see themselves in the worst possible light) creating a well-recognized reluctance to seek aid. (Fisher, The Psychotherapeutic Professions and the Law of Privileged Communications (1964) 10 Wayne L.Rev. 609, 617; Slovenko, *supra*, 6 Wayne L.Rev. 175, 188; see also Rappeport, Psychiatrist-Patient Privilege (1963) 23 Md.L.J. 39, 46–47.) This reluctance is alleviated by the psychiatrist's assurance of confidentiality.

Second, the guarantee of confidentiality is important in eliciting the full disclosure necessary for effective treatment. To carry out the cure, the doctor must first diagnose the disease. Candor is essential to psychiatric diagnosis. This diagnostic process requires "a searching evaluation of the given personality in the light of his past experiences and current relationships" (Heller, Some Comments to Lawyers of the Practice of Psychiatry (1957) 30 Temp. L.Q. 401), requiring intensive examination of "innate and constitutional factors, the history of the individual's emotional, educational, cultural, vocational and medical backgrounds, the influence of sexual and aggressive instincts, so-called ego or personality strength, judgment and reality-testing." (*Id.* at p. 402.) Summarily stated, "The process involves a prying into the most hidden aspects of personality, a prying which discloses matters theretofore unknown even to the conscious mind of the patient." (Slovenko, *supra,* 6 Wayne L. Rev. 175, 185.)

The assurance of confidentiality is essential to bringing about full disclosure since the psychiatric patient approaches treatment with conscious and unconscious inhibitions to revealing his innermost thoughts. (Goldstein and Katz, *supra,* 36 Conn.B.J. 175, 178; Guttmacher and Weihofen, Privileged Communications Between Psychiatrist and Patient (1952) 28 Ind.L.J. 32, 34.) "Every person, however well-motivated, has to overcome resistances to therapeutic exploration. These resistances seek support from every possible source and the possibility of disclosure would easily be employed in the service of resistance." (Goldstein and Katz, *supra,* 36 Conn.Bar J. 175, 179; see also, 118 Am. J.Psych. 734, 735.) Until a patient can trust his psychiatrist not to violate their confidential relationship, "the unconscious psychological control mechanism of repression will prevent the recall of past experiences." (Butler, Psychotherapy and Griswold: Is Confidentiality a Privilege or a Right? (1971) 3 Conn.L.Rev. 599, 604.)[1]

Third, even if full disclosure is accomplished, assurance that the confidential relationship will not be breached is necessary to maintain the patient's trust of his psychiatrist, the very means by which treatment is effected. "[T]he essence of much psychotherapy is the contribution of trust in the external world and ultimately in the self, modelled upon the trusting relationship established during therapy." (Dawidoff, The Malpractice of Psychiatrists, 1966 Duke L.J. 696, 704.) Patients will be helped only if they can form a trusting relationship with the psychiatrist. (*Id.* at p. 704, fn. 34; Burnham, Separation Anxiety (1965) 13 Arch.Gen.Psychiatry 346, 356; Heller, *supra,* 30 Temp.L.Q. 401, 406.) Conversely, all authorities appear to agree treatment will be frustrated if the trust relationship cannot be developed because of collusive communication between the psychiatrist and others. (See, e. g., Ralph Slovenko (1973) Psychiatry and Law, p. 61; Cross, Privileged Communications Between Participants in Group Psychotherapy (1970) Law and the Social Order, 191, 199; Hollender, The Psychiatrist and the Release of Patient Information (1960) 116 Am.J.Psychiatry 828, 829.)

Therefore, given the importance of confidentiality to the practice of psychiatry, it becomes clear the duty to warn imposed by the majority will cripple the use and effectiveness of psychiatry: many people, potentially violent—yet susceptible to treatment—will be deterred from seeking it; those seeking aid will be inhibited from making the self-revelation necessary to effective treatment; finally, requiring the psychiatrist to violate the patient's trust by forcing the doctor to disseminate confidential statements will destroy the interpersonal relationship by which treatment is effected.

The law recognizes the psychiatrist's ability to lessen a patient's propensity for violence. Indeed, this ability is so well established that the majority, in its second reason for imposing a duty to warn, concludes that because the psychiatrists' conduct caused Poddar to discontinue treatment, the psychiatrists actually "contributed to the danger" that Poddar would act violently. (*Ante,* p. 135 of 118 Cal.Rptr., p. ____ of ____ P.2d.)

By imposing such duty on psychiatrists, the majority contributes to society's danger. Given the majority's recognition that under existing psychiatric procedures only a relatively few receiving treatment will ever present a serious risk of violence (*ante,* p. 136 of 118 Cal.Rptr., p. ____ of ____ P.2d.), the newly imposed duty will likely result in a *net increase* in violence—inconsistent with the policies of preventing future violence and of weighing the consequence to the community.

The majority overlooks the widespread impact of its new duty by pointing out that only a few psychiatric patients will ever really create a serious risk of violence and by assuming that the number of necessary warnings will similarly be few. (*Ante,* p. 136 of 118 Cal.Rptr., p. ____ of ____ P.2d.). This assumption strays from reality.

The psychiatric community recognizes that the process of determining potential violence in a patient is far from exact, being wrought with complexity and uncertainty. (See, Rector, *Who Are the Dangerous?* (July 1973) Bull. of the Amer. Acad. of Psych. and the Law 186; Kozol, Boucher, and Garofalo, *The Diagnosis and Treatment of Dangerousness* (1972) 18 Crime and Delinquency 371; Justice and Birkman, *An Effort to Distinguish the Violent From the Nonviolent* (1972) 65 So. Med.J. 703.) In fact, precision has not even been attained in predicting who of those having already committed violent acts will again become violent, a task recognized to be of simpler proportion. (Kozol, Boucher, and Garofalo, *supra,* 18 Crime and Delinquency 371, 384.)

This predictive uncertainty is fatal to the majority's underlying assumption that the number of disclosures will necessarily be small. As noted, above psychiatric patients are encouraged to discuss all thoughts of violence. And, as the majority concedes, they often express such thoughts. However, unlike this court, the psychiatrist does not enjoy the benefit of hindsight in seeing which few, if any, of his patients will ultimately become violent. Now, operating under the majority's duty, the psychiatrist—with each patient and each visit—must instantaneously calculate potential violence. The difficulties researchers have encountered in accurately predicting violence will be heightened for the practicing psychiatrist dealing for brief periods in his office with heretofore nonviolent patients. And, given the decision not to warn must always be made at the psychiatrist's civil peril, one can expect all doubts will be resolved in favor of warning.

Relying on sections 1013, 1014, and 1024 of the Evidence Code, the majority suggests that, in any event, the new duty's harmful impact on the community has already been balanced by the Legislature in favor of warning. However, this conclusion is faulty, failing to differentiate between the *permissive* language of section 1024 and the *mandatory* duty of the majority.

Section 1014 of the Evidence Code provides that "the patient, whether or not a party, has a privilege to refuse to disclose, and to prevent another from disclosing, a confidential communication between patient and psychotherapist . . . ." Section 1013 expressly provides that the patient is the holder of the privilege. Section 1024 provides, "There is no privilege under this article if the psychotherapist has reasonable cause to believe that the patient is in such mental or emotional condition as to be dangerous to himself or to the person or property of another and that disclosure of the communication is necessary to prevent the threatened danger."

Section 1024 is solely permissive. When a psychiatrist has determined to his satisfaction that some sort of formal disclosure must be made to protect the patient or others, section 1024 precludes the patient from invoking the section 1014 privilege to prevent him from doing so.[2] Clearly, section 1024 neither imposes—nor contemplates—a legal duty mandating the psychiatrist to warn, and the impact of *requiring* him to warn is much greater than that of *allowing* him to do so.

Our sympathy for the victim of violent acts of the mentally ill should not blind us to the needs of the mentally ill or to the ultimate goal of reducing the level of violence. Because the majority's holding will severely impair the ability of the doctor to treat effectively, resulting in a net increase in violence, I cannot concur in the majority's new rule.

Duty of Police to Warn

Although the police defendants get lost in the course of the majority's opinion, the holding concludes the officers may also be liable for failing to warn.

The ground for imposing liability on the police officers is unclear. The holding is so broad it may be understood, in light of the facts of this case, as meaning that the mere release of Poddar gave rise to the duty to warn. The majority not only imposes a new duty on police officers, but may also have held that jail and prison officials must now warn of potential violence whenever a prisoner is released pursuant to bail order, parole, or completion of sentence.

It is disturbing that the majority should take, by ambiguous statement and without discussion, the very broad step of imposing on a peace officer the near impossible duty to notify potential victims of threatened violence. The majority states that duty is dependent on considerations of policy—but the policy goes unexplained.

Conclusion

It appears the tragedy of Tatiana Tarasoff has led the majority of our court to unfairly penalize the professions of psychiatry and law enforcement, to the detriment of society.

I would permit plaintiffs to proceed against the psychiatrists for failure to warn on the theory the psychiatrist's conduct in terminating treatment increased the risk of violence. Absent such conduct, I would disallow a cause of action for failure to warn based solely on the existence of the prior psychiatrist-patient relationship. Finally, I conclude no justification has been shown for imposing the inordinate duty to warn on the police officers.

McCOMB, J., concurs.

NOTES

Notes to the Majority Opinion (Justice Tobriner)

1. The criminal prosecution stemming from this crime is reported in People v. Poddar (1974) 10 Cal.3d 750, 111 Cal.Rptr. 910, 518 P.2d 342.
2. The therapist defendants include Dr. Moore, the psychologist who examined Poddar and decided that Poddar should be committed; Dr. Gold and Dr. Yandell, psychiatrists at Cowell Memorial Hospital who concurred in Moore's decision; and Dr. Powelson, chief of the department of psychiatry, who countermanded Moore's decision and directed that the staff take no action to confine Poddar. The police defendants include Officers Atkinson, Brownrigg and Halleran, who detained Poddar briefly but released him; Chief Beall, who received Moore's letter recommending that Poddar be confined; and Officer Teel, who, along with Officer Atkinson, received Moore's oral communication requesting detention of Poddar.
3. Plaintiffs' complaints allege that defendants failed to warn Tatiana's parents of the danger to Tatiana from Poddar. The complaints do not specifically state whether defendants warned Tatiana herself. Such an omission can properly be cured by amendment. As we stated in Minsky v. City of Los Angeles: "It is axiomatic that if there is a reasonable possibility that a defect in the complaint can be cured by amendment or that the pleading liberally construed can state a cause of action, a demurrer should not be sustained without leave to amend. (3 Witkin, Cal.Procedure, Pleading, § 844, p. 2449; accord La Sala v. American Sav. & Loan Assn. (1971), 5 Cal.3d 864, 876, 97 Cal. Rptr. 849, 489 P.2d 1113; Lemoge Electric v. County of San Mateo (1956) 46 Cal.2d 659, 664, 297 P.2d 638; Beckstead v. Superior Court (1971) 21 Cal.App.3d 780, 782. 98 Cal.Rptr. 779.) We believe a cause of action has been stated here." (11 Cal.3d 113, 118–119, 113 Cal.Rptr. 102, 107, 520 P.2d 726, 731).
4. See Merrill v. Buck (1962) 58 Cal.2d 552, 562, 25 Cal.Rptr. 456, 375 P.2d 304; Biakanja v. Irving (1958) 49 Cal.2d 647, 650, 320 P.2d 16; Walnut Creek Aggregates Co. v. Testing Engineers Inc. (1967) 248 Cal.App.2d 690, 695, 56 Cal.Rptr. 700.
5. This rule derives from the common law's distinction between misfeasance and nonfeasance, and its reluctance to impose liability for the latter. (See Harper & Kime, The Duty to Control the Conduct of Another (1934) 43 Yale L.J. 886, 887.) Morally questionable, the rule owes its survival to "the difficulties of setting any standards of unselfish service to fellow men, and of making any workable rule to cover possible sitnations where fifty people might fail to rescue. . . ." (Prosser, Torts (4th ed. 1971) § 56, p. 341.) Because of these practical difficulties, the courts have increased the number of instances in which affirmative duties are imposed not by direct rejection of the common-law rule, but by expanding the list of special relationships which will justify departure from that rule. (See Prosser, *supra*, § 56, at pp. 348–350.)
6. A line of cases discussing the liability of a defendant who negligently provides an instrumentality by which a third

person injures the plaintiff presents issues similar to the present case, although distinguishable in that such cases require the defendant only to take reasonable precautions to safeguard his own property. In Richards v. Stanley (1954) 43 Cal.2d 60, 271 P.2d 23, defendant left the ignition keys in her car; a thief stole the car and, driving negligently, injured the plaintiff. Relying on the rule that "Ordinarily, . . . in the absence of a special relationship between the parties, there is no duty to control the conduct of a third person so as to prevent him from causing harm to another" (43 Cal.2d at p. 65, 271 P.2d at p. 27), the court affirmed a judgment for defendant. A year later, however, in Richardson v. Ham (1955) 44 Cal.2d 772, 285 P.2d 269, the court held that defendants who left a bulldozer unlocked could be held liable for damage caused after trespassers started the vehicle and then abandoned it to run amuck. Distinguishing Richards v. Stanley, the court stated that the "extreme danger created by a bulldozer in uncontrolled motion and the foreseeable risk of intermeddling fully justify imposing a duty on the owner to exercise reasonable care to protect third parties from injuries arising from its operation by intermeddlers." (44 Cal.2d at p. 776, 285 P.2d at p. 271.) In Hergenrether v. East (1964) 61 Cal.2d 440, 39 Cal.Rptr. 4, 393 P.2d 164, the court further limited the scope of Richards v. Stanley, and imposed liability upon a defendant, who parked his truck in a "skid row" area with the ignition keys in the truck, for damages caused by the reckless driving of a thief. Again the court distinguished *Richards* on the ground that "[S]pecial circumstances which impose a greater potentiality of foreseeable risk or more serious injury, or require a lesser burden of preventative action, may be deemed to impose an unreasonable risk on, and a legal duty to, third persons." (61 Cal.2d at p. 444, 39 Cal.Rptr. at p. 6, 393 P.2d at p. 166.) The cases thus exemplify an evolution from a rule of "no duty" to a rule in which imposition of a duty of care depends upon the foreseeability of serious injury and the burden of precautions. (See Schwartz v. Helms Bakery Limited (1967) 67 Cal.2d 232, 240242, 60 Cal.Rptr. 510, 430 P.2d 68.)

7. The pleadings establish the requisite relationship between Poddar and both Dr. Moore, the psychotherapist who treated Poddar, and Dr. Powelson, who supervised that treatment. Plaintiffs also allege that Dr. Gold personally examined Poddar, and that Dr. Yandell, as Powelson's assistant, approved the decision to arrange Poddar's commitment. These allegations are sufficient to raise the issue whether a doctor-patient or psychotherapist-patient relationship, giving rise to a possible duty by the doctor or therapist reasonably to warn threatened persons of danger arising from the patient's mental illness, existed between Gold or Yandell and Poddar. (See Harney, Medical Malpractice (1973) p. 7.)

8. When a "hospital has notice or knowledge of facts from which it might reasonably be concluded that a patient would be likely to harm himself *or others* unless preclusive measures were taken, then the hospital must use reasonable care in the circumstances to prevent such harm." (Vistica v. Presbyterian Hospital (1967) 67 Cal.2d 465, 469, 62 Cal. Rptr. 577, 580, 432 P.2d 193, 196.) (Emphasis added.) A mental hospital may be liable if it negligently permits the escape or release of a dangerous patient (Underwood v. United States (5th Cir. 1966) 356 F.2d 92; Fair v. United States (5th Cir. 1956) 234 F.2d 288). Greenberg v. Barbour (E.D.Pa. 1971) 322 F.Supp. 745, upheld a cause of action against a hospital staff doctor whose negligent failure to admit a mental patient resulted in that patient assaulting the plaintiff.

9. Kaiser v. Suburban Transp. System (1965) 65 Wash.2d 461, 398 P.2d 14, 401 P.2d 350; see Freese v. Lemmon (Iowa 1973) 210 N.W.2d 576 (concurring opinion of Uhlenhopp, J.)

10. Ellis v. D'Angelo (1953) 116 Cal.App.2d 310, 253 P.2d 675, upheld a cause of action against parents who failed to warn a babysitter of the violent proclivities of their child; Johnson v. State of California (1968) 69 Cal.2d 782, 73 Cal.Rptr. 240, 447 P.2d 352, upheld a suit against the state for failure to warn foster parents of the dangerous tendencies of their ward; Morgan v. County of Yuba (1964) 230 Cal.App.2d 938, 41 Cal.Rptr. 508, sustained a cause of action against a sheriff who had promised to warn decedent before releasing a dangerous prisoner, but failed to do so.

11. Fleming and Maximov note that "While [section 1024] supports the therapist's less controversial *right* to make a disclosure, it admittedly does not impose on him a *duty* to do so. But the argument does not have to be pressed that far. For if it is once conceded . . . that a duty in favor of the patient's foreseeable victims would accord with general principles of tort liability, we need no longer look to the statute for a source of duty. It is sufficient if the statute can be relied upon . . . for the purpose of countering the claim that the needs of confidentiality are paramount and must therefore defeat any such hypothetical duty. In this more modest perspective, the Evidence Code's 'dangerous patient' exception may be invoked with some confidence as a clear expression of legislative policy concerning the balance between the confidentiality values of the patient and the safety values of his foreseeable victims." (Emphasis in original.) Fleming & Maximov, The Patient or His Victim: The Therapist's Dilemma (1974) 62 Cal.L. Rev. 1025, 1063.

12. Moore argues that after Powelson countermanded the decision to seek commitment for Poddar, Moore was obliged to obey the decision of his superior and that he therefore should not be held liable for any dereliction arising from his obedience to superior orders. Plaintiffs in response argue that Moore's duty to members of the public endangered by Poddar should take precedence over his duty to obey Powelson. Since plaintiffs' complaints do not set out the date of Powelson's order, the specific terms of that order, or Powelson's authority to overrule Moore's decisions respecting patients under Moore's care, we lack sufficient factual background to adjudicate this conflict.

13. No more specific immunity provision of the Government Code appears to address the issue.

14. Section 815.2 of the Government Code declares that "[a] public entity is liable for injury proximately caused by an act or omission of an employee of the public entity within the scope of his employment if the act or omission would, apart from this section, have given rise to a cause of action against that employee or his personal representative." The section further provides, with exceptions not applicable here, that "a public entity is not liable for an injury resulting from an act or omission of an employee of the public

entity where the employee is immune from liability." The Regents, therefore, are immune from liability only if all individual defendants are similarly immune.

15. We dismissed, in *Johnson,* the view that immunity continues to be necessary in order to insure that public employees will be sufficiently zealous in the performance of their official duties. The California Tort Claims Act of 1963 provides for indemnification of public employees against liability, absent bad faith, and also permits such employees to insist that their defenses be conducted at public expense. (See Gov.Code, §§ 825–825.6, 995–995.2.) Public employees thus no longer have a significant reason to fear liability as they go about their official tasks. We also, in *Johnson,* rejected the argument that a public employee's concern over the potential liability of his or her employer serves as a basis for immunity. (Johnson v. State of California, *supra,* 69 Cal.2d at pp. 790–793, 72 Cal.Rptr. 240, 447 P.2d 352.)
16. By analogy, section 830.8 of the Government Code furnishes additional support for our conclusion that a failure to warn does not fall within the zone of immunity created by section 820.2. Section 830.8 provides: "Neither a public entity nor a public employee is liable . . . for an injury caused by the failure to provide traffic or warning signals, signs, markings or devices described in the Vehicle Code. Nothing in this section exonerates a public entity or public employee from liability for injury proximately caused by such failure if a signal, sign, marking or device . . . was necessary to warn of a dangerous condition which endangered the safe movement of traffic and which would not be reasonably apparent to, and would not have been anticipated by, a person exercising due care." The Legislature thus concluded at least in another context that the failure to warn of a latent danger is not an immunized discretionary omission. (See Hilts v. County of Solano (1968) 265 Cal.App.2d 161, 174, 71 Cal.Rptr. 275.)
17. Section 5201 of the Welfare and Institutions Code provides: "Any individual may apply to the person or agency designated by the county for a petition alleging that there is in the county a person who is, as a result of mental disorder a danger to others, or to himself, or is gravely disabled, and requesting that an evaluation of the person's condition be made." We believe that defendant therapists' power to recommend confinement as provided by section 5201 suffices to place them within the class of persons protected by section 856 of the Government Code. They are persons who can "determin[e] in accordance with [section 5201] whether to confine a person for mental illness."
18. Because Dr. Gold and Dr. Yandell were Dr. Powelson's subordinates, the analysis respecting whether they are immune for having failed to obtain Poddar's confinement is similar to the analysis applicable to Dr. Moore.
19. Welfare and Institutions Code section 5008, subdivision (i), defines "peace officer" for purposes of the Lanterman-Petris-Short Act as a person specified in sections 830.1 and 830.2 of the Penal Code. Campus police do not fall within the coverage of section 830.1 and were not included in section 830.2 until 1971.
20. Defendant Powelson points out that plaintiffs do not allege that Powelson knew Tatiana or plaintiffs, nor that his alleged malice or oppression was directed toward them. Such an allegation, however, is not essential to a cause of action for punitive damages. In Toole v. Richardson-Merrell Inc. (1967) 251 Cal.App.2d 689, 60 Cal.Rptr. 398, the court upheld an award of punitive damages against the manufacturer of a dangerous drug. Rejecting the contention that proof of a deliberate intention by the manufacturer to injure the users was essential to punitive damages, the court stated that "malice in fact, sufficient to support an award of punitive damages on the basis of malice as that term is used in Civil Code section 3294, may be established by a showing that the defendant's wrongful conduct was wilful, intentional, and done in reckless disregard of its possible results." (251 Cal.App.2d at p. 713, 60 Cal. Rptr. at p. 415.)

Notes to the Minority Opinion (Justice Clark)

1. One survey indicated that five of every seven people interviewed said they would be less likely to make full disclosure to a psychiatrist in the absence of assurance of confidentiality. (See, Comment, Functional Overlap Between the Lawyer and Other Professionals: Its Implications for the Doctrine of Privileged Communications (1962) 71 Yale L.J. 1226, 1255.)
2. This purpose is made simplistically clear in the Law Revision Commission's comment accompanying section 1024: "Although this exception might inhibit the relationship between the patient and his psychotherapist to a limited extent, it is essential that appropriate action be taken if the psychotherapist becomes convinced during the course of treatment that the patient is a menace to himself or others *and the patient refuses to permit the psychotherapist to make the disclosure necessary to prevent the threatened danger*" (Italics added).

INDEX